Your Essential Revision Guide

# MRCOG PART ONE

Your Essential Revision Guide

# MRCOG PART ONE

The official companion to the
Royal College of Obstetricians and
Gynaecologists revision course

**Edited by**
Alison Fiander and Baskaran Thilaganathan

A machine-readable catalogue record for this publication is available from the British Library [www.bl.uk/catalogue/listings.html]

ISBN 978-1-906985-40-0

Published by the RCOG Press at the
Royal College of Obstetricians and Gynaecologists
27 Sussex Place, Regent's Park
London NW1 4RG

Registered Charity No. 213280

RCOG Press Editor: Fiona Courtenay-Thompson

Artwork by Oxford Designers & Illustrators
(David Morris, Elaine Leggett and Sue Aldridge)

Index: Cath Topliff MSocInd(Adv)

Design & typesetting: Christopher Wakeling / Typographic Design Unit

Printed in the UK by Bell & Bain Ltd, 303 Burnfield Road, Thornliebank, Glasgow G46 7UQ

# Contents

# About the authors

**Nazar N Amso**  PhD FRCOG FHEA
Senior Lecturer, Department of Obstetrics and
Gynaecology, University Hospital of Wales, Cardiff, UK

**Gul Bano**  MD FRCP
Senior Lecturer in Clinical Endocrinology, St George's
Hospital NHS Trust, London, UK

**Rosemary Bland**  PhD
Associate Professor in Molecular Endocrinology,
Warwick Medical School, University of Warwick,
Coventry, UK

**Mary Board**  MA DPhil(Oxon)
Biochemistry Lecturer, St Hilda's College, University
of Oxford, Oxford, UK

**Annette Briley**  MSc
Consultant Midwife/Clinical Trials Manager, Maternal
and Fetal Research Unit, Division of Women's Health,
King's College, London, UK

**Fiona Broughton Pipkin**  MA DPhil(Hon) FRCOG
Professor of Perinatal Physiology, Faculty of Medicine
and Health Sciences, University of Nottingham,
Nottingham, UK

**Daniel Brudney**  MRCP(UK)
Specialty Registrar, Department of Microbiology, Royal
Free Hospital, London, UK

**Sharon Cookson**  PhD
Postdoctoral Research Assistant, University of Oxford,
Nuffield Department of Obstetrics and Gynaecology,
John Radcliffe Hospital, Oxford, UK

**Arri Coomarasamy**  MD MRCOG
Senior Lecturer in Reproductive Medicine and
Gynaecology, University of Birmingham, UK, and
Subspecialist in Reproductive Medicine and Surgery,
Consultant Gynaecologist, Birmingham Women's
Hospital, Edgbaston, Birmingham, UK

**Rohan D'Souza**  MD MRCOG FCPS DNB DGO DFP
Clinical Fellow, Maternal and Fetal Medicine,
St George's Hospital NHS Trust, London, UK

**Alison Fiander**  FRCOG
Professor and Chair, Department of Obstetrics and
Gynaecology, School of Medicine, Cardiff University,
Cardiff, UK

**Raji Ganesan**  MD FRCPath
Consultant in Histopathology, Department of Cellular
Pathology, Birmingham Women's NHS Foundation
Trust, Edgbaston, Birmingham, UK

**Phillip E Hay**  FRCP
Reader in HIV/Genitourinary Medicine, Department
of Genitourinary Medicine, St George's, University of
London, London, UK

**Kevin Hayes** MRCOG
Consultant and Senior Lecturer, St George's, University of London, London, UK

**Mark Heining** FRCA
Consultant in Anaesthesia, Nottingham University Hospitals NHS Trust, Nottingham, UK

**Des Holden** PhD MRCOG
Consultant in Obstetrics, Royal Sussex County Hospital and Honorary Senior Lecturer, Brighton and Sussex Medical School, Brighton, East Sussex, UK

**Susan Hopkins** FRCPI MScEpi
Consultant in Infectious Diseases, Department of Microbiology, Royal Free Hospital, London, UK

**Asma Khalil** MRCOG
Senior Research Fellow in Feto-Maternal Medicine, University College London, UK

**Khalid S Khan** MD MRCOG
Professor of Women's Health and Clinical Epidemiology, Barts and the London School of Medicine, Queen Mary, University of London, UK

**Diana Lawrence-Watt** PhD
Emeritus Professor of Human Anatomy, Brighton and Sussex Medical School, Brighton, Sussex, UK

**Fiona Lyall** MBA PhD
Professor of Maternal and Fetal Health, School of Medicine, University of Glasgow, Yorkhill Hospitals, Glasgow, UK

**Michael Marsh** MD FRCOG
Consultant in Obstetrics and Gynaecology, King's College Hospital, London, UK; Honorary Senior Lecturer, King's College School of Medicine, London, UK; Honorary Senior Lecturer, Institute of Psychiatry, London, UK

**Helen Mason**
Senior Lecturer, Basic Medical Sciences Division, Faculty of Medicine and Biomedical Sciences, St George's, University of London, London, UK

**Anthony E Michael** PhD
Reader in Reproductive Science and Deputy Head of Graduate School, Academic Section of Obstetrics and Gynaecology, Division of Clinical Development Sciences, Faculty of Medicine and Biomedical Sciences, St George's, University of London, London, UK

**Vivek Nama** MD MRCOG
Clinical Research Fellow, Department of Obstetrics and Gynaecology, St George's Medical School, London, UK

**Aris T Papageorghiou** MRCOG
Consultant in Fetal Medicine and Obstetrics, Fetal Medicine Unit, Department of Obstetrics and Gynaecology, St George's Hospital NHS Trust, London, UK

**Neil Pugh** PhD F InstP
Consultant Physicist, Honorary Senior Lecturer, College of Medicine, University of Wales, Cardiff, UK

**Philip Rice** MRCPath
Department of Medical Microbiology, St George's Hospital, London, UK

**Ian Sargent** PhD
Professor of Reproductive Science, University of Oxford, Nuffield Department of Obstetrics and Gynaecology, John Radcliffe Hospital, Oxford, UK

**Ram Sharma** PhD
Lecturer, Centre for Learning Anatomical Sciences, Division of Medical Education, School of Medicine, University of Southampton, Southampton General Hospital, Southampton, UK

**Andrew H Shennan** MD FRCOG
Professor of Obstetrics, Maternal and Fetal Research
Unit, Division of Women's Health, King's College
London, UK

**Andrew Sizer** MPH MD PhD MRCOG DFFP
Consultant in Obstetrics and Gynaecology,
Royal Shrewsbury Hospital, Shrewsbury, UK
and Senior Lecturer, Keele University School
of Medicine, Keele, UK

**Katrina Tatton-Brown** MD
Consultant in Clinical Genetics, South West Thames
Regional Genetics Service, Department of Genetics,
St George's Hospital NHS Trust, London, UK

**Baskaran Thilaganathan** MD FRCOG
Director, Fetal Medicine Unit, Department of
Obstetrics and Gynaecology, St George's Hospital
NHS Trust, London, UK

# Acknowledgements

We would like to thank the team of dedicated freelance copy editors, without whom the completion of this book would not have been possible: Martina Habeck, Elisabeth Rees-Evans and Katharine Timberlake. Especial thanks are due to Fiona Courtenay-Thompson, who managed the whole editorial project with enormous skill and patience.

We would also like to acknowledge the contribution of Alex Landau of the RCOG Examination Department, and the talented artists of Oxford Designers and Illustrators, particularly David Morris, Elaine Leggatt and Sue Aldridge, who interpreted the authors' requirements with skill and flair. Their results speak for themselves.

### Chapter 10

The authors wish to thank the following for their contribution and critical review of the manuscript, in their areas of expertise: Dr John Alcolado (Reader/ Honorary Consultant Physician, University Hospital of Wales: electrocardiography), Dr Andrew Wood (Consultant Radiologist, University Hospital of Wales: X-rays, CT and MRI), Mr Andrew Bryant (radio-therapy physicist, Velindre Hospital, Cardiff: radio-therapy), Dr Neil Warren (Lecturer, Welsh Institute for Minimal Access Therapy-WIMAT, Cardiff University: electrosurgery) and Mr Anthony Griffiths (Consultant Obstetrician and Gynaecologist, University Hospital of Wales: electrosurgery).

### Chapters 16 and 17

The author is grateful to Professor Whitehead of the Department of Physiology, St George's, University of London, for the use of tables and diagrams.

### Chapter 33

The authors are most grateful to Dr Paul Silcocks, Clinical Senior Lecturer, Nottingham Clinical Trials Support Unit, for reading and making helpful comments on the manuscript.

# Abbreviations used in the book

| | |
|---|---|
| $^{125}I$ | iodine-125 |
| $^{131}I$ | iodine-131 |
| $^{137}Cs$ | caesium-137 |
| $^{177}Lu$ | lutetium-177 |
| $^{192}Ir$ | iridium-192 |
| 2,3-DPG | 2,3-diphosphoglycerate |
| 5α-DHT | 5α-dihydrotestosterone |
| $^{90}Y$ | yttrium-90 |
| α-FP | alphafetoprotein |
| β-hCG | beta-human chorionic gonadotrophin |
| θ | scattering angle |
| ρ | density of a material |
| ABPA | allergic bronchopulmonary aspergillosis |
| ACE | angiotensin-converting enzyme |
| ACTH | adrenocorticotrophic hormone |
| ADP | adenosine diphosphate |
| AFP | alphafetoprotein |
| AMP | adenosine monophosphate |
| ANP | atrial natriuretic peptide |
| AP | accessory proteins |
| APC | adenomatous polyposis coli |
| APC | antigen-presenting cell |
| APECED | autoimmune polyendocrinopathy, candidiasis and ectodermal dystrophy |
| APS | autoimmune polyendocrinopathy syndrome |
| APUD | amine precursor uptake and decarboxylation |
| ASD | atrial septal defect |
| ATM | ataxia telangiectasia mutated |
| ATP | adenosine triphosphate |
| AVP | arginine vasopressin |
| AVSD | atriventricular septal defect |
| ADH | antidiuretic hormone |

| | |
|---|---|
| B cell | bursa-equivalent cell |
| BAC | bacterial artificial chromosome |
| BMD | bone mineral density |
| B-mode ultrasound | brightness mode ultrasound |
| BMUS | British Medical Ultrasound Society |
| bNOS | brain nitric oxide synthase |
| BSO | bilateral salpingo-oophorectomy |
| C | carbon atom |
| c | (in the context of ultrasound) speed of a sound wave |
| CaBP | $Ca^{2+}$-binding protein (nur in figure) |
| CaMK | $Ca^{2+}$/calmodulin-dependent kinase |
| cAMP | cyclic adenosine monophosphate |
| CaSR | $Ca^{2+}$-sensing receptor |
| CCA | common carotid artery |
| CCR | chemokine C-C motif receptor |
| CDK2 | cyclin-dependent kinase 2 |
| cDNA | complementary DNA |
| cffDNA | cell-free fetal DNA |
| CEMACH | Confidential Enquiry into Maternal and Child Health |
| CEMD | Confidential Enquiry into Maternal Deaths |
| CGH | comparative genomic hybridisation |
| CGIN | cervical glandular intraepithelial neoplasia |
| cGMP | cyclic guanosine monophosphate |
| CHD | coronary heart disease |
| CIN | cervical intraepithelial neoplasia |
| CMACE | Centre for Maternal and Child Enquiries |
| CMV | cytomegalovirus |
| CNS | central nervous system |
| CO | carbon monoxide |

| | | | |
|---|---|---|---|
| CoA | coenzyme A | CaBP | $Ca^{2+}$-binding protein (nur in figure) |
| $^{125}I$ | iodine-125 | CaMK | $Ca^{2+}$/calmodulin-dependent kinase |
| $^{131}I$ | iodine-131 | cAMP | cyclic adenosine monophosphate |
| $^{137}Cs$ | caesium-137 | CaSR | $Ca^{2+}$-sensing receptor |
| $^{177}Lu$ | lutetium-177 | CCA | common carotid artery |
| $^{192}Ir$ | iridium-192 | CCR | chemokine C-C motif receptor |
| 2,3-DPG | 2,3-diphosphoglycerate | CDK2 | cyclin-dependent kinase 2 |
| 5α-DHT | 5α-dihydrotestosterone | cDNA | complementary DNA |
| $^{90}Y$ | yttrium-90 | cffDNA | cell-free fetal DNA |
| α-FP | alphafetoprotein | CEMACH | Confidential Enquiry into Maternal and Child Health |
| β-hCG | beta-human chorionic gonadotrophin | | |
| θ | scattering angle | CEMD | Confidential Enquiry into Maternal Deaths |
| ρ | density of a material | | |
| ABPA | allergic bronchopulmonary aspergillosis | CGH | comparative genomic hybridisation |
| | | CGIN | cervical glandular intraepithelial neoplasia |
| ACE | angiotensin-converting enzyme | | |
| ACTH | adrenocorticotrophic hormone | cGMP | cyclic guanosine monophosphate |
| ADP | adenosine diphosphate | CHD | coronary heart disease |
| AFP | alphafetoprotein | CIN | cervical intraepithelial neoplasia |
| AMP | adenosine monophosphate | CMACE | Centre for Maternal and Child Enquiries |
| ANP | atrial natriuretic peptide | | |
| AP | accessory proteins | CMV | cytomegalovirus |
| APC | adenomatous polyposis coli | CNS | central nervous system |
| APC | antigen-presenting cell | CO | carbon monoxide |
| APECED | autoimmune polyendocrinopathy, candidiasis and ectodermal dystrophy | CoA | coenzyme A |
| | | COPD | chronic obstructive pulmonary disease |
| APS | autoimmune polyendocrinopathy syndrome | COX | cyclooxygenase |
| | | Cox2 | cyclooxygenase type II |
| APUD | amine precursor uptake and decarboxylation | CRH | corticotrophin-releasing hormone |
| | | CRH-BP | corticotrophin-releasing hormone binding protein |
| ASD | atrial septal defect | | |
| ATM | ataxia telangiectasia mutated | CRT | conformal radiotherapy |
| AVP | arginine vasopressin | CT | computed tomography |
| AVSD | atriventricular septal defect | CTG | cardiotocography |
| ADH | antidiuretic hormone | CVS | chorionic villus sampling |
| B cell | bursa-equivalent cell | CYP | cytochrome P450 |
| BAC | bacterial artificial chromosome | CYP11A1 | cholesterol side chain cleavage enzyme |
| BMD | bone mineral density | CYP17A | steroid 17α-hydroxylase |
| B-mode ultrasound | brightness mode ultrasound | CYP19 | aromatase |
| | | DC | dendritic cell |
| BMUS | British Medical Ultrasound Society | DCC | defective in sister chromatid cohesion |
| bNOS | brain nitric oxide synthase | DCT | distal convoluted tubule |
| BSO | bilateral salpingo-oophorectomy | DEET | N,N-diethyl-m-toluamide |
| C | carbon atom | dex | dexamethasone |
| c | (in the context of ultrasound) speed of a sound wave | DEXA | dual energy X-ray absorptiometry |
| | | DHA | docosahexaenoic acid |

DHEA    dehydroepiandrosterone
DHEAS   dehydroepiandrosterone sulphate
DOPA    dihydroxyphenylalanine
DPPC    dipalmitoylphosphatidylcholine
$E_1$    estrone
$E_2$    17-beta-estradiol
$E_3$    estriol
EBM    evidence-based medicine
ECG    electrocardiogram
EDTA    ethylenediaminetetraacetic acid
EFSUMB    European Federation of Societies for Ultrasound in Medicine and Biology
EIA    enzyme immunoassay
eNOS    endothelial nitric oxide synthase
EPO    erythropoietin
ER    endoplasmic reticulum
ERPC    evacuation of retained products of conception
Fab    antigen-binding fragment
FAD    flavin adenine dinucleotide
$FADH_2$    reduced form of flavin adenine dinucleotide
FBM    fetal breathing movement
Fc    crystallisable fragment
$f_d$    Doppler frequency shift
FHR    fetal heart rate
FISH    fluorescence in situ hybridisation
FSH    follicle-stimulating hormone
$f_t$    frequency of a transmitted signal
G    (in DNA and RNA sequences) guanine
G protein    guanine-nucleotide-binding protein
G0    quiescent state
G1    gap 1
G2    gap 2
GABA    γ-aminobutyric acid
GBS    group B streptococci
GDM    gestational diabetes mellitus
GDP    guanosine diphosphate
GH    growth hormone
GHRH    growth-hormone-releasing hormone
GI    gastrointestinal
Gi    inhibitory G protein
GLP-1    glucagon-like peptide 1
GLUT3    glucose transporter type 3
GM-CSF    granulocyte–macrophage colony-stimulating factor

GnRH    gonadotrophin-releasing hormone
Gs protein    stimulatory G protein
GTP    guanosine triphosphate
Gy    gray
H0    null hypothesis
$H_2CO_3$    carbonic acid
$H_2O_2$    hydrogen peroxide
$H_2PO_4^-$    dihydrogen phosphate
$HbA_{1c}$    glycated haemoglobin
HbF    fetal haemoglobin
hCG    human chorionic gonadotrophin
HCl    hydrochloric acid
$HCO_3^-$    bicarbonate ion
HDL    high-density lipoprotein
HLA    human leucocyte antigen
HNPCC    hereditary nonpolyposis colon cancer
$HPO_4^{2-}$    hydrogen phosphate
HPV    human papilloma virus
HRT    hormone replacement therapy
HSD    hydroxysteroid dehydrogenase
HSL    hormone-sensitive lipase
HSP    heat shock protein
HSV    herpes simplex virus
IACR    International Association of Cancer Registries
ICA    internal carotid artery
ICAM    intercellular cell adhesion molecule
IDBP    intracellular vitamin-D-binding protein
IFN    interferon
Ig    immunoglobulin
IGF    insulin-like growth factor
IL    interleukin
ILT    immunoglobulin-like transcript
IMRT    intensity-modulated radiation therapy
inh    inhibin
iNOS    inducible nitric oxide synthase
$IP_3$    inositol trisphosphate
$IP_4$    inositol tetrakisphosphate
IUCD    intrauterine contraceptive device
IVC    inferior vena cava
IVC    inferior vena cava
IVF    in vitro fertilisation
IVIg    intravenous immunoglobulin
K    dissociation constant

| | |
|---|---|
| KIR | killer cell immunoglobulin-like receptor |
| KOH | potassium hydroxide |
| KTP | potassium titanyl phosphate |
| KUB X-ray | kidney, ureter and bladder X-ray |
| LDL | low-density lipoprotein |
| Leu | leucine |
| LGV | lymphogranuloma venereum |
| LH | luteinising hormone |
| LTV | long-term variability |
| MAO | monoamine oxidase |
| MAP | mitogen-activated protein |
| MB | mamillary bodies |
| MELAS | mitochondrial encephalomyopathy with lactic acidosis and stroke-like episodes |
| MERFF | myoclonic epilepsy with ragged red fibres |
| Met | methionine |
| MHC | major histocompatibility complex |
| MHRA | Medicines and Healthcare products Regulatory Agency |
| MLCK | myosin light chain kinase |
| MLPA | multiplex ligation-dependent probe amplification |
| M-mode ultrasound | movement mode ultrasound |
| MMR | measles, mumps and rubella |
| MRI | magnetic resonance imaging |
| mRNA | messenger RNA |
| MRSA | meticillin-resistant Staphylococcus aureus |
| mVDR | membrane-bound vitamin D receptor |
| NAAT | nucleic acid amplification test |
| $NAD^+$ | oxidised form of nicotinamide adenine dinucleotide |
| NADH | reduced form of nicotinamide adenine dinucleotide |
| $NADP^+$ | oxidised form of nicotinamide adenine dinucleotide phosphate |
| NADPH | reduced form of nicotinamide adenine dinucleotide phosphate |
| $NaHCO_3$ | sodium bicarbonate |
| NCAM | neural cell adhesion molecule |
| Nd:YAG | neodymium-doped yttrium aluminium garnet |

| | |
|---|---|
| $NH_4^+$ | ammonium ion |
| NICE | National Institute for Health and Clinical Excellence |
| NK | natural killer |
| NNRTI | nonnucleoside reverse transcriptase inhibitor |
| NO | nitric oxide |
| NPT2 | inorganic phosphate cotransporter type II |
| NRTI | nucleoside reverse transcriptase inhibitor |
| NSAID | nonsteroidal anti-inflammatory drug |
| NT | nuchal translucency |
| OC | optic chiasm |
| OGTT | oral glucose tolerance test |
| $OH-$ | hydroxyl ion |
| P (encircled) | phosphate group |
| PAPP-A | pregnancy-associated plasma protein A |
| PAS | periodic acid–Schiff stain |
| $PCO_2$ | partial pressure of carbon dioxide |
| PCR | polymerase chain reaction |
| PDH | pyruvate dehydrogenase |
| PECAM | platelet endothelial cell adhesion molecule |
| PGD | prostaglandin D |
| PGE | prostaglandin E |
| $PGF_{2\alpha}$ | prostaglandin $F_{2\alpha}$ |
| PGH | prostaglandin H |
| PGI | prostaglandin I |
| $PGI_2$ | prostacyclin |
| pH value | negative logarithm to the base 10 of the H+ concentration |
| pheH | phenylalanine hydroxylase |
| Pi | inorganic phosphate |
| PID | pelvic inflammatory disease |
| $PIP_2$ | phosphatidyl bisphosphate |
| pK value | negative logarithm to the base 10 of the dissociation constant K |
| PKC | protein kinase C |
| PLC | phospholipase C |
| PMCA | plasma membrane $Ca^{2+}$-ATPase |
| $Po_2$ | partial pressure of oxygen |
| $PO_3^{4-}$ | phosphate ion |
| POF | premature ovarian failure |
| Pol II | polymerase II |

POMC    pro-opiomelanocortin
PPNG    pelicillinase-producing Neisseria
        gonorrhoeae
PRF     prolactin-releasing factor
PSA     prostate-specific antigen
PTH     parathyroid hormone
PTHR    parathyroid hormone receptor
PTHrP   parathyroid-hormone-related peptide
PUL     pregnancy of unknown location
PUV     pregnancy of 'uncertain viability'
PVN     paraventricular nucleus
QF-PCR  quantitative fluorescence polymerase
        chain reaction
RBC     red blood cell
RCT     randomised controlled trial
ROC     receiver operating characteristic
RPR     rapid plasma reagin
rRNA    ribosomal RNA
RXR     retinoid X receptor
s or SD standard deviation
$s^2$   variance
SDS     sodium dodecyl sulphate
SE      standard error
SEM     standard error of the mean
SHBG    sex hormone-binding globulin
SO      supraoptic nucleus
SPA     spiral artery
spp.    two or more species
ssp.    subspecies
StAR    steroidogenic acute regulator
STBM    syncytiotrophoblast microparticle
STI     sexually transmitted infection
STR     short tandem repeat
STV     short-term variability
Sv      sievert
t       (in the context of pulsed ultrasound)
        pulse duration
T       (in DNA sequences) thymine
T       (in the context of pulsed ultrasound)
        pulse repetition period
T cell  thymus-derived cell
$T_3$   triiodothyronine
$T_4$   thyroxine
TAG     triacylglycerol

TALH    thick ascending loop of Henle
Tc cell cytotoxic T cell
TCA     tricarboxylic acid
TCR     T cell receptor
TGC     time-gain compensation
TGF-β   transforming growth factor beta
Th1 cell T helper cell type 1
Th2 cell T helper cell type 2
TIB     thermal index in bone
TIC     thermal index in the cranium
TIS     thermal index in soft tissues
TK      tyrosine kinase
TNF-α   tumour necrosis factor alpha
TPHA    Treponema pallidum
        haemagglutination
Tr cell regulatory T cell
TRAP    tartrate-resistant acid phosphatase
TRH     thyrotrophin-releasing hormone
tRNA    transfer RNA
TRPV5   epithelial $Ca^{2+}$ channel 1
TRPV6   epithelial $Ca^{2+}$ channel 2
TSH     thyroid-stimulating hormone
TSH     thyroid-stimulating hormone
TTPA    Treponema pallidum particle
        agglutination
TSH     thyroid-stimulating hormone
U       (in RNA sequences) uracil
$uE_3$  unconjugated estradiol
uNK     uterine natural killer cell
UPD     uniparental disomy
v       velocity of a moving object
VCAM    vascular cell adhesion molecule
VDR     vitamin D receptor
VDRL    venereal disease research laboratory
VEGF    vascular endothelial growth factor
VIN     vulvar intraepithelial neoplasia
VIP     vasoactive intestinal peptide
VLDL    very-low-density lipoprotein
VSD     ventricular septal defect
VZIG    varicella zoster immune globulin
VZV     varicella zoster virus
WBC     white blood cell
Z       acoustic impedance

## Organisms

| | | | |
|---|---|---|---|
| B. burgdorferi | Borrellia burgdorferi | M. marinum | Mycobacterium marinum |
| B. hermsii | Borrellia hermsii | M. microti | Mycobacterium microti |
| B. pseudomallei | Burkholderia pseudomallei | M. pneumoniae | Mycoplasma pneumoniae |
| B. recurrentis | Borrellia recurrentis | M. tuberculosis | Mycobacterium tuberculosis |
| C. albicans | Candida albicans | M. ulcerans | Mycobacterium ulcerans |
| C. difficile | Clostridium difficile | N. gonorrhoeae | Neisseria gonorrhoeae |
| C. diphtheriae | Corynebacterium diphtheriae | N. meningitidis | Neisseria meningitides |
| C. glabrata | Candida glabrata | P. aeruginosa | Pseudomonas aeruginosa |
| C. krusei | Candida krusei | P. carinii | Pneumocystis carinii |
| C. pneumoniae | Chlamydia pneumoniae | P. falciparum | Plasmodium falciparum |
| C. psittaci | Chlamydia psittaci | P. malariae | Plasmodium malariae |
| C. tetani | Clostridium tetani | P. ovale | Plasmodium ovale |
| C. trachomatis | Chlamydia trachomatis | P. vivax | Plasmodium vivax |
| C. tropicalis | Candida tropicalis | S. agalactiae | Streptococcus agalactiae |
| E. coli | Escherichia coli | S. anginosus | Streptococcus anginosus |
| E. faecalis | Enterococcus faecalis | S. aureus | Staphylococcus aureus |
| E. faecium | Enterococcus faecium | S. bovis | Streptococcus bovis |
| G. vaginalis | Gardnerella vaginalis | S. capitis | Staphylococcus capitis |
| L. mono-cytogenes | Listeria monocytogenes | S. dysgalactiae | Streptococcus dysgalactiae |
| L. interrogans | Leptospira interrogans | S. epidermidis | Staphylococcus epidermidis |
| M. abscessus | Mycobacterium abscessus | S. equisimilis | Streptococcus equisimilis |
| M. africanum | Mycobacterium africanum | S. haemolyticus | Staphylococcus haemolyticus |
| M. avium | Mycobacterium avium | S. milleri | Streptococcus milleri |
| M. bovis | Mycobacterium bovis | S. mitis | Streptococcus mitis |
| M. chelonae | Mycobacterium chelonae | S. mutans | Streptococcus mutans |
| M. fortuitum | Mycobacterium fortuitum | S. paratyphi | Salmonella paratyphi |
| M. genitalium | Mycoplasma genitalium | S. pneumoniae | Streptococcus pneumoniae |
| M. genitalium | Mycoplasma genitalium | S. pyogenes | Streptococcus pyogenes |
| M. hominis | Mycoplasma hominis | S. saprophyticus | Staphylococcus saprophyticus |
| M. hominis | Mycoplasma hominis | T. carateum | Treponema carateum |
| M. intracellulare | Mycobacterium | T. pallidum | Treponema pallidum |
| M. kansasii | Mycobacterium kansasii | T. pallidum | Treponema pallidum |
| M. leprae | Mycobacterium leprae | T. vaginalis | Trichomonas vaginalis |
| M. leprae | Mycobacterium leprae | T. vaginalis | Trichomonas vaginalis |
| | | U. urealyticum | Ureaplasma urealyticum |

# Preface

I am delighted to welcome this additional aid to learning for the MRCOG Part 1 examination. The expertise and experience of the authors is clear and allows doctors using this book to be secure in the knowledge that it contains up-to-date, accurate information. The examples of questions are drawn directly from the RCOG questions bank and add significantly to the interpretation of the text.

Attaining the Part 1 MRCOG is a rite-of-passage that many of us remember and that we, at the RCOG, want to ensure helps trainees understand the importance of the underlying clinical sciences in our specialties. This book will be an aid in the first part of a successful Obstetrics and Gynaecology career.

I am sure you will find this book a useful addition to your studies.

**Professor Wendy Reid** FRCOG
**Vice President, Education**
**Royal College of Obstetricians and Gynaecologists**

# Introduction

CHAPTER 1

# Taking the Part 1 MRCOG examination

*Alison N Fiander*

## Introduction

The Part 1 MRCOG examination underwent modernisation between 2005 and 2007. This chapter deals with the background to the changes and their implementation. It also discusses extended matching questions (EMQs) as forming a component of the examination since September 2007 and describes further changes to the examination format that come into effect from March 2012.

## Background

The decision to modernise the Part 1 MRCOG in 2005 came after it was noted that pass rates were falling and that the examination was perceived as a difficult basic science hurdle tending to lack obvious clinical relevance.

However, basic sciences are vitally important to the clinical practice of obstetrics and gynaecology and are therefore an essential element of the examination. While some subjects, such as surgical anatomy of the pelvis, are static, others are continually changing. For example, rapid advances in bioscience since the 1980s, including ultrasound, *in vitro* fertilisation, prenatal diagnosis, clinical epidemiology and evidence-based medicine, are already impacting upon clinical practice and need to be reflected in both the syllabus and in the examination. Advances in gene therapy and stem cell science will begin to impact on practice in the next decade and these also need to be taken into account.

Set against this background, a working group was convened in 2005, chaired by Professor W Ledger FRCOG, to determine the fitness for purpose of the existing Part 1

MRCOG examination and to make recommendations regarding the syllabus, content and format of a new Part 1 MRCOG examination. The working group identified the need for a clearly defined syllabus, with a core knowledge at Part 1 MRCOG as a prerequisite for progressing to the Part 2 examination. The group also saw the need to map the basic clinical sciences in Part 1 MRCOG to the new core curriculum for training in obstetrics and gynaecology.

The revised Part 1 MRCOG syllabus and examination is concerned with preparing a doctor to become a specialist in obstetrics and gynaecology in an age of new bioscience, as well as being an aid to direct learning. It acknowledges that the practising clinician must be able to evaluate and incorporate new scientific tools into clinical practice and advise patients of the utility of new techniques. It recognises that knowledge is the single best determinant of expertise in a subject.

### Findings of the Part 1 MRCOG working group

The working group reviewed the undergraduate curricula of a sample of UK medical schools to try and see why candidates were finding the Part 1 MRCOG examination increasingly difficult. It found a tendency towards incorporation of basic sciences into integrated curricula with a move towards basic science being taught by clinicians rather than scientists and towards problem-based learning and an applied knowledge base. In addition, there seemed to be a trend towards an overall reduction in the basic science content of the curricula. These findings suggested that Part 1 MRCOG candidates, who should have been revising basic science in preparation for the examination, were in fact studying some of it for the first time. The working group also reviewed the Part 1 MRCOG question bank and considered that some of the questions were out of date, while others lacked obvious clinical relevance or were somewhat obscure.

The working group made the following recommendations:

- To end exemption from the Part 1 MRCOG examination.
- To define a detailed syllabus for Part 1 as part of the overall MRCOG core curriculum.
- To update the question bank ensuring quality and clinical relevance.
- To revise the distribution of questions and add new areas to be examined.
- To include extended matching questions (EMQs).
- To use standard setting to determine the pass mark.

## Implementation of Part 1 MRCOG working group recommendations

### ENDING PART 1 MRCOG EXEMPTION

Exemption ended at the end of 2006 in recognition of the fact that the new Part 1 MRCOG examination formed an integral part of the overall core curriculum in obstetrics and gynaecology and that it was impossible to guarantee that the Part 1 syllabus was covered by other examinations.

### PART 1 MRCOG SYLLABUS

The aim of revising the Part 1 MRCOG syllabus was to make it clearer and better defined, to map it to the modules and domains of the core curriculum and to update it to include new bioscience topics such as clinical trial design, molecular biology and genomics.

The Part 1 syllabus and other relevant information can be found on the RCOG website at: www.rcog.org.uk/education-and-exams/examinations/exam-part-one.

### PART 1 MRCOG QUESTION BANK REVIEW

As a result of the review of the Part 1 MRCOG question bank in 2006, out of date questions were updated and obscure questions and those lacking obvious clinical relevance to obstetrics and gynaecology were removed. New questions were developed, particularly in the new areas to be examined, and extended matching questions (EMQs) were added.

### DISTRIBUTION OF QUESTIONS

A small reduction in the number of questions for certain subjects, such as anatomy, embryology, endocrinology, biochemistry and physiology, allowed an increase in other areas, such as statistics and epidemiology. New topics were also introduced, such as clinical trial design and analysis, molecular and cell biology, genomics and the regulation of gene expression.

The following pie charts show the new distribution of questions for paper 1 and paper 2 (Figure 1.1), although this will vary slightly from sitting to sitting. The charts also indicate the new question areas that have been included in the Part 1 MRCOG examination since September 2007.

FIGURE 1.1 **Distribution of questions in the Part 1 MRCOG examination (these may vary slightly from sitting to sitting)**

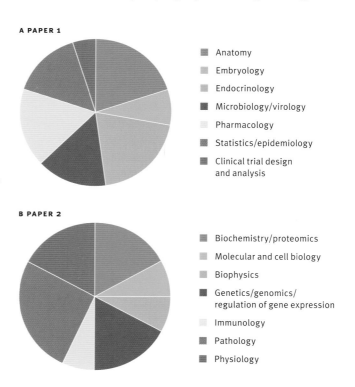

A PAPER 1

- Anatomy
- Embryology
- Endocrinology
- Microbiology/virology
- Pharmacology
- Statistics/epidemiology
- Clinical trial design and analysis

B PAPER 2

- Biochemistry/proteomics
- Molecular and cell biology
- Biophysics
- Genetics/genomics/ regulation of gene expression
- Immunology
- Pathology
- Physiology

## INCLUSION OF EXTENDED MATCHING QUESTIONS

EMQs have been incorporated into the Part 1 MRCOG examination since September 2007 and at present contribute 20% of the examination marks.

The examination comprises two papers, each of two hours duration separated by a break. Each paper contains 48 multiple choice questions (MCQs) each with five items (240 items in total) and 20 EMQs (1–3 items per option list). Figure 1.2 shows the current composition of the Part 1 MRCOG examination.

The current value of each correct MCQ answer remains the same: one mark for each true/false answer. Each correct EMQ answer is worth three marks. Time management is important and it is suggested that the candidate spends approximately 96 minutes on the MCQs and 24 minutes on the EMQs.

### STANDARD SETTING

Standard setting to determine the pass mark is already undertaken for the Part 1 MRCOG examination. The aim of standard setting is to improve the fairness and validity of the examination and to set levels of competence required for success. Standard setting produces a criterion-referenced pass mark by assessing the difficulty of individual papers using a modified Angoff method.

FIGURE 1.2  **Composition of the Part 1 MRCOG examination**

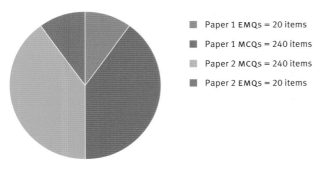

- Paper 1 EMQs = 20 items
- Paper 1 MCQs = 240 items
- Paper 2 MCQs = 240 items
- Paper 2 EMQs = 20 items

**PAPER 1**
Anatomy, embryology, endocrinology, microbiology, virology, pharmacology, statistics, epidemiology, clinical trial design and analysis

**PAPER 2**
Biochemistry, proteomics, molecular and cell biology, biophysics, genetics, genomics, regulation of gene expression, immunology, pathology, physiology

## Extended matching questions

### WHY?

EMQs have been incorporated into both the Part 1 and the Part 2 MRCOG examinations for a number of reasons. They test understanding of a subject in greater depth than MCQs by assessing the candidate's knowledge of the relationship between facts. Therefore candidates who have an in-depth knowledge will pass, while those who do not will fail.[1] They also tend to define clinical relevance more quickly and reduce the inherent 'clues' of MCQ formats.

EMQs have been used in the Part 2 MRCOG examination since 2006 and have demonstrated improved discrimination compared with MCQs in defining pass and fail candidates. Both EMQs and MCQs are computer marked with complete accuracy.

### WHAT?

EMQs comprise three parts: a list of options or answers, a lead-in statement or instructions and 1–3 items or questions. This can be seen in the blank EMQ template in appendix 3. The option list is lettered to reflect the candidate's EMQ answer sheet (appendix 4) and will often be in alphabetical or numerical order for ease of reference. The lead-in statement puts the question into context and tells the candidate what to do. The items are numbered to match the answer sheet.

### HOW?

The recommended way of approaching EMQs is to read the lead-in statement first, followed by the items. The candidate should think about the answer and then select the most appropriate option from the list. Reading the list of options first may be confusing, as the list will contain incorrect options and distractors. EMQs can be written with a single list of options or can be combined into a table format thereby increasing the number of elements of the syllabus examined by a single item, as well as looking at a candidate's ability to link knowledge.[2]

The candidate is reminded to select the single option that fits best, even if they feel that there are several possible options. As with the MCQ paper, if two or more boxes are marked on the same question, no mark will be awarded, even if one of the options chosen is the correct one. It is therefore important to ensure that any mistakes are fully erased so that they will not be picked up by the computer. Although the candidate's answer sheet will provide 20 possible answers, the option lists may not use all of these. Most option lists will provide 10–14 options.

It is worth noting that EMQs have been allocated more time than MCQs in recognition that they take longer to read and consider. As with MCQs, there is no negative marking for EMQs so it is worth attempting every question. It is recommended that candidates practise both question formats before taking the examination. Examples of EMQs and MCQs for Part 1 MRCOG are given for each chapter in this book and can also be found on the RCOG website and in *EMQs for the MRCOG Part 1*.[3]

While the introduction of EMQs has been effective in increasing the depth of knowledge tested in the Part 1 MRCOG, from March 2012 they will be replaced by single best answer questions (SBAQs). SBAQs are similar in format to EMQs. They consist of a lead-in statement and five options from which the candidate is required to select the most appropriate answer. Given the lower scoring tariff for an SBAQ compared with an EMQ, this development will allow a greater range of knowledge to be tested within similar time constraints without compromising the profundity of knowledge being tested. Benefiting from the relative breadth of MCQs and the relative depth of EMQs in this way, the introduction of SBAQs will be instrumental in producing a more clinically relevant and more reliable Part 1 MRCOG examination.

## Multiple choice questions

MCQs continue to form the major part of the Part 1 MRCOG examination. They allow wide subject coverage ensuring efficient use of examination time and perform consistently and reliably well.

Appendix 5 shows a blank MCQ template with a stem or lead-in statement and then 5 items, each of which require a true (T) or false (F) answer. Appendix 6 shows an MCQ answer sheet. As with EMQs, the candidate is reminded that there is no negative marking and it is recommended that every question is attempted.

## Blueprinting

Blueprinting ensures even subject and domain coverage and that the examination is neither too predictable nor unpredictable. It confirms that subject areas comprising core knowledge for the specialty are suitably covered to test trainees comprehensively. The new MRCOG core curriculum allows examinations to be blueprinted and maps the Part 1 MRCOG examination as a component part (together with the Part 2 MRCOG examination) of the overall process of assessment for future specialists in obstetrics and gynaecology. The Part 1 MRCOG examination has been blueprinted since 2007.

## Summary

In summary, the Part 1 MRCOG examination has been modernised to ensure that it remains fit for purpose, assessing basic clinical sciences as relevant to the clinical practice of obstetrics and gynaecology. A new detailed syllabus has been developed and the question bank updated to ensure questions are relevant. Extended matching questions have been incorporated into the Part 1 MRCOG examination alongside traditional multiple choice questions The forthcoming introduction of SBAQs from March 2012, meanwhile, will further improve the examination's relevance and reliability.

REFERENCES

1. McCoubrie P. Improving the fairness of multiple-choice questions: a literature review. *Med Teach* 2004;26:709–12.

2. Duthie S, Fiander A N, Hodges P D. Extended matched questions: a new component of the Part 1 examination leading to membership of the Royal College of Obstetricians and Gynaecologists. *The Obstetrician & Gynaecologist* 2007;9:189–94.

3. Duthie J, Hodges P. *EMQs for the MRCOG Part 1*. London: RCOG Press; 2007.

# Anatomy

# CHAPTER 2

# Anatomy of the pelvis, femoral triangle and inguinal canal

*Diana Lawrence-Watt*

## Bones of the pelvis

The bones of the pelvis present an impressive skeletal ring between the heads of the femurs and the fifth lumbar vertebra. The pelvis consists of the sacrum and right and left hip, or innominate, bones. All three bones allow the pelvis to undertake its role of bearing the weight of the body as well as responding to the musculature that acts upon it. Each hip bone is formed by the fusion of three bones: the ilium, ischium and pubis. These bones unite within the cavity of the acetabulum, which receives the head of the femur. Fusion between the ilium and the pubis is also evidenced by the presence of the iliopubic eminence.

### GREATER AND LESSER PELVIS

The pelvis itself is arbitrarily divided into two regions, described as the greater pelvis and the lesser pelvis. The greater pelvis is formed by the iliac blades on both sides and by the base of the sacrum posteriorly. The lesser pelvis is the region that describes the true 'basin', having an inlet and an outlet as well as the muscular pelvic floor. The pelvic inlet, the boundaries of which are described as the pelvic brim, has obstetric significance in relation to measurements taken in obstetric practice (Figure 2.1). The pelvic brim consists of the promontory and ala of the sacrum posteriorly, the arcuate and pectineal lines laterally and anterolaterally respectively, with the anterior boundary of the inlet being formed by the superior pubic rami, the body of pubis and the pubic symphysis.

FIGURE 2.1 **Female bony pelvis**

**A** Anteroposterior diameter from the midpoint of the sacral promontory to the upper border of the pubic symphysis, usually measured between the third sacral segment and posterior surface of the symphysis
**B** Transverse diameter measured between two similar points on opposite sides of the pelvic brim
**C** Oblique diameter measured from the iliopubic eminence to the lowest point of the contralateral sacroiliac joint

### PELVIC INLET AND OUTLET

As well as providing the bony elements of the birth canal, the lesser pelvis gives attachments to many ligaments and to elements of the pelvic floor. It also contains the pelvic viscera. The outlet of the pelvis is formed by four elements of bone: the coccyx posteriorly, the pubic symphysis anteriorly and the two ischial tuberosities laterally. The strong sacrotuberous ligaments stretch between the sacrum/coccyx and the ischial tuberosities, with the result that the outlet of the pelvis is described as rhomboid in shape. The inlet of the pelvis has a wide, transverse oval opening, whereas the outlet presents a more oval diameter in its anteroposterior relationship.

These anatomical correlates are reflected during labour. The fetal head enters the pelvic inlet positioned with the longer, anteroposterior dimension across the widest and therefore transverse diameter of the pelvis. At the pelvic outlet, the fetal head is positioned anteroposteriorly in relation to the pelvic outlet, this being the widest diameter of both head and outlet. The shape of both the pelvic outlet and inlet are therefore important considerations in labour, because the cross-sectional shape of the birth canal differs at these anatomical levels.

The shape of the pelvic outlet corresponds to three wide arches, formed by the subpubic arch anteriorly and the two greater sciatic notches posteriorly. Spanning across the posterior region on each side are the sacrotuberous and sacrospinous ligaments, which convert the sciatic notches into foramina. These foramina are occupied by muscles and important vessels and nerves. The presence of the sacrotuberous and sacrospinous ligaments and the mobile coccyx ensure that the posterior part of the pelvic outlet is a relatively flexible structure.

### PELVIC ARTICULATIONS AND LIGAMENTS

The articulations of the pelvis are the sacroiliac joint, the pubic symphysis and the joint between the sacrum and the mobile coccyx. Although the sacroiliac joint is described as a plane joint with very limited movement, the joint surfaces are anything but flat. In fact, they interdigitate by a series of depressions and elevations, fitting into each other to restrict movement of the joint and affording it great strength.

The main ligaments of the sacroiliac joint are the ventral sacroiliac ligament, the dorsal sacroiliac ligament and the interosseus ligament. The ventral sacroiliac ligament should not be truly described as a ligament as it is in fact a thickening of the joint capsule.

The dorsal sacroiliac ligament, consisting of quite weak bands of tissue, arises from the intermediate and lateral crests of the sacrum, which pass down to the posterior superior iliac spine and the inner lip of the iliac crest. The lower part of this ligament, arising from the third and fourth sacral segments and passing to the posterior superior iliac spine, may form a separate structure termed the long posterior sacroiliac ligament. Some of the fibres of the posterior sacroiliac ligament, when present, may also merge with the sacrotuberous ligament.

The ligament of the sacroiliac joint that deserves most comment is the interosseous ligament, the strongest ligament uniting the hip bones to the sacrum. The interosseous ligament occupies the space between the bony elements at the back of the joint. It is covered by the dorsal sacroiliac ligament, from which it is separated by the dorsal primary rami of the sacral nerves and vessels. Consisting of deep and superficial strata, fibres from the deep layer pass from depressions on the sacrum to depressions on the tuberosity of the ilium. The most notable fibres of the superficial layers frequently form the short posterior iliac ligament, which spans between the superior articular process and the lateral crest of the first two segments of the sacrum to the ilium.

The pubic symphysis forms a secondary cartilaginous joint that unites the two pubic bones via a fibrocartilaginous disc and the superior and arcuate pubic ligaments. The latter is separated from the urogenital diaphragm by an interval, through which the deep vein of the clitoris enters into the pelvis.

### PELVIC ARTICULATIONS IN PREGNANCY

In pregnancy, all joints of the pelvis afford a greater degree of movement than in the nonpregnant state. This movement is more pronounced in the sacroiliac joint, which can result in increased strain on the ligaments following pregnancy.

## Functional anatomy of the abdominal wall

Supporting and compressing the abdominal contents are the muscles of the anterior abdominal wall: the external and internal oblique, transversus and rectus abdominis. The oblique muscles act in compression, their contraction being important in birth when expelling the fetus from the uterus.

## EXTERNAL OBLIQUE

The external oblique muscle arises from the outer surfaces of the lower eight ribs, these fibres interdigitating with fibres of the serratus anterior and latissimus dorsi. Fibres from the lower two ribs pass vertically down to the anterior part of the iliac crest, whereas fibres from the other ribs pass downwards and medially, becoming aponeurotic level with the tip of the ninth costal cartilage. The fibres of the two external oblique muscles meet in the midline of the body, interdigitating to form the linea alba, a tendinous raphe that extends vertically from the xiphoid process to the pubic symphysis.

The linea alba is formed by the fibres of all three muscles from each side of the body – the two oblique muscles and the transversus abdominis. It is interrupted by the umbilicus, which transmits the umbilical vessels, the urachus and the vitelline duct during fetal life but closes soon after birth. The median umbilical ligament on the deep surface of the abdominal wall represents the remnants of the urachus. The medial umbilical ligaments represent the remnants of the umbilical arteries. The umbilical vein regresses to give rise to the ligamentum teres, which ascends from the umbilicus to the liver between the two layers of the falciform ligament.

The lower fibres of the aponeurosis of the external oblique muscle, which stretches from the anterior superior iliac spine to the pubic tubercle, is thickened and folded in on itself to form the inguinal ligament. This infolding forms the floor of the inguinal canal.

From the medial end of the inguinal ligament, fibres pass backwards and medially to the pectineal line to constitute the lacunar ligament. The base of this ligament forms the medial boundary of the femoral ring.

## INTERNAL OBLIQUE

The thinner internal oblique muscle arises from the lumbar fascia, the lateral part of the inguinal ligament and the anterior part of the iliac crest. Posterior fibres ascend vertically to the lower ribs, where they are continuous with fibres of the external intercostal muscle. Fibres arising from the iliac crest pass upwards and medially and meet in the midline, contributing to the linea alba. Fibres from the inguinal ligament arch downwards and medially, crossing over the round ligament and becoming aponeu-

rotic. These fibres insert behind the round ligament to the pubic crest and medial part of the pectineal line, together with similar fibres from the transversus abdominis, thus constituting the falx inguinalis or conjoint tendon.

The falx inguinalis lies behind the superficial inguinal ring of the inguinal canal to strengthen an otherwise weak point in the abdominal wall. Medially, the falx is continuous with the anterior wall of the rectus sheath. Occasionally it may be continuous laterally with a band of aponeurotic fibres, the interfoveolar ligament, which extends from the lower border of the transversus abdominis to the superior ramus of the pubis. This band gives additional strength to the falx inguinalis.

## TRANSVERSUS ABDOMINIS

Arising deep from the internal oblique muscle, from the same origin as that of the internal oblique muscle, are the fibres of the transversus abdominis, oriented horizontally across the abdomen to meet in the midline in the linea alba. The aponeuroses in the upper approximately fourth-fifths of the muscle pass behind the rectus abdominis, while the fibres of the lower part, those arising from the inguinal ligament and iliac crest, lie in front of the rectus abdominis. Additionally, fibres from the transversus muscle originate from the inner aspect of the lower six costal cartilages and interdigitate with the muscular fibres of the diaphragm.

As with the internal oblique muscle, the fibres that take origin from the inguinal ligament pass downwards and medially over the round ligament and contribute to the conjoint tendon, which inserts behind the round ligament to the pubic crest and pectineal line. The rectus abdominis originates from the crest and tubercle of the pubis and broadens as it ascends to insert on the costal cartilages of the fifth, sixth and seventh ribs.

## RECTI MUSCLES

The two recti muscles are separated from each other by the linea alba and both present three transverse tendinous intersections, one related to the level of the xiphoid process, one at the umbilicus and one midway between the xiphoid process and the umbilicus.

The recti muscles each lie within the rectus sheath, formed by the aponeurosis of the two oblique muscles and the transversus abdominis. As the aponeurosis of the internal oblique muscle on each side approaches the lateral border of the rectus muscle it divides into two laminae, one passing deep to the rectus muscle and the other superficial to the muscle. The aponeurosis of the transversus abdominis lies posterior to the rectus muscle and that of the external oblique muscle lies anterior to it. Hence the anterior wall of the rectus sheath is formed of the aponeurosis of the external oblique muscle plus half the thickness of the internal oblique muscle. The posterior wall is formed by half the thickness of the internal oblique aponeurosis and the aponeurosis of the transversus abdominis. Medial to the recti muscles the layers from each side reunite with each other to form the linea alba.

This is the arrangement of the rectus sheath from midway between the pubic symphysis and umbilicus to the superior part of the muscle. Below this point all three aponeuroses pass over the recti muscles, resulting in a deficiency of the posterior wall of the sheath below this point, where it is formed only by the transversalis fascia, which lies deep to the transversus abdominis. The difference in the thickness of the posterior wall of the sheath above and below the division of the internal oblique aponeurosis is evidenced by the presence of the arcuate line. This line is the point where the transversus abdominis and half the thickness of the internal oblique aponeurosis pass deep to the recti muscles. The arcuate line is also the point where the inferior epigastric vessels gain access to the rectus sheath. The transversalis fascia is thin and lies between the transversus abdominis and the parietal layer of peritoneum.

### CAESAREAN SECTION

In caesarean section, the incision through the abdominal wall is made transversely, two fingers' breadth above the pubic symphysis. The transverse incision through the skin, subcutaneous fat and rectus sheath is so directed as to prevent cutting across the segmental areas of skin, or dermatomes, of the anterior abdominal wall, which is innervated by the lower six intercostal nerves travelling in the neurovascular plane between the transversus and the internal oblique muscle. Each intercostal nerve finally enters the rectus sheath, having supplied the muscles of the abdominal wall as well as the area of skin, or dermatome, specific to each nerve. A transverse incision appears to result in less scarring as compared with a vertical incision and is less likely to cause rupture of the recti muscles and sheath.

## Inguinal canal

The inguinal canal (Figure 2.2), situated between the abdominal cavity and the labia majora, is obliquely placed between the deep and superficial inguinal rings and transmits the round ligament of the uterus and the ilioinguinal nerve. The canal is located just superior to the medial half of the inguinal ligament.

The floor of the inguinal canal is formed of the infolded inguinal ligament uniting with the transversalis fascia, with arching fibres of both the transversus abdominis and the internal oblique muscle forming its roof. Contraction of these overarching fibres is increased when there is an increase in intra-abdominal pressure. The anterior wall of the canal is formed of skin, superficial fascia and the external oblique aponeurosis. Muscle fibres of the internal oblique muscle also contribute to the most lateral part of the anterior wall, specifically where it lies opposite the deep inguinal ring. The posterior wall of the canal, formed by the transversalis fascia, would be exceptionally weak if it were not reinforced by the conjoint tendon and the reflected part of the inguinal ligament.

The inguinal ligament is an expansion of the lateral crus of the superficial inguinal ring, which passes upwards and medially to merge with the rectus sheath, passing behind the external oblique muscle but in front of the conjoint tendon. Both the conjoint tendon and the reflected part of the inguinal ligament strengthen the weak part of the abdominal wall caused by the canal, although the oblique orientation of the canal also aids in this strengthening.

### DEEP AND SUPERFICIAL INGUINAL RINGS

The deep inguinal ring is formed in the transversalis fascia, midway between the anterior superior iliac spine and the pubic symphysis. Transversus abdominis fibres arch over it superiorly and the inferior epigastric vessels are an immediate medial relation to this ring. When intra-abdominal pressure is raised, contraction of internal oblique fibres is increased so that they act as a valve

FIGURE 2.2 **Femoral sheath and inguinal canal**

Cut margin of external
oblique aponeurosis

Transversalis fascia
forming anterior layer
of femoral sheath

Round ligament in inguinal
canal with covering
from internal oblique
aponeurosis

Lacunar ligament
(medial relation
of femoral ring)

Falciform margin of
saphenous opening

mechanism on the deep inguinal ring, closing it down. The superficial ring is placed above the inguinal ligament, just lateral to the pubic tubercle, and is formed by an opening in the aponeurosis of the external oblique muscle. The margins of this opening are thickened to form the lateral and medial crura of the ring.

## ROUND LIGAMENT

The round ligament passes through the transversalis fascia at the deep inguinal ring, although the ring is not visible externally as the fascia at this point forms a covering or sleeve – the internal spermatic fascia – over the round ligament. As the ligament and internal fascial layer pass through the internal oblique muscle, the round ligament gains another covering from this layer, termed the cremasteric fascia. Even in the female (although more so in the male) this covering contains a few muscle fibres, forming the cremaster muscle. Finally, as the round ligament and its gained coverings pass through the external

oblique aponeurosis, it is clothed with its outer layer, the external spermatic fascia, derived from this aponeurosis and giving rise to a third layer covering the ligament. Accompanying the round ligament and its coverings through the canal is the ilioinguinal nerve.

## ILIOINGUINAL NERVE

From the anterior primary ramus of L1, the ilioinguinal nerve emerges from the lateral border of the psoas major, crosses the quadratus lumborum, perforates the transversus abdominis close to the anterior part of the iliac crest and runs in this neurovascular plane until it pierces the internal oblique muscle. At this point, it enters the inguinal canal, emerging through the superficial inguinal ring, to be distributed to the skin on the medial aspect of the thigh as well as the skin covering the mons pubis and the related part of the labia majora. In its course it also supplies the fibres of the internal oblique and transversus abdominis muscles, which contribute to the conjoint tendon. Damage to the ilioinguinal nerve will therefore weaken the conjoint tendon, potentially inducing the development of a direct hernia.

## Femoral triangle

The superficial fascia of the inguinal region is thick and is distinguishable as two separate layers: the superficial layer, which is continuous with the superficial fascia of the abdomen, and the deep layer. Between the two lie the superficial inguinal lymph nodes and the long saphenous vein. The deep layer fuses with the deep fascia of the thigh, the fascia lata, just below the inguinal ligament. The deep layer also contributes to the saphenous opening because it merges with the fascia forming the opening as well as the fascia forming the femoral sheath. The fascia lata is thick both proximally and laterally in the thigh, forming the iliotibial tract. The saphenous opening transmits the great saphenous vein and in this region the fascia lata is divided into two layers.

### SUPERFICIAL LAYER OF THE FASCIA LATA

The superficial layer of the fascia lata is lateral to the saphenous opening and is attached to the entire length of the inguinal ligament, to the anterior superior iliac spine and to the pectineal line of the pubis. It is reflected inferolaterally from the pubic tubercle and forms the falciform margin of the saphenous opening. The deep layer of the fascia lata is medial to the saphenous opening, being continuous with the superficial layer at the lower margin of the opening. It continues upward to cover the adductor muscles and passes behind the femoral sheath, merges with it and ends by attaching to the pectineal line. The superficial layer of the fascia lata is therefore anterior to the femoral sheath, whereas the deep layer is posterior.

### FEMORAL SHEATH

The femoral sheath itself is formed by the continuation of the transversalis fascia in front of the femoral vessels and by the fascia covering the iliacus muscle behind these vessels. These two layers terminate by fusing with fascia on the outer layers of the femoral vessels; hence the entire sheath is funnel shaped and wider at its proximal end.

The lateral wall of the femoral sheath is pierced by the femoral branch of the genitofemoral nerve. The medial wall is perforated by the great saphenous vein as it drains into the femoral vein. The femoral sheath lies within the femoral triangle, the boundaries of which are superiorly the inguinal ligament, laterally the medial border of the sartorius and medially the medial border of the adductor longus. The lateral border of the adductor longus contributes to the floor of the femoral triangle, as do the iliacus, the psoas major and the pectineus.

The femoral sheath lies within the femoral triangle and contains, from medial to lateral, the femoral canal, vein and artery. The immediate lateral relation of the sheath is the femoral nerve. The femoral canal contains lymph vessels and deep inguinal lymph nodes. Its proximal opening is the femoral ring, the medial aspect of which is formed by the lacunar ligament. The round ligament of the uterus passes over the femoral vein, just above the femoral ring, as the round ligament enters the deep inguinal ring. Just lateral to this, the inferior epigastric vessels enter the rectus sheath and travel up the sheath on its posterior wall to anastomose with the superior epigastric vessels. Although the femoral ring allows expansion of the femoral vein, it causes a weak area of the abdominal wall. This area of weakness can result in herniation of abdominal contents through this space – a femoral hernia. As the femoral ring is larger in women, because of the greater width of the female pelvis and smaller femoral vessels relative to the male, femoral hernias are more common in women than men.

## Muscles of the pelvis

The musculature of the pelvis (Figure 2.3) is divided into two distinct groups. The first group is formed of the obturator internus and the piriformis and clothes the inside of the pelvic walls. The second group, which is of greater relevance to the practice of obstetrics and gynaecology, is formed of the levator ani and the coccygeus and constitutes the pelvic diaphragm or floor.

The pelvic diaphragm is covered on both its superior and inferior surfaces by investing fascia, which is continuous above with the fascia covering the pelvic viscera and below with the fascia of the perineum. The levator ani is attached to two bony points: the inner surface of

FIGURE 2.3  **Pelvic diaphragm**

Tendinous arch
of levator ani

Coccygeus

Puborectalis

Obturator internus

Pubococcygeus

Iliococcygeus

the pubic bone and the medial aspect of the spine of the ischium. Between these two points, the fibres take origin from the fascia overlying the obturator internus.

## PUBOVAGINALIS

Fibres of the two levator muscles meet in the median plane. There is variability in the direction of the fibres, giving rise to different named parts of levator depending on the direction of its fibres. The most anterior fibres originate from the body of the pubis and, passing in an anteroposterior direction to the perineal body (situated in the midline between the urogenital triangle and the anal triangle), pass across the sides of the vagina, forming the pubovaginalis (a supplementary but significant sphincter of the vagina) before inserting to the anterior surface of the coccyx. Fibres that arise more laterally pass backwards, downwards and medially, finally meeting fibres from the opposite side to form the puborectalis. The puborectalis forms a sling of muscle around the junction of the rectum and anus. The fibres of the puborectalis intermingle with the deep fibres of the external anal sphincter and the perineal body.

## LEVATOR ANI

Those fibres of the levator ani that lie in an anteroposterior direction give rise to the pubococcygeus part of the muscle. The fibres that arise from the medial aspect of the ischial spines pass from lateral to medial to form the part of the levator ani named the iliococcygeus. Between the two bony points that give origin to the levator muscle, the body of the pubis and the ischial spines, fibres arise from the fascia covering the obturator internus. The levator muscle also has a fascial covering, the superior fascia of the pelvic diaphragm, and this contributes to the fascia covering the obturator internus above the levator attachment, giving rise to the structure referred to as tendinous arch of levator ani. However, some explanation is necessary here, as this structure differs from the tendinous arch of the pelvic fascia, which is more medially placed and gives rise to the attachment of the lateral supporting ligament of the urinary bladder. The medial borders of the levator muscle meet in a median raphe, although the two sides of the muscle are held apart in the midline by the structures that pass through the diaphragm to exit the pelvis.

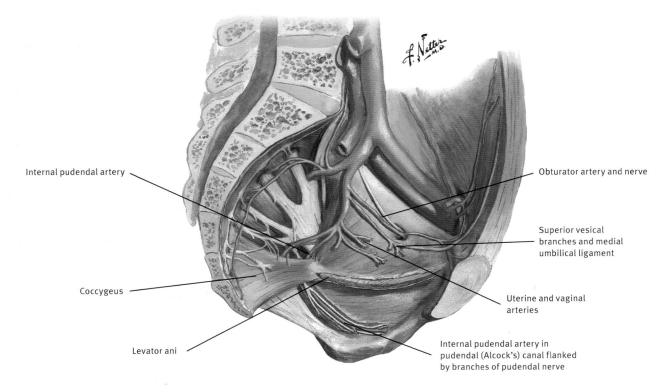

Internal pudendal artery

Obturator artery and nerve

Superior vesical branches and medial umbilical ligament

Coccygeus

Uterine and vaginal arteries

Levator ani

Internal pudendal artery in pudendal (Alcock's) canal flanked by branches of pudendal nerve

## COCCYGEUS

Completing the muscular diaphragm of the pelvic floor is the coccygeus, arising from the ischial spine and the deep surface of the sacrospinous ligament to insert to the coccyx and lateral margin of the fifth sacral segment. Both the levator muscle and the coccygeus support the pelvic viscera, with the levator muscle constricting the rectum and vagina. Damage to the pelvic floor muscles occurs during birth. As the pubovaginalis portion of the levator muscle is attached to the perineal body, rupture of the latter can divide the levator muscles and may later predispose to uterovaginal prolapse. The lower surface of the levator ani is clothed by the inferior fascia of the pelvic diaphragm and forms the medial wall of the ischioanal fossa.

## Vessels of the pelvis

The abdominal aorta divides into the right and left common iliac arteries at the level of the vertebral disc between L4 and L5 (Figure 2.4). Owing to the position of the aorta, the right common iliac artery is approximately 1 cm longer than the left and crosses directly in front of L5. Both common iliac arteries are covered in parietal peritoneum, which separates the vessels from the small intestine. Fibres of the superior hypogastric plexus form a meshwork over the common iliac arteries and the psoas muscle lies laterally to each.

Posteriorly, the right common iliac artery is related to the termination of both common iliac veins, which unite to form the inferior vena cava. The left artery is antero-lateral to its corresponding vein. Level with the sacroiliac joint, both of the common iliac arteries divide into their internal and external divisions. The external iliac artery continues towards the thigh related to the medial border of the psoas major, and enters the thigh by passing under the inguinal ligament midway between the pubic symphysis and the anterior superior iliac spine: the mid-inguinal point that lies approximately 1 cm medial to the midpoint of the inguinal ligament.

## COURSE OF THE INTERNAL ILIAC ARTERY

At the point of their division into the external and internal arteries, the internal arteries are crossed anteriorly by the ureters as they enter the pelvis. Arising anterior to the sacroiliac joint, the internal iliac arteries continue to the level of the upper margin of the greater sciatic notch, where they divide into anterior and posterior divisions. The posterior division passes through the upper part of the greater sciatic foramen to divide into its terminal branches of the superior gluteal, lateral sacral and iliolumbar arteries. The anterior division continues into the pelvis to give off numerous branches, taking a course towards the spine of the ischium. Related immediately anterior to this division is the ureter, the ovarian artery and accompanying venae comitantes, the fimbriated end of the uterine tube and the ovary.

The internal iliac veins lie behind the internal iliac arteries. The external iliac veins lie below and medial to the external iliac arteries, with the right external vein positioned posteromedial to the right external artery as the vein continues into the pelvis. The obturator nerve emerges from the medial aspect of psoas major, lying first at the division of the common iliac vessels into their internal and external branches (Figure 2.4) and then on the side wall of the pelvis above the obturator vessels as the nerve and vessels pass through the obturator canal to gain access to the medial compartment of the thigh.

## BRANCHES OF THE INTERNAL ILIAC ARTERY

The internal iliac arteries give rise to many branches within the pelvis. The original stem of the umbilical artery persists in the adult and crosses the lateral wall of the pelvis on the levator ani. This part of the umbilical artery remains patent and gives rise to one or several superior vesical branches, which supply the superior aspect of the bladder. These vessels also give branches to supply the distal end of the ureter.

The distal end of the original umbilical artery, having become fibrous, ascends towards the umbilicus and,

being covered in parietal peritoneum, raises a fold of peritoneum on each side of the inner surface of the anterior abdominal wall, known as the medial umbilical ligament. The obturator artery enters the obturator canal by passing forward on the lateral wall of the pelvis, 2–3 cm below the pelvic brim, to enter the obturator canal. The obturator nerve, which emerges from the medial aspect of psoas, is an immediate superior relation to the artery as both pass through the canal to leave the pelvis. The uterine artery, first lying on the fascia overlying the levator muscle , turns medially in its course towards the cervix, crossing above and in front of the ureter, which it also supplies. The artery then ascends in the broad ligament of the uterus to the junction of the body of the uterus and the uterine tube, where its branches turn laterally to anastomose with those of the ovarian artery (Figure 2.5).

### FIGURE 2.5  **Lymph vessels and nodes of the pelvis and genitalia**

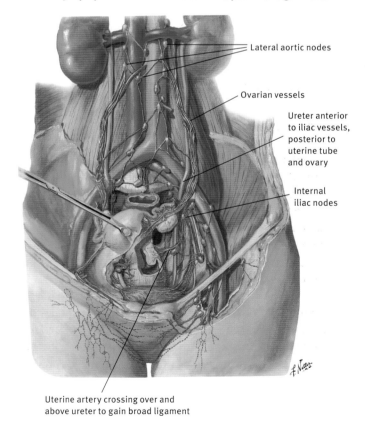

Lateral aortic nodes

Ovarian vessels

Ureter anterior to iliac vessels, posterior to uterine tube and ovary

Internal iliac nodes

Uterine artery crossing over and above ureter to gain broad ligament

Blood supply to the vagina usually arises as branches from the uterine artery. These branches from the uterine artery supply the mucous membrane of the vagina as well as supplying the related parts of the bladder and rectum. The vaginal branches, together with uterine branches, contribute to the azygous system of vessels supplying the vagina.

The middle rectal and inferior vesical arteries may arise in common from the internal iliac artery. The middle rectal artery is often elusive but, when present, it supplies the muscular wall of the lower part of the rectum. The inferior vesical artery supplies the fundus of the bladder as well as giving small branches to the distal part of the ureter.

The terminal branches of the internal iliac artery are the internal pudendal artery and the inferior gluteal artery, the latter being the larger terminal division. The internal pudendal artery leaves the pelvis through the lower part of the greater sciatic foramen, between the coccygeus and the piriformis, and winds around the spine of the ischium, sandwiched between the medially placed pudendal nerve and the laterally placed nerve to the obturator internus. The internal pudendal artery enters the perineum through the lesser sciatic foramen to enter the pudendal (or Alcock's) canal within the perineum.

### PUDENDAL CANAL

Located on the lateral wall of the ischioanal fossa, the fascial sheath of the pudendal canal forms the roof and lateral wall of the fossa. The sheath fuses with the lower part of the obturator fascia as well as being continuous with the inferior fascia of the pelvic diaphragm and the falciform process of the sacrotuberous ligament (which extends from the ischial tuberosity along the ischial ramus). In the canal, the pudendal artery is accompanied by two veins and the pudendal nerve. The artery lies between the two terminal branches of the pudendal nerve – the dorsal nerve of the clitoris above and the perineal nerve below – at the anterior end of the canal.

The inferior rectal artery branches from the internal pudendal artery at the start of the pudendal canal. Just superior to the ischial tuberosity it emerges from the medial wall of the sheath, crossing the ischioanal fossa to supply the skin and muscles of the anal region. At the anterior end of the pudendal canal, the perineal artery arises from the internal pudendal artery, travelling through the inferior fascial layer of the urogenital diaphragm to enter the superficial perineal space. The inferior gluteal artery, the larger terminal branch of the internal iliac artery, leaves the pelvis posterior to the internal pudendal artery. The inferior gluteal artery also passes between the piriformis and the coccygeus via the lower part of the greater sciatic foramen, to supply the gluteal region and structures in the posterior aspect of the thigh.

### LYMPHATIC DRAINAGE OF THE PELVIS

As with all other regions of the body, lymph vessels and nodes draining the pelvis are associated with the major regional blood vessels and their branches. Lymph from the pelvis passes to the nodes studded along the internal iliac veins. From here the lymph is carried into the paravertebral or lateral aortic nodes situated on the lateral aspects of the verterbral bodies. These latter nodes receive lymph from the ovaries, kidneys and adrenal glands as well as from the muscles of the posterior abdominal wall. From here lymph is carried into the cisterna chyli, positioned posterior to the aorta at the level of L1–2, and continues from here into the thoracic duct. The internal iliac lymph nodes receive lymph from all of the pelvic viscera and deep perineum, as well as the gluteal region. (For lymphatic drainage of the uterus and vagina see chapter 4.)

## Innervation of the pelvic region – somatic and autonomic

### LUMBAR PLEXUS

Both the lumbar plexus and the sacral plexus contribute to the innervation of the pelvis. The lumbar plexus is formed from the anterior primary rami of T12 / L1–L4. The plexus is formed within the substance of the psoas major. The lumbar plexus gives rise to both the femoral nerve, through the posterior divisions of L2, 3 and 4, and the obturator nerve from the anterior divisions of these nerve roots. The femoral nerve emerges from the lateral aspect of the psoas major and runs on the iliacus. The nerve runs between the psoas major and the iliacus until it reaches the inguinal ligament, where it becomes related to the anterior surface of the iliopsoas as this muscle passes under the inguinal ligament. Superiorly it is therefore separated from the distal end of the external iliac artery and the proximal end of the femoral artery by the psoas but once it enters the thigh it lies immediately lateral to the femoral artery.

The femoral nerve divides into anterior and posterior divisions in the thigh, supplying the muscles and skin in this region. Within the pelvis, the femoral nerve supplies various small branches to the iliacus. From its medial aspect, near the inguinal ligament, it supplies the nerve to the pectineus, which passes behind the femoral sheath and enters the anterior surface of the pectineus.

The obturator nerve emerges from the medial border of the psoas muscle. At the brim of the pelvis it lies behind the common iliac vessels and continues lateral to the internal iliac vessels on the obturator internus, passes above the obturator artery and into the obturator canal above this vessel. The obturator nerve exits the pelvis to supply the adductor muscles and the skin on the medial aspect of the thigh. As the obturator nerve within the pelvis supplies the parietal peritoneum in the vicinity of the ovary, pain arising in this organ may be referred to the medial aspect of the thigh.

The lumbar plexus gives rise to four other nerves: the subcostal, the iliohypogastric, the ilioinguinal and the genitofemoral. Both the subcostal and the iliohypogastric nerves cross the quadratus lumborum, pierce the transversus abdominis and run in the neurovascular plane between the transversus abdominis and the internal oblique. They supply the transversus abdominis and the internal oblique muscle and the skin of the lower part of the abdomen. The genitofemoral nerve lies on the anterior surface of the psoas muscle, where it divides into its femoral and genital branches. The femoral branch of the genitofemoral nerve passes below the inguinal ligament to supply the skin overlying the femoral triangle. The genital branch passes through the deep inguinal ring to supply the fibres of the cremaster muscle.

## SACRAL PLEXUS

Uniting the lumbar plexus to the sacral plexus is the lumbosacral trunk, L4–5. This large trunk, which is related to the medial aspect of the psoas muscle, crosses the pelvic brim anterior to the sacroiliac joint and joins the ventral primary ramus of S1. The sacral plexus is formed from the lumbosacral trunk and the anterior primary rami of S1–4. The plexus lies on the piriformis, behind the internal iliac vessels, the ureter and the gut. The constituent nerves form into an upper and lower group to exit the greater sciatic foramen and supply the structures of the lower limb. The upper group of nerves, L4–S2 and part of S3, form the sciatic nerve, whereas the lower division of the plexus, mainly S3–4 with a small contribution from S2, forms the pudendal nerve. Within the pelvis, the sacral plexus supplies the piriformis and the levator ani, the former via the nerve that exits at S1–2 and enters the anterior surface of the muscle, and the latter through branches derived from S4.

## PUDENDAL NERVE

Of particular note to obstetric anatomy is the pudendal nerve, S2–4. This nerve leaves the pelvis through the greater sciatic foramen, winds around the ischial spine medial to the internal pudendal artery and just deep to the sacrospinous ligament to gain the perineum through the lesser sciatic foramen and enter the pudendal canal to innervate the vulva and perineum.

As with the internal pudendal artery, the pudendal nerve gives off the inferior rectal nerve, which crosses the ischioanal fossa to supply the external anal sphincter, the lining of the distal end of the anal canal and the perianal skin. The pudendal nerve further divides into two terminal branches in the perineum – the perineal nerve and the dorsal nerve of the clitoris (discussed further in chapter 3). The pudendal nerve is important therefore in maintaining sphincter function and, through innervation of the muscles of the region, providing muscular support to the viscera. The positioning of the nerve, deep to the sacrospinous ligament and close to the point of the ischial spine, makes it accessible for a pudendal nerve block to relieve pain during instrumental delivery. The ischial spine and sacrospinous ligament can be palpated vaginally and the pudendal needle is passed through the sacrospinous ligament to the pudendal nerve. The pudendal nerve also supplies sensory branches to the lower part of the vagina through sensory fibres in the inferior rectal nerve and posterior labial branches of the perineal nerve.

## SYMPATHETIC AND PARASYMPATHETIC DIVISIONS

Within the pelvis, both sympathetic and parasympathetic divisions of the autonomic nervous system have to be considered.

The sympathetic division, being the thoracolumbar outflow, has a contribution from both thoracic and lumbar levels. Thoracic sympathetic fibres gain access to the abdomen and pelvis via the greater and lesser splanchnic nerves. These are preganglionic branches that arise in the thorax but have entered the abdomen through the crura of the diaphragm and synapse in the ganglia related to the main aortic branches. The greater splanchnic nerve carries preganglionic sympathetic fibres from the fifth to ninth or tenth thoracic sympathetic ganglia. Additionally, this nerve also carries visceral afferent fibres. Passing through the crura of the diaphragm, fibres from the greater splanchnic nerve mainly contribute to the coeliac ganglion. The lesser splanchnic nerve from the ninth and tenth or eleventh thoracic sympathetic ganglia mainly passes to the aorticorenal ganglion in the abdomen.

In the lumbar region the sympathetic chain consists of four ganglia, which lie on the lateral aspect of the lumbar vertebrae. Sympathetic fibres from this part of the chain are distributed into the pelvis via the superior hypogastric plexus – often erroneously named the pre-sacral nerves (erroneously because they form a meshwork rather than a single nerve).

### *Superior hypogastric plexus*

The superior hypogastric plexus lies anterior to the bifurcation of the aorta. From the plexus, sympathetic fibres are carried into the pelvis as two main trunks – the right and left hypogastric nerves – each lying medial to the internal

FIGURE 2.6 A **Autonomic nerves and ganglia of the abdomen**

Superior hypogastric plexus

Right and left hypogastric nerves to inferior hypogastric plexus iliac artery and its branches. The superior hypogastric plexus also contains parasympathetic fibres, which arise from the pelvic splanchnic nerves (S2–4) (Figure 2.6 A) and ascend from the inferior hypogastric plexus. However, it is more usual for these parasympathetic fibres to ascend to the left-hand side of the superior hypogastric plexus and cross the branches of the sigmoid and left colic vessel branches, as these parasympathetic branches are distributed along the branches of the inferior mesenteric artery. The hypogastric nerves send sympathetic fibres to the ovarian and ureteric plexuses, the fibres of which orig-inate within the renal and aortic sympathetic plexuses.

## Inferior hypogastric plexus

The inferior hypogastric plexus, or pelvic plexus as it is also known, is a continuation of the right and left hypogastric nerves in the pelvis. This plexus is also joined by parasympathetic fibres from the pelvic splanchnic nerves, derived from S2–4 of the sacral plexus. These fibres supply parasympathetic innervation to the pelvic viscera and the hindgut. The inferior hypogastric or pelvic plexus is situated within the fascia surrounding the rectum, with fibres passing from here into the pelvic floor in order to reach the pelvic viscera. Fibres of this plexus lie on either side of the rectum, the cervical and vaginal fornices and the posterior aspect of the bladder. They also send fibres into the broad ligament. The plexus is derived from fibres of the lower three thoracic (T10–12) and upper two lumbar segments (L1–2) of the spinal cord as well as the preganglionic parasympathetic fibres from the pelvic splanchnic nerves.

The fibres of the pelvic/inferior hypogastric plexus that gain access to the broad ligament give rise to the uterovaginal plexus (Figure 2.6 B). Some fibres from this

FIGURE 2.6 B **Innervation of the female reproductive organs (schema)**

Greater splanchnic nerve

Lesser splanchnic nerve

Ovarian artery/plexus

Superior hypogastric plexus

Uterovaginal and inferior hypogastric plexuses

Pelvic splanchnic nerve

Pudendal nerve

**KEY**
= = Sympathetic
= = Parasympathetic
— Afferent fibres

Netter Anatomy Illustrations from www.netterimages.com
© Elsevier Inc. All rights reserved.

part of the plexus travel with both vaginal and uterine arteries, while others pass directly to the cervix. Those travelling with the uterine artery supply the body of the uterus, the upper part of the broad ligament and the uterine tubes and communicate with branches from the ovarian plexus. Fibres travelling with the vaginal arteries are distributed to the walls of the vagina as well as the erectile tissue of the vestibule and the clitoris.

While the sympathetic fibres within the inferior hypogastric/pelvic plexus are responsible for uterine contraction and vasoconstriction and the parasympathetic fibres produce opposing effects, it should be remembered that hormonal regulation of the uterus may alter or even override the effects of the two autonomic divisions.

The afferent fibres, which accompany many of the efferent fibres to the viscera, are the sensory components of autonomic function and elicit visceral reflexes. Afferent fibres also include pain fibres and such general visceral afferent fibres are reported to be carried in the pelvic splanchnic nerves. Pain fibres from the body of the uterus pass back to the hypogastric plexus and lumbar splanchnic nerves to the lower thoracic and upper lumbar levels of the spinal cord. Afferent fibres of the cervix and upper part of the vagina, however, pass via the pelvic splanchnic nerves, while afferents from the lower vagina and perineum travel in the pelvic splanchnic nerves.

# CHAPTER 3

# Anatomy of the bladder, ureter, urethra, anus and perineum

*Diana Lawrence-Watt*

## Pelvic viscera

The pelvic viscera within the female are surrounded by visceral peritoneum, resulting in several named spaces anterior and posterior to the various organs. Additionally, folds of fascia or parietal peritoneum are represented by named ligaments that transmit blood vessels and nerves to the pelvic viscera (Figure 3.1).

## Urinary bladder

The position of the urinary bladder depends on whether it is full or empty. The empty bladder lies completely within the lesser pelvis but rises into the abdominal cavity when filled or distended.

The fundus of the bladder is triangular in outline and is related to the anterior wall of the vagina. It is covered

FIGURE 3.1 **Pelvic viscera**

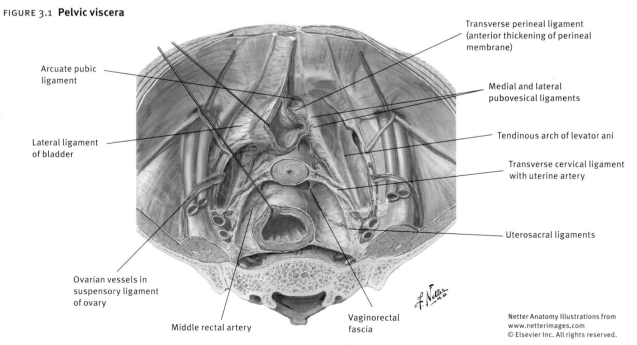

Arcuate pubic ligament

Lateral ligament of bladder

Ovarian vessels in suspensory ligament of ovary

Middle rectal artery

Transverse perineal ligament (anterior thickening of perineal membrane)

Medial and lateral pubovesical ligaments

Tendinous arch of levator ani

Transverse cervical ligament with uterine artery

Uterosacral ligaments

Vaginorectal fascia

**23**

FIGURE 3.2 **Urinary bladder**

Parietal peritoneum

Parietal peritoneum

Vesicouterine pouch

Rectouterine pouch

Levator ani

Perineal body

in parietal peritoneum that has been reflected from the anterior abdominal wall. The apex of the bladder is directed towards the pubic symphysis. The neck of the bladder lies on the pelvic floor, within the fascia that surrounds the urethra.

The superior surface of the female bladder is not entirely covered in peritoneum as this thin layer of tissue is reflected from it to form the quite shallow vesico-uterine pouch. From this pouch, the peritoneum covers the uterus and the posterior fornix of the vagina. The peritoneum is then reflected from the uterus to the middle part of the rectum, where it forms the deep recto-uterine pouch (Figure 3.2).

### LIGAMENTS OF THE BLADDER

Laterally, the bladder is actually connected to the pelvic fascia. The pelvic fascia is a thickening and condensation of fibrous tissue that forms the lateral true ligaments of the bladder.

Just before the lateral ligaments approach the deep surface of the pubic bone, they diverge to form two thickened bands, one lying more medial to the other. These

bands are called the pubovesical ligaments. The medial pubovesical ligament attaches to the inside aspect of the pubic bone, close to the midpoint of the symphysis. From here it passes downwards and backwards to form the floor of the retropubic space. The pubovesical ligaments play a significant role in supporting the bladder neck and in urinary continence.

The apex of the bladder is continuous with the urachus (a fibrous cord covered in a fold of peritoneum), forming the median umbilical ligament and representing the closure of the upper end of the vesico-urethral canal present during embryonic development.

### MUSCLES AND MEMBRANES OF THE BLADDER

The bladder wall consists of the detrusor muscle. This is a smooth muscle disposed into three layers: outer and inner longitudinal layers, with a middle circular layer interposed between them. The middle layer is relatively thin over most of the bladder but is thickened at the neck of the bladder where it gives rise to sphincter vesicae around the internal urethral orifice.

Inside the bladder, the mucous membrane is loosely

FIGURE 3.3 **Urinary bladder and surrounding anatomy**

Trigone of bladder
(smooth triangular area)

Levator ani

Round ligament
of uterus

Vagina

Ureteric orifice

Obturator internus

Urethrael sphincter

Urethra

Deep perineal fascia

Superficial perineal fascia

attached to the smooth muscle walls, allowing the membrane to be thrown into folds when the bladder is contracted and to become smooth when the bladder is distended.

On the posterior wall of the bladder lies the trigone (Figure 3.3). The trigone is derived from the fusion of the distal ends of the two ureters into the posterior wall of the bladder. The ureters, unlike the bladder, are mesodermal in origin and the appearance of the trigone reflects the different developmental origins of the ureters and the bladder. The inferior point of the trigone arises in embryonic development from the fusion of the two mesonephric ducts into the posterior wall of the bladder, these ducts also being of mesodermal origin. The lower point of the trigone in the fully developed bladder is related to the outlet of the urethra at the internal urethral orifice. The mucous membrane covering the trigone is more firmly attached to the underlying muscle. The trigone does not exhibit the folds characteristic of the other regions of the bladder as it does not expand.

## INNERVATION OF THE BLADDER

The parasympathetic and sympathetic fibres to the bladder are contained within the pelvic plexus. The efferent parasympathetic fibres from the pelvic splanchnic nerves convey motor fibres to the detrusor muscle, but also convey inhibitory fibres to sphincter vesicae. The urethral sphincter, which forms the urogenital diaphragm (Figure 3.3), is supplied by the pudendal nerve.

## Urethra

The urethra (Figure 3.3) is a 4–6 cm long muscular tube that runs from the internal urethral orifice of the bladder to the external urethral orifice lying in the vestibule immediately anterior to the opening of the vagina. The two opposing walls of the urethra are in contact with each other at all times, apart from when urine passes through. The urethra itself is firmly attached to the anterior wall of the vagina.

The epithelium of the urethra is thrown into folds. The largest fold of the posterior wall is termed the urethral crest. Numerous small mucous secreting glands open into the urethra. At the distal end of the urethra on each side, several of these glands group together and open into a duct known as the paraurethral duct. The paraurethral duct runs downwards in the submucosal tissue and opens on the lateral aspect of each side of the external urethral orifice.

### MUSCLES, MEMBRANES AND BLOOD SUPPLY

The smooth muscle of the urethra is continuous with the smooth muscle of the bladder. However, in the urethra it is arranged as internal longitudinal and external circular fibres. The circular fibres at the proximal end of the urethra give rise to sphincter vesicae, or the internal sphincter, whereas those related to the external urethral orifice form the urethral sphincter.

The mucous membrane of the urethra is continuous with that of the bladder. The proximal end of the urethra is composed of transitional epithelium. At a more distal level the urethral epithelium is of a non-keratinised stratified squamous nature. Below the mucous layer there is a thin layer of erectile tissue containing smooth muscle fibres and elastic connective tissue, as well as a plexus of veins.

Blood supply to the urethra is via the perineal branches of the internal pudendal artery. Blood drains via similar venous branches. The urethra receives autonomic innervation via the pelvic plexus.

### RUPTURE OF THE URETHRA

If rupture of the urethra occurs, urine escapes below the level of the urogenital diaphragm but deep to the membranous layer of the superficial fascia. However, as both these layers are attached to the ischiopubic rami and are also continuous with each other around the superficial transverse perineal muscles, urine cannot pass laterally or posteriorly. Additionally, urine cannot escape into the lesser pelvis as the opening into this is closed by the perineal membrane. Consequently, the only route the urine can take is via the areolar tissue of the mons pubis and the anterior abdominal wall.

## Ureters

Formed in embryonic life from a bud from the distal end of the mesonephric duct, the ureters are approximately 25 cm in length and lie behind the parietal peritoneum.

Each ureter commences at the pelvis of the kidney, descends on the psoas major and crosses in front of the slender genitofemoral nerve. The ovarian arteries and accompanying veins in turn cross anterior to the ureters as they descend towards the pelvis. The ureters enter the pelvis anterior to either the end of the common iliac artery or the proximal end of the internal iliac artery (see Chapter 2, Figure 2.5), following the lateral wall of the pelvis towards the greater sciatic notch. Level with the ischial spine, the ureters turn medially in the fascia of the pelvic floor to reach the lateral aspect of the bladder. The ureters are crossed superiorly by the uterine vessels as these vessels enter the substance of the broad ligament at the level of the cervix.

At the level of the internal iliac artery, the ovaries are immediately anterior to the ureters. Just above the lateral fornix of the vagina, the ureters pass forwards and are usually described at this point as being placed 2 cm lateral to the supravaginal region of the cervix. Inclining medially, each ureter enters the posterior wall of the bladder, which is related at this point to the anterior aspect of the vagina. However, as the uterus itself is often placed to one side of the median plane, it is often the case that one ureter has a greater relationship to the front of the vagina than the other.

The ureters are described as having three coats: an outer, an inner and an intermediate. At its proximal end, the outer fibrous coat is continuous with the capsule of the kidney and distally merges into the wall of the bladder as the ureters enter the posterior bladder wall. The intermediate muscular coat consists of inner longitudinal and outer circular smooth muscle layers in the upper two-thirds of each ureter. A further outer longitudinal layer of smooth muscle cells is added to this coat in the distal one-third of each ureter (although at this level the inner longitudinal layer of muscle is less well developed). It is important to note that at all levels of the ureters, connective tissue interlaces the smooth muscle and definition of the muscle into distinct layers is not always obvious. The inner mucous coat of each ureter is thrown into longitudinal folds consisting of fibrous and elastic tissue and is covered in a transitional epithelial layer.

## BLOOD SUPPLY AND INNERVATION

Each ureter receives its blood supply through an anastomosis of several arteries. The proximal end is supplied by the renal artery and during its course it also receives supply from the ovarian, common iliac and superior vesical arteries. The nerve supply is through branches from the renal, aortic, presacral and pelvic autonomic plexuses.

## Perineum

The perineum overlies the diamond-shaped inferior pelvic aperture (Figure 3.4). The four points of the diamond are the pubic symphysis anteriorly, the coccyx posteriorly and the ischial tuberosities laterally. The region is divided into two triangles by an arbitrary line through the ischial tuberosities. The area anterior to this line is described as the urogenital triangle. The area posterior to this line is described as the anal triangle. The muscles of these two areas are often described separately but they unite at the perineal body and therefore constitute a single unit.

## MUSCLES OF THE PERINEUM

The muscles of the urogenital region are normally described as two groups: superficial and deep. The superficial group of muscles consists of the bulbospongiosus, the right and left ischiocavernosus and the right and left transverse perineal muscles. The vagina and urethra open on to the surface of the skin of the vestibule, bounded by the labia minora laterally. The labia minora join anterior to the clitoris, thereby defining the anterior boundary of the vestibule.

The deep group of muscles consists of the urethral sphincter and the deep transverse perineal muscles. These muscles occupy the deep perineal pouch. Collectively these deep muscles form the structure called the urogenital diaphragm. The urogenital diaphragm, analogous to the pelvic diaphragm, is formed of muscles sandwiched between two layers of fascia. The muscles in this case are the urethral sphincter and the deep transverse perineal muscles. The upper layer of fascia forms the superior fascia of the urogenital diaphragm. The lower layer of fascia is described as the inferior, and thicker,

FIGURE 3.4 **Muscles of the perineum**

FIGURE 3.5 **Urethra and surrounding anatomy**

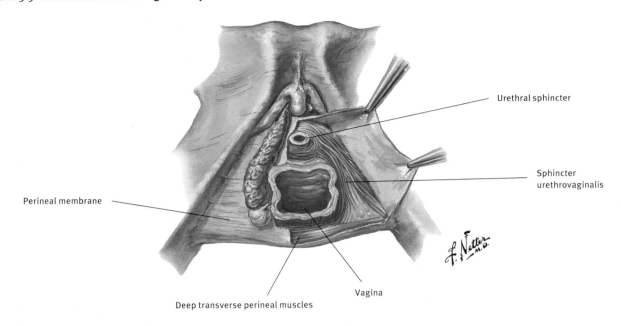

Urethral sphincter

Sphincter urethrovaginalis

Perineal membrane

Vagina

Deep transverse perineal muscles

layer of fascia of the urogenital diaphragm, also called the perineal membrane. The space between the two layers of fascia is the deep perineal pouch. This pouch contains the muscles just described and also the urethra and urethral glands and various vessels and nerves.

## PERINEAL MEMBRANE

The perineal membrane is pierced by the vagina, urethra, blood vessels and nerves. The outer coat of the vagina fuses with the perineal membrane as it passes through (Figure 3.5). The membrane stretches horizontally across the pubic arch and has a thickened apex. This thickened region is referred to as the transverse perineal ligament. Between this ligament and the arcuate pubic ligament (which spans across the inferior aspect of the pubic symphysis), the deep dorsal vein of the clitoris enters the pelvis and the dorsal nerve of the clitoris passes out of the pelvis to supply the clitoris.

## BLOOD SUPPLY TO THE PERINEUM

The main arterial supply to the perineum (Figure 3.6) is via the internal pudendal artery, one of the two termi-

nal branches of the anterior division of the internal iliac artery. This artery exits the pelvis to enter the gluteal region via the greater sciatic foramen. It winds its way around the ischial spine, accompanied by the medially placed pudendal nerve, to gain entry into the perineum. Here, the artery is confined to the proximal end of the pudendal (or Alcock's) canal, a fascial compartment related to the deep surface of the ischial tuberosity and the ischiopubic rami. The pudendal canal forms the lateral boundary of the ischioanal fossa, which is bounded medially by the external anal sphincter and the inferior fascia of the pelvic diaphragm.

The roof and lateral wall of the pudendal canal is formed by the lower part of the fascia of the obturator internus, extending both upwards to blend with the inferior fascia of the pelvic diaphragm and downwards to become the sacrotuberous ligament. Branches from both the internal pudendal artery and the pudendal nerve escape from the medial aspect of the pudendal canal to supply the region.

The inferior rectal artery leaves the pudendal canal near its proximal end and traverses medially across the ischioanal fossa to supply the anal canal and skin of the region. A more distal branch of the internal pudendal artery is the perineal artery, which branches from the internal pudendal artery near the anterior end of the pudendal canal. The perineal artery supplies branches both deep to and superficial to the perineal membrane, supplying both skin and muscle in this region.

The branches of the perineal artery are as follows: the posterior labial branches, which supply the labia; the artery to the bulb of the vestibule, which supplies the erectile tissue of the bulb of the vestibule; the deep artery of the clitoris, which supplies the corpus cavernosum; and the dorsal artery of the clitoris, which supplies the dorsum, glans and the prepuce of the clitoris.

### INNERVATION OF THE PERINEUM

The pudendal nerve supplies similar branches to the internal pudendal artery (Figure 3.7 A). The inferior rectal nerve supplies the external anal sphincter, the lower part of the anal canal and the perianal skin and accompanies the inferior rectal artery.

The perineal nerve accompanies the perineal artery and divides into posterior labial and muscular branches. The posterior labial branches usually pass superficial to the perineal membrane but the perineal nerve also sup-

plies branches that pass deep to this membrane. The deep branch of the perineal nerve supplies the ischiocavernosus and the dorsal nerve of the clitoris. The dorsal nerve of the clitoris passes deep to the perineal membrane and runs forward to supply the clitoris.

### PUDENDAL NERVE BLOCK

The pudendal nerve also supplies sensory branches to the distal part of the vagina via the inferior rectal nerve and posterior labial branches. To reduce pain during delivery, the pudendal nerve can be blocked. This is achieved by inserting a needle through the sacrospinous ligament into the pudendal nerve, which runs deep to this ligament (Figure 3.7 B).

## Anal region

The boundaries of the anal triangle are the posterior aspect of the perineal membrane and laterally the ischial tuberosities and sacrotuberous ligament. Central to this region is the anal canal, with the ischioanal fossae positioned laterally (Figure 3.8).

FIGURE 3.6 **Arteries of the perineum**

Dorsal artery of clitoris

Deep artery of clitoris

Internal pudendal artery and branch (artery to bulb of vestibule)

Perineal artery

Internal pudendal artery in pudendal (Alcock's) canal

Inferior rectal artery

FIGURE 3.7 A  **Innervation of external genitalia and perineum**

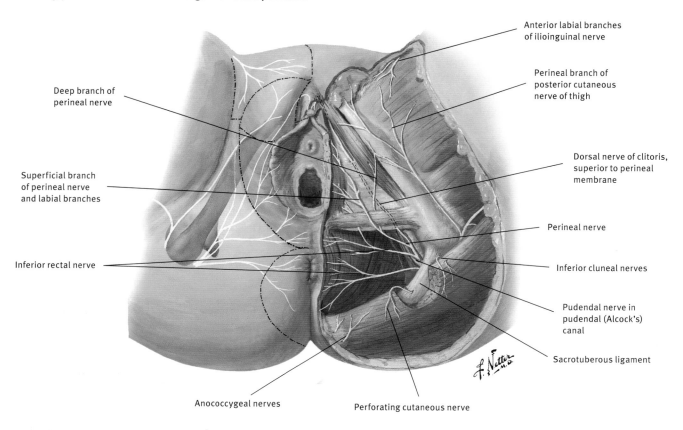

Anterior labial branches
of ilioinguinal nerve

Perineal branch of
posterior cutaneous
nerve of thigh

Deep branch of
perineal nerve

Dorsal nerve of clitoris,
superior to perineal
membrane

Superficial branch
of perineal nerve
and labial branches

Perineal nerve

Inferior cluneal nerves

Inferior rectal nerve

Pudendal nerve in
pudendal (Alcock's)
canal

Sacrotuberous ligament

Anococcygeal nerves

Perforating cutaneous nerve

FIGURE 3.7 B  **Pudendal nerve block**

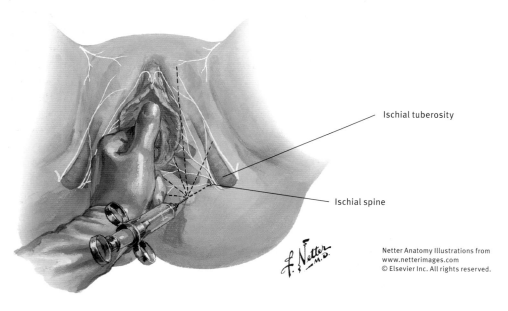

Ischial tuberosity

Ischial spine

FIGURE 3.8 **Muscles of the anal region**

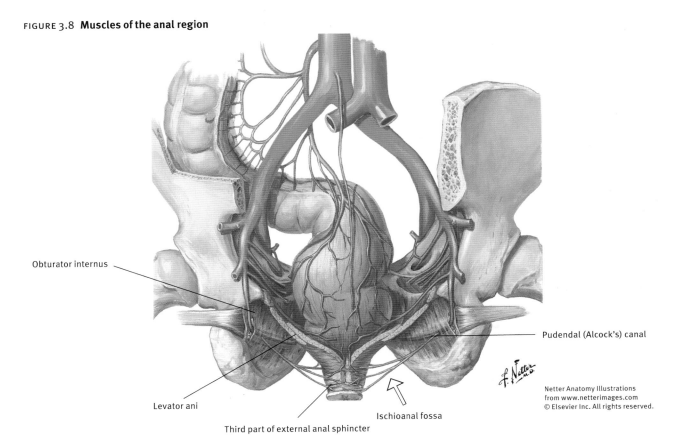

Obturator internus

Levator ani

Third part of external anal sphincter

Ischioanal fossa

Pudendal (Alcock's) canal

The muscles of the urogenital region and the anal region meet in the perineal body. The perineal body is a fibromuscular node between the urogenital region and the anal region where the muscles of the two regions unite to form a functional unit. Fibres of levator ani also contribute to the perineal body.

## ANAL CANAL

The anal canal is approximately 3–4 cm long and is surrounded by muscles that act as sphincters to close the canal. The upper part of the anal canal is lined by mucous membrane, which is thrown into longitudinal folds. These folds are termed the anal columns. The anal columns are characterised at their distal end by having anal valves and anal sinuses.

Both internal and external sphincters line the anal canal. The internal anal sphincter surrounds the upper three-quarters of the anal canal and its lower extremity is the white line. The white line is the transition point between the internal anal sphincter and the subcutaneous part of the external anal sphincter.

The external anal sphincter surrounds the lower part of the anal canal, overlapping the internal anal sphincter but inserted into skin at the lower end of the canal. The externus muscle can be divided into deep, superficial and subcutaneous regions. Deep fibres of the external anal sphincter interdigitate with fibres of the puborectalis and with the muscles of the deep perineal pouch via the perineal body. Superficial fibres of the external anal sphincter are inserted to the coccyx and contribute fibres to the anococcygeal ligament, a body of fibrous and muscular tissue separating the anus from the coccyx.

The subcutaneous part of the sphincter is a thin, horizontal band around the distal part of the anal canal. It lies below the internal anal sphincter with some fibres attaching to the anococcygeal ligament and the perineal body. This part of the sphincter does not have any bony attachments.

# Anatomy of the uterus, vagina, ovaries and breast

*Diana Lawrence-Watt*

## Uterus

The bulk of the tissue of the uterus is smooth muscle. In the nonpregnant state it weighs approximately 40 g but in pregnancy its weight increases to approximately 800 g, owing to both hypertrophy and hyperplasia of the smooth muscle fibres.

While the body of the uterus is composed of smooth muscle fibres, the cervix is composed mainly of dense connective tissue. This connective tissue acts to hold the fetus in the uterus, allowing the smooth muscle of the uterus to stretch and undergo hypertrophy.

The junction between the cervix and the uterus undergoes dilation and thinning in pregnancy. This thinner part of the wall is the region that can be incised in caesarean section.

The uterus is entirely located in the lesser pelvis, between the bladder and the rectum (Figure 4.1). The uterine tubes enter the uterus on either side, at the junction of the fundus and the body.

The uterus is a moveable organ and is held by four ligaments. These are discussed in detail below. In addition to the ligaments, folds of peritoneum form structures related to the uterus. However, these folds have a very

FIGURE 4.1 **Pelvic viscera and perineum**

Rectovaginal fold

Uterovesical fold

External anal sphincter

Deep transverse perineal muscle

Body of clitoris

Ischiocavernosus

limited role in holding the uterus in its pelvic location. Anteriorly, the uterovesical fold of peritoneum is reflected on to the upper surface of the bladder from the uterus at the junction of the cervix and uterine body. The recto-vaginal fold of peritoneum is reflected on to the surface of the rectum from the posterior fornix of the vagina and forms the floor of the rectouterine pouch. This pouch is bounded anteriorly by the posterior wall of the uterine body, posteriorly by the rectum and laterally by folds of peritoneum passing from the cervix to the posterior walls of the lesser pelvis.

## UTEROSACRAL LIGAMENTS

The folds of peritoneum extending posteriorly from the cervix to the walls of the lesser pelvis contain a substantial amount of smooth muscle and fibrous tissue. These folds are attached to the anterior surface of the sacrum and form the true ligaments of the uterus: the uterosacral ligaments (Figure 4.2).

## BROAD LIGAMENT

Related to either side of the uterus is the broad ligament (Figure 4.2). This is a fold of peritoneum that contains the uterine tubes, the round ligament of the uterus and the ligament of the ovary.

From the side of the uterus, the broad ligament reaches the lateral wall of the pelvis and results in a septum that interposes between the anterior region of the pelvis containing the bladder and the posterior region of the rectum. The ovary is attached to the posterior layer of the broad ligament via the mesovarium.

The suspensory ligament of the ovary is the part of the broad ligament that extends from the infundibulum of the uterine tube and upper pole of the ovary to the lateral wall of the pelvis. The suspensory ligament contains the ovarian vessels, nerves and lymphatics and continues over the external iliac vessels as a distinct fold. The term mesometrium is used for the part of the broad ligament

FIGURE 4.2 **Ligaments of the uterus**

Round ligament

Broad ligament

Ligament of ovary

Mesovarium

Uterosacral ligament

Suspensory ligament of ovary

FIGURE 4.3 **Uterus and adnexa**

Internal os

Cervical canal with palmate folds

External os

Vaginal fornix

Mesometrium with uterine vessels

Endometrium

Myometrium

Transverse cervical (cardinal) ligament with uterine vessels

that extends from the pelvic floor upwards to the ovary and the ligament of the ovary.

The uterine artery, a branch of the anterior division of the internal iliac artery, is carried between the layers of the broad ligament. Having crossed above the ureter as it inclines medially to gain the posterior wall of the bladder, the uterine artery passes approximately 1.5 cm lateral to the cervix. The artery then travels superiorly within the substance of the broad ligament to anastomose with branches of the ovarian artery, affording a rich anastomotic supply from both arteries to the uterine tube.

### TRANSVERSE CERVICAL LIGAMENT

From its origin at the internal iliac artery, the uterine artery travels within the substance of the transverse cervical, or cardinal, ligament (Figure 4.3). This ligament is attached to the lateral aspect of the cervix and the lateral wall of the pelvis and gives considerable support to the uterus.

The transverse cervical ligament is one of the ligaments that are instrumental in retaining the position of the uterus within the pelvis. The name here is confusing as it is not truly ligamentous but rather a condensation of dense connective tissue that has formed around the neurovascular structures extending from the lateral walls

of the pelvis to the pelvic viscera. Nevertheless, this 'ligament' is very firmly fused to the fascia surrounding the cervix and upper part of the vagina and passes backwards and upwards to the root of the internal iliac vessels.

The transverse cervical ligament supports the cervix and upper vagina, helping to maintain the angle between the axis of the vagina and the anteverted uterus. Inferiorly it is continuous with the superior fascia of the pelvic diaphragm.

### ROUND LIGAMENT

The round ligament of the uterus (Figure 4.2) may also play some role in maintaining the uterus in an anteverted position. The round ligament initially courses between the layers of the broad ligament. It then passes through the deep inguinal ring to enter the inguinal canal and end in the tissue of the labia majora, accompanied by the ilioinguinal nerve as it passes through the inguinal canal.

## Cervix and vagina

The cervix forms the cylindrical lower one-third of the uterus. The internal os is the communication between the cervix and the uterus. The external os is the communication between the cervix and the vagina (Figure 4.3). The cervix forms a less extensible region around the lower end of the uterus and may give some support to prevent expulsion of the fetus before term.

The cervical mucosa is very different from the endometrium of the uterus, undergoing very little morphological change during the endometrial cycle. During pregnancy, the cervix increases its vascularity and is less rigid than in the nonpregnant state. The mucous secretion of the cervix thickens during pregnancy, serving as a mechanical barrier to infection. In late pregnancy the dense collagen of the cervix loosens owing to uptake of fluid by mucopolysaccharides. This loosening of the cervix allows the lower section to shorten as the upper section expands.

The vagina is a muscular canal that lies between the cervix and the vestibule and opens on to the perineum. The vaginal part of the cervix continues into the anterior wall of the vagina producing two recesses: the anterior and posterior fornices. The posterior fornix is closely

related to the peritoneal cavity and is covered in peritoneum. This peritoneum is reflected on to the rectum, forming the rectouterine pouch.

## Blood supply and lymphatic drainage of the uterus, cervix and vagina

Although the main blood supply to the uterus is from the uterine arteries, an azygous system of arteries exists to supply the uterus, cervix and vagina with a very rich arterial supply (Figure 4.4). This network of vessels has contributions from the uterine, vaginal and internal pudendal arteries.

Lymph from the uterus mainly passes to the internal iliac nodes. However, there may be some communication with superficial inguinal nodes as lymph vessels may pass via the round ligaments to these nodes. Malignant cells from the uterus can track to the superficial inguinal nodes via such a route.

FIGURE 4.4 **Blood supply to the uterus and ovaries**

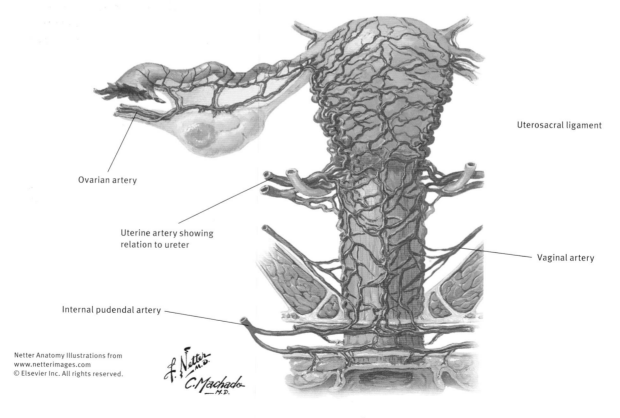

Ovarian artery

Uterine artery showing relation to ureter

Internal pudendal artery

Uterosacral ligament

Vaginal artery

## Uterine tubes and ovaries

The uterine tubes and ovaries are situated in the upper margin of the broad ligament (Figure 4.5). Each uterine tube is approximately 10 cm long. The medial end of each tube opens into the superior angle of the cavity of the uterus and the lateral end opens into the peritoneal cavity close to the ovary. The lateral end is fimbriated and the fimbriae lead into a funnel-shaped region, or infundibulum, of the tube. The infundibulum in turn leads into the ampulla and then into the isthmus of the tube. The intramural part of the tube passes through the superolateral aspect of the uterine wall to open into the upper part of the uterine cavity.

The ovaries are situated on each side of the uterus, close to the lateral wall of the lesser pelvis. Each one is attached to the posterosuperior aspect of the broad ligament by a short pedicle of peritoneum called the mesovarium. In nulliparous women, the ovary is vertical and has medial and lateral surfaces and tubal and uterine extremities. The ovary occupies a depression, called the ovarian fossa, on the lateral wall of the pelvis. The ovarian fossa is bounded by the obliterated umbilical artery anteriorly and by the ureter and internal iliac artery posteriorly. The tubal extremity is related to the external iliac vein.

Attached to the tubal extremity of the ovary are the fimbriae of the uterine tube and a fold of peritoneum known as the suspensory ligament of the ovary. This suspensory ligament, which contains the ovarian vessels and nerves, passes superiorly over the external iliac vessels.

The lateral surface of the ovary is in contact with the parietal peritoneum, which lines the ovarian fossa and separates the ovary from the extraperitoneal tissue and obturator vessels and nerves. The medial surface of the ovary is mainly covered by the uterine tube. The ovarian bursa is the peritoneal recess between the medial aspect of the ovary and the mesosalpinx, the latter being the mesentery of the fallopian tube.

## Autonomic nerve supply to the uterus and adnexa

During pregnancy and parturition, the neural pathways are of great importance and are highlighted in Figure 4.6 (see chapter 2 for more detailed discussion of the uterine nerve supply).

Sensory fibres from the uterine body and fundus travel with sympathetic fibres via the hypogastric plexuses to thoracic cord levels 11 and 12. Sensory fibres from the cervix and upper vagina travel via the pelvic splanch-

FIGURE 4.5  **Uterus, ovaries and uterine tubes**

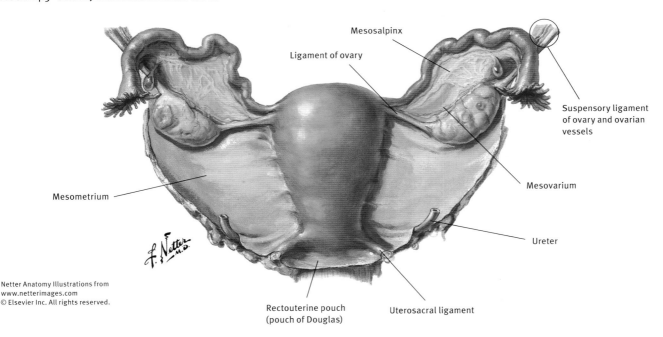

Mesosalpinx

Ligament of ovary

Suspensory ligament of ovary and ovarian vessels

Mesovarium

Mesometrium

Ureter

Rectouterine pouch
(pouch of Douglas)

Uterosacral ligament

FIGURE 4.6 **Neuropathways in parturition**

— Sensory fibres from body and fundus of uterus accompany sympathetic fibres via hypogastric plexuses to T11 and 12

- - - Sensory fibres from cervix and upper vagina accompany pelvic splanchnic nerve S2, 3 and 4

– – Sensory fibres from lower vagina and perineum accompany somatic fibres via pudendal nerve to S2, 3 and 4

— Motor fibres to body and fundus of uterus (sympathetic)

- - - Motor fibres to lower uterus, cervix and upper vagina (parasympathetic)

– – Motor fibres to lower vagina and perineum via pudendal nerve (somatic)

nic nerves to S2, 3 and 4. Sensory fibres from the lower vagina and perineum are also distributed to S2, 3 and 4 but via the pudendal nerve.

Motor fibres to the uterine body and fundus are sympathetic in origin, arising from the superior hypogastric plexus. Motor fibres to the lower segment of the uterus and the upper part of the vagina are parasympathetic in origin and travel via the pelvic splanchnic nerves. Motor fibres to the lower vagina and perineum are somatic fibres, travelling via the pudendal nerve.

## Breast

The base of the breast extends from the second rib to the sixth rib and overlies the investing fascia of the pectoralis major. The majority of the tissue of the breast in the non-pregnant state is composed of fat. During pregnancy, the glandular content of the breast increases owing to milk production within the lactiferous ducts.

## STRUCTURE AND DEVELOPMENT OF THE BREAST

The breast is divided into approximately 20 fat-filled lobules, each of which contains a lactiferous duct. Each lactiferous duct extends in a radial manner towards the nipple, where it opens on to the surface (Figure 4.7). Also opening around the nipple are the areolar glands. These glands secrete an oily, protective lubricant, particularly during pregnancy and lactation.

The lobules of the breast are separated from each other by a fibrous tissue suspensory ligament, which extends from the deep fascia covering pectoralis major to the dermis of the skin. Additional fibres extend from the connective tissue of the breast to the skin and these may pull on the skin if the organ is swollen with excess tissue fluid. This pulling results in a *peau d'orange* appearance of the skin of the breast.

During puberty, the ducting system of the breast becomes fully established. Alveolar parts of the ducts make their appearance at this time, although during puberty the increase in breast size is attributed to an increase in fat deposition. During pregnancy, both the ducts and the alveoli of the glands further develop to produce milk. Following pregnancy the breast returns to its normal prepregnant state via a process of apoptosis and the action of macrophages on these tissues. Postmenopause, the breast atrophies further as the suspensory ligaments become less taut due to the withdrawal of estrogens. The breast at this time of life therefore begins to sag.

## BLOOD SUPPLY AND LYMPHATIC DRAINAGE OF THE BREAST

The breast is supplied with blood mainly from the lateral thoracic artery, a branch of the axillary artery, through lateral mammary branches. Lateral mammary branches may also arise from lateral cutaneous branches of the posterior intercostal arteries. Medial mammary branches arise from the internal thoracic artery, a branch of the first part of the subclavian artery.

Lymphatic drainage of the breast is extensive, with more than 75% occurring via the axillary nodes. The various groups of these axillary nodes cluster around the pectoralis minor and the axillary vessels. The remaining drainage is via the para-aortic nodes. Drainage can also occur across the midline and below the diaphragm via interconnecting lymph channels.

FIGURE 4.7 **Anterolateral dissection of the breast**

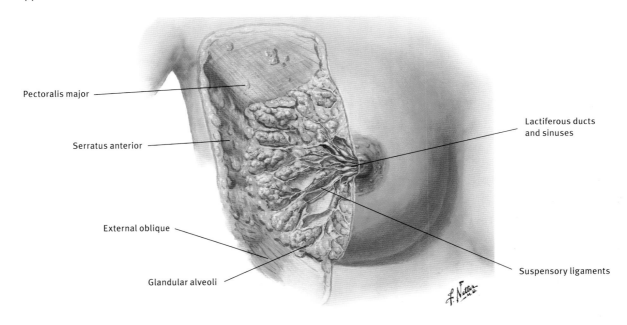

Pectoralis major

Serratus anterior

External oblique

Glandular alveoli

Lactiferous ducts and sinuses

Suspensory ligaments

## Sample questions relating to the anatomy of the abdomen and pelvis

### EXTENDED MATCHING QUESTIONS

### Questions 1–7

■ *This question relates to the anatomy of the abdomen and pelvis. For each item below, choose the* **single** *correct number for X from the list of options (A–J). Each option may be used once, more than once, or not at all.*

OPTIONS

▷ **A** 1
▷ **B** 2
▷ **C** 3
▷ **D** 4
▷ **E** 5
▷ **F** 6
▷ **G** 7
▷ **H** 8
▷ **I** 9
▷ **J** 12

1 ▶ The sacrum is made of X vertebrae

2 ▶ The sacrum contains X foramen

3 ▶ The female urethra is X cm long

4 ▶ The hip bone is made of X bones

5 ▶ There are X tendinous insertions of the rectus abdominus

6 ▶ The external oblique muscle arises from the lower X ribs

7 ▶ The rectus sheath has X vessels

### Questions 8–11

■ *This question relates to the nerves of the pelvis. For each item below, choose the* **single** *best option from the list of options (A–N). Each option may be used once, more than once or not at all.*

OPTIONS

▷ **A** L4
▷ **B** L4–5
▷ **C** L4–S1
▷ **D** L4–S3
▷ **E** L5–S1
▷ **F** L5–S2
▷ **G** S1
▷ **H** S1–2
▷ **I** S1–3
▷ **J** S1–4
▷ **K** S2
▷ **L** S2–3
▷ **M** S2–4
▷ **N** S3–4

8 ▶ The pelvic splanchnic nerves originate from here

9 ▶ Innervation of the piriformis muscle

10 ▶ The sciatic nerve originates from this cord level

11 ▶ The pudendal nerve originates from this cord level

### Questions 12–20

■ *This question relates to the histology of the female genital tract. For each item below, choose the* **single** *best option from the list of options (A–H). Each option may be used once, more than once or not at all.*

OPTIONS

▷ **A** Stratified squamous epithelium
▷ **B** Columnar epithelium
▷ **C** Ciliated cells
▷ **D** Secretory cells
▷ **E** Cuboidal epithelium
▷ **F** Transitional cells
▷ **G** Pseudostratified columnar epithelium
▷ **H** Smooth muscle cells

12 ▶ Composes the bladder mucosa

13 ▶ Covers the clitoris

14 ▶ Present in the distal fallopian tube

15 ▶ Lines the endocervix

16 ▶ Present in the medial fallopian tube

17 ▶ Covers the ovary

18 ▶ Lines the uterus

19 ▶ Covers the vagina

20 ▶ Covers the endocervix

## MULTIPLE CHOICE QUESTIONS

21 ▶ Regarding the pelvic nerves:

A ▷ They are part of the autonomic nervous system
B ▷ The sacral plexus gives off the pudendal nerve
C ▷ The sciatic nerve is formed by the L4–S2 roots
D ▷ The sciatic nerve passes through the lesser sciatic foramen
E ▷ The sciatic nerve supplies the anterior aspect of the knee

22 ▶ The obturator nerve:

A ▷ is formed by the L2–5 roots
B ▷ lies along the floor of the pelvis
C ▷ exits the pelvis through the obturator canal
D ▷ splits into anterior, medial and posterior parts on leaving the pelvis
E ▷ supplies muscles of the anterior thigh

23 ▶ Regarding the arteries of the pelvis:

A ▷ The umbilical artery supplies the posterior portion of the bladder
B ▷ The pelvic ureters are supplied by the superior vesical artery
C ▷ The inferior vesicle artery originates from the posterior internal iliac artery
D ▷ The vaginal artery originates from the anterior part of the internal iliac artery
E ▷ The lower rectum is supplied by the inferior rectal artery

24 ▶ Concerning the urinary system:

A ▷ The ureters cross the bifurcation of the common iliac arteries on entering the pelvis
B ▷ The ureters are retroperitoneal along their whole length
C ▷ The renal arteries supply the ureters along their entire length
D ▷ The ureters pass above the uterine artery
E ▷ The ureters drain lymph to the internal iliac lymph nodes

25 ▶ Concerning the vagina:

A ▷ The lateral two walls of the vagina are in contact with each other
B ▷ The bulbospongiosus muscle compresses the vagina
C ▷ The superior third of the vagina is supplied by the vaginal arteries
D ▷ The pudendal nerve provides somatic innervation to the whole vagina
E ▷ Sympathetic innervation is derived from the lumbar splanchnic nerves

26 ▶ Concerning the female reproductive system:

A ▷ The cervix drains lymph into to the internal iliac lymph nodes
B ▷ The cervical canal has its widest part at the internal os
C ▷ The round ligament is posterior to the ovarian ligament
D ▷ The cervix is more muscular than the uterus
E ▷ The broad ligament is formed by peritoneum

27 ▶ Concerning the female reproductive system:

A ▷ The mesometrium suspends the ovary
B ▷ The cardinal ligaments provide a major support for the uterus
C ▷ The uterosacral ligaments attach to the lateral part of the sacrum
D ▷ The rectouterine pouch (pouch of Douglas) is the lowest part of the pelvis
E ▷ The uterus drains blood into the external iliac vein

# Biochemistry

# CHAPTER 5

# Cell and molecular biology

*Fiona Lyall*

## Structure and function of the cell and its organelles

Two types of cell exist:

- Prokaryotic cells, such as bacteria, have a simple internal organisation and no defined nucleus.
- Eukaryotic cells, which comprise all plant and animal cells, have a more complex internal structure with a clearly defined membrane surrounding the nucleus.

Eukaryotic cells are typically 10–100 micrometres across – about ten times the size of prokaryotic cells. Despite their differences, prokaryotic and eukaryotic cells have certain structures in common and perform many complicated tasks in basically the same way. This chapter focuses on eukaryotic cells.

To maintain their integrity, eukaryotic cells have a plasma membrane that surrounds their watery interior. The plasma membrane consists of a bilayer of phospholipids, with cholesterol embedded within it to make the membrane more rigid. Only plants and fungi have cell walls surrounding the plasma membrane.

The plasma membrane does not only separate the inside of the cell from the outside environment, it also has other functions. For example, protein transporters embedded in it allow transport of water-soluble molecules across the membrane. The plasma membrane also contains receptors that bind circulating signalling molecules and hormones. Activation of receptors through such binding results in the transient reorganisation of certain proteins (the so-called signal transduction proteins) inside the cell. This in turn leads to a chain of events called cell signalling, which can trigger a variety of processes within the cell.

The majority of eukaryotic cells, including human cells, also contain internal membranes that enclose organelles within the cell (Figure 5.1). Most organelles, the nucleus being one of the exceptions, only have a single membrane. These membranes allow individual organelles to control their own internal ionic composition such that it will differ from that of the cytosol (the area outside the organelles but within the plasma membrane). Thus, the internal structure of the cell is highly organised to support the function of the cell and, ultimately, of the body.

### NUCLEUS

The nucleus is the largest organelle. It contains the cell's chromosomes and is the place where almost all DNA

FIGURE 5.1 **Diagram of a human cell showing major organelles**

Nuclear pore
Plasma membrane
Peroxisome
Microfilaments
Chromatin
Mitochondrion
Nucleus
Nucleolus
Lysosome
Rough endoplasmic reticulum
Ribosome
Vesicles
Smooth endoplasmic reticulum
Microtubules
Golgi complex
Fusion, exocytosis and discharge of vesicle contents

replication and RNA synthesis occurs.

The nucleus is separated from the cytoplasm by a double membrane called the nuclear envelope. The nuclear envelope isolates and protects the cell's DNA from various molecules that could accidentally damage its structure or interfere with its processing. Pores in the nuclear membranes regulate the movement of substances between nucleus and cytoplasm. In many cells the outer nuclear membrane is continuous with the rough endoplasmic reticulum.

The nucleus contains a suborganelle called the nucleolus and it is within this suborganelle that most of the cell's ribosomal RNA is synthesised.

## ENDOPLASMIC RETICULUM

The endoplasmic reticulum is a network of interconnected internal membranes. There are two varieties: rough and smooth.

The rough endoplasmic reticulum is so called because it has ribosomes attached to its outer surface; the smooth endoplasmic reticulum does not.

The smooth endoplasmic reticulum is the site where synthesis of fatty acids and phospholipids occurs. Many cells have little smooth endoplasmic reticulum but in liver cells it is abundant. Enzymes in the smooth endoplasmic reticulum of liver cells modify and detoxify molecules such as pesticides and carcinogens and exposure to large amounts of such chemicals results in a large increase in endoplasmic reticulum volume in liver cells.

Ribosomes bound to the rough endoplasmic reticulum synthesise organelle and membrane proteins as well as all proteins to be secreted from the cell. Secretory proteins pass through the rough endoplasmic reticulum membrane and accumulate in the inner cavity of the rough endoplasmic reticulum before being transported to their destination. Rough endoplasmic reticulum is particularly abundant in cells that are specialised in the production of secreted proteins such as antibodies (for example plasma cells) or digestive enzymes (for example pancreatic acinar cells).

Most proteins leave the rough endoplasmic reticulum within minutes after their synthesis in small membrane-bound transport vesicles. These vesicles bud off from the rough endoplasmic reticulum and transport the proteins to the lumen of the Golgi complex.

## GOLGI COMPLEX

The Golgi complex is also surrounded by a membrane. Within different regions of the Golgi complex, different enzymes modify secreted proteins and membrane proteins in different ways depending on the structure and ultimate destination of the proteins.

After modification, the proteins are transported out of the Golgi complex in a second set of transport vesicles. Some vesicles will contain proteins destined for the plasma membrane, while others contain proteins for lysosomes or other organelles.

## MITOCHONDRIA

Mitochondria are found in nearly all eukaryotic cells, and there are usually several or many in each cell. These organelles burn glucose for fuel in the process of cellular respiration to produce ATP. Essentially, they are the 'power house' of the cell.

Mitochondria have a smooth outer membrane and a convoluted inner membrane, which are separated by an intermembrane space. The convolutions of the inner membrane are called cristae and the space inside the inner membrane is the mitochondrial matrix. As glucose is burned for fuel, a mitochondrion shunts various chemicals back and forth across the inner membrane (from the matrix to the intermembrane space and vice versa).

Mitochondria contain their own DNA, which, in contrast to the nuclear DNA, is inherited through the mother.

## LYSOSOMES AND PEROXISOMES

Lysosomes and peroxisomes can be likened to the 'disposal system' of a cell because they remove substances the cell no longer requires, including old organelles.

Lysosomes and peroxisomes are surrounded by a single membrane and are rich in digestive enzymes. For example, lysosomes can contain more than three dozen enzymes for degrading proteins, nucleic acids and polysaccharides. All lysosome enzymes work at acidic pH values; thus, the internal pH value is maintained at around 4.8. The cell would not be able to house such destructive enzymes if they were not contained in a membrane-bound system to protect the rest of the cell.

Many materials degraded by lysosomes are brought into the cell by one of the following processes:

- endocytosis (materials are taken up by invagination of a part of the plasma membrane to form a small membrane-bound vesicle)
- phagocytosis (larger particles such as bacteria are enveloped by the plasma membrane and internalised).

Peroxisomes contain several oxidases that oxidise organic substances. This process generates the toxic molecule hydrogen peroxide ($H_2O_2$), which is then converted to $O_2$ and $H_2O$ by the enzyme catalase. The peroxisome is the main organelle for oxidising fatty acids, which are precursors for key synthetic pathways. Toxic molecules in the blood are also cleared by peroxisomes, particularly in liver and kidney cells.

## CYTOSOL AND CYTOSKELETON

The cytosol of the cell does not only contain the cell organelles, it also contains the cytoskeleton. The cytoskeleton is made up of three classes of fibres: microtubules (20 nm diameter), microfilaments (7 nm diameter) and intermediate filaments (10 nm diameter). The cytoskeleton gives the cell rigidity and strength, thereby allowing it to maintain its shape, and changes in its organisation underpin a cell's ability to migrate.

Finally, the cytosol also contains many particles such as glycogen-containing granules.

## Cell signalling

In multicellular organisms, a complex intercellular communication network exists that coordinates metabolism, differentiation, growth and repair. The term cell signalling refers to the communication between cells by means of signalling molecules. Released by the signalling cell or bound to its surface, signalling molecules produce a response in a target cell that has receptors for that particular signalling molecule. The process of converting an extracellular signal into a response in the target cell is known as signal transduction.

Extracellular signalling by means of secreted molecules can be classified as endocrine, paracrine and autocrine, depending on the distance travelled by the signalling molecule:

- Endocrine signalling involves the release of hormones from endocrine glands; the hormones are then carried in the bloodstream to a distant target site (Figure 5.2 A).
- In paracrine signalling the signalling molecule produced by a cell acts only on cells very close to it (Figure 5.2 B); neurotransmitters work by paracrine signalling.
- In autocrine signalling a cell responds to a signalling molecule that it has released itself (Figure 5.2 C); many growth factors operate like this and it is commonly seen in tumour growth.

In a fourth method of extracellular signalling, the signalling molecules are membrane-bound proteins that can interact with receptors on adjacent cells (Figure 5.2 D).

Most types of animal cell have a characteristic set of

FIGURE 5.2 **Extracellular signalling methods**

**A** Endocrine signalling

Endocrine gland secreting hormone into bloodstream

Blood vessel

Hormone released at distant site

Target cell

**B** Paracrine signalling

Target cell

**C** Autocrine signalling

**D** Cell signalling via membrane-attached proteins

Signal cell      Target cell

high-affinity receptors allowing them to respond to a range of signalling molecules. The effect of some signalling molecules varies depending on the cell type they encounter. For example, acetylcholine increases the contraction of skeletal muscle but decreases the contraction force of heart muscle and thereby the heart rate. Cells can also modulate their response to a particular ligand by altering the number of cell-surface receptors for that ligand.

Some chemical signalling mechanisms are rapid and transient. Examples include insulin secretion in response to raised blood glucose levels and neurotransmission, a process that is even faster than insulin secretion. Some signalling processes are slow in onset and long-lasting such as estradiol production by the ovaries at the onset of puberty.

Many signalling molecules are required just to allow the cell to survive and further signalling molecules are required to enable the cell to proliferate. When deprived of survival signalling molecules, cells may undergo programmed cell death (apoptosis).

## SIGNALLING MOLECULES

The binding of ligands to receptors leads to increases or decreases in the concentration of second-messenger molecules such as cyclic adenosine monophosphate (cAMP), cyclic guanosine monophosphate (cGMP), diacylglycerol, inositol trisphosphate (IP$_3$) and Ca$^{2+}$. These in turn modify various cell functions.

### *Inositol trisphosphate and diacylglycerol*

IP$_3$ and diacylglycerol are produced through hydrolysis of inositol phospholipids (phosphoinositides), which are mainly located in the inner half of the plasma membrane. The inositol phospholipid known as phosphatidyl bisphosphate (PIP$_2$) is the most important member of this class of lipids in terms of cell signalling, even though it accounts for less than 10% of the total inositol lipids and less than 1% of all the phospholipids in the cell membrane. The breakdown of PIP$_2$ starts with the binding of a signalling molecule to its receptor in the plasma membrane.

FIGURE 5.3 **Phospholipase C signalling pathway**

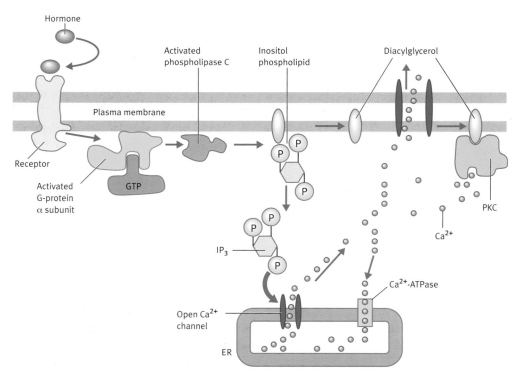

ER = endoplasmic reticulum | GTP = guanosine triphosphate | IP$_3$ = inositol trisphosphate | P = phosphate group | PKC = protein kinase C

The activated receptor stimulates a guanine-nucleotide-binding protein (G protein) known as $G_q$, which in turn activates an inositide-specific phospholipase C called phospholipase C-β. This enzyme cleaves $PIP_2$ into two products (Figure 5.3):

- $IP_3$
- diacylglycerol.

These two molecules act as mediators for separate signalling pathways.

$IP_3$ is small and water-soluble. It diffuses into the cytosol, where it binds to and opens $IP_3$-gated $Ca^{2+}$ release channels in the endoplasmic reticulum (Figure 5.3) or, in muscle cells, ryanodine receptors in the sarcoplasmic reticulum. In fact, in many cell types both forms of $Ca^{2+}$ receptors are present. To end the $Ca^{2+}$ response, $Ca^{2+}$ is pumped back out of the cytosol and $IP_3$ is broken down by phosphatases within the cell.

Some of the $IP_3$ is also phosphorylated to form inositol tetrakisphosphate ($IP_4$), which may promote the refilling of the intracellular $Ca^{2+}$ stores and/or mediate slower or longer-lived responses within the cell.

Diacylglycerol remains attached to the plasma membrane and has two potential fates. First, it can be cleaved to give arachidonic acid, which can be used as a precursor in the synthesis of eicosanoids. Second, and more importantly, it can act as a second messenger. The initial rise in $Ca^{2+}$ brought about by $IP_3$ causes an enzyme called protein kinase C (C because it is $Ca^{2+}$-dependent) to move from the cytosol to the plasma membrane, where it is activated by diacylglycerol (Figure 5.3).

Protein kinase C is a serine/threonine protein kinase that regulates the function of other proteins by phosphorylating their serine and/or threonine residues. In addition, protein kinase C can alter the transcription of specific genes. In one pathway, the enzyme catalyses the phosphorylation of mitogen-activated protein (MAP) kinase, which in turn phosphorylates and activates the transcription factor Elk-1. Together with another protein (the serum response factor), Elk-1 binds to the serum response element, a short DNA sequence in the promoter region of the target gene. This leads to transcription of the gene. In another pathway, activation of protein kinase C results in the release of nuclear factor kappa B, which moves into the nucleus also to activate the transcription of specific genes.

As diacylglycerol is rapidly metabolised, sustained activation of protein kinase C for longer-term responses depends on a second wave of diacylglycerol production. This time, diacylglycerol is released by phospholipase-mediated cleavage of phosphatidylcholine, the major phospholipid in the cell.

### Eicosanoids

Eicosanoids are signalling molecules that are continuously made in the plasma membrane of all mammalian tissues. They are synthesised from 20-carbon fatty acid chains (mainly arachidonic acid), which in turn are cleaved from membrane phospholipids by phospholipases. There are four major groups of eicosanoids:

- prostaglandins
- prostacyclins
- thromboxanes
- leucotrienes.

The first three are collectively known as prostanoids. The generation of prostanoids is catalysed by the enzyme prostaglandin $H_2$ synthase, also known as cyclooxygenase (COX), whereas formation of leucotrienes occurs via a lipoxygenase pathway.

Detailed information on the prostaglandin synthetic pathway is provided in chapter 6. In the current context, it is important to note that there are two main forms of COX, known as COX-1 and COX-2. These two enzymes have similar functions but are the products of different genes. In general, COX-1 is found in tissues that produce prostaglandins constantly, such as the stomach mucosa, whereas COX-2 is only expressed at sites of inflammation and so is inducible. A third type of COX, COX-3, is formed by alternative splicing of the gene encoding COX-1.

Prostaglandins and leucotrienes are important stimulators of the myometrium during labour (see chapter 6 for a discussion of the regulation of myometrial contractility). The increase in prostaglandin levels during labour is thought to be caused by induction of COX-2 in fetal membranes. Bacterial products and proinflammatory cytokines can also increase expression of COX-2 and hence prostaglandin synthesis. In addition, high concentrations of prostanoids have been reported during menstruation, in particular in conditions associated with painful menstruation, such as menorrhagia, dysmenorrhoea and endometriosis.

The synthetic pathways of eicosanoids can be targeted by therapeutic drugs. For example, corticosteroid drugs such as cortisone inhibit phospholipase and are used to treat inflammatory conditions such as arthritis. Nonsteroidal anti-inflammatory drugs (NSAIDs), including aspirin and ibuprofen, block the first oxidation step of arachidonic acid that is catalysed by COX.

Older NSAIDs such as indometacin inhibit both COX-1 and COX-2. Newer NSAIDs are selective for COX-2. In general, the more COX-2-selective an NSAID is, the better its adverse effect profile. For example, COX-2-selective inhibitors are just as effective in the treatment of menstrual pain as NSAIDs but have fewer gastrointestinal adverse effects.

Aspirin inhibits both COX-1 and COX-2 (it is actually much more active against COX-1 than COX-2; hence its poor adverse effect profile). Unlike most NSAIDs, which are competitive antagonists, aspirin functions by permanently acetylating the active site of the COX enzyme. It can be used at a low dose to inhibit platelet thromboxane synthesis with little effect upon vascular endothelial prostacyclin synthesis. This may be of value in thromboprophylaxis and in the management of pre-eclampsia.

Low doses of aspirin permanently disable platelet COX as the platelets pass through the hepatic portal system. Since the platelet has no nucleus, it cannot synthesise a new supply of COX and so platelet thromboxane synthesis is permanently inhibited. Most of the aspirin is then inactivated within the liver. The small amount of aspirin that then passes into the general circulation may acetylate vascular endothelial COX but, since these cells have a nucleus, they can synthesise a new supply of COX and maintain prostacyclin synthesis.

### Nitric oxide and carbon monoxide

Most signalling molecules are hydrophilic molecules but some are small enough to pass straight into the cell where they can directly exert their effects. One such example is the gas nitric oxide (NO). NO is produced from L-arginine by the enzyme NO synthase in the presence of co-factors and $O_2$; the by-product is L-citrulline. There are three main forms of this enzyme:

- endothelial NO synthase (eNOS)
- inducible NO synthase (iNOS)
- brain NO synthase (bNOS).

These enzyme isoforms are the products of different genes that share about 50–60% sequence homology. Many cells express more than one form of NO synthase.

eNOS was first described in endothelial cells. It is constitutively expressed and is dependent on $Ca^{2+}$ and calmodulin. NO has a very short half-life (5–10 seconds) and is converted to nitrates and nitrites in the blood. Endothelial cells on blood vessels release NO in response to increased shear stress or agents such as acetylcholine. The released NO diffuses to the underlying smooth muscle, where it reacts with iron in the active site of the enzyme guanylate cyclase to produce the intracellular mediator cGMP. The effects of guanylate cyclase are rapid and result in muscle relaxation. Thus, continual release of NO from blood vessels is one of the main mechanisms for keeping blood pressure at its normal level.

In pregnancy, blood pressure falls and it is thought that the associated vasodilation is partly mediated by increased NO release. NO is also important in the regulation of blood flow within the placenta and eNOS is expressed on the entire syncytiotrophoblast surface, just as it is expressed on blood vessels. Placental eNOS is thought to inhibit the aggregation of neutrophils and platelets present in maternal blood in the intervillous space.

The expression of iNOS is induced in response to inflammatory signals such as bacterial cell-wall products, which include lipopolysaccharides and cytokines such as interferon gamma or tumour necrosis factor alpha. It is induced in activated macrophages and neutrophils. NO released from these cells helps them to kill invading microorganisms. The activity of iNOS is independent of $Ca^{2+}$ and calmodulin.

bNOS was first described in the brain. Like eNOS, it is constitutively expressed and is dependent on $Ca^{2+}$ and calmodulin for activity.

NO is released by many types of nerve cell to convey signals to neighbouring cells. For example, NO released by autonomic nerves in the penis causes local blood-vessel dilatation resulting in penile erection. In reproductive biology, NO has also been implicated in the control of myometrial quiescence, in the onset of labour and in cervical ripening, although the evidence for some of these functions is certainly not conclusive.

The effects of NO on blood vessels also explain the efficacy of glyceryl trinitrate in the treatment of angina, for which it has been used for nearly 100 years. Glyceryl trinitrate is converted to NO, which relaxes blood vessels in the heart. Glyceryl trinitrate has also been used in an attempt to prevent preterm labour by relaxing myometrial smooth muscle and to ripen the cervix.

Carbon monoxide (CO) is another gas that stimulates guanylate cyclase. CO is produced by the enzymes haem oxygenase 1 and 2. Haem oxygenase 1 is inducible, while haem oxygenase 2 is constitutively expressed. It is now known that CO, like NO, is important in maintaining vasodilatation in the placenta.

## Calcium

Cells maintain low concentrations of free $Ca^{2+}$ (100 nmol/l) despite much higher concentrations in the extracellular fluid (10 mmol/l) and endoplasmic reticulum. Increases in intracellular $Ca^{2+}$ concentrations are one way in which extracellular signals are transmitted across the plasma membrane. When $Ca^{2+}$ channels are transiently opened in the plasma or endoplasmic reticulum membranes, intracellular $Ca^{2+}$ concentrations rise to about 50 micromoles/l and activate $Ca^{2+}$-responsive proteins in the cell. Resting $Ca^{2+}$ concentrations are kept very low by several means. $Ca^{2+}$-ATPases in the plasma membrane pump $Ca^{2+}$ out of the cell. Nerve and muscle cells, which use $Ca^{2+}$ to a greater extent for signalling, have an additional $Ca^{2+}$ pump ($Na^+,Ca^{2+}$-exchanger) in the plasma membrane, which couples $Na^+$ influx to $Ca^{2+}$ efflux.

In the endoplasmic reticulum, there is yet another $Ca^{2+}$-ATPase that takes up $Ca^{2+}$ from the cytosol. Mitochondria can also pump $Ca^{2+}$ inside; a low-affinity, high-capacity $Ca^{2+}$ pump in the inner mitochondrial membrane uses the electrochemical gradient generated across the membrane during electron transport in oxidative phosphorylation. This pump only operates when $Ca^{2+}$ levels are extremely high, usually as a consequence of cell damage. $Ca^{2+}$-binding proteins in the cytoplasm and in the endoplasmic reticulum offer additional $Ca^{2+}$ buffering capacity.

Calmodulin is a $Ca^{2+}$-binding protein found in all eukaryotic cells. It mediates many $Ca^{2+}$-regulated processes and undergoes a conformational change when bound to $Ca^{2+}$. When this happens, the $Ca^{2+}$–calmodulin complex can bind to various target proteins and alter their activity. Among the $Ca^{2+}$–calmodulin targets are various enzymes (such as eNOS and bNOS) and membrane transport proteins. Most effects of $Ca^{2+}$–calmodulin are, however, indirect and are mediated by $Ca^{2+}$–calmodulin-dependent protein kinases; an example for such an enzyme is myosin light chain kinase, which activates smooth muscle contraction.

Two pathways of $Ca^{2+}$ signalling have been well defined. One is used mainly by excitable cells. When nerve-cell membranes are depolarised by an action potential, voltage-gated $Ca^{2+}$ channels open and $Ca^{2+}$ enters the cell, leading to the secretion of neurotransmitters. In the other pathway, binding of extracellular signalling molecules to cell-surface receptors ultimately leads to the opening of channels in the endoplasmic reticulum and a rise in the intracellular $Ca^{2+}$ concentration. The opening of these channels is brought about by the intermediate molecule $IP_3$.

## Cyclic adenosine monophosphate

cAMP is synthesised from ATP by the plasma-membrane-bound enzyme adenylate cyclase (also known as adenylyl cyclase) and is rapidly and continually destroyed by cAMP phosphodiesterases. cAMP-mediated phosphorylation and dephosphorylation can increase or decrease the activity of many different enzymes. The effects of cAMP are mediated via activation of cAMP-dependent protein kinases (also known as protein kinases A).

The cellular response to cAMP varies depending on the cell type. For example, increased cAMP levels in the liver stimulate glycogen breakdown; in adipocytes they stimulate the production of fatty acids and in ovarian cells they induce the formation of estradiol and progesterone.

## Cyclic guanosine monophosphate

The synthesis of cGMP is catalysed by guanylate cyclase, which converts guanosine triphosphate (GTP) to cGMP. Membrane-bound guanylate cyclase is activated by peptide hormones such as atrial natriuretic peptide, while soluble guanylate cyclase is activated by NO to stimulate cGMP synthesis.

cGMP relaxes smooth muscle. It also activates protein kinase G enabling it to phosphorylate a number of substrates.

cGMP is degraded by phosphodiesterases. Sildenafil (Viagra®; Pfizer, New York, NY, USA) enhances the vasodilatory effects of cGMP by inhibiting phosphodiesterase 5.

## CELL-SURFACE RECEPTORS

Cell-surface receptors belong to one of four major classes. Each will be discussed in detail.

### G-protein-coupled receptors

Ligand binding to a G-protein-coupled receptor activates a G protein, which in turn activates a target enzyme that either generates a second messenger or modulates an ion channel. In fact, most G proteins regulate the concentrations of the intracellular signalling molecules cAMP or $Ca^{2+}$ by targeting adenylate cyclase or phospholipase C, respectively.

Receptors linked to G proteins comprise the largest family (over 100 members) of cell-surface receptors. They all have a similar structure consisting of a polypeptide chain that threads back and forth through the plasma membrane seven times.

The G proteins themselves are fully known as trimeric GTP-binding regulatory proteins. They are called trimeric because they are made up of alpha, beta and gamma subunits. The nature of the alpha subunit determines the action of the G protein. For example, stimulatory G proteins ($G_s$ proteins) have an alpha s subunit that activates adenylate cyclase, resulting in the production of cAMP; inhibitory G proteins ($G_i$ proteins) have an alpha i subunit that inhibits adenylate cyclase and thus blocks the production of cAMP; $G_q$ proteins have an alpha q subunit that activates phospholipase C, thereby triggering the production of the second messengers $IP_3$ and diacylglycerol.

The detailed mechanism of G protein activation is shown in Figure 5.4 using adenylate cyclase activation as an example. The inactive $G_s$ protein is bound to the inside surface of the cell membrane and the alpha unit binds

FIGURE 5.4 **G-protein-coupled activation of adenylate cyclase**

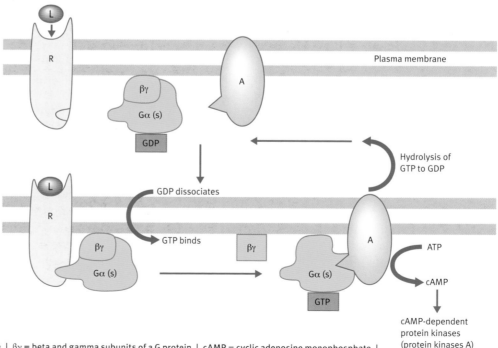

A = adenylate cyclase | βγ = beta and gamma subunits of a G protein | cAMP = cyclic adenosine monophosphate | Gα (s) = alpha subunit of a stimulatory G protein | GDP = guanosine diphosphate | GTP = guanosine triphosphate | L = ligand | R = receptor

guanosine diphosphate (GDP). When a ligand binds to the receptor, the conformation of the receptor is altered exposing a binding site for the $G_s$ protein. Assembly of the ligand–receptor–$G_s$ protein complex is brought about by diffusion of the subunits within the membrane and results in the alpha subunit switching its affinity from GDP to GTP.

Binding of GTP instead of GDP causes the dissociation of the alpha subunit from the beta and gamma subunits and this in turn exposes the alpha subunit's binding site for adenylate cyclase. The alpha subunit now binds to and activates adenylate cyclase, resulting in the conversion of ATP to cAMP.

When the ligand dissociates, the receptor returns to its original conformation. The alpha subunit will eventually hydrolyse the attached GTP to GDP by its inherent enzymatic activity, allowing the alpha subunit to reassociate with the beta and gamma subunits so that the system returns to the original inactivated state.

Many hormones, neurotransmitters and local mediators (for example epinephrine, serotonin and glucagon) signal through G-protein-coupled receptors. In some cases, the same ligand can stimulate or inhibit cAMP production depending on the receptor to which it binds. For example, when adrenaline binds to beta-adrenergic receptors, it activates adenylate cyclase; by contrast, binding to alpha-2-adrenergic receptors inhibits the enzyme. This is because beta-adrenergic and alpha-2-adrenergic receptors are coupled to different G proteins, the former to $G_s$ and the latter to $G_i$.

Several bacterial toxins also act via G-protein-coupled receptors. Cholera toxin is an enzyme that alters the alpha subunit of $G_s$ so that it can no longer hydrolyse GTP. The constitutive stimulation of adenylate cyclase results in the prolonged production of cAMP in intestinal epithelial cells, causing a large efflux of $Na^+$ and $H_2O$ and leading to the symptoms of severe diarrhoea that are characteristic of cholera.

FIGURE 5.5 **Cell-surface receptors**

**A** Ion channel receptors

**B** Tyrosine-kinase-linked receptors

**C** Receptors with intrinsic enzyme activity

cGMP = cyclic guanosine monophosphate | GTP = guanosine triphosphate | L = ligand | P = phosphate group | R = receptor | TK = tyrosine kinase

Pertussis toxin (produced by the bacterium *Bordetella pertussis*, which colonises the respiratory tract and causes whooping cough) alters the alpha i subunit to prevent its interaction with G-protein-coupled receptors, so that the subunit cannot inhibit adenylate cyclase. This increases cAMP concentration and thus affects normal cellular signalling. It is not known whether this contributes to the cough itself but it does facilitate adherence to the tracheal epithelium.

### Ion channel receptors

Ligand binding to an ion channel receptor changes the conformation of the receptor (Figure 5.5 A). This allows specific ions to flow through the receptor, thus altering the electric potential across the membrane. An example of this type of receptor is the acetylcholine receptors at nerve–muscle junctions.

### Tyrosine-kinase-linked receptors

Ligand binding to a tyrosine-kinase-linked receptor results in the formation of a receptor dimer from two monomeric receptors (Figure 5.5 B). The cytosolic portion of the dimeric transmembrane receptor then binds to, and activates, the cytosolic enzyme tyrosine kinase. The activated tyrosine kinase in turn phosphorylates tyrosine residues in the receptor. As a result, substrate proteins that bind to the phosphotyrosine residues are phosphorylated.

Tyrosine-kinase-linked receptors are also known as the superfamily of cytokine receptors, with ligands including erythropoietin and the interferons.

### Receptors with intrinsic enzyme activity

The fourth group of cell-surface receptors are those that have their own intrinsic enzyme activity in their cytosolic domain (Figure 5.5 C). Again, ligand binding tends to induce dimerisation of the receptor. One example is the enzyme guanylate cyclase, which generates the second messenger cGMP. Another example is receptors with intrinsic tyrosine kinase activity. The latter example includes some receptors for growth factors, such as nerve growth factor and platelet-derived growth factor, and the receptor for insulin.

An important downstream signalling molecule that is activated through receptor tyrosine kinases is the GTP-binding protein Ras. Ras belongs to the same superfamily of intracellular switch proteins as does the alpha subunit of G proteins. However, while the alpha subunit acts as part of a trimeric protein, Ras is a monomeric GTPase. Activation of Ras induces a kinase cascade that ends in the activation of MAP kinase. This serine/threonine kinase can enter the nucleus, where it phosphorylates many proteins including transcription factors.

## Cell–cell adhesion

In multicellular organisms, many cells have the ability to connect with each other tightly for the purpose of communication. A number of integral membrane proteins called cell adhesion molecules enable cells to adhere to each other and to the extracellular matrix. We will see later that cells are also able to interact with each other and communicate locally via specialised cell junctions.

The major classes of cell adhesion molecules are cadherins, immunoglobulins, selectins and integrins.

### CADHERINS

Cadherins cause adhesion via homophilic (self–self) binding to other cadherins in a $Ca^{2+}$ dependent manner. Cadherins hold cells together, enable the segregation of cell collectives into discrete tissues during development, maintain tissue integrity and are expressed in a temporal and spatial manner during embryonic development. Most cadherins function as transmembrane linker proteins, with the cytoplasmic domain interacting with the cytoskeleton (actin and intermediate filaments) of the cells they join together.

### IMMUNOGLOBULIN-LIKE MOLECULES

Immunoglobulin-like adhesion molecules comprise a large group of molecules that are generated from a comparably small number of genes by alternative splicing. Collectively, they have both homophilic and heterophilic binding properties. The best-studied members of this group are the neural cell adhesion molecules (NCAMs),

FIGURE 5.6 **Leucocyte diapedesis**

ICAM-1 = intercellular cell adhesion molecule 1  |  IL-8 = interleukin-8

which are expressed predominantly in nervous tissue, and the intercellular cell adhesion molecules (ICAMs) 1, 2 and 3. This family also includes platelet endothelial cell adhesion molecule 1 (PECAM-1) and vascular cell adhesion molecule 1 (VCAM-1).

### INTEGRINS

Integrins are a diverse and large group of heterodimeric glycoproteins. The two subunits, alpha and beta, both participate in binding. Integrins participate in cell–cell adhesion and facilitate communication between the cytoskeleton and the extracellular matrix, allowing each to influence the orientation and structure of the other. Events such as clustering of integrins activate a number of intracellular signalling pathways.

Some integrins exist in active and inactive states. For example, a group of integrins responsible for the binding of white blood cells to the endothelium are normally inactive, allowing the leucocytes to circulate freely. In response to inflammatory mediators, these integrins become activated and mediate a process termed extravasation or diapedesis (Figure 5.6). Defects in the expression of certain integrins can result in diseases characterised by abnormal inflammatory responses.

### SELECTINS

The selectins (E-, P- and L-selectin) are primarily expressed by leucocytes and endothelial cells and, like integrins, they are important in many host-defence mechanisms involving those cells. In contrast to other cell adhesion molecules, selectins bind to carbohydrate residues located on the cell surface and the resulting binding forces are relatively weak.

Figure 5.6 illustrates how cell adhesion molecules allow the endothelium and circulating cells in the bloodstream to signal to each other. Shown is the fate of a circulating neutrophil that has been attracted by interleukin-8 released from a site of inflammation. Selectin-mediated interactions result in the formation of weak (transitory) bonds between the neutrophil and endothelial cells, promoting the rolling of the white blood cell along the endothelium towards the site of inflammation. Integrins expressed at the site of inflammation bind more tightly to the neutrophil and stop it in place, while ICAM-1 helps secure the adhesion to the endothelium. As a result, the cell leaves the bloodstream via the endothelium and moves into the inflamed tissue, where it can release leucotrienes (to cause vasoconstriction and increase vascular permeability), free radicals and proteases as part of the inflammatory response.

## Cell junctions

Cells are also able to interact with each other and communicate locally via specialised cell junctions. There are four major classes of junctions:

- tight junctions
- adherens junctions and desmosomes
- hemidesmosomes
- gap junctions.

The former three are adhering junctions, whereas gap junctions are communicating junctions.

Tight junctions essentially form an impermeable seal between two cells. In the gastrointestinal tract, tight junctions prevent the escape of digestive enzymes from the lumen into the intracellular space.

Adherens junctions and desmosomes bind the plasma membrane of adjacent cells at various spots, which gives strength and rigidity to the entire tissue.

Hemidesmosomes are junctions that connect a cell's intermediate filaments to the underlying extracellular matrix. These junctions firmly anchor epithelial cells, thereby increasing the rigidity of epithelial tissues.

Gap junctions are specialised cell–cell junctions that are formed from a mirror image of protein units (connexons) located in the plasma membranes of two cells. As a result, the cytoplasms of these cells are connected by narrow water-filled channels. These channels allow passage of small signalling molecules, such as $Ca^{2+}$ and cAMP, but not of large molecules such as proteins.

In the myometrium, gap junctions provide low-resistance pathways between smooth muscle cells, thereby increasing their electrical coupling to allow increased coordination of myometrial contractility. During pregnancy, gap junctions are present at very low numbers in the myometrium; however, labour is associated with an increase in the number and size of gap junctions. This has led to the idea that gap junctions are essential, but not sufficient, for effective labour and delivery.

## Cell cycle, cell growth and division and cancer

### CELL DIVISION

To know when to divide, cells use their own internal clock known as the cell cycle (Figure 5.7). During each cycle, a series of events occurs in an orderly sequence. DNA is duplicated during the synthesis phase (S phase). The two DNA copies are then moved to opposite ends of the cell.

**FIGURE 5.7 Cell cycle and cell cycle checkpoints**

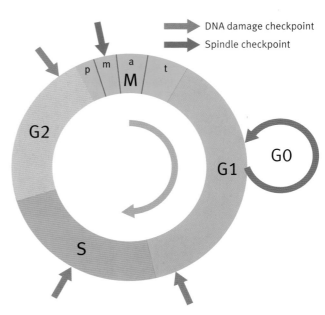

a = anaphase | G0 = quiescent phase | G1 = gap 1 | G2 = gap 2 | m = metaphase | M = mitosis | p = prophase | S = synthesis phase | t = telophase

Halving of the genome is called mitosis (M phase). Mitosis is divided into several stages:

- During prophase the chromosomes condense.
- During metaphase sister chromatids produced by DNA replication during the S phase become aligned in the centre of the cell.
- During anaphase the sister chromatids separate and move to opposite poles of the mitotic apparatus/spindle.
- During telophase the nuclear envelope breaks down and reforms around the segregated chromosomes. The final physical division of the cytoplasm to yield two daughter cells is called cytokinesis.

The period between M and S is called gap 1 (G1). The period between S and M is called gap 2 (G2). Both gap phases allow time for cell growth. The gaps also enable the cells to monitor the internal and external environment before committing to the S phase and then to mitosis. Nondividing cells exit the cell cycle and enter the quiescent state (G0).

## CELL CYCLE CONTROL

Progress through the cell cycle involves important check-points (Figure 5.7):

- DNA damage checkpoints detect DNA damage before and during the S phase. If damage is detected, the activity of a protein called cyclin-dependent kinase 2 (CDK2) is inhibited and progression through the cell cycle is stopped. If the damage to the DNA is not repairable (for example using the DNA repair proteins BRCA1 and BRCA2), the cell undergoes apoptosis.
- Spindle checkpoints check that spindle fibres attach to kinetochores. If any fibres fail to attach, apoptosis occurs.

Several proteins have a key role in the regulation of the cell cycle. For example, a protein called adenomatous polyposis coli (APC) activates a transcription factor known as Myc, which induces the transcription of a number of genes for movement from G1 to the S phase of the cell cycle.

The protein p53 can detect DNA damage and inhibit the cell cycle by blocking CDK2. In addition, p53 has a key role in apoptosis.

Finally, the protein ataxia telangiectasia mutated (ATM) also detects DNA damage and stops the cell cycle (with help from p53) if required. In addition, ATM maintains normal telomere length, thereby counteracting the tendency of the chromosome to shorten with each round of replication.

## DEVELOPMENT OF CANCER

Multiplication of cells is tightly regulated. It exceeds cell death in children so that they can increase in size to become adults. In adulthood, the half-life of cells varies a lot depending on the function of the cell. For example, intestinal cells have a half-life of a few days before being renewed, red blood cells have a half-life of about 100 days, liver cells rarely die and brain cells are slowly lost over a lifetime with no or very little renewal.

If the regulatory mechanisms that control cell growth and apoptosis break down, a clone of cells (tumour) can begin to appear in an area where this is not wanted. There are over 200 types of human cancer:

- Carcinomas are derived from endoderm or ectoderm.
- Sarcomas are derived from mesoderm.
- Leukaemias are a class of sarcomas that grow as individual cells in the blood.

### Oncogenes and tumour suppressors

The types of protein involved in normal cell growth that can lead to cancer when mutated are as follows (Figure 5.8 provides an overview of these proteins):

- Growth factors or their receptors, signal transduction proteins and transcription factors can acquire gain-of-function mutations that turn the affected gene (the proto-oncogene) into an oncogene. Mutated oncogene alleles are usually dominant.
- Cell cycle control proteins usually act as tumour repressors and loss-of-function mutations in these proteins can make it more likely that a cell becomes a tumour cell. Mutated tumour repressor alleles tend to be recessive.

Virus-encoded proteins can also cause cancer by acting on growth factor receptors.

FIGURE 5.8 **Proteins involved in cell growth and cancer development**

E = effector, e.g. tyrosine kinase  |  G = growth factor  |
R = growth-factor receptor  |  S = signal transduction protein

Over 50% of cancers have mutations in the tumour suppressor protein p53, rendering p53 unable to function. This allows faulty mutant cells to continue through the cell cycle and to escape apoptosis. Both *p53* alleles must be mutated for the function of the protein to fail.

APC also acts as a tumour suppressor protein. Absence of a functional APC protein results in inappropriate activation of the transcription factor Myc, resulting in uncontrolled cell proliferation. Again, both alleles of the *APC* gene must be mutated for this to occur, as one normal copy of the gene can result in the production of sufficient APC protein.

### Transformation of a normal cell into a cancer cell

Some individuals inherit cancer-causing mutations in the germline but most cancers are caused by mutations in somatic cells (any cell other than a germ cell) and such mutations usually accumulate over years. The accumulation of a few right up to perhaps 20 mutations may be required to start off a cancer; hence, cancer is often a disease of the aged.

The example of colorectal cancer illustrates this point. Individuals with an inherited *APC* mutation are at increased risk of developing colorectal cancer. However, APC only has a role in the first stage of the development of cancer, namely the development of colorectal polyps. If the tumour is removed at the polyp stage, the prognosis is good. If not, polyp cells can accumulate further mutations starting with mutation of *Ras* into an oncogene and followed by other changes including loss of function of a tumour suppressor protein called defective in sister chromatid cohesion (DCC) and loss of function of p53. Another common genetic lesion in colorectal cancer involves mutations in the so-called mismatch repair proteins, which have a role in DNA repair.

This example shows that lesions in a single gene are generally not transforming. Instead, transformation usually involves the suppression of apoptosis followed by a series of other events that eventually lead to malignancy.

### Oncogenic viruses

Some viruses can cause cancer by subverting normal cell control mechanisms. At some point in evolution, these viruses have incorporated normal cellular proto-oncogenes into their genome, and these proto-oncogenes have subsequently been mutated to become oncogenes. For example, the Harvey sarcoma virus contains the *Ha-ras* gene, which differs from the human *Ras* gene by the presence of a single point mutation. Overexpression of *Ha-ras* has been identified in human bladder tumours.

Another example is the viral Src (v-Src) protein produced by Rous sarcoma virus (Src is short for sarcoma). This protein is a constitutively active mutant of the cellular Src (c-Src) protein, a protein tyrosine kinase that, like Ras, is involved in signal transduction. The v-Src protein is produced at much higher levels than c-Src and continuously and inappropriately phosphorylates a number of target proteins.

Retroviruses such as Harvey sarcoma virus and Rous sarcoma virus contain an RNA genome. In a host cell, they first hijack the cell's replication process to make a DNA copy of their own viral RNA. The DNA is then inserted into the cell's chromosomal DNA giving rise to the replication of the viral genome and the production of viral proteins, including oncogenes.

Many DNA viruses also contain oncogenes and, unlike retroviruses, they need the oncogenes for their own survival. Examples include the family of human papillomaviruses, which cause genital warts and other benign tumours of epithelial cells.

## TUMOUR GROWTH AND SPREAD

### Growth properties of cancer cells

Cancer cells are usually less well differentiated than normal cells and may start to lose their specific functions and instead exhibit features of rapidly growing cells. They can exist in one of three states:

- They go constantly through the cell cycle.
- They are in a quiescent state (G0), able to re-enter the cell cycle at any time.
- They are no longer able to divide but continue to contribute to the size of the tumour.

Drugs such as cisplatin, which belongs to the family of platinum compounds, only affect dividing cells. However, in some tumours, such cells may constitute as little as 5% of the total tumour mass. Cisplatin does not affect the ability of tumour cells to spread and is indiscriminate in affecting all rapidly dividing cells; hence its associated adverse effects such as hair loss, nausea and suppression of bone marrow function. The drug has to be given at a dose that still allows enough normal cells to survive so the treated person can recover.

### Metastasis

Tumours that do not spread are benign; an example would be a wart. An important feature of malignancy is the ability to spread. The process of spreading and establishment in secondary sites is called metastasis.

Metastatic cells break their adhesive contacts with other cells and are also able to overcome the movement restraint provided by the basal lamina (basement membrane). The basal lamina is a fibrous network of collagens and proteoglycans that support epithelial and other cells. Many tumour cells secrete plasminogen activator, which in turn converts plasminogen to the active protease plasmin. Plasmin then digests the basal lamina allowing some of the tumour cells to enter and travel in the bloodstream.

To colonise another site, the tumour cell must attach to the endothelium at the site of metastasis and migrate across it to the tissue below. Fewer than one in 10 000 cancer cells that escape into the bloodstream survive. Those that do have acquired many new characteristics that allow them to grow in a tissue from which they did not originate.

Paradoxically, a number of primary tumours can secrete substances that inhibit metastasis of secondary tumours. In these cases, removal of the primary tumour can actually promote the metastatic process.

### Angiogenesis

To grow beyond a mass of about 2 mm in diameter (about $10^6$ cells), a tumour requires a blood supply or it will not be able to sustain further growth. Many tumours therefore release growth factors such as vascular endothelial growth factor (VEGF), basic fibroblast growth factor or transforming growth factor alpha. These growth factors can stimulate a process known as angiogenesis.

Angiogenesis involves degradation of the basement membrane of an adjacent capillary, migration of the endothelial cells towards the tumour and ultimately the formation of a new capillary that can supply nutrients to the tumour.

Current cancer research includes the search for treatments that can stop angiogenesis. Approaches include:

- blocking signals from the tumour; for example, the drug bevacizumab is approved to treat colon cancer by intercepting VEGF signals
- blocking VEGF receptors on endothelial cells
- using small-molecule drugs that can get inside endothelial cells and interfere with tyrosine kinase
- targeting the enzymes that clear the pathway for blood vessels to extend
- targeting oncogenes to prevent angiogenesis from starting.

## DNA, RNA, the genetic code and protein synthesis

DNA contains all the information required to build the entire body. During transcription, DNA is copied into RNA, which has three roles in protein synthesis. Messenger RNA (mRNA) carries the message from DNA and specifies the correct order of amino acids during protein synthesis. Next, during translation, the amino acids are assembled into proteins. This requires the help of transfer RNA (tRNA), which interprets the message on the mRNA, and of ribosomal RNA (rRNA).

### STRUCTURE OF DNA AND RNA

DNA and RNA are very similar in structure. Both are made up of nucleotides, which have three components:

- a nitrogen-containing base, which is either a purine or a pyrimidine; in DNA, the four bases are adenine, guanine, thymine and cytosine; in RNA, uracil replaces thymine; adenine and guanine are purines and consist of a pair of fused nitrogen-containing rings, whereas cytosine, thymine and uracil are pyrimidines and consists of a single nitrogen-containing ring.
- a five-carbon sugar (pentose); in RNA the sugar is a ribose, whereas in DNA the sugar is a deoxyribose
- a phosphate group linked to the pentose by a phosphodiester bond.

FIGURE 5.9 **Structure of DNA**

**A** Building blocks of DNA

**B** DNA double helix

A = adenine | C = cytosine | G = guanine | P = phosphate group | S = sugar molecule | T = thymine

Each nucleotide has two distinctive ends: a 5-prime end, where a phosphate group is attached to carbon atom number 5 of the sugar ring, and a 3-prime end, where a hydroxyl group is attached to carbon atom number 3 of the sugar.

DNA molecules can contain up to several hundred million nucleotides. Figure 5.9 shows how the nucleotides link together to form nucleic acids.

DNA consists of two polynucleotide strands wound together to form a double helix. The two strands in the DNA backbone run antiparallel to each other: one of the DNA strands is built in the 5-prime to 3-prime direction, while the other runs in the opposite direction. The two sugar–phosphate backbones are on the outside of the double helix and the base pairs are on the inside.

The strands are held together through base pairing between the two strands. Adenine always pairs with thymine through two weak hydrogen bonds and cytosine

FIGURE 5.10 **DNA replication at a replication fork**

A = adenine | C = cytosine | G = guanine | T = thymine

FIGURE 5.11 **Transcription**

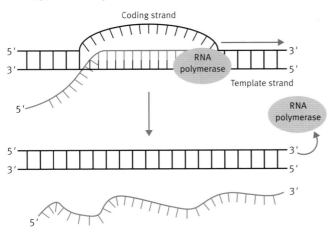

always pairs with guanine through three weak hydrogen bonds. When two strands are paired as shown in Figure 5.9 they are said to be complementary.

By contrast, RNA can be fewer than 100 to thousands of nucleotides long and is usually single-stranded.

## DNA SYNTHESIS

DNA replication begins with the unwinding of the DNA double helix by proteins called helicases, which break the hydrogen bonds. The junction between the unwound part and the open part is called a replication fork (Figure 5.10).

One of the template strands is the leading strand. DNA polymerase adds the complementary nucleotides and binds the sugars and phosphates. It follows the helicase as it unwinds and continuously forms new DNA. The leading strand is oriented in the 3-prime to 5-prime direction and DNA polymerase travels from the 5-prime to the 3-prime end of the new strand. It cannot add nucleotides in the opposite direction.

The other side of the ladder is the lagging strand, oriented in the 5-prime to 3-prime direction. DNA polymerase also adds complementary nucleotides on this side but it is now travelling in the opposite direction (moving away from the helicase). As a result, the lagging strand is made in many discontinuous segments rather than continuously as for the leading strand. This process results in the creation of several fragments, called Okazaki fragments, which are then joined together by DNA ligase.

During replication, DNA synthesis occurs simultaneously at many points along the original strand (multiple replication forks). It would take a long time to go from one end of the parent DNA to the other; thus it is more efficient to open up several points at the same time.

## RNA SYNTHESIS

To allow the DNA template to be copied into mRNA, the two DNA strands must first unwind (denature). Transcription begins with RNA polymerase binding to the promoter region (upstream of the coding region) in the DNA (Figure 5.11). As in DNA replication, transcription proceeds in the 5-prime to 3-prime direction, but during RNA synthesis uracil replaces thymine. The single DNA strand that is copied to form the new strand is called the template strand and the strand that is not used is called the coding strand. Once the mRNA is released, the DNA strands reanneal.

Transcription can involve many RNA polymerases on a single DNA template, so that many RNA molecules can be produced during copying.

## GENE SPLICING

The DNA sequence in genes contains exons (the DNA regions that are being transcribed to the final functional mRNA molecule) and introns (noncoding sequences). Following the production of an identical RNA transcript of the original DNA sequence, the introns are removed by a process known as splicing (Figure 5.12) and the exons are joined together. Although exons can include the sequences that code for amino acids, some exons are also noncoding.

The process of alternative splicing (Figure 5.12) allows a single gene to be translated into multiple proteins that are similar but have their own distinct function, such as targeting a particular cell. For example, alternative splicing of the VEGF transcription product results in the production of a family of VEGF variants that take on various roles in vasculogenesis and angiogenesis.

## PROTEIN SYNTHESIS

Proteins are chains of polypeptides, which in turn are chains of amino acids. Amino acids are held together by

FIGURE 5.12 **Gene splicing**

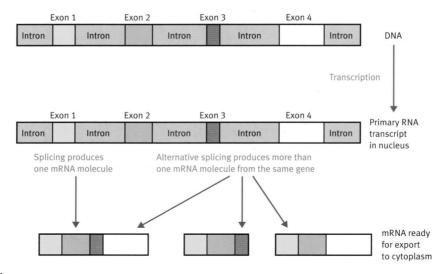

mRNA = messenger RNA

strong peptide bonds. mRNA contains the code for the amino acid sequence.

To understand translation, it is important to first understand the genetic code (the rules by which mRNA is made, or translated, into proteins). Within an mRNA molecule, each triplet of nucleotides is called a codon. Each codon specifies an amino acid. The code is degenerate, meaning that more than one codon can specify the same amino acid but no codon specifies more than one amino acid.

Protein synthesis (translation) also requires tRNA and rRNA. The tRNA deciphers the code, with each amino acid having its own tRNA. One end of the tRNA molecule has a binding site for a particular amino acid and the other side contains the anticodon that can base-pair with the codon. As protein synthesis proceeds, the correct tRNA with its attached amino acid is added to the growing polypeptide chain (Figure 5.13). However, this also requires the help of the ribosome. The ribosome is a multiunit structure containing rRNA and proteins. As the ribosome moves along, the free tRNA that has donated an amino acid leaves the ribosome and is free to receive another amino acid. The next tRNA molecule then adds an amino acid and the polypeptide chain grows. At the end, the complete polypeptide is released and the ribosome drops off. Multiple ribosomes move along the mRNA, so that multiple copies of the polypeptide can be made more quickly.

The sequence of amino acids in a polypeptide chain is called the primary structure of a given protein. The term secondary structure refers to the folding of the polypeptide chain into one of two geometric arrangements, an alpha helix or a beta sheet stabilised by hydrogen bonds. The term tertiary structure refers to the folding of the polypeptide chain into an overall arrangement and this is achieved through hydrophobic interactions and disulphide bonds. The term quaternary structure refers to the arrangement of multiple polypeptide chains (subunits) in multimeric proteins.

## POST-TRANSLATIONAL MODIFICATION

After translation, proteins can undergo chemical modification such as the addition of an acetyl group (acetylation), which affects the lifespan of the protein, addition of a phosphate group (phosphorylation), which is used to regulate the activity of a protein, and addition of carbohydrate chains (glycosylation). Many secreted proteins and membrane proteins are glycosylated.

FIGURE 5.13 **Protein synthesis**

A = adenine | Ala = alanine | C = cytosine | G = guanine | Leu = leucine |
Met = methionine | mRNA = messenger RNA; tRNA = transfer RNA | U = uracil

## Laboratory techniques

### SOUTHERN BLOTTING

Southern blotting (Figure 5.14) is used to detect the presence and amount of a particular sequence of DNA in a sample that contains many other DNA sequences, such as total cellular DNA. This technique was named after its inventor, Edwin Southern. The names of other blotting methods were chosen in reference to Edwin Southern's surname.

### NORTHERN BLOTTING

Northern blotting is a very similar technique. It is used to detect the presence and amount of a particular RNA sequence in a sample containing a mixture of RNA molecules.

### WESTERN BLOTTING

Western blotting is used to detect the presence and amount of a specific protein in a tissue sample. This technique employs gel electrophoresis (the movement of proteins through a gel matrix exposed to an electric current, with smaller proteins travelling faster leading to separation of the proteins) and immunoblotting with a specific antibody raised against the protein of interest.

Tissues are homogenised first to solubilise the proteins. The proteins are then denatured with reducing agents to break disulphide bonds and allow separation by molecular weight. They are also coated in sodium dodecyl sulphate (SDS), which gives them a negative charge.

Once the proteins have been separated and transferred to a membrane, the antibody is added. For example, a typical primary antibody for the detection of COX-1 in myometrial tissue homogenates would be antihuman COX-1 from goat (in other words, human COX-1 protein had been injected into goats to raise antibodies against the human protein). Thereafter, a secondary antibody is added. This could be an antigoat antibody from mouse, rabbit or another species (except goat or human).

The secondary antibody is linked to a radioactive, chromogenic, fluorescent or chemiluminescent tag. For example, if the tag is horseradish peroxidase, addition of a chemiluminescent substrate will result in the emission of light, which can be detected by a photographic film. The stronger the detection signal, the more protein is present.

FIGURE 5.14 **Southern blotting**

Blotting paper with weight on top

Gel is face up and DNA fragments transfer by capillary action

1. DNA fragments are separated by size on an agarose gel by electrophoresis

2. DNA fragments are blotted onto a nitrocellulose membrane

3. DNA fragments are fixed to the membrane

4. The membrane is exposed to a DNA probe containing the sequence to be detected; the probe is labelled with a radioactive or fluorescent tag

5. Depending on the tag used, DNA that binds the probe is detected on an X-ray film via either radioactivity or light given off

\* DNA molecular weight markers

## POLYMERASE CHAIN REACTION

Polymerase chain reaction (PCR) is used to amplify a specific sequence of DNA or RNA, which can be present in a mixture with other DNA or RNA fragments. If RNA rather than DNA is being amplified, it must first be transcribed into complementary DNA (cDNA) by the enzyme reverse transcriptase.

The key ingredients in a PCR reaction are the four nucleotides (adenine, thymine, cytosine and guanine), a heat-stable DNA polymerase called *Taq* polymerase and primers. Primers are short nucleic-acid sequences that are complementary to the template-strand DNA. When the primer sequence is attached to the template strand, the *Taq* polymerase can then continue to add on further nucleotides. With this method, the number of DNA strands grows exponentially.

PCR can be used to amplify very small amounts of DNA and has many applications in genetic testing, forensics and scientific research.

## DNA MICRORARRAYS

DNA microarrays enable the simultaneous analysis of the expression of thousands of genes. Essentially, a DNA microarray is a collection of thousands of DNA spots (short oligonucleotides) that are bound to a solid surface. These microarrays can be purchased commercially and can be custom-made to include genes belonging to particular gene families that the researcher is interested in looking at.

Expression of the genes of interest can be assayed by synthesising fluorescently labelled cDNA from mRNA that has been isolated from cells exposed to different conditions. For example, a researcher might isolate mRNA from cultured myometrial cells that have been exposed to mechanical stretch and from cultured control cells that have been left untreated. The mRNA from each culture would then be converted into cDNA by reverse transcription. Subsequently, the DNA from each experiment would be labelled with a dye and added to separate microarray plates. That way, the researcher could see which genes in the cells were affected by the mechanical stretch.

## BIOINFORMATICS

Bioinformatics is the term used to describe the computer methods for storing, distributing and analysing the huge number of DNA sequences that have been reported.

Several databanks around the world, one of the main ones being GenBank at the National Institutes of Health, USA, store all newly reported DNA sequences and allow scientists from all over the world access via the Internet. Researchers who have sequenced a DNA fragment can enter their sequence into such a databank and determine if their sequence is similar to any other sequences that have already been submitted. If so, and if the function of the encoded protein is already known, this will give them a hint on the function of the DNA they have sequenced. For example, mutations in the *BRCA1* gene convey a high risk of developing breast cancer. When this gene was sequenced and entered into a DNA databank, it was discovered that it was very similar to a yeast gene that produces a cell cycle checkpoint protein.

## PROTEOMICS

Proteomics is the large-scale study of proteins and, in particular, their structures and function. The term proteomics was chosen to make an analogy with genomics, the study of genes. After genomics, proteomics is the next step in the study of a biological system.

However, proteomics is far more complex than genomics and provides a more accurate understanding of how the body works. This is primarily because an organism's genome is constant, whereas its proteome (the entire complement of proteins) varies from cell to cell and changes continuously. Protein expression is different in different parts of the body, at different stages of development and under different environmental conditions. On top of this, about 25 000 genes have been identified so far in humans but there are probably more than 500 000 proteins derived from these genes. This is the result of events such as alternative splicing and post-translational modification (for example glycosylation, phosphorylation). It is also important to note that the level of transcription of a gene does not necessarily reflect the level of expression of the respective protein; mRNA can be degraded rapidly or not translated efficiently, so that large amounts of mRNA can result in only small amounts of protein. Finally, many proteins are only functional if they form complexes with other proteins or RNA molecules. Proteomics therefore also involves the study of protein interactions.

A number of methods are available in the field of proteomics. The traditional method for the study of protein interactions is yeast two-hybrid analysis, which detects physical interactions (such as binding) between two proteins or between a single protein and a DNA molecule. Other methods employed in proteomics include protein microarrays (similar to DNA microarrays).

Proteomics has a crucial role in the development of new drugs. If a protein is thought to be involved in a disease, information on its three-dimensional structure can be used to design drugs that interfere with, or block, the action of the protein. For example, in Alzheimer's disease, elevations in beta-secretase levels result in the creation of beta-amyloid, which is the principal constituent of the brain plaques that are associated with the development of dementia. Drugs targeting the enzyme beta-secretase decrease the production of beta-amyloid and so slow the progression of the disease.

Proteomics is also important in the discovery of disease biomarkers that can be used for diagnostic purposes.

# CHAPTER 6

# Steroids and prostaglandins

*Anthony E Michael*

## Introduction

Steroids and prostaglandins are both classes of lipid hormones. However, they differ fundamentally in their molecular substrates, synthetic pathways, cellular receptors, mechanisms and speed of action, and physiological responses. The cellular actions of placental steroid hormones and prostaglandins on the myometrium need to be coordinated carefully to ensure timely delivery of the infant at term. This chapter covers these topics and ends with a discussion of the cellular mechanisms underlying the control of myometrial contractions.

## Steroid hormones

### STEROID SYNTHESIS AND METABOLISM

#### Origins, transport and metabolism of cholesterol

As shown in Table 6.1, steroid hormones can be broadly classified as:

- corticosteroids (synthesised in the adrenal cortex)
- gonadal steroids (synthesised in the ovary or testis).

All steroid hormones are derived from cholesterol by the sequential removal of carbon groups and addition of oxygen-containing groups (Figure 6.1).

Four major sources of cholesterol are used for steroid hormone biosynthesis:

- *de novo* cholesterol biosynthesis (from acetate)
- plasma membrane
- intracellular lipid droplets (containing cholesteryl esters, such as cholesteryl oleate)
- plasma lipoproteins (primarily low-density lipoprotein cholesterol).

The rate-determining step in the synthesis of steroid hormones is the removal of the 6-carbon side chain from the 27-carbon substrate cholesterol to generate the first 21-carbon steroid, pregnenolone (Figure 6.2). This reaction is catalysed by the cytochrome P450 (CYP)-based cholesterol side chain cleavage enzyme (CYP11A1, previously named P450$_{SCC}$), which is located in the inner

TABLE 6.1 **Classification of steroid hormones**

| Class of steroid | Number of carbon atoms | Major physiological example |
|---|---|---|
| **CORTICOSTEROIDS** [a] | | |
| Mineralocorticoids | 21 | Aldosterone |
| Glucocorticoids | 21 | Cortisol |
| Androgens | 19 | DHEA |
| **GONADAL STEROIDS** [b] | | |
| Progestins | 21 | Progesterone |
| Androgens | 19 | Testosterone |
| Estrogens | 18 | Estradiol |

[a] Made in zones of the adrenal cortex | [b] made in the ovary or testis | DHEA = dehydroepiandrosterone

FIGURE 6.1 **Overview of steroid hormone biosynthesis**

**A** Structure of cholesterol

**B** Synthesis of steroid hormones from cholesterol

In part B of this figure, C = carbon atom

FIGURE 6.2 **Metabolism of cholesterol to pregnenolone**

C = carbon atom | CYP11A1 ($P450_{scc}$) = cholesterol side chain cleavage enzyme

mitochondrial membrane facing the matrix. The relevance of this fact is that the lipid substrate cholesterol has to be transported across the aqueous space that lies between the outer and the inner mitochondrial membranes. The intracellular trafficking of cholesterol to the CYP11A1 enzyme relies on the actions of:

- steroidogenic acute regulator (StAR) protein
- mitochondrial peripheral benzodiazepine receptors.

Cellular levels of StAR increase following stimulation of steroidogenic cells by luteinising hormone, follicle-stimulating hormone, human chorionic gonadotrophin or adrenocorticotrophic hormone. The StAR protein then acts as a ligand for the mitochondrial peripheral benzodiazepine receptors, which bring the mitochondrial membranes into apposition by activating voltage-dependent anion channels to mediate $Cl^-$ efflux from the aqueous intermembrane space.

The significance of StAR in steroidogenesis is underscored in pregnancies complicated by lipoid congenital adrenal hyperplasia. In this condition, failure of StAR in the fetal adrenal glands prevents transport of cholesterol into the mitochondria of the adrenocortical cells, leading to the accumulation of cholesteryl esters within engorged lipid droplets in the adrenal cortex. As a consequence, the fetal adrenal glands fail to make any of the corticosteroid hormones. This rare condition is usually lethal *in utero*. If affected infants are delivered, they have problems inflating their lungs (because of the absence of fetal glucocorticoids *in utero*) and enter a salt-wasting crisis (because of the absence of aldosterone).

### Steroidogenic enzymes

Although the pathways for steroid biosynthesis seem to be complex, they revolve around just two classes of enzyme:

- CYP enzymes
- hydroxysteroid dehydrogenase (HSD) enzymes.

The function of the CYP enzymes is to catalyse the hydroxylation reactions required to increase the solubility of the steroid hormones in aqueous media (blood, extracellular fluid and urine). In addition, some of the CYP enzymes – specifically CYP11A1 and steroid 17α-hydroxylase (CYP17A or $P450_{c17}$) – also act as lyase

FIGURE 6.3  **Operation of steroidogenic enzymes: cytochrome P450 enzymes**

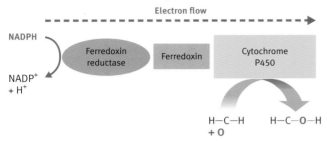

NADP$^+$ = oxidised form of nicotinamide adenine dinucleotide phosphate  |
NADPH = reduced form of NADP

enzymes to cleave single carbon bonds.[1] The hydroxylase function of CYP enzymes relies on the transport of electrons from the reduced form of the nucleotide co-factor nicotinamide adenine dinucleotide phosphate (NADPH) to the haem centre of the CYP enzyme via ferredoxin reductase and ferredoxin (Figure 6.3).

The HSD enzymes (3β-HSD and 17β-HSD) are oxidoreductase enzymes that belong to the superfamily of short-chain alcohol dehydrogenases. As such, the HSD enzymes catalyse the oxidation of secondary alcohol groups and/or the reduction of ketone groups on steroid hormones at designated carbon positions (Figure 6.4). In addition, 3β-HSD acts as a $\Delta^5,\Delta^4$ isomerase to convert the weak steroids pregnenolone and dehydroepiandrosterone to the more potent steroid metabolites progesterone and androstenedione, respectively. During this reaction, the double bond between carbon positions 5 and 6 (signified by the symbol $\Delta^5$) of the steroid B ring is relocated to carbon positions 4 and 5 (signified by the symbol $\Delta^4$) of the A ring (Figure 6.5 A). By contrast, the 17β-HSD enzymes act primarily as reductase enzymes, reducing

FIGURE 6.4  **Operation of steroidogenic enzymes: hydroxysteroid dehydrogenase enzymes**

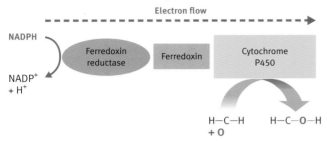

NAD(P)$^+$ = oxidised form of nicotinamide adenine dinucleotide (phosphate)  |
NAD(P)H = reduced form of NAD(P)

FIGURE 6.5  **Steroid metabolism by hydroxysteroid dehydrogenase enzymes**

**A**  3β-Hydroxysteroid dehydrogenase

**B**  17β-Hydroxysteroid dehydrogenase

DHEA = dehydroepiandrosterone  |  HSD = hydroxysteroid dehydrogenase  |
NAD$^+$ = oxidised form of nicotinamide adenine dinucleotide  |
NADH = reduced form of NAD  |  NADP$^+$ = reduced form of NAD phosphate  |
NADPH = reduced form of NADP

the ketone at carbon position 17 on androstenedione and estrone to the more potent beta-alcohol group at carbon position 17, characteristic of testosterone and estradiol (Figure 6.5 B).

### Tissue-specific patterns of steroidogenesis

The pathway of steroid biosynthesis within a given steroidogenic tissue depends on the precise pattern of CYP and HSD expression in that tissue:

- In testis Leydig cells, CYP11A1, CYP17A, 3β-HSD and 17β-HSD act in sequence to synthesise testosterone (Figure 6.6 A).
- In the theca cells of ovarian follicles, CYP11A1, CYP17A and 3β-HSD act in sequence to synthesise androstenedione (Figure 6.6 B).
- In the follicular granulosa cells, follicle-stimulating hormone upregulates the enzyme aromatase (CYP19 or P450$_{AROM}$), which converts androstenedione from the theca cells into estrone. Estrone can subsequently be reduced by 17β-HSD to the more potent estrogen, estradiol (Figure 6.6 C).

## FIGURE 6.6 Tissue-specific steroidogenic pathways

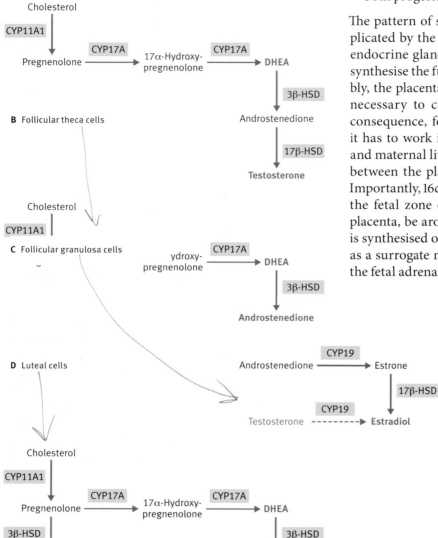

**A** Testis Leydig cells

**B** Follicular theca cells

**C** Follicular granulosa cells

**D** Luteal cells

CYP11A1 = cholesterol side chain cleavage enzyme | CYP17A = steroid 17α-hydroxylase | CYP19 = aromatase | DHEA = dehydroepiandrosterone | HSD = hydroxysteroid dehydrogenase

- In the steroidogenic cells of the corpus luteum, CYP11A1, 3β-HSD, CYP17A, CYP19 and 17β-HSD are all expressed, enabling the luteal cells to synthesise both progesterone and estradiol (Figure 6.6 D).

The pattern of steroid synthesis in the placenta is complicated by the fact that the placenta is an 'incomplete endocrine gland': it lacks the key enzymes required to synthesise the full range of steroid hormones. Most notably, the placenta does not express the CYP17A enzyme necessary to convert progestins to androgens. As a consequence, for the placenta to synthesise estrogens, it has to work in concert with the fetal adrenal gland and maternal liver, with steroids passing back and forth between the placenta, fetal and maternal circulations. Importantly, 16α-hydroxyandrostenedione secreted from the fetal zone of the fetal adrenal cortex can, in the placenta, be aromatised to estriol, a unique steroid that is synthesised only by the placenta and that can be used as a surrogate marker to assess the functional status of the fetal adrenal gland.

## Steroid metabolism and clearance

After their secretion, steroid hormones can undergo extensive metabolism at peripheral sites, including skin, bone and adipose tissue. For example, to induce virilisation of the external genitalia, testosterone must be converted within the genital skin fibroblasts to the androgen metabolite 5α-dihydrotestosterone by the steroid 5α-reductase 2 enzyme. By contrast, to cause closure of the epiphyses of the long bones, testosterone must be metabolised within the bone by CYP19 to generate estradiol, which acts on the epiphyses via the estrogen receptor, rather than the androgen receptor.

To be cleared from the body, steroid hormones have to be rendered more hydrophilic (water-soluble) so that they can pass out into the urine or faeces. This two-step process, catalysed primarily in the liver, typically involves the sequential actions of:

- CYP or HSD enzymes, which create polar hydroxyl (alcohol) groups
- conjugating enzymes (typically glucuronyltransferases or sulphotransferases), which catalyse condensation reactions to add polar or charged chemical groups (such as glucuronides and sulphates, respectively) to the polar hydroxyl/alcohol groups.

## STEROID HORMONE ACTIONS

### Steroid hormone receptors

Owing to their hydrophobicity, steroid hormones can pass easily through the plasma membrane of target cells and so exert their actions via intracellular receptors that serve as ligand-dependent transcription factors.[2] There are five different steroid hormone receptors, each of which binds a distinct class of steroid hormone with relatively high affinity (Table 6.2).

All steroid hormone receptors are composed of the same four functional domains:

- ligand-binding domain, which binds the steroid hormone in a hydrophobic binding pocket
- DNA-binding domain, which typically comprises a pair of zinc fingers to bind DNA
- dimerisation domain (located within the ligand-binding domain), which facilitates interactions between pairs of activated steroid receptors
- transactivating factor domains, which interact with proteins in the preinitiation transcription complex.

In the vacant state, steroid receptors may reside in either the cytoplasm or the nucleus. Following the binding of a steroid ligand, the activated receptors translocate into the nucleus, where they bind DNA to modulate the transcription of target genes.[2] Steroid receptors always act as molecular dimers, which can either be homodimers (for example glucocorticoid–glucocorticoid receptors) or heterodimers (for example glucocorticoid–progesterone receptors). The dimeric receptors either possess or

TABLE 6.2 **Classification of the steroid hormone receptors**

| Receptor name | Conventional abbreviation | Physiological ligand |
|---|---|---|
| Progesterone receptor | PR | Progesterone |
| Mineralocorticoid receptor [a] | MR | Aldosterone (and deoxycorticosterone) |
| Glucocorticoid receptor [b] | GR | Cortisol |
| Androgen receptor | AR | 5α-DHT (and testosterone) |
| Estrogen receptor | ER | Estradiol (and estrone) |

[a] Also referred to as type 1 corticosteroid receptor | [b] also referred to as type 2 corticosteroid receptor | 5α-DHT = 5α-dihydrotestosterone

recruit (via their transactivating domains) enzymes that remodel chromatin in such a way as to either increase or decrease the rate of transcription of the target genes.

### Steroid hormone actions

Dimeric receptors bind to DNA at specific nucleotide sequences (termed steroid response elements) that are typically found in the promoter region of the target gene. The dimeric receptors are then able to interact with receptor-interacting proteins, which can act either as co-repressor or as coactivator proteins:

- Co-repressor proteins recruit histone deacetylase enzymes, which remove the acetyl groups from the neighbouring histone proteins. This has the effect

of allowing the DNA to remain in the annealed, condensed state, thereby repressing the transcription of the target genes.
- Coactivator proteins recruit histone acetyltransferase enzymes, which exert the opposite action of acetylating the histones to decondense and open the DNA, thereby increasing the rate of gene transcription.

Owing to the complexity of their genomic mode of action, the speed of action of steroid hormones is relatively slow. Typically, it takes steroid hormones anything between 6 hours and several days to effect a change in cellular function by changing the repertoire of genes expressed in the target cell.

## Prostaglandins

### PROSTAGLANDIN SYNTHESIS AND METABOLISM

### Arachidonic acid

All prostaglandins are synthesised from arachidonic acid, a polyunsaturated fatty acid (Figure 6.7).[3] In the cell, this polyunsaturate is typically found esterified to membrane phospholipids. Hence, the simplest way for arachidonic acid to be liberated for prostaglandin synthesis is by the action of phospholipase $A_2$ on membrane phospholipids to generate free arachidonate and the residual lysophospholipid molecules. The rate-determining cleavage of arachidonate by phospholipase $A_2$ is inhibited by lipocortin, which is in turn upregulated by the anti-inflammatory glucocorticoid steroids (for example cortisol and dexamethasone).

### Cyclooxygenase enzymes

Once liberated, arachidonate is acted upon by the enzyme cyclooxygenase (COX, also called prostaglandin $H_2$ synthase) to synthesise prostaglandin $G_2$, an intermediate that is rapidly converted to prostaglandin $H_2$ (Figure 6.7). There are two forms of COX enzyme:

- COX-1, a constitutively active isoenzyme
- COX-2, a hormone-responsive/inducible isoenzyme.

Both COX enzymes are inhibited by indometacin and

FIGURE 6.7 **Prostaglandin synthesis from membrane phospholipids**

COX = cyclooxygenase | PGD synthase = prostaglandin D synthase |
$PGD_2$ = prostaglandin $D_2$ | PGE synthase = prostaglandin E synthase |
$PGE_2$ = prostaglandin $E_2$ | PGF synthase = prostaglandin F synthase |
$PGF_{2\alpha}$ = prostaglandin $F_{2\alpha}$ | $PGH_2$ = prostaglandin $H_2$ |
PGI synthase = prostaglandin I synthase | $PGI_2$ = prostaglandin $I_2$ |
$PLA_2$ = phospholipase $A_2$

TABLE 6.3  **Classification of the major prostaglandin receptors and the predominant signalling pathways activated by each class of receptor**

| Prostaglandin | Receptor | Conventional abbreviation | Second messenger |
|---|---|---|---|
| $D_2$ | D-prostanoid receptor | DP receptor | ↑ cAMP |
| $E_2$ | E-prostanoid receptor subtype 1 | $EP_1$ receptor | ↑ $Ca^{2+}$ |
| $E_2$ | E-prostanoid receptor subtype 2 | $EP_2$ receptor | ↑ cAMP |
| $E_2$ | E-prostanoid receptor subtype 3 | $EP_3$ receptor | ↓ cAMP |
| $E_2$ | E-prostanoid receptor subtype 4 | $EP_4$ receptor | ↑ cAMP |
| $F_{2\alpha}$ | F-prostanoid receptor | FP receptor | ↑ $IP_3$ / ↑ $Ca^{2+}$ |
| $I_2$ | I-prostanoid receptor | IP receptor | ↑ cAMP |

↑ = increased  |  ↓ = decreased  |  cAMP = cyclic adenosine monophosphate  |  $IP_3$ = inositol trisphosphate

other nonsteroidal anti-inflammatory drugs, such as aspirin.

### Prostaglandin synthase enzymes

Once generated by the COX enzymes, prostaglandin $H_2$ can be metabolised by a range of prostaglandin synthase enzymes to generate various prostaglandins, each with a distinct array of actions. Specifically, prostaglandin $H_2$ can be acted upon by the prostaglandin D, prostaglandin E, prostaglandin F and prostaglandin I synthases to generate prostaglandin $D_2$, prostaglandin $E_2$, prostaglandin-$F_{2\alpha}$ and prostaglandin $I_2$ (prostacyclin), respectively (Figure 6.7).

### Prostaglandin metabolism

The biological activity of each prostaglandin relies on the presence of an alcohol group at carbon position 15. Hence, oxidation of this alcohol to a 15-carbon ketone by 15-hydroxyprostaglandin dehydrogenase results in the rapid inactivation of prostaglandins. The 15-hydroxyprostaglandin dehydrogenase enzyme is highly expressed in the lungs, such that around 65% of prostaglandins are inactivated with each pass through the pulmonary circulation. The susceptibility of prostaglandins to oxidative inactivation catalysed by 15-hydroxyprostaglandin dehydrogenase limits the actions of these lipid hormones to autocrine and paracrine effects on neighbouring cells.

### PROSTAGLANDIN ACTIONS

Given that prostaglandins are lipid hormones synthesised from a fatty-acid substrate, they would intuitively be expected to have free access to the interior of target cells and hence to exert their actions via intracellular (probably nuclear) receptors, as is the case for steroid hormones. However, despite their lipid structure, prostaglandins exert their effects on target cells via G-protein-coupled receptors on the cell surface.

Specific information on the prostaglandin $F_{2\alpha}$ and prostaglandin $E_2$ receptors can be found in Table 6.3. By way of overview:

FIGURE 6.8  **Balanced control of myometrial contractions**

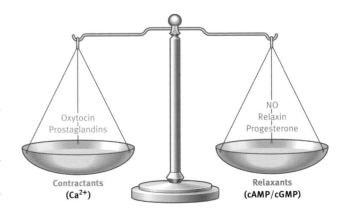

cAMP = cyclic adenosine monophosphate  |  cGMP = cyclic guanosine monophosphate  |  NO = nitric oxide

73

- Prostaglandin $F_{2\alpha}$ generally acts via the F-prostanoid receptor to exert its cellular effects via the phospholipase C–inositol trisphosphate–$Ca^{2+}$ signalling pathway.
- Prostaglandin $E_2$ can activate a series of four distinct E-prostanoid receptors, which generally transduce their signals via changes in the intracellular concentration of cyclic adenosine monophosphate (cAMP) and the activity of the cAMP-dependent protein kinase.

The ability of prostaglandin $F_{2\alpha}$ and prostaglandin $E_2$ to activate different signal transduction pathways probably accounts for the fact that their cellular actions are generally opposite and antagonistic. Through activation of protein kinases via second-messenger molecules/ions, prostaglandins are able to alter the function of pre-existing proteins and elicit cellular responses within seconds or minutes (rather than hours or days).

FIGURE 6.9 **Uterine oxytocin–prostaglandin $F_{2\alpha}$ spiral**

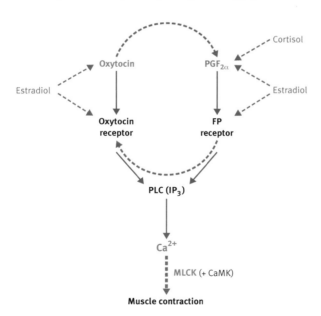

cAMK = $Ca^{2+}$/calmodulin-dependent kinase ∣ IP$_3$ = inositol trisphosphate ∣ MLCK = myosin light chain kinase ∣ PGF$_{2\alpha}$ = prostaglandin $F_{2\alpha}$ ∣ PLC = phospholipase C

## Regulation of myometrial contractility

The regulation of myometrial contractions involves a yin–yang balance between contractant molecules, which serve to increase myometrial contractions, and relaxant molecules, which antagonise the contractants so as to decrease the frequency and/or force of myometrial contractions (Figure 6.8). The contractant molecules include:

- oxytocin, a peptide molecule that originates from the uterus, rather than the posterior lobe of the pituitary gland
- prostaglandins, specifically prostaglandin $F_{2\alpha}$.

Both of these hormones activate phospholipase C (via the oxytocin receptor and F-prostanoid receptor, respectively), leading to an increase in the intracellular $Ca^{2+}$ concentration and activation of both myosin light chain kinase and $Ca^{2+}$/calmodulin-dependent protein kinase to increase the force of myometrial muscle contractions (Figure 6.9). The stimulation of myometrial contractions is augmented by the fact that oxytocin can stimulate uterine prostaglandin synthesis, while prostaglandin $F_{2\alpha}$ can, in turn, upregulate the expression of oxytocin receptors, culminating in a positive feedback loop that drives myometrial contractions (Figure 6.9). In addition, this loop is subject to modulation by steroid hormones, specifically by estradiol and cortisol. These steroids increase the expression of the genes that encode oxytocin, the oxytocin and F-prostanoid receptors and the enzymes required to synthesise prostaglandins.

The relaxant molecules act in opposition to oxytocin and prostaglandins and are therefore often referred to as anticontractant hormones. The relaxant/anticontractant pathways operate primarily via the cyclic-nucleotide second messengers cAMP and cyclic guanosine monophosphate (cGMP), which activate the cAMP-dependent and cGMP-dependent protein kinases to dephosphorylate the myosin light chain and limit the force of contractions.

The major myometrial relaxant is progesterone, which impairs the synthesis and action of both oxytocin and prostaglandin $F_{2\alpha}$ via a combination of classic genomic and nonclassic (hence rapid) nongenomic pathways. In addition, progesterone increases the intracellular cAMP concentration and decreases the operation of gap junctions (impairing the ability of the myometrial myocytes to act as a functional syncytium).[4] The actions of progesterone are supplemented by the relaxant actions of:

- nitric oxide, which seems to relax the myometrium independently of its ability to stimulate soluble guanylyl cyclase and elevate cGMP levels
- relaxin, which increases cAMP levels
- prostacyclin, which also increases cAMP levels.

At term, the decline in placental output of progesterone, and hence in the ratio of progesterone to estradiol, causes a switch in the steroidal control of the myometrium from predominantly relaxant actions to the contractant actions that are required for the onset of labour.

## Summary and revision

In conclusion, although steroids and prostaglandins are related in being classes of lipid hormone, they differ fundamentally in several respects. These include the precise nature of the molecular substrates, the enzymes required for hormone biosynthesis, the cellular receptors through which steroids and prostaglandins act, their mechanisms and speed of action and, most importantly, the physiological responses that steroid hormones and prostaglandins elicit.

### REFERENCES

1. MILLER W L. Molecular biology of steroid hormone synthesis. *Endocr Rev* 1988;9:295–318.

2. CARSON-JURICA M A, SCHRADER W T, O'MALLEY B W. Steroid receptor family: structure and functions. *Endocr Rev* 1990;11:201–20.

3. SMITH W L. Prostanoid biosynthesis and mechanisms of action. *Am J Physiol* 1992;263:F181–91.

4. MESIANO S. Myometrial progesterone responsiveness. *Semin Reprod Med* 2007;25:5–13.

# Fluid and acid–base balance

*Mark Heining*

## Fluid and electrolyte balance in pregnancy

During the course of a normal pregnancy, extracellular fluid accumulates:

- plasma volume rises typically from 3 to 4.5 litres
- interstitial-fluid volume rises typically from 11 to 15 litres.

The intracellular fluid volume also rises minimally.

These changes account for about 6–8 kg of the weight gain experienced during pregnancy. There is an accompanying accumulation of $Na^+$ and $K^+$, so that there is no overall significant change in the concentrations of these ions.

Because of the accumulation of $H_2O$ in the plasma compartment during a normal pregnancy, there is a fall in the concentration of plasma albumin and therefore a fall in the colloid osmotic pressure of plasma. This results in an imbalance in the so-called Starling forces, which control the movement of fluid across the capillary membrane:

- intravascular pressure pushes fluid out of the vessel
- colloid osmotic pressure tends to keep it in.

As a result of the drop in colloid osmotic pressure during pregnancy, accumulation of interstitial fluid and development of oedema become more likely, especially during the third trimester when arterial pressure rises.

It should be noted that in certain disease states, most importantly pre-eclampsia, there may be a fall in plasma volume.

## Acid–base balance

### SOME DEFINITIONS

Understanding of the acid–base balance is helped greatly by a clear understanding of the relevant terminology.

### Acids and bases

An acid is a proton donor, meaning that it tends to give up $H^+$ ions. A base is a proton acceptor, meaning that it tends to take up $H^+$ ions. It follows that acids and bases may be anions, cations or electrically neutral.

For example, ammonium ($NH_4^+$) is an anionic acid in equilibrium with ammonia ($NH_3$):

$$NH_4^+ \rightleftarrows NH_3 + H^+$$

Dihydrogen phosphate ($H_2PO_4^-$) is a cationic acid in equilibrium with hydrogen phosphate ($HPO_4^{2-}$):

$$H_2PO_4^- \rightleftarrows HPO_4^{2-} + H^+$$

Hydrochloric acid (HCl) is a neutral acid in equilibrium with $H^+$ and $Cl^-$:

$$HCl \rightleftarrows H^+ + Cl^-$$

These are all acids because they tend to give up $H^+$ ions.

### pH value

The pH value of a solution is the negative logarithm to the base 10 of the $H^+$ concentration and is a dimensionless quantity (it has no units). This means that the higher the $H^+$ concentration (the more acidic the solution), the lower the pH value.

### Acidaemia and acidosis

These terms are often used interchangeably in everyday clinical practice and this can be a source of confusion. Strictly speaking, acidaemia means that the blood is more acidic than normal, while acidosis refers to the underlying process (for example ketoacidosis, lactic acidosis) that may cause acidaemia. Alkalaemia and alkalosis have comparable meanings.

### ACID LOAD

The normal pH value of the blood and extracellular fluid is about 7.4, with a range of about 7.35–7.45. Because of the logarithmic derivation of the pH value, this represents an $H^+$ concentration in the order of nmol/l. Table 7.1 shows how physiological pH values in the normal range correspond to the concentration of $H^+$.

Clearly, the pH value is normally controlled within a narrow range. The importance of this must be appreciated in the context of the amount of $H^+$ production that takes place in the body:

- 15 000 mmol/day from $CO_2$ production
- 50–150 mmol/day from the production of phosphoric acid and sulphuric acid
- 1000 mmol/day from lactic acid production.

The impact of this on the overall pH value of the extracellular fluid is minimised by three mechanisms:

TABLE 7.1 **Physiological pH values and corresponding concentrations of hydrogen ions**

| pH | $H^+$ concentration (nmol/l) |
| --- | --- |
| 7.0 | 100 |
| 7.2 | 63 |
| 7.4 | 40 |
| 7.6 | 25 |
| 7.8 | 16 |

- very quick response (within seconds) – buffer systems in the blood, proceeding with the speed of a chemical reaction
- quick response (within minutes) – changes in ventilation
- slow response (within days) – renal mechanisms for the adjustment of $H^+$ excretion.

### BUFFERS

A buffer system is a system that tends to minimise changes in the pH value of a solution. It normally consists of a weak acid with its conjugate base (this is what remains when $H^+$ has left the acid molecule). An example would be:

$$R\text{–}COOH \rightleftarrows R\text{–}COO^- + H^+$$
$$\text{(acid)} \qquad \text{(conjugate base)}$$

Addition of further $H^+$ ions will cause the reaction to shift towards the left, resulting in the formation of more undissociated acid because the conjugate base tends to combine with the extra $H^+$ ions, while the reverse happens if $H^+$ ions are removed from the system. The buffering power of a system is greatest when half the buffering groups are undissociated and half are dissociated; that is, when $[R\text{–}COOH]$ equals $[R\text{–}COO^-]$. The pH value at this point equals the pK value of the system, with the pK value being the negative logarithm to the base 10 of the dissociation constant, K.

The most important buffers in extracellular fluid are the bicarbonate ($HCO_3^-$) system and haemoglobin. Other proteins also contribute some buffering power.

### Bicarbonate as a buffer

Carbonic acid ($H_2CO_3$) is a relatively strong acid, so the $HCO_3^-$ system is a relatively weak buffer. Its importance lies in the link between $H_2CO_3$, $HCO_3^-$ and dissolved $CO_2$:

$$CO_2 + H_2O \rightleftarrows H_2CO_3 \rightleftarrows H^+ + HCO_3^-$$

Hence the contribution of ventilation and $CO_2$ excretion to the acid–base balance.

The relationship between the components of the $HCO_3^-$ buffer system can be described by the following equation, where K is the dissociation constant of $H_2CO_3$, $\alpha$ is the solubility coefficient for $CO_2$ in plasma and $PCO_2$ is the partial pressure of $CO_2$:

$$[H^+] = K \times \alpha PCO_2 / [HCO_3^-]$$

Taking negative logarithms yields the following equation:

$$pH = pK + \log [HCO_3^-]/\alpha PCO_2$$

This is the Henderson–Hasselbach equation, sometimes more familiar in the following form:

$$pH = pK + \log [base]/[acid]$$

It follows that by knowing any two of the three variables $[H^+]$, $[HCO_3^-]$ and $PCO_2$, the third may be calculated. This is important when interpreting results given by bench blood gas machines, as some machines calculate $HCO_3^-$ concentration while others measure it.

### Haemoglobin as a buffer

The importance of the haemoglobin buffer system lies in the fact that haemoglobin is present in high concentration and has multiple acidic and basic groups such as carboxyl (–COOH) and amino (–NH$_2$) groups, respectively. The former will release $H^+$ ions if the solution becomes more basic, while the latter will take up $H^+$ ions (forming –NH$_3^+$) if the solution becomes more acidic.

Reduced haemoglobin is a weaker acid than oxygenated haemoglobin and hence it is a more effective buffer. Therefore, as haemoglobin releases $O_2$ in the tissues, more $H^+$ ions are buffered. As more $H^+$ ions are buffered, more $CO_2$ will dissolve in the plasma to maintain $H_2CO_3$ concentration. This aids $CO_2$ transport and is known as the Haldane effect.

### CARBON DIOXIDE CARRIAGE

$CO_2$ is carried in blood in three ways.

A small amount is carried in simple solution, with the dissolved $CO_2$ being in equilibrium with $H_2CO_3$ and hence with $HCO_3^-$:

$$CO_2 + H_2O \rightleftarrows H_2CO_3 \rightleftarrows H^+ + HCO_3^-$$

A slightly larger amount forms carbamino compounds with plasma proteins:

$$R\text{-}NH_2 + CO_2 \rightleftarrows R\text{-}NHCOO^- + H^+$$

The $H^+$ ion may in turn be buffered.

Finally, the majority enters red blood cells, where three things happen:

- $CO_2$ stays in simple solution, as in plasma
- $CO_2$ forms carbaminohaemoglobin, facilitated by the reduction in haemoglobin, the Haldane effect and the extra buffering of $H^+$ ions by the high concentration of haemoglobin
- significant amounts of $H_2CO_3$ are formed in a reaction catalysed by the enzyme carbonic anhydrase (present in large amounts in red blood cells); $H_2CO_3$ in turn splits into $H^+$ and $HCO_3^-$; the $H^+$ ions are buffered by haemoglobin and the $HCO_3^-$ ions diffuse out of the red blood cell into the plasma, in exchange for $Cl^-$ ions.

Note that, just as the reduction of haemoglobin aids $CO_2$ carriage in the Haldane effect, an increase in the $CO_2$ content of the red blood cell aids $O_2$ release from haemoglobin in the Bohr effect. In the case of $O_2$ transfer in the placenta, there is a 'double Bohr effect' because $CO_2$ leaves the fetal side of the membrane and accumulates on the maternal side; maternal haemoglobin is more likely to release $O_2$, fetal haemoglobin more likely to bind $O_2$.

### CLINICAL STATES OF ACID–BASE DISTURBANCE

Clinical states of acid–base disturbance are important since many physiological processes (such as enzyme activity and membrane stability) may be affected by changes in the pH value. In the following discussion, the suffixes -aemia and -osis will be used in their correct meanings as outlined at the beginning of this chapter.

Acidaemia and alkalaemia may both be caused by primarily respiratory or primarily metabolic processes, although the term metabolic needs to be interpreted flexibly. There are therefore four situations to describe:

- **Acidaemia arising from respiratory acidosis.** This is caused by underventilation with consequent build-up of $CO_2$.
- **Alkalaemia arising from respiratory alkalosis.** This is caused by overventilation with a consequent fall in $CO_2$ concentration. Such a situation may occur by voluntary hyperventilation or by overvigorous artificial ventilation during anaesthesia or intensive care.

- **Acidaemia arising from metabolic acidosis.** The term metabolic refers to more than just metabolic processes (such as lactic acidosis or diabetic ketoacidosis) that cause increased production of acid. It may also refer to increased ingestion of acid (as in salicylate overdose) or failure to excrete acid (as in renal failure).
- **Alkalaemia arising from metabolic alkalosis.** 'Metabolic' is an even less appropriate term here because no metabolic process leads to a build-up of alkali. Metabolic alkalosis therefore refers to loss of acid (as in severe vomiting) or injudicious intake of alkali (as in overuse of alkali in the symptomatic management of peptic ulcers or overzealous use of intravenous $HCO_3^-$ in the management of metabolic acidosis).

Clearly, the management of these situations depends on an understanding of the underlying processes and this in turn depends on accurate understanding of the information given by commercial blood gas machines.

### INTERPRETATION OF BLOOD GASES

Normal ranges of blood gas values vary slightly from one machine to another and from one population to another. Approximate values are provided in Table 7.2.

In all the acid–base disturbances described earlier, physiological processes will tend to compensate for the acid–base imbalance, so that the change in pH value will be smaller than predicted by the extent of the primary process. For example, a metabolic acidosis will normally be partially compensated by increased ventilation, which produces a respiratory alkalosis.

The success of treatment depends mainly on the correct identification of the primary disturbance (see also Box 7.1 and Table 7.3). An obvious starting point is to remember that compensation is rarely complete; the measured pH value will have changed in the direction of the primary disturbance. For example, a pH value that is

---

**BOX 7.1 Interpretation of blood gases**

**1. Remember this equation:**

$$\triangleright \quad CO_2 + H_2O \rightleftarrows H^+ + HCO_3^-$$

It satisfactorily explains acid–base disorders and their physiological compensation. If $H^+$ is generated, the reaction shifts to the left; if $CO_2$ is generated, the reaction shifts to the right.

**2. Remember normal blood gas values:**

- pH = 7.35–7.45
- $PCO_2$ = 4.5–5.8 kPa
- $[HCO_3^-]$ = 23–28 mmol/l

**3. Then follow this algorithm:**

- Start with the pH value: is it acidosis or alkalosis?
- Then $CO_2$: if the partial pressure is high, it is respiratory acidosis or at least has a respiratory component. If it is not high, then it is not respiratory acidosis.
- Lastly $HCO_3^-$: if the concentration is low, this confirms the presence of metabolic acidosis and vice versa.
- If $CO_2$ and $HCO_3^-$ values are going in opposite directions (that is, one is higher and the other is lower than normal), it is a mixed disorder.

---

TABLE 7.2 **Normal blood gas values**

| Parameter | Normal range |
|---|---|
| pH | 7.35–7.45 |
| $PO_2$ | 12.5–14.3 kPa |
| $PCO_2$ | 4.5–5.8 kPa |
| $[HCO_3^-]$ | 23–28 mmol/l |
| Standard $[HCO_3^-]$ | 24–30 mmol/l |

$[HCO_3^-]$ = bicarbonate concentration | $PO_2$ = partial pressure of $O_2$ | $PCO_2$ = partial pressure of $CO_2$ | standard $[HCO_3^-]$ = bicarbonate concentration under standard conditions ($PCO_2$ = 40 mmHg, 37 degrees C, saturated with $O_2$)

TABLE 7.3 **Interpretation of blood gases**

| Parameter measured | Acidosis | Alkalosis |
|---|---|---|
| pH | Low | High |
| $PCO_2$ (respiratory component) | High | Low |
| $[HCO_3^-]$ (metabolic component) | Low | High |

$[HCO_3^-]$ = bicarbonate concentration | $PCO_2$ = partial pressure of $CO_2$

more acidic than normal is usually caused by an acidosis as the primary event, whereas a pH value that is more alkaline than normal is usually caused by an alkalosis as the primary event.

Next, the $PCO_2$ should be inspected. If low, this indicates a respiratory alkalosis; if high, there is a respiratory acidosis. Either may be the primary event or a compensatory response.

The presence of a metabolic disturbance may be indicated by a change in the $HCO_3^-$ concentration: it falls in metabolic acidosis and rises in metabolic alkalosis. Again, either may be a primary or compensatory event.

When looking at the clinical context, it is worth remembering that respiratory compensation (for a primary metabolic event) occurs within a few seconds or minutes, whereas metabolic compensation depends on changes in the excretion of renal $HCO_3^-$ and therefore takes hours to days.

However, over-reliance on the $HCO_3^-$ concentration as an indicator of metabolic disturbance can be misleading, particularly if there is a mixed respiratory and metabolic acidosis or if a quantitative measurement of metabolic disturbance is required. Hence, over the years, a variety of other measurements has been introduced, including standard $HCO_3^-$, anion gap, buffer base and base excess.

Nowadays, base excess is regarded as the most useful quantitative index of metabolic acid–base derangement. The normal range is from –2 (slightly acidic) to +2 (slightly alkaline); there are no units. Severe metabolic acidosis is considered to be present when the base excess is more negative than –10. A negative base excess is sometimes called a base deficit.

## CLINICAL CORRECTION OF AN ACID–BASE DISTURBANCE

Changes in the pH value affect many physiological processes, mainly enzyme activity and stability of excitable membranes (including those of nerves, striated muscle and cardiac muscle). Management of any acid–base disturbance therefore depends on the clinical context and the severity of the resulting physiological abnormality.

Respiratory acidosis, as already mentioned, is caused by hypoventilation. If treatment is clinically indicated, this is by taking over ventilation (by positive-pressure or negative-pressure ventilation) or by treatment of the cause (for example, the use of naloxone hydrochloride in an overdose of opioid).

Metabolic acidosis is treated by treatment of the underlying cause. For example, there is the standard management of diabetic ketoacidosis (involving rehydration and administration of insulin), or restoration of cardiac output in lactic acidosis arising from shock. If very severe and there are convincing clinical indications, treatment with intravenous sodium bicarbonate ($NaHCO_3$) may be needed. Great care is necessary with dose as it is easy to give too much and there is always a risk of causing intracellular alkalosis.

Both metabolic alkalosis and respiratory alkalosis are rare and difficult to treat.

## ACID–BASE BALANCE IN PREGNANCY

Pregnancy is associated with a slight respiratory alkalosis. A compensatory fall in $HCO_3^-$ concentration occurs, which reduces the change in pH value, but the low $PCO_2$ is necessary to maintain a diffusion gradient for $CO_2$ across the placenta.

During labour, maternal hyperventilation and respiratory alkalosis become more extreme. Because of the relatively short timescale, compensation by renal mechanisms does not occur and so the consequences of alkalosis are more marked.

Alkalosis causes a leftward shift of the oxyhaemoglobin dissociation curve and therefore an increased affinity of maternal haemoglobin for $O_2$. This may lead to a fall in the partial pressure of $O_2$ in the umbilical vein and even metabolic acidosis (owing to anaerobic metabolism) in the fetus. Additionally, the increased proportion of deoxygenated haemoglobin in the fetus allows more $CO_2$ to remain in solution and thus contributes to respiratory acidosis. Extreme maternal hyperventilation during labour may therefore contribute to both metabolic acidosis and respiratory acidosis in the fetus.

### Fetal acid–base abnormalities

As suggested, acidaemia in the fetus is nearly always a mixed respiratory and metabolic disturbance, with blood gas measurements showing a low pH value, a raised $PCO_2$, a low $HCO_3^-$ concentration and a raised base deficit (negative base excess). Treatment consists of correction of any underlying cause or aggravating factor, such as maternal shock.

### Maternal acid–base abnormalities

Pregnant women do not only have a 'physiological' alkalosis but they may also be subject to the usual abnormalities that occur in nonpregnant individuals. If acidaemia is present, the cause may be (among other things) diabetic ketoacidosis, dehydration or shock. Again, the management is correction of the cause by administration of fluids, administration of insulin if indicated or arrest of haemorrhage.

Treatment with $NaHCO_3$ is rarely necessary, especially since the associated hazards are well documented and the affected women are mostly fit and able to correct acidosis once organ perfusion is restored.

CHAPTER 8

# Calcium homeostasis and bone

*Rosemary Bland*

## Calcium homeostasis

$Ca^{2+}$ is essential for a number of physiological mechanisms such as muscle contraction, intra- and extracellular signalling (as a second messenger; see chapter 5), activation of enzymes (as a co-factor), stabilisation of membrane potentials and nerve excitability and, of course, normal bone and tooth formation (Table 8.1). Consequently, circulating levels of $Ca^{2+}$ are tightly regulated.

The adult body contains around 1.2 kg of $Ca^{2+}$. Approximately 99% of this is stored in the skeleton as hydroxyapatite, the mineral component of bone. About 1% is present intracellularly, although it is important to remember that $Ca^{2+}$ does not occur free in the cytoplasm but is sequestered in intracellular organelles such as the endoplasmic reticulum, mitochondria and, in skeletal muscle, the sarcoplasmic reticulum and is available for rapid release if required.

The intracellular $Ca^{2+}$ concentration is approximately 100 nmol/l. The concentration gradient across the cells is maintained by the plasma membrane $Ca^{2+}$-ATPase (PMCA) and, in some cells, the $Na^+,Ca^{2+}$-exchanger (also known as NCX). Extracellular $Ca^{2+}$ accounts for only 0.1% of total body $Ca^{2+}$. This equates to a normal serum concentration of approximately 2.5 mmol/l (normal range 2.2–2.6 mmol/l).

TABLE 8.1 **Physiological functions of calcium**

| Function | Notes |
|---|---|
| Bone mineralisation | $Ca^{2+}$ is a component of hydroxyapatite, the mineral component of bones |
| Tooth formation | $Ca^{2+}$ is a constituent of the mineral component of teeth |
| Muscle contraction | Binding of $Ca^{2+}$ to troponin allows myosin to bind actin |
| Enzyme co-factor | $Ca^{2+}$ is required by blood clotting enzymes[a] |
| First extracellular messenger | $Ca^{2+}$ binds to a membrane-bound receptor |
| Second intracellular messenger | $Ca^{2+}$ regulates a number of intracellular signalling proteins |
| Secretion and exocytosis | $Ca^{2+}$ is used for neurotransmitter release from synapses and is required for exocytosis |
| Stabilisation of membrane potentials | $Ca^{2+}$ is essential for the maintenance of membrane potentials and for depolarisation |
| Regulation of cellular division, proliferation and apoptosis | $Ca^{2+}$ modifies many intracellular signalling pathways |

[a] For example, the chelating agent EDTA is added to blood collection tubes to bind to $Ca^{2+}$ and thereby inhibit these enzymes, so as to stop the blood clotting

BOX 8.1 **Quick guide to the control of calcium homeostasis**

The concentration of serum $Ca^{2+}$ is detected by the $Ca^{2+}$-sensing receptor on the parathyroid glands. In response to low serum $Ca^{2+}$ concentrations, parathyroid hormone (PTH) is released. It acts on the bone to stimulate bone resorption. In the kidney, PTH promotes resorption of $Ca^{2+}$ and excretion of phosphate ($PO_4^{3-}$). It also increases the activity of the enzyme 25-hydroxyvitamin $D_3$ 1α-hydroxylase, which catalyses the conversion of calcidiol to its active metabolite calcitriol.

Calcitriol increases bone turnover, increases absorption of $Ca^{2+}$ from the intestine and enhances $Ca^{2+}$ and $PO_4^{3-}$ reabsorption in the kidney, resulting in an increase in serum $Ca^{2+}$ concentration. $Ca^{2+}$ and calcitriol provide negative feedback to the parathyroid gland to inhibit further secretion of PTH.

Calcitonin, produced in the thyroid gland, acts to decrease the serum $Ca^{2+}$ concentration and is secreted in response to hypercalcaemia. It inhibits renal $Ca^{2+}$ and $PO_4^{3-}$ reabsorption and osteoclastic bone resorption.

Fibroblast growth factor 23, a phosphaturic hormone, is released from bone cells (mostly osteocytes) in response to stimulation by calcitriol and seeks to limit calcitriol-induced increases in serum $PO_4^{3-}$ concentration.

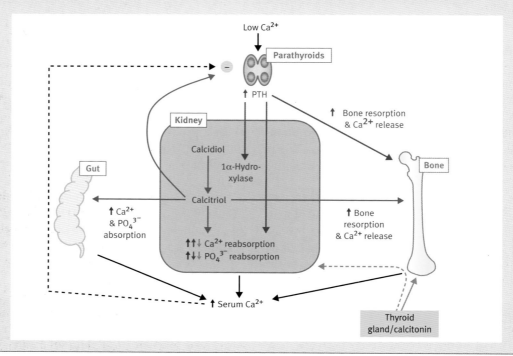

Approximately 45% of serum $Ca^{2+}$ circulates in the free ionised form, which is biologically active. The remaining 55% circulates in a bound form, with about 10% bound to anions, including lactate, phosphate ($PO_4^{3-}$) and bicarbonate, and about 45% bound to plasma proteins (mainly albumin). Consequently, a change in albumin levels will alter the ratio of free to bound $Ca^{2+}$. Values are therefore quoted as 'total adjusted' $Ca^{2+}$ (the value for total $Ca^{2+}$ has been corrected for albumin levels).

**IMPORTANT POINT**

**$Ca^{2+}$**

Clinicians usually order a total $Ca^{2+}$ value to evaluate $Ca^{2+}$ status but it is the free, ionised $Ca^{2+}$ that is biologically active. Conditions that alter the balance between free and bound $Ca^{2+}$ will not alter the total $Ca^{2+}$ concentration but will change the physiological responses. For example, in acidosis the $H^+$ ions compete with the $Ca^{2+}$ ions for the binding of plasma protein, so acidosis increases the concentration of free serum $Ca^{2+}$ without altering the levels of total $Ca^{2+}$. The biochemistry of people with acidosis therefore seems to be normal even though they are hypercalcaemic.

TABLE 8.2  **Current UK Reference Nutrient Intake for calcium**

| Age | Reference Nutrient Intake (mg/day) |
| --- | --- |
| Infant | 525 |
| 1–3 years | 350 |
| 4–6 years | 450 |
| 7–10 years | 550 |
| 11–18 years | 800 (women), 1000 (men) |
| Adults | 700 |
| Lactating women | 1250 |

TABLE 8.3  **Organs that regulate calcium homeostasis**

| Organ | Function |
| --- | --- |
| Kidney | Response to $Ca^{2+}$, PTH, vitamin D and calcitonin |
| | Activation of vitamin D |
| | Regulation of $Ca^{2+}$ and $PO_4^{3-}$ reabsorption and excretion |
| Bone[a] | Storage (buffer) of $Ca^{2+}$, $PO_4^{3-}$ and $Mg^{2+}$ |
| Parathyroid glands | Response to changes in serum $Ca^{2+}$ (express the CaSR) |
| | Synthesis and secretion of PTH |
| Gastrointestinal tract | Absorption of $Ca^{2+}$ and $PO_4^{3-}$ |
| Thyroid glands | Response to changes in serum $Ca^{2+}$ (express the CaSR) |
| | Synthesis and secretion of calcitonin |

[a] Bone remodelling is regulated by PTH, calcitonin and vitamin D |
CaSR = $Ca^{2+}$-sensing receptor | PTH = parathyroid hormone | $PO_4^{3-}$ = phosphate

$Ca^{2+}$ is obtained from the diet. Ideally, adults should have an intake of approximately 1000 mg/day, although the current UK Reference Nutrient Intake for adults (detailed in Table 8.2) is set slightly lower at 700 mg/day. This figure should be higher in adolescents and in pregnant and lactating women because of the increased requirements for $Ca^{2+}$ for bone growth and milk formation.

Absorption of $Ca^{2+}$ from the diet is relatively inefficient, with only 20–30% of dietary intake being taken up by the body. Absorption varies with age (increased in children and decreased with advanced age), intestine function, diet (lactose increases absorption, oxalates and phytates decrease absorption by binding to the ingested $Ca^{2+}$) and vitamin D availability. $Ca^{2+}$ absorption can occur throughout the gastrointestinal tract but the majority (60–70%) of all ingested $Ca^{2+}$ is absorbed in the small intestine.

The control of $Ca^{2+}$ homeostasis (Box 8.1) and the maintenance of serum $Ca^{2+}$ levels require a complex interaction between $Ca^{2+}$, hormones (vitamin D, parathyroid hormone and calcitonin) and four main organs (the intestine, parathyroid glands, the kidneys and bone; see Table 8.3). This is described in more detail in the following sections.

## MECHANISM OF CALCIUM ABSORPTION AND EXCRETION

$Ca^{2+}$ is absorbed from the intestine via transcellular or paracellular routes (Figure 8.1). Transcellular absorption involves entry of $Ca^{2+}$ into the cell via the epithelial $Ca^{2+}$ channel 2 (TRPV6) in the microvilli of the brush border.

Bound to $Ca^{2+}$-binding proteins (calmodulin and calbindin), $Ca^{2+}$ then moves through the cell to the basolateral membrane. Export into the extracellular fluid of the lamina propria occurs by exocytosis or by the PMCA. Paracellular transport also requires the presence of $Ca^{2+}$-binding proteins.

All of the free (ionised) $Ca^{2+}$ and the $Ca^{2+}$ bound to anions is filtered by the glomerulus and most (99%) of the filtered $Ca^{2+}$ is reabsorbed (Figure 8.2). $Ca^{2+}$ is reabsorbed by passive paracellular (80%) and active transcellular (20%) processes. Transcellular transport requires the presence of epithelial $Ca^{2+}$ channel 1 (TRPV6) in the apical membrane.

## CALCIUM BALANCE

The $Ca^{2+}$ balance depends on the amount of $Ca^{2+}$ absorbed minus the amount of $Ca^{2+}$ excreted, as well as the balance between the amount buffered in the bone and the concentration in the extracellular fluid. Generally, children have a positive $Ca^{2+}$ balance, in adults the balance should be neutral (input equals output) and postmenopausal women and the elderly usually have a negative $Ca^{2+}$ balance.

FIGURE 8.1 **Calcium absorption from the intestine**

CaBP = Ca²⁺-binding protein | PMCA = plasma membrane Ca²⁺-ATPase | TRPV6 = epithelial Ca²⁺ channel

Adapted with permission from Nussey S, Whitehead SA. *Endocrinology: An Integrated Approach.* Oxford: BIOS Scientific Publishers; 2001.

A disruption in $Ca^{2+}$ homeostasis can result in hypocalcaemia or hypercalcaemia and it is important to remember that changes in $Ca^{2+}$ homeostasis will usually alter $PO_4^{3-}$ status.

## Hormones that regulate serum $Ca^{2+}$ levels

The three main hormones that regulate serum $Ca^{2+}$ levels are parathyroid hormone (PTH) and vitamin D, which increase serum $Ca^{2+}$ concentrations, and calcitonin, which reduces serum $Ca^{2+}$ concentrations. Table 8.4 contains a summary of the characteristics and functions of these hormones.

### PARATHYROID HORMONE

PTH is a peptide hormone that is synthesised in the parathyroid glands. These glands (normally four) are located on the posterior of the thyroid gland. They originate from the pharyngeal pouches, are small (3–8 mm long, 2–5 mm wide, 1.5 mm deep with a weight of less than 40 mg each) and are supplied by branches of the inferior thyroid arteries. The parathyroid glands contain two cell types: oxyphil cells, which have no known function, and chief cells, which synthesise and secrete PTH.

FIGURE 8.2 **Reabsorption of calcium along the nephron**

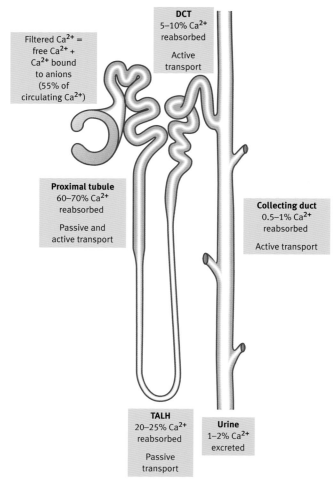

DCT = distal convoluted tubule | TALH = thick ascending loop of Henle

### *Synthesis and release of parathyroid hormone*

PTH is synthesised as a 115-amino-acid compound called prepro-PTH. Cleavage reactions produce PTH, an 84-amino-acid molecule that is stored in vesicles until required. The release of PTH is initiated by the $Ca^{2+}$-sensing receptor (CaSR) in response to hypocalcaemia. PTH secretion occurs within seconds and the parathyroids contain sufficient PTH to maintain secretion for approximately 60 minutes. If prolonged PTH secretion (secretion for hours to days) is required, PTH synthesis is increased.

TABLE 8.4 **Summary of the characteristics and physiological functions of the main hormones that regulate calcium homeostasis**

| Hormone | Hormone type | Receptor | Site of synthesis | Signal for synthesis and/or secretion | Physiological actions | Net effect on $Ca^{2+}$ homeostasis |
|---|---|---|---|---|---|---|
| PTH | Peptide | G-protein-coupled receptor (PTHR1) | Chief cells in the parathyroid glands | Low $Ca^{2+}$ | Bone: ↑ bone resorption<br><br>Kidney: ↑ $PO_4^{3-}$ excretion<br><br>Kidney: ↓ $Ca^{2+}$ excretion<br><br>Kidney: ↑ vitamin D activation | ↑ Serum $Ca^{2+}$<br><br>↓ Serum $PO_4^{3-}$ |
| Vitamin D (calcitriol) | Secosteroid | Nuclear receptor (VDR)<br><br>A member of the steroid/thyroid receptor superfamily | Hydroxylated (activated) in the proximal convoluted tubules of the kidney<br><br>Extra-renal activation of vitamin D can also occur | Low $Ca^{2+}$<br><br>Low $PO_4^{3-}$<br><br>PTH | Bone: ↑ bone formation and mineralisation<br><br>Bone: ↑ bone remodelling<br><br>GI tract: ↑ $Ca^{2+}$ absorption<br><br>Kidney: ↑ $Ca^{2+}$ and $PO_4^{3-}$ reabsorption | ↑ Serum $Ca^{2+}$<br><br>↑ Serum $PO_4^{3-}$ |
| Calcitonin | Peptide | G-protein-coupled receptor | C cells in the parathyroid glands | High $Ca^{2+}$ | Kidney: ↑ $PO_4^{3-}$ excretion<br><br>Kidney: ↓ $Ca^{2+}$ reabsorption<br><br>Bone: inhibits osteoclast function | ↓ Serum $Ca^{2+}$ |

↑ = increase  |  ↓ = decrease  |  GI = gastrointestinal  |  $PO_4^{3-}$ = phosphate  |  PTH = parathyroid hormone  |  PTHR1 = PTH receptor type 1  |  VDR = vitamin D receptor

If the hypocalcaemia is not corrected and PTH secretion needs to be sustained for days or even months, proliferation of the parathyroid gland cells increases and this results in hyperplasia and unregulated synthesis and release of PTH (secondary hyperparathyroidism).

### Parathyroid-hormone receptors

PTH binds to the PTH receptor (PTHR), which is a G-protein-coupled receptor. Ligand binding activates cyclic adenosine monophosphate (cAMP) as a second messenger and results in the phosphorylation of intracellular proteins. There are at least two PTHR subtypes, PTHR1 and PTHR2. The first 34 amino acids of PTH bind to PTHR1 and it has classically been assumed that the biological activity of PTH is only attributable to these 34 amino acids. The function of other fragments of the PTH peptide is currently under investigation.

> **IMPORTANT POINT**
>
> **Parathyroid hormone receptors**
>
> If the receptor subtype is not specified, reference is probably made to PTHR1.

### Physiological actions of parathyroid hormone

PTH acts on the bone and kidney. In bone, it causes bone resorption and, thereby, $Ca^{2+}$ and $PO_4^{3-}$ release. PTH binds to PTHRs on the osteoblasts, resulting in osteoblast-mediated activation of osteoclast differentiation. *In vitro* studies have also shown inhibition of collagen synthesis by PTH-activated osteoblasts.

In the kidney, PTH has three main actions. In the distal convoluted tubule, it increases $Ca^{2+}$ reabsorption possibly by increasing the transport of $Ca^{2+}$ that is mediated by TRPV5. In the proximal and distal convoluted tubules, PTH inhibits the reabsorption of $PO_4^{3-}$ and so increases $PO_4^{3-}$ excretion. In the proximal tubule, it blocks $PO_4^{3-}$ resorption by reducing expression of the $Na^+$-dependent inorganic phosphate co-transporter type II (NPT2). PTH also increases the renal activation of vitamin D by increasing expression and activity of the enzyme 25-hydroxyvitamin $D_3$ 1α-hydroxylase (CYP27B1; 1α-hydroxylase).

### Hyperparathyroidism

Hyperparathyroidism results from excess synthesis and release of PTH and is associated with increased bone resorption. There are two main forms: primary and secondary hyperparathyroidism.

Primary hyperparathyroidism is caused by a defect of the parathyroid glands, normally a benign tumour. Malignant tumours are rare and may be associated with multiple endocrine neoplasia syndrome. Primary hyperparathyroidism is characterised by increased levels of PTH and calcitriol and decreased levels of $PO_4^{3-}$ and hypercalcaemia. The increase in calcitriol levels and the decrease in $PO_4^{3-}$ levels indicate that the kidneys are functioning. Individual cells respond normally to feedback signals but the increase in cell numbers means that, on balance, PTH is synthesised and released in excess.

Primary hyperparathyroidism is one of the most frequent causes of hypercalcaemia and is the third most common endocrine disorder after diabetes and hyperthyroidism (prevalence one in 500–1000).

Secondary hyperparathyroidism occurs as a result of defective feedback control. Most commonly, the primary defect is in the kidneys and the development of secondary hyperparathyroidism is usually associated with chronic kidney disease.

In renal disease, the kidney is unable to respond normally to PTH, so renal reabsorption of $Ca^{2+}$ is not stimulated and vitamin D activation is not promoted. As a result, $Ca^{2+}$ absorption from the intestine cannot be increased on demand. One consequence of this is that the bone is the only place where PTH can act to increase serum $Ca^{2+}$ levels. The resulting loss of $Ca^{2+}$ from the bone causes high bone turnover, bone demineralisation (osteomalacia) and renal osteodystrophy. As a consequence of the failure to increase serum $Ca^{2+}$ levels and the lack of vitamin D signalling, the normal negative feedback on the parathyroid glands is absent and they continue to produce and secrete PTH. This results in hyperplasia and eventually the parathyroid glands lose their sensitivity to $Ca^{2+}$ and vitamin D.

Ultimately, secondary hyperparathyroidism will progress to tertiary hyperparathyroidism, which is almost exclusively associated with end-stage renal disease and should be treated in the same way as primary hyperparathyroidism.

### Calcium-sensing receptor

The CaSR is a G-protein-coupled receptor that is sensitive to serum $Ca^{2+}$ concentrations in the physiological range. The receptor was originally cloned from bovine parathyroid glands but is known to be expressed in a number of tissues including the kidneys, the intestine, vascular smooth muscle cells and bone. Synthetic allosteric activators of the CaSR (calcimimetics) for the treatment of hyperparathyroidism and CaSR antagonists (calcilytics) for the potential treatment of osteoporosis have been developed.

Several disorders related to mutations in the CaSR exist. Familial hypocalciuric hypercalcaemia and neonatal severe hyperparathyroidism are associated with loss-of-function mutations and autosomal dominant hypoparathyroidism is associated with an activating mutation.

### Parathyroid-hormone-related peptide

PTH-related peptide (PTHrP, also known as PTH-like peptide) is able to bind to PTHR1 (the first 34 amino acids of PTHrP are similar to those of PTH and the first 13 amino acids of the two peptides are almost identical) and therefore mimics PTH actions. It is produced by many cells including cancer cells and is often responsible for hypercalcaemia associated with malignancy. Its physiological functions are not completely understood. It regulates chondrocyte development and therefore endochondral bone formation, placental $Ca^{2+}$ transport and fetal development.

## VITAMIN D

The classification of vitamin D as a vitamin is incorrect because we make most of the vitamin D that we require and vitamin D is a pleiotrophic secosteroid. Dietary intake of vitamin $D_2$ may account for 10–20% of our vitamin D levels but the majority (80–90%) is synthesised in the skin as vitamin $D_3$. The final activation step occurs predominantly in the proximal convoluted tubule of the kidney, although extrarenal synthesis can also occur.

Vitamin D is required for normal bone remodelling and it increases serum levels of $Ca^{2+}$ and $PO_4^{3-}$ mainly by increasing their intestinal absorption. A number of different vitamin D metabolites exist. The metabolite that is considered to be the biologically active molecule is $1\alpha,25$-dihydroxyvitamin $D_3$ (calcitriol). All vitamin D metabolites are transported in blood bound to vitamin-D-binding protein. The major circulating form of vitamin D is 25-hydroxyvitamin $D_3$ (calcidiol), which is considered to be a good surrogate marker of vitamin D status. It is the metabolite of vitamin D that is usually measured clinically. The average serum concentrations of vitamin D are 7.5–100 nmol/l for 25-hydroxyvitamin $D_3$ and 48–156 pmol/l for calcitriol.

**IMPORTANT POINT**

**Active vitamin D metabolites**

Although calcitriol is currently considered to be the only vitamin D metabolite with biological activity, there is increasing evidence that other metabolites may also have some biological activity.

### Vitamin D synthesis

The first step in vitamin D synthesis requires modification of 7-dehydrocholesterol in the keratinocytes to

FIGURE 8.3  **Synthesis of vitamin D**

Sunlight[a]

7-Dehydrocholesterol

Dietary vitamin $D_2$

Vitamin $D_3$

25-Hydroxylase

Calcidiol

$1\alpha$-Hydroxylase

Calcitriol

[a] Ultraviolet light (290–320 nm)

vitamin $D_3$ (cholecalciferol), a reaction that is mediated by ultraviolet light (sunlight). Vitamin D activation then occurs via a number of hydroxylation reactions. Vitamin $D_2$ (dietary vitamin D) and vitamin $D_3$ are hydroxylated in the liver by 25-hydroxylase into calcidiol, which is further hydroxylated into calcitriol in the proximal convoluted tubule of the kidney by the enzyme 1α-hydroxylase, a mitochondrial cytochrome P450 enzyme (Figure 8.3). In contrast to 25-hydroxylase activity, which depends on substrate availability, the activity of 1α-hydroxylase is very tightly regulated and is increased by PTH, low $Ca^{2+}$ levels, low $PO_4^{3-}$ levels and calcitonin and is inhibited by calcitriol. Calcitriol is further metabolised (and inactivated) by 24-hydroxylase, an enzyme that is present in all vitamin D target tissues and induced by calcitriol.

The ability to activate vitamin D varies with sunlight exposure, age, ethnic status and mineral status and requires a functional liver and kidneys. Vitamin D insufficiency (less than 50 nmol/l) and deficiency (less than 15–20 nmol/l) are common throughout the world. Populations living at northern and southern latitudes have lower levels of vitamin D than people living nearer the equator. Elderly people often have insufficient vitamin D as they have lower 1α-hydroxylase activity and reduced mobility may result in decreased exposure to sunlight. Asian and black populations are also vitamin-D-deficient. To some extent, this can be attributed to a combination of dietary factors, reduced sunlight exposure (among those living in regions of low ultraviolet radiation intensity and among those who are required to wear clothing covering most of their skin) and reduced 1α-hydroxylase activity.

Vitamin D can also be activated at a number of extrarenal sites. The role of extrarenal activation is not yet fully understood (it does not seem to contribute to circulating levels of calcitriol). Extrarenal activation is thought to participate in a number of nonclassic (unrelated to $Ca^{2+}$ homeostasis) actions of vitamin D and to act in a paracrine/autocrine fashion.

> **IMPORTANT POINT**
>
> **Vitamin D availability and storage**
>
> The inactive metabolites of vitamin D (vitamin $D_2$, vitamin $D_3$ and calcidiol) are stored in body fat and can be released when required. This allows for storage of excess vitamin D produced during the summer, when sunlight is available, for release and activation during winter months.

### Vitamin D receptor and vitamin D signalling

Vitamin D acts via a nuclear receptor. Vitamin D is lipophilic and it had been thought that vitamin D and other steroid hormones crossed cell membranes by diffusion. Although this may occur, it is now apparent that there are specific transport proteins in the cell membrane (Figure 8.4). Megalin, a large glycoprotein, has been identified as the membrane transporter for calcidiol and calcitriol. If required, calcidiol is hydroxylated to calcitriol in the mitochondria. Calcitriol translocates to the nucleus (bound to intracellular vitamin-D-binding proteins), where it binds to the vitamin D receptor (VDR). The ligand-bound VDR and its heterodimer partner, retinoid X receptor, bind to specific DNA sequences known as vitamin D response elements and, under the regulation of a number of accessory proteins, function as a transcription factor (Figure 8.4).

There is evidence that vitamin D is also able to act via a nongenomic pathway and a membrane receptor.

### Physiological actions of vitamin D

Vitamin D is classically known to mediate $Ca^{2+}$ homeostasis but a role has now also emerged as a potent regulator of a number of other cellular functions. Vitamin D regulates the development of cells within the immune system and plays a role in the modulation of inflammation. It has antiproliferative and prodifferentiation properties and has been shown to induce apoptosis and impair progression through the cell cycle in a number of cancer cell types.

Vitamin D affects $Ca^{2+}$ homeostasis by acting on the bone, the intestine and the kidney. In bone, calcitriol regulates osteoblast activity to increase bone mass and calcification. Vitamin D is also required for chondrocyte development. Consequently, vitamin D deficiency results

FIGURE 8.4 **Vitamin D signalling**

AP = accessory proteins  |  IDBP = intracellular vitamin-D-binding protein  |  mRNA = messenger RNA  |  mVDR = membrane-bound VDR  |  Pol II = polymerase II  |  RXR = retinoid X receptor  |  VDR = vitamin D receptor

in defective bone mineralisation and growth plate abnormalities (rickets in children and osteomalacia in adults). Vitamin D also promotes osteoclast differentiation and so promotes bone resorption. By increasing the development and function of both osteoblasts and osteoclasts, vitamin D increases the rate of bone remodelling.

$Ca^{2+}$ absorption in the intestine, as outlined in Figure 8.1, also requires adequate calcitriol levels. Vitamin D signalling increases the expression of TRPV6, calbindins, calmodulin and PMCA and can increase intestinal $Ca^{2+}$ absorption three-fold.

In the kidney, vitamin D has three main actions. It increases $Ca^{2+}$ reabsorption in the proximal and distal convoluted tubules. It increases $PO_4^{3-}$ reabsorption in the proximal convoluted tubule and inhibits activation of vitamin D by inhibition of 1α-hydroxylase. In chronic kidney disease, mineral homeostasis is disrupted. The reduced activity of renal 1α-hydroxylase leads to reduced levels of calcitriol and eventually triggers secondary hyperparathyroidism and renal bone disease (renal osteodystrophy). Vascular calcification (arteriosclerosis) is also common in people with chronic kidney disease and is responsible for increased morbidity and mortality.

## Vitamin D deficiency and rickets

Vitamin D deficiency can be of nutritional origin (poor diet or malabsorption), although this is rare, or caused by failure to synthesise vitamin D. Vitamin D activation may be limited in liver or kidney disease and insufficient vitamin D production is also associated with ultraviolet light deficiency (lack of sunlight).

Vitamin D deficiency causes rickets in children and osteomalacia in adults. These are conditions of decreased mineralisation of the bones, attributable to a lack of both $Ca^{2+}$ and vitamin D and sometimes $PO_4^{3-}$.

In rickets, there is a failure to mineralise endochondral bone in the growth plate, which results in elongation of the growth plate and delayed calcification. Weight bearing produces deformity of the limbs. Other likely bone defects include soft skull bones (craniotabes), delayed closure of the anterior fontanel, Harrison sulcus (indentation of the chest wall; pigeon chest) and thickening of the ankles, knees and wrists. Affected children also suffer from bone pain, increased fractures, defects in tooth formation and muscle weakness.

In osteomalacia, there is a failure to mineralise newly formed osteoid. This leads to increased osteoid width and decreased bone mineralisation. Bones appear thin on X-ray and the most common feature is osteopenia/osteoporosis. Occasionally, Looser zones may be apparent, which suggests osteomalacia. A bone biopsy may be needed to confirm the diagnosis.

Vitamin D resistance also presents as vitamin D deficiency. Two rare genetic conditions exist: vitamin D resistance type 1 or pseudovitamin D resistance, which is caused by a defect in the 1α-hydroxylase gene, and vitamin D resistance type 2 or hereditary vitamin-D-resistant rickets, where there is a defect in the gene encoding VDR.

### CALCITONIN

Calcitonin is a peptide hormone that is produced by the C cells (parafollicular cells) in the thyroid gland in response to increased circulating $Ca^{2+}$ levels. Calcitonin acts on the kidneys and bone but, in contrast to PTH and vitamin D, it decreases serum $Ca^{2+}$ levels.

### Calcitonin synthesis, receptors and release

Post-transcriptional processing of the calcitonin gene leads to the production of calcitonin and calcitonin-gene-related peptide. However, the physiological actions of calcitonin and calcitonin-gene-related peptide are distinct. This contrasts with the situation regarding PTH and PTHrP, which are the products of different genes but have some similar actions.

Calcitonin-gene-related peptide is a potent vasodilator but it also functions as a neurotransmitter. By contrast, calcitonin is released in response to hypercalcaemia, binds to a G-protein-coupled receptor and activates cAMP signalling.

### Physiological actions of calcitonin

Calcitonin acts on the bone and kidney. In the kidney, calcitonin inhibits reabsorption of $PO_4^{3-}$ and $Ca^{2+}$ in the proximal tubule, promoting their excretion. In bone, it acts on the osteoclasts, causing them to shrink and reduce bone resorption and so preventing the release of $Ca^{2+}$ and $PO_4^{3-}$. Interestingly, calcitonin seems to have a relatively minor role in $Ca^{2+}$ homeostasis in humans.

---

**IMPORTANT POINT**

**Hormone action**

For each hormone you should know:

- the type of receptor through which it works
- where and how it is synthesised
- the signal for synthesis/release
- the target organ
- the biological action and physiological consequence.

---

## Phosphate

As we have already seen, $Ca^{2+}$ homeostasis is closely related to that of $PO_4^{3-}$ but this chapter is not going to discuss the regulation of $PO_4^{3-}$ homeostasis in detail. $PO_4^{3-}$ ions are stored in bone and bone reabsorption and remodelling release $PO_4^{3-}$ in addition to $Ca^{2+}$. Likewise, $Ca^{2+}$-containing foods generally also contain $PO_4^{3-}$, so an increase of dietary $Ca^{2+}$ will often increase dietary $PO_4^{3-}$. Absorption of $PO_4^{3-}$ from the diet is efficient, with about 80% of ingested $PO_4^{3-}$ being absorbed.

$PO_4^{3-}$ is required for the formation of high-energy compounds (for example ATP and creatinine phosphate) and second messengers (for example cAMP, inositol phosphates) and for the phosphorylation of enzymes. It is also a component of DNA, RNA, bone and membrane phospholipids.

Approximately 86% of $PO_4^{3-}$ is stored in the bone and 14% is present intracellularly; the extracellular concentration of $PO_4^{3-}$ is very low (0.03–0.1%). The normal serum concentration of $PO_4^{3-}$ is 0.8–1.4 mmol/l and, in contrast to $Ca^{2+}$, only 10% of serum $PO_4^{3-}$ is bound.

It is important to remember that the kidney is the only organ capable of excreting $PO_4^{3-}$. Hence, people with chronic kidney disease are at risk of hyperphosphataemia.

### FIBROBLAST GROWTH FACTOR 23

Both bone reabsorption and an increase in vitamin D will lead to increases in the serum levels of $PO_4^{3-}$ as well as $Ca^{2+}$. It is therefore important that there is a mechanism to prevent vitamin-D-mediated hyperphosphataemia. Fibroblast growth factor 23 is a recently discovered $PO_4^{3-}$-regulating hormone (a phosphatonin). The phosphaturic molecule is produced by mineralised tissues, in particular osteocytes and possibly osteoblasts, in response to stimulation with vitamin D. It acts by reducing the expression of NPT2 in the apical membrane of the proximal tubule, which in turn increases $PO_4^{3-}$ excretion in urine.

## Pregnancy and calcium balance

Pregnancy and lactation are periods of increased $Ca^{2+}$ requirement to enable the growth of fetal tissues and the production of milk, and are a huge drain on the mother's mineral resources. The fetus contains approximately 20–30 g of $Ca^{2+}$ and is relatively hypercalcaemic compared with the mother (the ratio of the fetal to maternal $Ca^{2+}$ concentration is 1.4 to 1.0). Most (80%) of the $Ca^{2+}$ accumulation in the fetus occurs in the third trimester, when ossification occurs.

$Ca^{2+}$ and $PO_4^{3-}$ are transferred to the fetal circulation against a concentration gradient by use of various $Ca^{2+}$ transporters. Many fetal tissues produce PTHrP, which plays a role in the regulation of placental $Ca^{2+}$ transport by modifying placental calbindin or the PMCA.

The fetus can also synthesise PTH by week 12 of gestation (PTH does not cross the placenta) but serum levels of this hormone remain low for the first 2–3 days postpartum. At birth, the newborn baby has low PTH and high calcitonin levels.

To cope with the requirements of the fetus, the mother has decreased/normal levels of PTH, increased levels of calcitonin and increased levels of vitamin D. $Ca^{2+}$ absorption from the intestine is also increased. These changes occur early in the pregnancy before the fetus requires significant amounts of $Ca^{2+}$. It is thought that this increases the mother's $Ca^{2+}$ stores in preparation for the fetal requirement. Maternal bone mineral density (BMD) varies throughout pregnancy with changes in both cortical BMD (generally increased) and trabecular BMD (generally decreased). Bone turnover also increases in the third trimester.

### FETAL DEVELOPMENT AND VITAMIN D

Studies have linked the vitamin D status of the mother to the development of the fetus. For example, studies of knockout mice that are deficient of the genes encoding VDR or 1α-hydroxylase have suggested that vitamin D is vital for fertility and fetal development. There is also a clear link between the development of diabetes (type 1 and type 2) and vitamin D levels in both the mother and the baby. This evidence has led to the suggestion that pregnant women, particularly Asian women, should receive vitamin D supplementation during pregnancy. A number of European countries also supplement children for the first few years of life.

## Bone

Bone is a metabolically active tissue that has a number of functions:

- support
- protection (e.g. skull and ribs)
- production of blood cells from the bone marrow
- attachment of muscle, tendons and ligaments
- storage (buffer) of minerals ($Ca^{2+}$, $PO_4^{3-}$ and $Mg^{2+}$).

### BONE STRUCTURE

Normal bone comprises a protein matrix (osteoid) and a mineral component. Osteoid makes up about 25% of bone content and is secreted by osteoblasts. It consists of type 1 collagen (90%) and noncollagenous proteins (glycoproteins and proteoglycans; approximately 10%). The mineral component (hydroxyapatite) makes up approximately 65% of bone content. Mineralisation requires high concentrations of $Ca^{2+}$ and $PO_4^{3-}$ for crystallisation to occur. The strength of bone is dependent on bone mineral content but the structure is also extremely important. It is highly organised and can be considered analogous to reinforced concrete in that it requires strength and rigidity but also flexibility to complement the brittleness of the hydroxyapatite. Collagen provides resilience and the mineral component rigidity.

There are two types of bone tissue: trabecular (also referred to as cancellous) and cortical (or compact). Trabecular bone is strong, lightweight and has a spongy appearance. By contrast, cortical bone is extremely strong but heavy and forms the outer (cortical) layer of the bone. In the axial skeleton, there is only a thin layer of cortical bone. Trabecular bone has a very large surface area that is significantly greater than that of cortical bone. As a result, it provides a large area for interaction with the extracellular fluid, which makes it more important than cortical bone in $Ca^{2+}$ and $PO_4^{3-}$ homeostasis.

Histologically, bone can be classified as woven bone (new bone) or lamellar bone (mature bone). Woven bone results from rapid osteoid production, such as occurs in fracture healing. The collagen structure is haphazard and the resulting bone is weak. Lamellar bone is remodelled woven bone; it is highly organised with collagen fibres that are arranged in parallel lamellae (sheets).

### BONE CELLS

There are three types of bone cells: osteoblasts, osteoclasts and osteocytes. Osteoblasts are the cell type responsible for bone production and arise from mesenchymal stem cells. They produce matrix components and mineralise osteoid. When inactive, they form flat bone-lining cells.

Osteoclasts reabsorb bone. They are multinucleated cells from the bone marrow lineage that act alone or in pairs. Attachment of the osteoclasts to the bone surface is essential for bone reabsorption.

Osteocytes are terminally differentiated osteoblasts trapped in the bone. They are located in lacunae (small cavities) and maintain contact with the surface by cellular extensions that pass through fluid-filled canaliculi (Figure 8.5). Their primary function is thought to be the response to mechanical strain.

## BONE REMODELLING

Bone remodelling occurs continuously on the surface of the bone to maintain good-quality bone and structural integrity. Remodelling can be periosteal (occurring at the periosteum–bone interface) and endosteal (occurring at the bone–bone marrow interface).

Remodelling occurs in small areas called osteons, as illustrated in Figure 8.5. The quiescent bone surface is lined with bone-lining cells (Figure 8.5 A). Osteocytes embedded in the bone are connected to each other and the bone surface via a series of canaliculi. Following a 'bone resorption' signal, mature osteoclasts develop. These break down the bone structure, destroying both the hydroxyapatite and osteoid and leaving small pits (Howship lacunae) in the bone surface (Figure 8.5 B). Osteoblast differentiation is triggered and osteoblasts then fill the resorption pits with osteoid (Figure 8.5 C), which is eventually mineralised. A complete cycle takes between 90 and 130 days.

Osteoclastic bone reabsorption and osteoblastic bone formation are normally tightly coupled. A disruption in this balance leads to altered bone mineral content and structure. For example, too much or too little bone may be produced (as in osteopetrosis or osteoporosis) or the structure may be modified (as in rickets and osteomalacia, where there is loss of mineral component).

A number of factors regulate bone remodelling and bone cell development and function, including hormones, cytokines and growth factors. Estrogen is vital for normal bone development in both men and women. It inhibits osteoclast function and osteoclastogenesis and may promote osteoblast survival. Its loss at the menopause is fundamental in the development of postmenopausal osteoporosis. Similarly, testosterone is required for bone strength in both men and women and hypogonadism accounts for approximately 20% of osteoporosis in men. Glucocorticoids (cortisol) are also required for

### FIGURE 8.5 Bone remodelling

A Quiescent phase

B Osteoclastic bone resorption

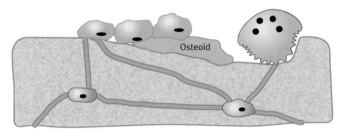

C Deposition of osteoid by osteoblasts and mineralisation of the new bone

bone development. However, excess levels of glucocorticoids are associated with decreased bone formation and increased bone loss as well as with decreased intestinal $Ca^{2+}$ absorption and increased renal $Ca^{2+}$ excretion.

TABLE 8.5  **Biochemical measures of bone turnover**

| Type of bone-cell activity measured | Serum markers | Urinary markers |
| --- | --- | --- |
| Bone formation and/or remodelling | Bone-specific alkaline phosphatase[a]<br><br>Osteocalcin[a]<br><br>Propeptides of type 1 collagen[a] | |
| Bone resorption | TRAP[b]<br><br>Type 1 collagen<br><br>Collagen cross-links | Hydroxyproline<br><br>Pyridinolines<br><br>Collagen cross-links |

[a] Produced by osteoblasts; raised levels indicate increased bone turnover, which usually reflects increased bone reabsorption produced by osteoclasts;
[b] raised levels indicate increased osteoclastic activity  |  TRAP = tartrate-resistant alkaline phosphatase produced by osteoclasts

## ASSESSMENT OF BONE REMODELLING AND BONE MINERAL DENSITY

BMD can be assessed by imaging and biochemical measurements. X-rays will often show defects in bone structure but dual energy X-ray absorptiometry (DEXA) is the diagnostic measure of BMD and bone mineral content (see Chapter 10 for further information on this technique). Areas of osteoblastic activity can be identified following injection of a radionucleotide (often technetium) that targets areas of bone remodelling.

Biochemical markers of bone turnover can measure either bone formation or bone resorption; they are listed in Table 8.5.

If it is important to identify at a cellular level the pathological changes that have occurred, then a bone biopsy can be taken. Bone biopsies are not performed unless necessary because the procedure is invasive and painful.

## OSTEOPOROSIS AND OSTEOPENIA

Osteoporosis, which means porous bones, is a common bone disease. One in two women and one in five men over the age of 50 years are at risk of an osteoporotic fracture. It is a combination of decreased BMD and a change in microarchitecture that can result in fractures following minimal trauma. Osteoporotic fractures are associated with increased morbidity and mortality.

Osteoporosis occurs when osteoclast resorption exceeds osteoblast bone formation. Consequently, in a normal bone-remodelling cycle, the resorption pits are not fully restored by the osteoblasts and microfractures are not effectively repaired. In osteoporosis, both collagen and mineral is lost, so in contrast to most other bone conditions, the remaining bone is normal but there is less of it.

Although osteoporosis is associated with bone pain, often the first sign of osteoporosis is a fracture. Compression fractures of the spine, which cause kyphosis, are a common feature of osteoporosis. Osteoporosis is frequently considered to be a female disease but it has been recognised recently that it is also common in men. The increased numbers of men being diagnosed with osteoporosis is in part attributable to increased life expectancy.

Osteopenia is identical to osteoporosis but there is less loss of bone mineral. Management involves the prevention of progression to osteoporosis. Often nothing is done, except to offer dietary and lifestyle advice (increase $Ca^{2+}$ intake, increase weight-bearing exercise, ensure the person is vitamin D-replete, reduce smoking and consumption of alcohol).

The possibility of identifying osteopenia, a forerunner to osteoporosis, raises the question of screening. Currently, DEXA scans are not performed unless there is a predisposition to osteoporosis, such as long-term steroid use, premature menopause, prolonged secondary amenorrhoea, a history of fragility fractures, radiological osteopenia, vertebral deformity or a family history of early and severe osteoporosis. If a screening programme were introduced, this would raise the question of what treatment to offer to those identified with osteopenia.

TABLE 8.6 **World Health Organization diagnostic criteria for osteoporosis**

| Category | T-score [a] |
|----------|-------------|
| Normal | Above –1.0 |
| Osteopenia | –1.0 to –2.5 |
| Osteoporosis | Below –2.5 |

[a] Defined as the number of standard deviations above or below the average bone mineral density value for a young healthy adult

### Diagnosis of osteoporosis and osteopenia

The World Health Organization diagnostic criteria for osteoporosis are outlined in Table 8.6. The diagnosis is made on the basis of the BMD value as determined by a DEXA scan.

### What determines whether a person develops osteoporosis?

It is important to realise that it is perfectly normal to lose bone mineral, and so BMD, as we age. Bone loss occurs at almost every skeletal site with age. It becomes a problem when the BMD falls so low that it increases the fracture risk. It is very important to prevent fractures as osteoporotic fractures are associated with increased morbidity and mortality. So what determines how much bone an individual loses?

During childhood and early adult life, bone formation is greater than bone resorption and over 90% of adult bone mass is acquired, with the rate of bone mass acquisition being greatest during the pubertal growth spurt (Figure 8.6). The bone mass accrued by the time full skeletal maturation is achieved is known as the peak bone mass, which is higher in men than in women. Bone mass then remains fairly constant until around 40 years of age, at which point bone formation becomes less efficient and bone loss begins to occur. The rate of bone loss in men and women is similar, with the exception of the period around the menopause, when the loss of estrogen accelerates the rate of loss in women (Figure 8.6). Both the rate of bone loss and the peak bone mass obtained are important factors that determine a person's chance of developing osteoporosis.

In women, the loss of estrogen at menopause is often

FIGURE 8.6 **Change in bone mass with age**

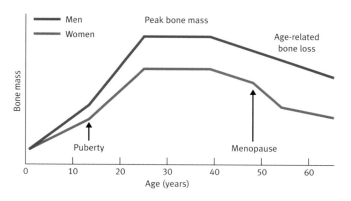

the main cause of osteoporosis development. In men, hypogonadism and prescribed corticosteroids account for around 40% of osteoporosis; however, osteoporosis in men is often idiopathic.

Risk factors associated with an osteoporotic fracture include low BMD, low body weight, cigarette smoking, alcohol consumption, poor nutrition, vitamin D and/or $Ca^{2+}$ deficiency, physical inactivity, sex hormone deficiency and some drugs (corticosteroids, heparin). Endocrine disorders including hypogonadism, hyperparathyroidism, hyperthyroidism and Cushing syndrome and some malignancies are also associated with bone loss. It is thought that genetic factors account for 50–80% of the variance in BMD.

Why is the loss of BMD so damaging? The loss of bone strength seen in osteoporotic bone is greater than that attributable to the loss of bone mineral content alone. This is because in osteoporosis there is also a change in the structure of trabecular bone. The complex cross-linking of the trabeculae gives bone added strength and a loss of this cross-linking results in an additional loss of structural integrity.

> **INTERESTING FACTS**
>
> **Osteoporosis**
>
> - Hip fractures in the UK cause as many deaths as breast cancer.
> - Men experience more osteoporotic fractures than prostate cancer.
> - Every 3 minutes someone in the UK has an osteoporotic fracture.

## Management of osteoporosis

Minimising any further loss of bone and prevention of fractures are the main management strategies in osteoporosis. Peak bone mass cannot be altered once it has been obtained; therefore, management should focus on:

- maintenance of current BMD and reduction in the rate of bone loss
  - lifestyle and dietary advice
  - drug treatment (most current osteoporosis drugs prevent further bone loss; anabolic drugs are likely to be important in the future)
- early detection (DEXA scan)
- prevention of fractures
  - minimising falls (good footwear, glasses, walking aids, muscle strength and balance)
  - lessening the impact of falls (hip protectors).

The National Institute for Health and Clinical Excellence (NICE) has produced guidelines for the prevention of primary and secondary osteoporotic fractures. At present, the drugs of choice are bisphosphonates. Selective estrogen receptor modulators, strontium ranelate and PTH are also covered by current NICE guidelines. Hormone replacement therapy, while effective, should not be prescribed for osteoporosis treatment unless other drugs are ineffective or not tolerated.

### Pregnancy, lactation and osteoporosis

Pregnancy and breastfeeding are a significant drain on the mother's $Ca^{2+}$ stores. For example, lactation requires 280–400 mg/day of $Ca^{2+}$ and clinical osteoporosis, while rare, can occur. However, pregnancy-induced osteoporosis is difficult to assess (imaging techniques include exposure to radiation). It is usually identified in the third trimester (41%) or postpartum (56%). The presenting signs and symptoms are similar to those of age-related osteoporosis: pain, loss of height and vertebral fractures. It is important to try and assess whether the osteoporosis is attributable to the pregnancy or whether the pregnancy has exacerbated a pre-existing condition. However, pregnancy-induced osteoporosis and lactation-induced osteoporosis usually resolve approximately 6 months after birth or weaning and neither presents an increased lifetime risk of osteoporosis.

### Juvenile osteoporosis

Osteoporosis is rare in children. However, if it does occur, it can have a significant impact on the peak bone mass, as most bone accretion occurs during childhood. The rate of bone mass increase is most rapid during the first 3 years of life and most $Ca^{2+}$ is deposited during puberty. In addition, as described earlier, the peak bone mass can determine the risk of developing osteoporosis and clinicians are concerned that current lifestyles of young and adolescent children will not promote the development of a good peak bone mass.

Although juvenile osteoporosis is often idiopathic, it can also be caused by an underlying condition (rheumatoid arthritis or an endocrine disorder), drugs (steroids are a particular risk factor) or lifestyle.

## Calcium homeostasis and teeth

When considering $Ca^{2+}$ homeostasis and abnormalities of bone, the teeth should not be forgotten. Teeth are embedded in bone and contain three types of mineralised tissues: enamel, dentine and cementum. The mineral component of teeth resembles hydroxyapatite and they contain cells similar to osteoblasts. Odontoblasts make dentine, cementoblasts produce cementum and ameloblasts synthesise enamel.

People with conditions that alter $Ca^{2+}$ homeostasis, such as pregnancy and chronic kidney disease, often have problems with teeth. Defects of the teeth are also seen in genetic skeletal disorders, such as osteogenesis imperfecta and osteopetrosis. Likewise, metabolic bone disorders (vitamin D deficiency, rickets, hypophosphataemia, Paget's disease and osteoporosis) are associated with defective tooth development and mineralisation.

## FURTHER READING

Nussey SS, Whitehead SA. The parathyroid glands and vitamin D. In: Nussey SS, White SA. *Endocrinology: An Integrated Approach*. Oxford: BIOS Scientific Publishers Ltd; 2001. p 171–212.

Shoback D, Sellmeyer D, Bikle DD. Metabolic bone disease. In: Gardner DG, Shoback D, editors. *Greenspan's Basic and Clinical Endocrinology*. 8th ed. San Francisco: McGraw-Hill; 2007. p 281–345.

The National Osteoporosis Society [www.nos.org.uk].

The International Osteoporosis Foundation [www.iofbonehealth.org].

# Human metabolism: carbohydrates, fats and proteins

*Mary Board*

## Introduction

In accordance with the principle of energy conservation, energy extracted from food is harnessed for energy-consuming processes such as mechanical work, biosynthesis, active transport and protein phosphorylation. The link between the metabolism of fuels and the consumption of energy is provided by the high-energy compound ATP (Figure 9.1) and metabolic pathways are strictly regulated to ensure maintenance of appropriate levels of ATP. The differing requirements of individual cells and tissues mean that the ways in which ATP supplies are maintained are quite diverse.

## Carbohydrate metabolism

Carbohydrates are the only fuels that can be respired anaerobically and, moreover, glucose represents the most accessible energy source for many cells and tissues, most notably the brain and the erythrocyte.

### FORMS OF CARBOHYDRATE

Dietary carbohydrate can be ingested in a wide variety of forms, ranging from simple mono- or disaccharides to huge polymers (polysaccharides) that contain hundreds or thousands of monosaccharide residues (Table 9.1). The mono- and disaccharides provide the body with readily available glucose and their ingestion produces a rapid increase in blood glucose level. By contrast, glucose polymers, which are most abundant in the form of storage

FIGURE 9.1 **Maintenance of ATP levels**

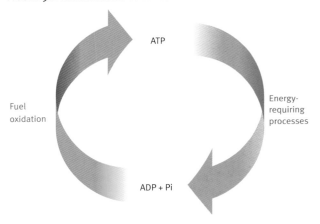

ADP = adenosine diphosphate | ATP = adenosine trisphosphate | Pi = inorganic phosphate

compounds such as plant starches or animal glycogen (Table 9.1), take much longer to be digested.

One way or another, all dietary carbohydrate can be converted to glucose. When glucose is removed from the blood because of its consumption by tissues, it is quickly replenished by breakdown of hepatic glycogen or by synthesis via hepatic gluconeogenesis.

### OVERVIEW OF GLUCOSE METABOLISM

Glucose is a versatile fuel: not only can it be consumed by all tissues but it can also be respired anaerobically, unlike fats or proteins. Aerobic and anaerobic respiration of glucose share the initial pathway of glycolysis in the cytosol. In the absence of $O_2$, glycolysis leads to the conversion

TABLE 9.1 **Examples of dietary carbohydrate**

| Carbohydrate | Monosaccharide components | Source |
|---|---|---|
| **MONOSACCHARIDES** | | |
| Glucose | Glucose | Fruit, honey |
| Fructose | Fructose | Fruit, honey |
| **DISACCHARIDES** | | |
| Lactose (milk sugar) | Glucose, galactose | Milk |
| Sucrose (table sugar) | Glucose, fructose | Cane sugar, prepared foods |
| **TRISACCHARIDES** | | |
| Trehalose | Glucose | Mushrooms |
| **POLYSACCHARIDES** | | |
| Amylose | Glucose (linear) | Plant starch |
| Amylopectin | Glucose (branched) | Plant starch |
| Glycogen | Glucose (branched) | Meat |

of 1 mole of glucose to 2 moles of lactate. This conversion brings about the formation of ATP via substrate-level phosphorylation and the production of the reduced co-factor nicotinamide adenine dinucleotide (NADH).

Aerobic respiration continues in the mitochondrion with the tricarboxylic acid (TCA) cycle and the electron transport chain and results in the complete oxidation of the glucose molecule to its combustion products, $CO_2$ and $H_2O$:

$$C_6H_{12}O_6 + 6\,O_2 \rightarrow 6\,CO_2 + 6\,H_2O$$

### ANAEROBIC METABOLISM

All glucose metabolism begins with the anaerobic cytosolic pathway of glycolysis (Figure 9.2). The pathway converts the six-carbon glucose molecule into two molecules of the three-carbon compound pyruvate, with the net production of 2 moles of ATP per mole of glucose by substrate-level phosphorylation.

Under anaerobic conditions, pyruvate is reduced to lactate (Figure 9.3). Indeed, the appearance of lactate in the bloodstream is often used as an indicator of the occurrence of anaerobic respiration. The molecule represents a metabolic dead end: the body has no use for lactate other

than to reconvert it to pyruvate. However, production of lactate from pyruvate by lactate dehydrogenase results in the regeneration of oxidised nicotinamide adenine dinucleotide ($NAD^+$) from NADH. This step is vital for the continued operation of glycolysis under anaerobic conditions because $NAD^+$ is a co-factor for the oxidation of glyceraldehyde-3-phosphate (Figure 9.2) and cytosolic supplies of $NAD^+$ are limited.

The glycolytic pathway can be reversed to bring about synthesis of glucose from noncarbohydrate sources (gluconeogenesis) in the liver. When this occurs, the irreversible reactions in Figure 9.2 (unidirectional arrows) must be bypassed by separate reactions catalysed in the reverse direction, whereas the reactions denoted by double arrows may be freely reversed.

### AEROBIC METABOLISM: PYRUVATE DEHYDROGENASE REACTION AND TRICARBOXYLIC ACID CYCLE

Under aerobic conditions, the product of the glycolytic pathway is pyruvate, which becomes the substrate for the remaining steps of the oxidative metabolism that take place within the mitochondrion. The three-carbon pyruvate molecule is converted to the two-carbon acetyl coenzyme A (CoA) molecule by the enzyme pyruvate

TABLE 9.2  **Steps contributing to ATP yield during anaerobic and aerobic respiration of glucose**

| Reduced co-factors produced (moles per mole glucose) | Route of ATP synthesis | Resulting ATP yield[a] (moles per mole glucose) |
|---|---|---|
| **GLYCOLYSIS** | | |
| | Substrate-level phosphorylation | 2 ATP |
| 2 NADH[b] | Oxidative phosphorylation | 5 ATP |
| **PDH REACTION** | | |
| 2 NADH | Oxidative phosphorylation | 5 ATP |
| **TCA CYCLE** | | |
| | Substrate-level phosphorylation[c] | 2 ATP |
| 6 NADH | Oxidative phosphorylation | 15 ATP |
| 2 FADH$_2$ | Oxidative phosphorylation | 3 ATP |

The blue bracket shows the scope of anaerobic respiration, the red bracket that of aerobic respiration; [a] estimated from empirical data; [b] NADH generated in the cytosol must be shuttled into the mitochondrion; [c] substrate-level phosphorylation during the succinyl coenzyme A synthetase reaction produces guanosine triphosphate, which can be used to synthesise ATP. I FADH$_2$ = reduced form of flavin adenine dinucleotide I NADH = reduced form of nicotinamide adenine dinucleotide I PDH = pyruvate dehydrogenase I TCA = tricarboxylic acid

dehydrogenase (PDH), in a reaction that produces NADH. Acetyl CoA is then consumed by the TCA cycle (Figure 9.4) and converted to two molecules of $CO_2$. The cycle also produces three molecules of NADH, one molecule of the reduced form of flavin adenine dinucleotide (FADH$_2$) and one molecule of guanosine triphosphate (GTP) per turn (Table 9.2). The reduced co-factors NADH and FADH$_2$ pass their electrons along the electron transport chain to elicit ATP synthesis and GTP may be converted to ATP.

The PDH reaction, which links the anaerobic and aerobic pathways, is irreversible and cannot be bypassed in the reverse direction. Thus, no pathway exists for the conversion of acetyl CoA into pyruvate. Moreover, while two carbon atoms enter the TCA cycle in the form of acetyl CoA, two carbon atoms are lost as $CO_2$, meaning that there is no net gain of carbon by any TCA cycle intermediate. Thus, there is no pathway for the synthesis of glucose from acetyl CoA. These observations achieve significance during starvation.

**ATP YIELD FROM GLUCOSE**

Aerobic respiration produces 30–32 moles of ATP per mole of glucose, compared with 2 moles of ATP obtained during anaerobic respiration. This means that aerobic respiration of glucose is 15–16 times more efficient than anaerobic respiration. Table 9.2 illustrates how the ATP yield is derived.

Quoted yields of ATP vary considerably from text to text. Some sources put ATP yields at 30–32 moles for aerobic respiration, others at 36–38 moles. This discrepancy represents more than just the usual inability of biochemists to agree among themselves. The higher figure is derived from theoretical considerations, where the amount of energy liberated when electrons travel along the electron transport chain is divided by the amount of energy required to synthesise an ATP molecule. Theoretical yields are 3 moles of ATP per mole of NADH and 2 moles of ATP per mole of FADH$_2$. The lower figure is based on empirical values, that is, those derived from experiment. Empirical yields for NADH and FADH$_2$ are 2.5 moles of ATP and 1.5 moles of ATP, respectively. These values are lower because some of the energy obtained from electron transport is used for the export of ATP from the mitochondrion as well as for the synthesis of ATP.

FIGURE 9.2 **Glycolysis**

\* Reactions responsible for the production of ATP by substrate-level phosphorylation | ADP = adenosine diphosphate | ATP = adenosine triphosphate | NAD+ = oxidised form of nicotinamide adenine dinucleotide | NADH = reduced form of NAD

## ANAEROBIC TISSUES

Several cells and tissues rely wholly or partly on anaerobic respiration, either in a constitutive manner or as circumstances dictate. Partially anaerobic tissues include the kidney medulla, which is poorly perfused by blood and therefore receives little $O_2$, and the cells of the retina, where

FIGURE 9.3 **Reduction of pyruvate to lactate**

$NAD^+$ = oxidised form of nicotinamide adenine dinucleotide |
NADH = reduced form of NAD

$O_2$ metabolism is not favoured lest it damage the light-sensitive pigments necessary for photoreception. More extreme examples are represented by the red blood cell and by vigorously exercising white (type 2) muscle fibres.

Red blood cells show great economy of volume to maintain a property of deformability, which allows them to travel unimpeded through narrow capillaries. One of the means by which this is achieved is the complete absence of intracellular organelles, including mitochondria. Thus, the red blood cell has zero capacity for oxidative metabolism and relies entirely on anaerobic conversion of glucose to lactate to meet its energy requirements.

By contrast, white muscle fibres do have mitochondria. These fibres compose fast-twitch muscles, which are the 'fight or flight' muscles responsible for escape from danger (or, more mundanely, for sports such as sprinting). The rapid response of such muscles, and the ATP requirement involved, precludes use of the aerobic route for ATP generation. This is not because the aerobic route is longer and more time-consuming but rather because the rate of $O_2$ diffusion into the muscle fibre is so slow by comparison with the rate of ATP consumption by the contracting muscle. However, the very rapid rates of the enzyme-catalysed reactions in the glycolytic pathway can be increased 1000-fold in an almost instantaneous manner and this is sufficient to cater for the muscle's energy requirements.

As with all anaerobic episodes, the only fuel that can be respired by white muscle fibres is glucose. The white muscle fibre has large stores of intracellular glycogen to produce glucose units for anaerobic respiration (Figure 9.5) and the breakdown of glycogen in contracting muscle is stimulated by adrenaline, among other factors. The muscle cannot produce free glucose from glycogen because it lacks the enzyme glucose-6-phosphatase; therefore, glycogen is broken down to the glycolytic intermedi-

FIGURE 9.4 **Tricarboxylic acid cycle**

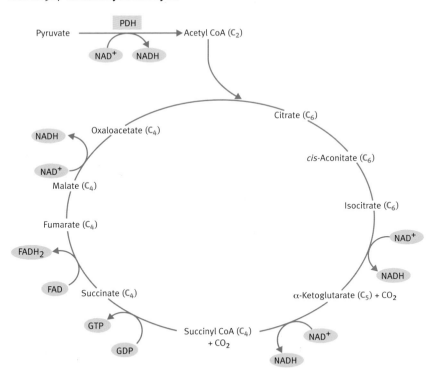

Products of the TCA cycle (per turn):
Reduced co-factors: $3 \times$ NADH, $1 \times$ FADH$_2$
High-energy compound: $1 \times$ GTP
Decarboxylation products: $2 \times CO_2$

Note that 2 moles of acetyl CoA are produced per mole of glucose and that oxidation of this acetyl CoA requires two turns of the cycle.
CoA = coenzyme A  |  GDP = guanosine diphosphate  |  GTP = guanosine triphosphate  |  FAD = oxidised form of flavin adenine dinucleotide  |
FADH$_2$ = reduced form of FAD  |  NAD$^+$ = oxidised form of nicotinamide adenine dinucleotide  |  NADH = reduced form of NAD  |
PDH = pyruvate dehydrogenase  |  TCA = tricarboxylic acid

FIGURE 9.5 **Fuels for anaerobically respiring muscle**

ate glucose-6-phosphate. The muscle may also take up glucose from the blood to fuel anaerobic ATP production. Ultimately, the source of blood glucose is likely to be liver glycogen.

## CARBOHYDRATE METABOLISM DURING STARVATION

During starvation, the body has access to huge fat reserves (which are metabolised to acetyl CoA) but to very little carbohydrate. Glycogen reserves are substantially depleted by the overnight fast and are undetectable after about 24 hours of fasting. This brings the body to something of a crisis because the brain has an absolute requirement for glucose. In the fed state, the brain consumes about 100 g/day of glucose and while this requirement can be reduced to about 25 g/day during starvation, it cannot be diminished any further. During such episodes, hepatic gluconeogenesis must maintain supplies of glucose.

FIGURE 9.6 **Release of glucogenic amino acids by muscle tissue during prolonged starvation**

Transamination reactions (1) convert the constituent amino acids of muscle protein into the transportable glucogenic amino acids alanine and glutamine; the liver transdeaminates (2) alanine and glutamine and their carbon skeletons can be used to synthesise glucose through the pathway of gluconeogenesis (3).

However, the irreversibility of the PDH reaction now presents something of a stumbling block: although the abundant fat stores allow the production of large amounts of acetyl CoA, this cannot be converted to pyruvate, which would be a gluconeogenic substrate. There is also no way of synthesising another gluconeogenic intermediate from acetyl CoA because two carbon atoms are lost during TCA cycle activity. The net result of these observations is that fat can never be converted to glucose under any circumstances.

It is interesting to note that plants, perhaps as a result of occupying an evolutionary pinnacle, do have means of converting fat into glucose (the glyoxylate shuttle).

Given that the brain's glucose requirement must be satisfied for its continued function, glucose must be synthesised from noncarbohydrate, nonfat precursors. This role is fulfilled by muscle protein and amino acids are released from wasting muscle relatively early on in starvation (Figure 9.6). Such wasting is not without its penalty, however, since loss of muscle protein leads to loss of function. Death from starvation (which occurs after around 60 days in a normal-sized adult) is most commonly caused by weakening of essential muscles.

## MAINTENANCE OF BLOOD GLUCOSE CONCENTRATIONS IN THE NORMAL AND DIABETIC STATE

The body expends a great deal of effort and energy in maintaining blood glucose levels within very narrow limits (Figure 9.7). For a healthy individual without diabetes, for whom glucose homeostasis is strictly controlled, fasting blood glucose might be as low as 4 mmol/l and postprandial levels might rise as high as 8 mmol/l but values do not vary outside these limits. Blood glucose is maintained during the first 24 hours of starvation by mobilisation of liver glycogen and thereafter by muscle protein breakdown, followed by gluconeogenesis. Blood glucose concentrations are maintained at around 4 mmol/l for the duration of starvation, until death occurs.

By contrast, uncontrolled diabetes can result in vast fluctuations in blood glucose concentration with severe consequences (Figure 9.7). The brain is perfectly able to function when the blood glucose concentration is 4 millimoles/l but loses this ability at 2 mmol/l, when a hypoglycaemic coma is very likely to result (Figure 9.7). When the blood glucose concentration is 2 mmol/l, there is still a total of 1.8 g of glucose present in the circulation (compared with 3.6 g at 4 mmol/l) but this glucose becomes much less accessible to the brain. These values are derived by assuming that an average-sized person has 5 l of blood (the molecular weight of glucose is 180 g). Here we can appreciate the importance of considering the concentration rather than the quantity of glucose. The brain takes up glucose by facilitated diffusion using the proteinaceous glucose transporter type 3 (GLUT3). GLUT3 has a $K_M$ for glucose of 1.6 mmol/l, meaning that the transporter will be saturated with glucose and working at maximal capacity at all normal concentrations of blood glucose. If the blood glucose concentration drops below 3 millimoles/l, however, the brain's glucose transporter is no longer saturated and is not able to satisfy the brain's glucose requirement. Such a situation is characteristic of hypoglycaemic coma caused, for example, by the presence of diabetes or by overconsumption of alcohol.

FIGURE 9.7 **Blood glucose levels**

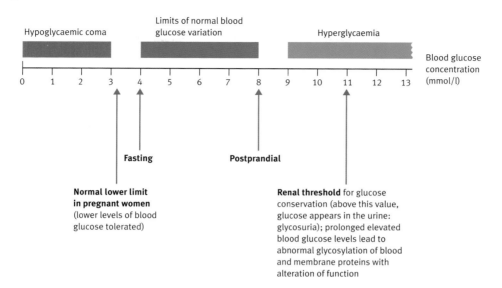

The Michaelis constant $K_M$, represents the substrate concentration at which an enzyme-catalysed reaction or a transport process reaches half-maximum velocity. If the $K_M$ is low, only a low substrate concentration is required for a process to occur at maximum velocity and vice versa. It is noteworthy that the glucose transporter in the brain has a lower $K_M$ than those present in any other cell or tissue. To a certain extent, this allows the brain preferential access to the glucose present in the bloodstream. (The $K_M$ is often quoted as an inverse index of the affinity of a transporter or enzyme for its substrate. This is not an equation that bears close scrutiny but it does provide a useful conceptual perspective: if the $K_M$ is low, the affinity is high and vice versa.)

## Fat metabolism

Fat molecules show great versatility in the uses to which they are put by the body. Table 9.3 outlines some of the diverse roles of fats. During the present chapter we will concern ourselves with their role in energy storage and oxidation.

In terms of both mass and caloric content, fat represents by far the largest energy depot in the body. Fat is stored as triacylglycerol (TAG or triglyceride) (Figure 9.8), which forms liquid droplets in the cytosol of the adipocyte. This represents a particularly efficient form of energy storage for many reasons. The fatty acid side chains of the TAG molecule are long and contain many hydrogen atoms, which behave as a reservoir of reducing potential for the production of the reduced co-factors NADH and $FADH_2$. These co-factors pass their electrons along the electron transport chain and elicit ATP production. This translates into an energy yield per unit weight for fat that is more than twice that for either carbohydrate or protein (Table 9.4).

The storage of TAGs in an anhydrous form (much different from the highly hydrated glycogen deposits in liver and muscle tissue) also contributes to the density and efficiency of energy storage. Moreover, fat can be stored in limitless quantities around the human physique. The adipocyte is a remarkably flexible cell that can shrink or expand to adopt a spherical shape to accommodate changing requirements for fat storage.

### MOBILISATION OF TRIACYLGLYCEROL

The TAG molecule (Figure 9.8) consists of a three-carbon glycerol backbone that is esterified to three fatty acid side chains and the free fatty acid molecule constitutes the accessible energy source for cells and tissues. The liberation of fatty acids from the TAG molecule is catalysed

TABLE 9.3  **Major roles of fats in the body**

| Role | Form |
|---|---|
| Energy storage | Triacylglycerol |
| Membrane formation | Phospholipids |
| Hormone synthesis | Eicosanoids (prostaglandins, thromboxanes, leucotrienes formed from essential fatty acids) |
| Intracellular signalling | Membrane phospholipids broken down to second messengers when hormone binds to its receptor |
| Regulation of gene transcription | Fatty acids (plus fat-soluble vitamins) |

TABLE 9.4  **Energy content of the main dietary components**

| Component | Energy yield (kJ/g) |
|---|---|
| Fat | 37 |
| Carbohydrate | 17 |
| Protein | 17 |

FIGURE 9.9  **Lipolysis and its control**

[a] Mediated by beta-3-adrenergic receptors  |  + indicates an increase in HSL activity  |  − indicates a decrease in HSL activity  |  ACTH = adrenocorticotrophic hormone  |  HSL = hormone-sensitive lipase  |  TAG = triacylglycerol

by the enzyme hormone-sensitive lipase (HSL) (Figure 9.9), in a reaction that is strictly controlled. Appropriate signals from adrenaline or glucagon ensure that fats are mobilised in response to a need for physical activity or during fasting, and the opposing signal from insulin conserves fat depots during the fed state.

It follows that the level of HSL activity has a strong impact on the level of plasma fatty acids and we can see the results of this association in Table 9.5. Many condi-

FIGURE 9.8  **Structure of triacylglycerol**

The presence of a double bond causes the fatty acid side chain to bend and adopt an angle of 135 degrees; such bends disrupt the packing of the side chains and thus the inclusion of unsaturated fatty acids is important in maintaining the fluidity of the TAG depot. [a] monounsaturated fatty acid  |  [b] saturated fatty acid  |  [c] polyunsaturated fatty acid  |  TAG = triacylglycerol

tions, such as fasting or exercising, produce an increase in the plasma concentration of fatty acids. A salutary note is sounded by the example of the racing driver (see the 'stress' entry in Table 9.5), who leads a stressful but sedentary lifestyle, which results in high levels of the stress hormone adrenaline. Adrenaline promotes the elevation of plasma fatty acid levels and prolonged elevation of blood fats is known to increase the risk of coronary heart disease (CHD). The propensity for atherosclerotic plaques to develop in the presence of high circulating levels of fats and cholesterol provides one of the links between CHD and the pursuit of a stressful lifestyle.

People with diabetes also have elevated plasma levels of fatty acids (Table 9.5). The absence or reduction of the antilipolytic insulin signal in diabetes causes HSL

TABLE 9.5  **Level of fatty acids in the blood under various conditions**

| Condition | Hormonal agent that influences HSL activity | Plasma fatty acids (mmol/l) |
|---|---|---|
| Normal (fed) | Balance between insulin and glucagon | 0.1–0.3 |
| Starvation[4] | Glucagon | 2.2[a] |
| Stress[5] | Adrenaline | 1.7[b] |
| Exercise[6] | Adrenaline | 1.0[c] |
| Diabetic coma[7] | Absence of insulin signal | 3.0 |
| Gestational diabetes mellitus[8] | Reduction of insulin signal | 0.7 |

[a] Value refers to a prolonged period of starvation (8 days)  |  [b] value refers to the example of the racing driver  |  [c] value refers to 15 minutes of exercise followed by 15 minutes of rest  |  HSL = hormone-sensitive lipase

to continue producing fatty acids even in the fed state (Figure 9.9). Again, this situation has its consequence in an increased risk of CHD among individuals with long-term diabetes. The term metabolic syndrome (or syndrome X) describes the frequent co-occurrence of type 2 diabetes, hypertension and CHD.

## TRANSPORT OF FATS

Fats of all kinds, being hydrophobic and insoluble, are transported in the blood in complexes with proteins (Table 9.6). Different lipoprotein complexes have different fat components and fulfil different functions. Thus, the lipid profile of the blood (that is, the relative concentrations of the different lipoprotein complexes) can provide an index of health. High levels of low-density lipoprotein

(LDL), often resulting from a high-fat diet but occasionally from a genetic disorder such as familial hypercholesterolaemia, are associated with an increased risk of CHD. By contrast, high levels of high-density lipoprotein (HDL), which imply active excretion of cholesterol, are associated with a lowered risk of CHD (Table 9.6).

Some dietary practices are considered to have a favourable impact on the lipid profile and to cause lowering of LDL and raising of HDL levels. Among these practices is the consumption of a diet rich in monounsaturated fats, such as olive oil (the Mediterranean diet) or certain nut oils including almond and walnut oils. Another is the pursuit of the Atkins diet,[1,2] a weight-reducing diet that involves the consumption of very little carbohydrate but unlimited quantities of fat and protein. This last observation is difficult to explain. It has been suggested that the

TABLE 9.6  **Lipoproteins in the circulation**

| Lipoprotein | Main fat constituent | Function |
|---|---|---|
| Chylomicron | Dietary TAG | Transports TAG from the intestine to other tissues for oxidation or storage (fed state) |
| VLDL | Endogenous TAG, cholesterol | Transports TAG produced in the liver to other tissues where it can be oxidised (fasting state) |
| LDL | Cholesterol and cholesteryl ester | Transports cholesterol from the liver to other tissues |
| HDL | Cholesteryl ester | Scavenges cholesterol from many tissues and takes it to the liver for excretion |
| Fatty acid–albumin | Fatty acid | Transports fatty acids from adipose tissue to other tissues where they can be oxidised (fasting state) |

HDL = high-density lipoprotein  |  LDL = low-density lipoprotein  |  TAG = triacylglycerol  |  VLDL = very-low-density lipoprotein

TABLE 9.7 **ATP production from oxidation of palmitate**

| Reduced co-factors/GTP produced (moles per mole palmitate) | ATP produced (moles per mole palmitate) |
|---|---|
| **7 × BETA-OXIDATION** | |
| 7 NADH | 17.5 |
| 7 FADH$_2$ | 10.5 |
| **8 × TCA CYCLE** | |
| 24 NADH | 60 |
| 8 FADH$_2$ | 12 |
| 8 GTP | 8 |
| **FATTY ACID ACTIVATION** | |
| None | −2 |
| **TOTAL** | |
| | 106 |

The 16-carbon palmitate molecule is converted to eight acetyl CoA molecules by seven rounds of the beta-oxidation pathway; the eight acetyl CoA molecules then undergo eight turns of the TCA cycle; the activation of palmitate, a reaction that adds the CoA moiety, consumes two ATP molecules per palmitate molecule. CoA = coenzyme A | GTP = guanosine triphosphate | FADH$_2$ = reduced form of flavin adenine dinucleotide | NADH = reduced form of nicotinamide adenine dinucleotide | TCA = tricarboxylic acid

high protein content of the Atkins diet has a satiating effect on the appetite. Thus, caloric intake by a person on the Atkins diet tends to be lower than that by control subjects. If the reduced caloric intake includes a reduced intake of fat, then there will be a corresponding reduction in lipoprotein particles carrying dietary fat and cholesterol (chylomicrons and LDLs).

## OXIDATION OF FATTY ACIDS

Many highly aerobic tissues, such as heart tissue and the red fibres of skeletal muscle, consume and oxidise fatty acids at a high rate. Once inside the cell, the fatty acid is activated by attachment of CoA. The fatty acyl CoA then constitutes the substrate for the beta-oxidation pathway.

Oxidation takes place inside the mitochondrion and repeated cycles of the beta-oxidation pathway (Figure 9.10) nibble away the hydrocarbon chain of the fatty acid. Each cycle produces one molecule of the two-carbon compound acetyl CoA as well as one molecule of FADH$_2$ and one molecule of NADH.

The shortened fatty acyl CoA rejoins the pathway for a repeat cycle. The acetyl CoA product is consumed by the TCA cycle in exactly the same way as that produced from pyruvate (Figure 9.4) and the reduced co-factors elicit ATP production (Table 9.7).

## INTEGRATION OF FAT AND CARBOHYDRATE METABOLISM

We have already observed the disparity between carbohydrate and fat stores in the body. Fat can be stored in seemingly limitless quantities, whereas glycogen reserves are very limited, lasting for only about 24 hours of starvation in the adult. This means that, after the first day of starvation, fat becomes the predominant fuel for the body, and it is a very energy-dense and efficient form of fuel.

However, fat has some limitations as a fuel source for the whole body with its diverse tissue-specific requirements. We have already seen that fat cannot be converted into glucose and is, therefore, useless in satisfying the brain's glucose requirement. Moreover, the brain itself cannot consume fatty acids as a fuel because lipoproteins do not cross the blood–brain barrier. Thus, oxidation of fatty acids cannot supply the 75% shortfall generated in the brain's energy requirements by its reduced glucose consumption during the starved state.

There is another factor to consider. When acetyl CoA is consumed by the TCA cycle, it must condense with an oxaloacetate molecule (Figure 9.4). To accommodate any extra acetyl CoA produced from increased rates of fat oxidation, levels of oxaloacetate must rise, too. Since glycogen has been depleted and oxaloacetate cannot be produced from acetyl CoA (owing to the loss of two $CO_2$ molecules earlier in the cycle), the carbon needed for oxaloacetate synthesis must derive from muscle protein (Figure 9.11).

## OXIDATION OF FATS DURING STARVATION: KETOGENESIS

An unusual situation exists inside liver cells because the liver is the only tissue performing significant rates of gluconeogenesis. During starvation, oxaloacetate is withdrawn from the TCA cycle in the liver to fuel glu-

### FIGURE 9.10  Beta-oxidation pathway

CoAS —C—C—C—C〜〜〜〜
         O  H  H
         ‖  |  |
            |  |
            H  H

Fatty acyl CoA (*n* carbons)

FAD ⟶ FADH₂    **Oxidation**

CoAS —C—C=C—C〜〜〜〜
         O     H
         ‖
               |
               H

H₂O    **Hydration**

CoAS —C—C—C—C〜〜〜〜
         O  H  H
         ‖  |  |
            |  |
            H  OH

NAD⁺ ⟶ NADH    **Oxidation**

CoAS —C—C—C—C〜〜〜〜
         O  H  O
         ‖  |  ‖
            |
            H

CoA    **Thiolysis**

CoAS —C—CH₃    +    CoAS —C—C〜〜〜〜
         O                     O
         ‖                     ‖

Acetyl CoA              Fatty acyl CoA
                        (*n*−2 carbons)

Repeated cycles of these four reactions convert the fatty acid with *n* carbons into $^n/_2$ moles of acetyl CoA. CoA = coenzyme A | FAD = oxidised form of flavin adenine dinucleotide | FADH₂ = reduced form of FAD | NAD⁺ = oxidised form of nicotinamide adenine dinucleotide | NADH = reduced form of NAD

coneogenesis (Figure 9.12). Since the liver also takes up fatty acids and rates of beta-oxidation remain high in this tissue, the imbalance between levels of acetyl CoA and oxaloacetate in the liver mitochondria is exaggerated (Figure 9.12). This imbalance stimulates the liver to channel excess acetyl CoA into ketogenesis.

The resulting ketone bodies are released into the blood for use by many tissues, most notably the brain. Ketone bodies supply about 75% of the brain's energy

### FIGURE 9.11  Metabolism during starvation: oxidation of fats by peripheral tissues

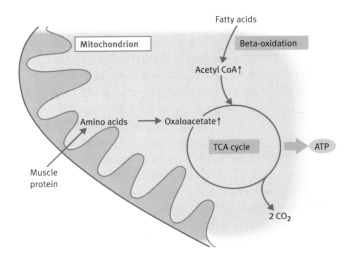

↑ = increased | CoA = coenzyme A | TCA = tricarboxylic acid

requirements during prolonged starvation. Ketone body production increases sharply after the first 24 hours of starvation and levels are sustained (at around 8 mmol/l) until death occurs.

### DIABETIC KETOACIDOSIS

An interesting complication arises for individuals with diabetes, in whom impaired control of HSL means that the plasma concentration and rates of oxidation of fatty acids persist at high levels even in the fed state. Since the rates of beta-oxidation and ketogenesis are little regulated other than by supply of their substrates (fatty acids and acetyl CoA, respectively), the loss of control of HSL leads to the uncontrolled production of ketone bodies. These compounds can achieve concentrations in the blood of people with diabetes that are several times higher than the normal maximum of 8 mmol/l.

Ketone bodies are acidic molecules, as are fatty acids. The acidic burden presented by the co-presence of ketone bodies and fatty acids in high concentrations can have an overwhelming effect on the buffering capacity of the blood, leading to a drop in pH (acidosis).

Diabetic ketoacidosis can be a severe condition, leading to a hypoxic coma. It is characteristic of type 1 diabetes, particularly when insulin therapy is interrupted or when a concurrent illness is present. The sequence of events is outlined in Figure 9.13. The drop in pH, although superficially small, disturbs many important interactions, perhaps most notably that of haemoglobin and $O_2$, which is pH-dependent. The erythrocyte attempts to rectify this situation by adjusting levels of 2,3-bisphosphoglycerate, a small molecule that mediates the affinity of haemoglobin for $O_2$.

Treatment for diabetic ketoacidosis, which centres on a slow infusion of insulin (given in the presence of glucose to avoid abrupt change in the blood glucose level), was in the past accompanied by administration of isotonic sodium bicarbonate if the blood pH was below 7. However, any clinical adjustment of the pH value must be made gradually to allow the erythrocyte time to readjust levels of 2,3-bisphosphoglycerate and this is a difficult balance to achieve. Hence, treatment with sodium bicarbonate is not a current practice. The dose of insulin administered is relatively low: sufficient to suppress hepatic glucose output but not high enough to stimulate glucose uptake by tissues.

## GESTATIONAL DIABETES MELLITUS

The consequences, outlined previously, of a loss or reduction of insulin control apply to any type of diabetes, but a word could profitably be said about the special case of gestational diabetes mellitus (GDM). Mild insulin resistance seems to affect all pregnant women and may be necessary to ensure that maternal uptake of glucose and other nutrients does not compromise fetal requirements. GDM represents a more severe situation but it is diffi-

cult to tell whether this disorder occurs at the extreme end of the normal insulin resistance spectrum in pregnancy or whether it represents an incipient form of type 2 diabetes.

There is some evidence to suggest that women who suffer from GDM, which normally persists only for the duration of pregnancy, may be at higher risk of developing type 2 diabetes later in life.[3] Some characteristics of GDM strongly resemble those of type 2 diabetes. Insulin levels are normal or raised but accompanied by high levels of plasma fatty acids and ketone bodies (high blood ketone body concentrations and ketonuria are often considered to be diagnostic for GDM). This indicates the presence of insulin resistance. Postprandial glucose levels in the blood are also greatly increased, presumably because of impaired uptake by maternal tissues.

The high glucose levels stimulate uptake by the fetus, which has a high metabolic requirement for this substrate. The rate of glucose uptake by the fetus is predictive of birth weight, and the raised blood glucose levels in GDM probably contribute to the fetal macrosomia that is associated with this condition.

## Protein metabolism

Rates of protein degradation are accelerated in two situations. The first concerns the consumption of a high-protein diet, when intake exceeds requirements, since excess protein cannot be stored. The second involves the increased breakdown of muscle protein during starva-

FIGURE 9.12 **Metabolism during starvation: gluconeogenesis and ketogenesis in the liver**

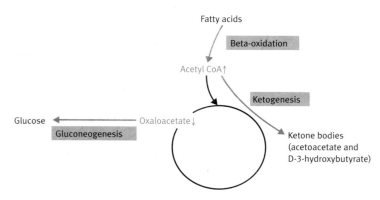

↑ = increased | ↓ = decreased | CoA = coenzyme A

## FIGURE 9.13  Metabolic disturbances in diabetic ketoacidosis

Loss of antilipolytic insulin signal

↓

High concentration of fatty acids,
high concentration of ketone bodies

↓

Drop in blood pH (from 7.4 to 6.9)

↓

Kidney excretes H$^+$, electrolytes and water;
osmotic diuresis develops as a result of
hyperglycaemia and glycosuria

↓

Dehydration

↓

Reduced blood flow

↓

Inefficient delivery of O$_2$ to peripheral tissues
(which begin to respire anaerobically,
producing lactate, which
contributes to the acidic burden)

↓

Hypoxia

↓

Subject takes huge gulping breaths ('air hunger')
in an attempt to rectify the hypoxia
and exhales CO$_2$

↓

Lowering of $P$CO$_2$ in blood

Clinical symptoms:
- hyperglycaemia and glycosuria
- ketonaemia and ketonuria
- low blood pH, K$^+$ and PO$_4^{3-}$
- low blood $P$O$_2$ and $P$CO$_2$

$P$CO$_2$ = partial pressure of CO$_2$ | $P$O$_2$ = partial pressure of O$_2$ |
PO$_4^{3-}$ = phosphate ion

## FIGURE 9.14  Removal of the alpha-amino group in amino acid metabolism

**A** Transamination

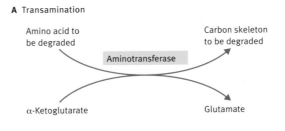

Amino acid to be degraded      Carbon skeleton to be degraded

Aminotransferase

α-Ketoglutarate      Glutamate

**B** Deamination

Glutamate dehydrogenase

NAD$^+$    NADH

Glutamate + H$_2$O ⇌ α-Ketoglutarate + NH$_4^+$

NAD$^+$ = oxidised form of nicotinamide adenine dinucleotide | NADH = reduced form of NAD | NH$_4^+$ = ammonium ion

The removal of the amino group is the first stage in amino acid metabolism. The amino group is incorporated into urea by the hepatic urea cycle and the remaining carbon skeleton contributes to one of the branches of metabolism already encountered in this chapter.

### REMOVAL OF THE ALPHA-AMINO GROUP

Amino acids undergo a combination of transamination reactions, where the amino group is transferred to a different carbon skeleton (Figure 9.14 A), and deamination, where the amino group is released as NH$_4^+$ (Figure 9.14 B). The transamination step is necessary to transfer the amino group from the target amino acid to α-ketoglutarate, thereby forming the amino acid glutamate. Glutamate is the substrate for the glutamate dehydrogenase reaction, which is able to accomplish the removal of the amino group in the form of NH$_4^+$.

One of the consequences of this sequence of reactions is that the pathway of amino acid degradation includes many aminotransferase enzymes with specificity for individual amino acids but only one enzyme (glutamate dehydrogenase) with deaminating activity.

tion, which is designed to release amino acids for glucose synthesis. In either event, proteins are degraded to their constituent amino acids.

Amino acids, the building blocks of proteins, contain the elements nitrogen, carbon, hydrogen and oxygen. The nitrogenous amino group is disposed of separately from the carbon skeleton. This separation is necessary to maintain nitrogen balance in the body and prevent accumulation of toxic nitrogenous compounds such as the ammonium ion (NH$_4^+$).

## UREA CYCLE

The urea cycle in the liver serves to detoxify $NH_4^+$. It incorporates 2 moles of nitrogen (1 mole derived from $NH_4^+$ and 1 mole from aspartate) into 1 mole of urea. Figure 9.15 shows the conversion achieved by the five reactions that constitute the urea cycle. The cycle consumes energy and spans both the cytosolic and the mitochondrial compartments. The product, urea, is a soluble, non-toxic vehicle for the transport of nitrogen atoms and is transported to the kidney for excretion.

Inborn errors of metabolism that result in deficiencies have been reported for all five enzymes that participate in the urea cycle. Such deficiencies result in hyperammonaemia and symptoms become manifest shortly after birth. The severity of the symptoms, which include swelling of the brain, lethargy and, ultimately, mental restriction, indicate the toxicity of $NH_4^+$ at high concentrations and justify the effort that the body expends in maintaining low concentrations.

The concentration of $NH_4^+$ does not normally exceed about 20 micromoles/l in the arterial and venous circulation (excluding the hepatic portal vein, where concentrations can be ten-fold higher). If concentrations are allowed to achieve values of 200 micromoles/l, then toxic symptoms appear. Even toxic concentrations are relatively low compared with those of most other blood-borne compounds and are insufficient to disturb the pH balance of the blood. Instead, high concentrations of $NH_4^+$ disturb some of the metabolic equilibria we have already met.

The two deamination reactions that convert glutamine to α-ketoglutarate produce $NH_4^+$, plus a reduced cofactor and a TCA cycle intermediate (Figure 9.16). Both reactions are reversible and can be displaced in the reverse direction if $NH_4^+$ concentrations exceed normal levels. The consequences of this displacement, however, are deleterious for the brain for a number of reasons. If the reactions shown in Figure 9.16 are displaced to the left-hand side, α-ketoglutarate and NADH are depleted and both of them are vital components of the oxidative metabolism on which the brain depends for energy generation. Levels of the neurotransmitter glutamate are also depleted, leading to functional impairment. Moreover, the ultimate product of the displacement, glutamine, accumulates and, by an unknown mechanism, leads to cell swelling.

### DEGRADATION OF AMINO-ACID CARBON SKELETONS

Each carbon skeleton has its individual pathway of degradation but there are seven eventual degradation products for all 20 amino acids. These products are shown in Figure 9.17 and all represent intermediates on pathways previously encountered in this chapter.

Given that one of the situations identified when amino acid degradation occurs at high rates is that of starvation, an important property of amino acids concerns whether or not they may contribute to glucose synthesis.

### GLUCOGENIC AND KETOGENIC AMINO ACIDS

Amino acids can be classified according to whether their carbon skeleton can contribute to the synthesis of glucose (glucogenic amino acids) or ketone bodies (ketogenic amino acids). Inspection of Figure 9.17 will show that any carbon skeleton converted to α-ketoglutarate or a later TCA cycle intermediate or to pyruvate can eventually become an intermediate of the gluconeogenic pathway and produce glucose. By contrast, amino acids that are converted to acetyl CoA or to acetoacetyl CoA cannot contribute to glucose synthesis (because of the loss of $CO_2$ from the cycle). Instead, this second group of carbon skeletons can produce ketone bodies.

FIGURE 9.15 **Synthesis of urea**

$$NH_4^+ + Bicarbonate + aspartate \ (amino \ acid) \xrightarrow[\quad]{3\ ATP \quad 2\ ADP + AMP} Urea + Fumarate \ (TCA \ cycle \ intermediate)$$

ADP = adenosine diphosphate | AMP = adenosine monophosphate | TCA = tricarboxylic acid

FIGURE 9.16  **Equilibria displaced by high concentrations of NH₄⁺**

GABA = γ-aminobutyric acid  |  NADH = reduced form of nicotinamide adenine dinucleotide  |  NH₄⁺ = ammonium ion  |  TCA = tricarboxylic acid

Both glucose and ketone bodies are important fuels during intermediate and prolonged starvation: both can be oxidised by many tissues (including the brain) to produce ATP. However, an especial significance attaches to the provision of glucose during starvation, because blood glucose levels must be maintained above 3 mmol/l to retain the accessibility of this substrate for the brain's glucose transporter.

Thus, when muscle protein breakdown accelerates during starvation, alanine and glutamine represent 60–70% of all amino acids released by muscle tissue. This does not reflect the composition of muscle protein, which is made up of a wide variety of the 20 amino acids available. Rather, it reflects the occurrence of transamination reactions within the muscle tissue that convert the constituent amino acids of muscle protein into alanine and glutamine. These two amino acids represent a stable means of transporting carbon to the liver, where the pathway of gluconeogenesis occurs (Figure 9.6).

Once in the liver, further rounds of transamination and deamination convert alanine and glutamine into pyruvate and α-ketoglutarate, respectively, which join the gluconeogenic pathway by the routes shown in Figure 9.18. Pyruvate is an intermediate on the cytosolic gluconeogenic pathway and is directly converted to glucose. α-Ketoglutarate is converted to oxaloacetate by

FIGURE 9.17  **Degradation of carbon skeletons derived from amino acid metabolism**

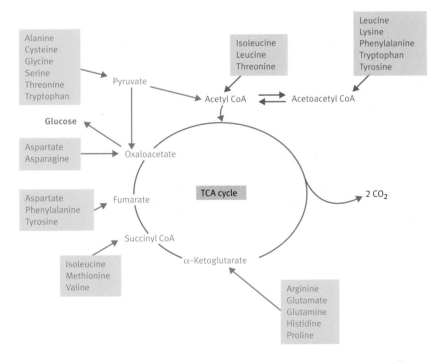

Glucogenic amino acids and intermediates are shown in red; ketogenic amino acids and intermediates are shown in blue.  |  CoA = coenzyme A  |  TCA = tricarboxylic acid

FIGURE 9.18 **Conversion of glucogenic amino acids to glucose**

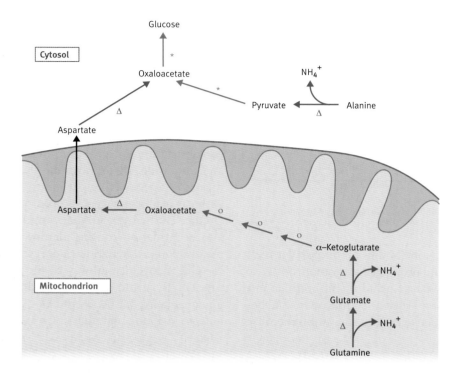

\* = gluconeogenic pathway | ○ = tricarboxylic acid cycle | ∆ = transamination reactions | $NH_4^+$ = ammonium ion

reactions of the TCA cycle and then must be transaminated to aspartate to leave the mitochondrion because the membrane is impermeable to oxaloacetate. Once in the cytosol, aspartate is transaminated to oxaloacetate, an intermediate on the gluconeogenic pathway.

Protein metabolism makes a vital contribution to the provision of glucose for the brain during starvation. This is an expensive process, however, since loss of muscle protein is accompanied by loss of function. To maximise the utility of glucogenic substrates, such as amino acids, starvation conditions are characterised by the adoption of a glucose-sparing strategy: tissues that are able to use substrates other than glucose do so during starvation and, thus, spare the precious glucose resources for the brain.

Quantitatively, the most significant among the tissues that adopt such a strategy is skeletal muscle, largely because of the huge mass it represents. During starvation, when plasma fatty acids are abundant but levels of glucose and insulin are low, muscle relies heavily on uptake

and oxidation of fatty acids and high rates of these processes serve to inhibit its uptake of glucose.

## INTEGRATION OF METABOLIC PATHWAYS IN THE LIVER DURING STARVATION

Owing to its role in glucose homeostasis, the liver bears the brunt of adaptation to starvation conditions. It is the only tissue that performs appreciable rates of gluconeogenesis and is the sole site of ketogenesis. We have seen that these two pathways are integrated (Figure 9.12) and that the balance between the gluconeogenic intermediate, oxaloacetate, and the ketogenic substrate, acetyl CoA, is crucial in determining rates of ketone body synthesis.

Now we can see that protein metabolism has an impact on this scheme, too. The supply of glucogenic amino acids, along with activation of gluconeogenesis by the hormones glucagon and cortisol, maintains appropriate rates of glucose synthesis (Figure 9.6).

FIGURE 9.19 **Molecular basis of phenylketonuria**

pheH = phenylalanine hydroxylase | DOPA = 3,4-dihydroxyphenylalanine

## Inborn errors of metabolism

A short word could profitably be said about inborn errors of metabolism, a disproportionate number of which seem to affect the metabolism of amino acids. We have already noted the effects of such disorders with respect to the urea cycle. Such conditions are characterised by genetic mutations that affect pathway enzymes. When the mutation produces an enzyme of greatly diminished activity, the result is that a substrate commonly present in the diet cannot be metabolised. A relatively common inborn error with potentially disastrous consequences is phenylketonuria.

### PHENYLKETONURIA

Phenylketonuria occurs in approximately one in 10 000 babies born in the UK and around 300 polymorphisms are thought to result in the same phenotype. The disorder is characterised by the absence or greatly diminished activity of the enzyme phenylalanine hydroxylase, with the result that the common amino acid, phenylalanine cannot be metabolised (Figure 9.19).

The consequences are various. Phenylalanine levels rise so that the amino acid takes part in unusual side reactions that produce phenylpyruvate, phenyllactate and phenylacetate (Figure 9.19). These compounds would normally be undetectable but appear in the urine when phenylketonuria is present.

The accumulation of phenylalanine itself interferes with uptake of many other amino acids by competition with the saturable amino acid transporter. This has a severe impact on the developing brain, which has a large requirement for amino acids for the synthesis of neurotransmitters and myelin and to promote growth. In addition, phenylpyruvate probably interferes with the oxidative metabolism by competing with pyruvate for mitochondrial uptake. Again, this has a severe impact on the brain, a highly oxidative tissue that relies heavily on the oxidation of pyruvate generated from glucose to fuel its energy requirements.

It is, unfortunately, rather predictable that the most severe symptoms suffered by those with untreated phenylketonuria concern gross mental restriction (IQ below 50). However, screening programmes mean that phenylketonuria is readily detected by means of the Guthrie test, which is carried out 6–14 days after birth. A spot of the baby's blood is used to supplement the medium of a bacterial strain that requires phenylalanine for growth. If the blood levels are above 240 micromoles/l, the bacteria flourish and phenylketonuria can be diagnosed.

Treatment involves the pursuit of a dietary regimen that excludes all but the minimal amounts of phenylalanine necessary for protein synthesis but includes sufficient amounts of tyrosine and other amino acids. Since accumulation of phenylalanine mainly affects the developing brain, the diet must be followed strictly until the age of around 11 years but can then be relaxed. It must be resumed during pregnancy to protect the fetal brain. Many commercial protein substitutes are available to control phenylalanine intake but noncompliance (possibly owing to the unpalatability of the protein substitutes) is common. As a consequence, many phenylketonuria sufferers, although diagnosed and treated, endure some degree of cognitive deficit.

Inspection of Figure 9.19 reveals that the metabolism of phenylalanine is closely linked to that of the amino acid tyrosine, a precursor for the pigment melanin. As a consequence of disruption of the melanin synthetic pathway, partial albinism accompanies the other symptoms of phenylketonuria. Other inborn errors of metabolism can also affect the pathways shown in Figure 9.19; lack of tyrosinase causes occulocutaneous albinism and lack of homogentisate 1,2-dioxygenase causes alkaptonuria.

FIGURE 9.20 **Fuel in the maternal–fetal unit**

FIGURE 9.21 **Summary of energy-yielding pathways in the newborn**

TAG = triacylglycerol

## Metabolic adaptation

Fuels used and metabolic pathways available vary hugely over the lifespan and a good example of this is the difference between fetal and neonatal metabolism.

### METABOLISM IN THE MATERNAL–FETAL UNIT

After an initial increase in insulin sensitivity in early pregnancy, mild insulin resistance develops in maternal tissues. Sensitivity can be reduced by 50–70% by the third trimester. This means that anabolic activities, such as lipogenesis and deposition of fat and glycogen by maternal tissues, are favoured in the first trimester but, by late pregnancy, nutrient uptake by the fetus is favoured at the expense of that by the mother.

During the late phase of pregnancy, maternal tissues take up little glucose but oxidise the abundant circulating fatty acids and ketone bodies at high rates (Figure 9.20). By contrast, the fetus consumes and oxidises glucose at high rates, aided by the maternal insulin resistance. Maternal blood glucose levels (which can rise steeply if GDM is present) are predictive of birth weight.

The fetus has little, if any, oxidative capacity for ketone bodies and fatty acids, although placental lipoprotein lipase activity increases in late gestation to allow storage

of fat in preparation for birth. Overall, fetal nutrition is oriented very much towards the consumption of glucose.

### METABOLISM IN THE NEWBORN BABY

The baby's metabolism matures enormously around the time of birth, with many metabolic pathways becoming active that cannot be detected in the fetus. The newborn liver is replete with glycogen and this, together with the emergent pathway of gluconeogenesis (inactive in the fetus), serves to regulate blood glucose levels (Figure 9.21).

The capacity of the liver for fatty acid oxidation also increases dramatically to meet energy requirements and supply the newly active ketogenic pathway with substrate. Hepatic lipogenic capacity, however, remains low during suckling, when fats are supplied through milk, and only increases markedly on weaning. The metabolic pathways available to newborn babies equip them for consumption of a relatively high-fat diet (human milk has a fat content of approximately 42 g/l). Lipoprotein lipase activity in tissues such as heart, skeletal muscle and brown adipose tissue increases dramatically during suckling to increase the availability of dietary fats to those tissues. This high enzymatic activity is maintained until weaning.

Dietary fats are vital for several purposes, other than energy generation. Human milk is rich in polyunsaturated fats, such as the omega-3 fatty acid α-linoleic acid. Long-chain derivatives of α-linoleic acid, such as docosahexaenoic acid (DHA), are crucial for development of the specialised membranes of the central nervous system. About two-thirds of the central nervous system content of DHA is laid down during the last trimester of gestation with the remaining third being incorporated during the first 3 months of life. Even a small interruption of DHA supply during these crucial periods can lead to impairment of cognitive development and compromise visual acuity.

Moreover, fatty acids are the fuel consumed by a specialised thermogenic organ, brown adipose tissue (Figure 9.21). Human newborns lack the appropriate muscular development to enable heat generation by shivering. Instead, they have large deposits of brown adipose tissue, especially in the interscapular region. Owing to the partial uncoupling of electron transport from ATP synthesis in brown adipose mitochondria, this tissue is able to harness the chemical energy contained in fatty acids for heat production (instead of for ATP generation) in a process of nonshivering thermogenesis (Figure 9.21).

## REFERENCES

1. STERN L, IQBAL N, SESHADRI P, CHICANO K L, DAILY D A, McGRORY J et al. The effects of a low-carbohydrate versus conventional weight loss diet in severely obese patients: one-year follow-up of a randomized trial. *Ann Intern Med* 2004;140:778–85.

2. YANCY W S Jr, OLSEN M K, GUYTON J R, BAKST R P, WESTMAN E C. A low carbohydrate, ketogenic diet versus a low fat diet to treat obesity and hyperlipidaemia. *Ann Intern Med* 2004;140:769–77.

3. OATS J N, BEISCHNER N A, GRAND P T. The emergence of diabetes and impaired glucose tolerance in women who had gestational diabetes. In: Weiss P A M, Coustan D R, editors. *Gestational Diabetes*. New York: Springer-Verlag; 1988. p.199–207.

4. ALBRINK M J, NEWIRTH R S. Effect of previous starvation on the response of plasma lipids and free fatty acids to a fat meal. *J Clin Invest* 1960;39:441–6.

5. TAGGART P, CARRUTHERS M. Endogenous hyperlipidaemia induced by emotional stress of racing driving. *Lancet* 1971;i: 363–6.

6. FRIEDBERG S J, HARLAN W R, TROUT D L, ESTES E H. The effect of exercise on the concentration and turnover of plasma non-esterified fatty acids. *J Clin Invest* 1960;39:215–20.

7. WATKINS P J, HILL D M, FITZGERALD M G, MALINS J M. Ketonaemia in uncontrolled diabetes. *Br Med J* 1970;4:522–5.

8. MEYER B, CALVERT D, MOSES R. Free fatty acids and gestational diabetes mellitus. *Aust N Z J Obstet Gynaecol* 1996;36:255–7.

# Sample questions relating to cell and molecular biology

## EXTENDED MATCHING QUESTIONS

### Questions 1–5

- *This question relates to the human cell cycle. For each phase below, select the **single** correct process from the list of options (A–H) by which it is characterised. Each option may be used once, more than once or not at all.*

OPTIONS

▷ **A**  RNA synthesis
▷ **B**  DNA synthesis
▷ **C**  Meiosis
▷ **D**  Mitosis
▷ **E**  Preparation for DNA synthesis
▷ **F**  Preparation for mitosis
▷ **G**  Preparation for meiosis
▷ **H**  Resting phase

**1** ▶  M phase

**2** ▶  S phase

**3** ▶  G0 phase

**4** ▶  G1 phase

**5** ▶  G2 phase

## MULTIPLE CHOICE QUESTIONS

**6** ▶  Regarding eukaryotic cell membranes:

   **A** ▷ Cholesterol makes the phospholipid bilayer of the plasma membrane become firm
   **B** ▷ Receptors for circulating molecules are found on the inside of the plasma membrane
   **C** ▷ Protein receptors are embedded within the plasma membrane
   **D** ▷ The Golgi complex has a single membrane surrounding it
   **E** ▷ The nucleus has a double membrane

**7** ▶  Regarding the nucleus of the cell:

   **A** ▷ It is the second largest organelle
   **B** ▷ The nuclear envelope is a single membrane
   **C** ▷ Messenger RNA is transported out of the nucleus
   **D** ▷ Ribosomal RNA is synthesised entirely within the nucleolus
   **E** ▷ The nucleus membrane is often continuous with the rough endoplasmic reticulum

**8** ▶  The following are synthesised inside the smooth endoplasmic reticulum:

   **A** ▷ Enzymes
   **B** ▷ Fatty acids
   **C** ▷ Glucose
   **D** ▷ Phospholipids
   **E** ▷ Proteins

**9** ▶  The rough endoplasmic reticulum:

   **A** ▷ has ribosomes attached to its surface
   **B** ▷ synthesises cell proteins
   **C** ▷ retains proteins for several days
   **D** ▷ is abundant in the pancreatic acinar cells
   **E** ▷ sends proteins to the smooth endoplasmic reticulum

**10** ▶  Human mitochondria characteristically:

   **A** ▷ metabolise proteins
   **B** ▷ have a smooth inner surface
   **C** ▷ contain cytosol
   **D** ▷ have reactions that occur in the intermembrane space
   **E** ▷ have DNA inherited through the mother only

**11** ▶  Regarding the cell's 'disposal system':

   **A** ▷ Lysosomes and peroxisomes have double membranes
   **B** ▷ Lysosomes and peroxisomes contain enzymes
   **C** ▷ Lysosomes have an internal pH of 3.0
   **D** ▷ Peroxisomes remove toxic molecules from the blood
   **E** ▷ Peroxisomes are the main organelle for oxidising fatty acids

**12** ▶ Regarding cell–cell signalling:

    **A** ▷ Endocrine signalling always relies on the bloodstream for transport

    **B** ▷ Neurotransmitters are a form of autocrine transmission

    **C** ▷ Self-signalling is known as autocrine signalling

    **D** ▷ Membrane-bound signalling proteins interact with receptors on a neighbouring cell

    **E** ▷ Gap junctions help retain cell rigidity

**13** ▶ Human eicosanoids:

    **A** ▷ are cell signalling molecules

    **B** ▷ are made in the mitochondria

    **C** ▷ are made by all cells

    **D** ▷ are all made from arachidonic acid

    **E** ▷ help myometrial relaxation

**14** ▶ Regarding cyclooxygenase (COX):

    **A** ▷ COX-1 is expressed at sites of inflammation

    **B** ▷ Aspirin temporarily inactivates platelet COX

    **C** ▷ Aspirin is more active against COX-1 than against COX-2

    **D** ▷ Aspirin is a COX antagonist

    **E** ▷ Fetal membranes release COX-2 during labour

**15** ▶ Regarding $Ca^{2+}$ as an intracellular messenger:

    **A** ▷ The intracellular concentration of free $Ca^{2+}$ is higher than the $Ca^{2+}$ concentration of the extracellular fluid

    **B** ▷ The endoplasmic reticulum has high levels of free $Ca^{2+}$

    **C** ▷ Mitochondria pump $Ca^{2+}$ in from the cytosol

    **D** ▷ $Ca^{2+}$-ATPases pump $Ca^{2+}$ out of cells

    **E** ▷ the $Ca^{2+}$–calmodulin complex directly activates smooth muscle contraction

**16** ▶ Regarding the molecular basis of cancer:

    **A** ▷ Oncogenes are present in tumour cells only

    **B** ▷ Proto-oncogenes are required for normal cell growth

    **C** ▷ Tumour cells have less mitotic activity than normal cells

    **D** ▷ *p*53 mutations are present in half of all cancers

    **E** ▷ Presence of the protein adenomatous polyposis coli (APC) is a cause of colorectal cancer

**17** ▶ Regarding neoplastic cells:

    **A** ▷ They are usually well differentiated

    **B** ▷ Carcinomas can be derived from endoderm

    **C** ▷ Sarcomas are derived from ectoderm

    **D** ▷ Metastatic tumour cells break down the basal lamina

    **E** ▷ Tumour masses of more than 1 mm need their own blood supply

**18** ▶ Regarding nucleic acids:

    **A** ▷ DNA is longer than RNA

    **B** ▷ RNA is single-stranded

    **C** ▷ DNA strands are held together by ionic bonds

    **D** ▷ uracil replaces guanine in RNA

    **E** ▷ DNA and RNA contain the same pentose sugar

**19** ▶ Regarding the synthesis of messenger RNA (mRNA):

    **A** ▷ The process is called translation

    **B** ▷ RNA polymerase is the main enzyme of this process

    **C** ▷ The base sequence of the mRNA transcript matches that of the template strand

    **D** ▷ Only one mRNA copy is produced from each part of DNA

    **E** ▷ Exons are removed from the mRNA

**20** ▶ Regarding protein synthesis:

    **A** ▷ The final step of forming proteins from messenger RNA is called transcription

    **B** ▷ The whole process requires mRNA, ribosomal RNA and transfer RNA

    **C** ▷ Transfer RNA carries three amino acids

    **D** ▷ Ribosomes have no role in the final part of protein synthesis, where messenger RNA acts as a blueprint for the sequence of amino acids

    **E** ▷ The tertiary structure of a protein depends on hydrophilic interactions between different parts of the amino acid sequence

# Sample questions relating to steroids and prostaglandins

## EXTENDED MATCHING QUESTIONS

### Questions 1–4

■ *This question relates to prostaglandins. For each prostaglandin below, select the* **single** *correct secondary messenger effect from the list of options (A–G). Each option may be used once, more than once or not at all.*

OPTIONS

▷ **A** Several effects
▷ **B** Increases the concentration of $Ca^{2+}$
▷ **C** Increases the concentration of cyclic adenosine monophosphate (cAMP)
▷ **D** Increases the concentrations of inositol trisphosphate and $Ca^{2+}$
▷ **E** Decreases the concentration of $Ca^{2+}$
▷ **F** Decreases the concentration of cAMP
▷ **G** Decreases the concentrations of inositol trisphosphate, increases $Ca^{2+}$

1 ▶ Prostaglandin $D_2$

2 ▶ Prostaglandin $E_2$

3 ▶ Prostaglandin $F_{2\alpha}$

4 ▶ Prostaglandin $I_2$

## MULTIPLE CHOICE QUESTIONS

5 ▶ Regarding the synthesis of steroids:

A ▷ The process involves two classes of enzyme
B ▷ Cytochrome P450 increases steroid solubility
C ▷ The pattern of enzyme expression determines the type of steroid produced
D ▷ The placenta can form the full range of steroids
E ▷ Estriol is unique to the fetus

6 ▶ Regarding steroid hormone receptors:

A ▷ Steroids cannot pass through the plasma membrane
B ▷ The ligand-binding domain has a hydrophilic binding site
C ▷ The DNA-binding domain contains sulphur bridges
D ▷ Steroid receptors exist on the plasma membrane and the nucleus membrane
E ▷ An activated steroid receptor translocates into the nucleus

7 ▶ The following are steroid receptors:

A ▷ Aldosterone receptor
B ▷ Androgen receptor
C ▷ Cortisol receptor
D ▷ Estrogen receptor
E ▷ Progesterone receptor

8 ▶ Regarding the synthesis of prostaglandins:

A ▷ All prostaglandins are synthesised from arachidonic acid
B ▷ Arachidonic acid is found in the cytosol
C ▷ Phospholipase $A_1$ releases free arachidonate
D ▷ Cyclooxygenase enzymes act on the free arachidonate
E ▷ Prostaglandin $G_2$ is the first prostaglandin formed

9 ▶ Regarding prostaglandins:

A ▷ They act via G proteins
B ▷ They act by freely transcending the plasma membrane
C ▷ They have fast response times
D ▷ Prostaglandin $F_{2\alpha}$ exerts its cellular effects via $Ca^{2+}$ signalling
E ▷ Prostaglandin $E_2$ transduces its signals via changes in the intracellular concentration of cyclic adenosine monophosphate (cAMP)

10 ▶ Regarding myometrial contractions:

A ▷ They are caused by oxytocin
B ▷ They are caused by prostaglandin $F_2$
C ▷ They are caused by hormones that increase the concentration of cyclic adenosine monophosphate (cAMP)
D ▷ Oxytocin suppresses uterine prostaglandin synthesis
E ▷ Prostaglandin $F_2$ increases the number of oxytocin receptors on the uterus

11 ▶ Regarding progesterone:

A ▷ It is the most important myometrial relaxant
B ▷ It increases the intracellular concentration of cyclic adenosine monophosphate (cAMP)
C ▷ It influences the action of oxytocin only
D ▷ Placental output is stable throughout pregnancy
E ▷ Prostacyclin opposes its actions

12 ▶ Regarding prostaglandins:

A ▷ They are a class of leucotrienes
B ▷ They share the common precursor arachidonic acid
C ▷ They increase the flux of $Ca^{2+}$ from the extracellular fluid into myometrial muscle to cause myometrial contractility
D ▷ Only prostaglandin $E_2$ can ripen the cervix
E ▷ During labour, the cervix is the most important location of prostaglandin release

# Sample questions relating to fluid and acid–base balance

## EXTENDED MATCHING QUESTIONS

### Questions 1–6

■ *This question relates to clinical states of acid–base disturbance. For each item below, choose the* **single** *best option from the list of options (A–H). Each option may be used once, more than once or not at all.*

#### OPTIONS

▷ **A** Acidosis
▷ **B** Alkalosis
▷ **C** Acidaemia
▷ **D** Alkalaemia
▷ **E** Respiratory alkalosis
▷ **F** Respiratory acidosis
▷ **G** Metabolic alkalosis
▷ **H** Metabolic acidosis

1 ▶ Causes the blood pH value to be lower than expected

2 ▶ Is caused by an increase in the partial pressure of $O_2$

3 ▶ Causes the blood pH value to be higher than expected

4 ▶ Causes a decrease in the partial pressure of $CO_2$

5 ▶ Causes an increase in the concentration of bicarbonate ions

6 ▶ Causes an increase in the partial pressure of $CO_2$

## MULTIPLE CHOICE QUESTIONS

7 ▶ During pregnancy:

A ▷ the $Na^+$ plasma concentration decreases
B ▷ the plasma volume increases from 3 to 4.5 l
C ▷ the interstitial-fluid volume remains unchanged
D ▷ the intracellular-fluid volume remains the same
E ▷ there is no change in the colloid osmotic pressure of plasma

8 ▶ Regarding the acid–base balance of the extracellular fluid:

A ▷ Acidosis occurs when the blood is more acidic than normal
B ▷ Buffers readjust the pH value of the extracellular fluid over a few hours
C ▷ Renal mechanisms that adjust $H^+$ excretion begin to work within minutes
D ▷ The buffer capacity of a buffer is greatest when it is all in either a weak alkaline or a weak acidic form
E ▷ The bicarbonate system is a strong buffer

9 ▶ Regarding the acid–base balance:

A ▷ Haemoglobin has multiple acidic and basic groups
B ▷ Oxygenated haemoglobin is a better buffer then deoxygenated haemoglobin
C ▷ $CO_2$ dissolves better in plasma if haemoglobin is oxygenated
D ▷ $CO_2$ that enters red blood cells can be catalysed by carbonic anhydrase to form carbonic acid
E ▷ Bicarbonate ions diffuse out of red blood cells in exchange for $Cl^-$ ions

**10 ▶** In labour:

**A** ▷ the mother tends to have an uncompensated respiratory acidosis

**B** ▷ maternal haemoglobin has an increased affinity for $O_2$

**C** ▷ there is a decrease in the concentration of deoxygenated haemoglobin in the fetus

**D** ▷ the fetus becomes acidotic because of its metabolism

**E** ▷ respiratory acidosis does not occur in the fetus

# Sample questions relating to $Ca^{2+}$ homeostasis and bones

## MULTIPLE CHOICE QUESTIONS

**1 ▶** The body uses $Ca^{2+}$ for the following processes:

**A** ▷ Muscle contraction

**B** ▷ Extracellular messenger

**C** ▷ Intracellular messenger

**D** ▷ Enzyme co-factor

**E** ▷ Stabilisation of membrane potentials

**2 ▶** The following play a role in $Ca^{2+}$ homeostasis:

**A** ▷ Bone

**B** ▷ Kidney

**C** ▷ Parathyroid glands

**D** ▷ Thyroid gland

**E** ▷ Gastrointestinal tract

**3 ▶** Regarding parathyroid hormone (PTH):

**A** ▷ Primary hyperparathyroidism is characterised by low serum concentrations of PTH and $Ca^{2+}$

**B** ▷ It promotes the renal excretion of phosphate

**C** ▷ It decreases the renal synthesis of calcitriol

**D** ▷ It is not synthesised by the fetus

**E** ▷ Secretion of PTH is increased by a decrease in serum Ca2+

**4 ▶** Regarding vitamin D:

**A** ▷ It is a polypeptide

**B** ▷ Fifty percent is acquired from the diet

**C** ▷ It is activated in the liver by $1\alpha$-hydroxylase

**D** ▷ It increases serum levels of $Ca^{2+}$ and $PO_4^{3-}$ by decreasing the rate of active secretion

**E** ▷ The major circulating form of vitamin D is 25-hydroxvitamin $D_3$ (calcidiol)

**5 ▶** Regarding vitamin D:

**A** ▷ It decreases the serum $Ca^{2+}$ concentration

**B** ▷ It decreases the serum phosphate concentration

**C** ▷ Calcitriol is metabolically active

**D** ▷ Calcidiol is metabolically active

**E** ▷ It is transported in the blood bound to vitamin-D-binding protein

**6 ▶** Regarding the synthesis of vitamin D:

**A** ▷ It requires ultraviolet light

**B** ▷ The first precursor to vitamin D is hydrocholesterol

**C** ▷ Vitamin $D_2$ and vitamin $D_3$ are hydroxylated to the same product

**D** ▷ Active vitamin D is formed in the distal convoluted tubule

**E** ▷ It is increased by low serum concentrations of phosphate

**7 ▶** Regarding the maternal and fetal $Ca^{2+}$ balance:

**A** ▷ In the fetus, 80% of $Ca^{2+}$ accumulation occurs in the first trimester

**B** ▷ Maternal bone mineral density decreases continually through pregnancy

**C** ▷ Low maternal vitamin D levels mean that the fetus is more likely to develop diabetes

**D** ▷ The neonate has low serum calcitonin

**E** ▷ The mother has high levels of parathyroid hormone

**8 ▶** Regarding the structure of bone:

**A** ▷ Seventy-five percent is matrix

**B** ▷ Ninety percent of matrix is type 1 collagen

**C** ▷ The mineral component contains $Ca^{2+}$

**D**◁ ➥ mineral component provides resilience

**E** ▷ Collagen provides rigidity

**9 ▶** Trabecular bone:

**A** ▷ is strong

**B** ▷ is heavy

**C** ▷ forms the outer part of bone

**D** ▷ is spongy in appearance

**E** ▷ has a high surface area

**10 ▶** In the metabolism of bone:

**A** ▷ osteoblasts produce bone

**B** ▷ osteoblasts respond to mechanical strain

**C** ▷ each osteoblast is constantly active

**D** ▷ osteoclasts reabsorb bone

**E** ▷ osteocytes produce matrix

11 ▶ Regarding bone remodelling:

  A ▷ A complete cycle takes 180 days
  B ▷ The process takes place deep in the bone
  C ▷ The process involves both osteoblast and osteoclasts
  D ▷ Hydroxyapatite is not destroyed
  E ▷ Gaps left by osteoclasts are filled with hydroxyapatite

12 ▶ Osteoporosis:

  A ▷ is associated with underactive osteoblasts
  B ▷ is only caused by a loss of estrogen
  C ▷ is diagnosed by a low score following a dual energy X-ray absorptiometry scan
  D ▷ does not occur in women below the age of 65 years
  E ▷ is associated with low body weight, cigarette smoking, alcohol consumption, poor nutrition and physical inactivity

13 ▶ Regarding osteopenia:

  A ▷ It is diagnosed if the bone mineral density is more than 2.5 standard deviations away from the mean value for a young healthy adult
  B ▷ The loss of bone mineral is greater than in osteoporosis
  C ▷ Increasing $Ca^{2+}$ intake is essential to prevent progression
  D ▷ It is more common in women with prolonged secondary amenorrhoea
  E ▷ It is more common in people with long-term steroid use

14 ▶ The following are true regarding osteoporosis:

  A ▷ Maximum bone mass is reached in puberty
  B ▷ Men have a higher maximum bone mass than women
  C ▷ Any decrease in bone mineral density is dangerous
  D ▷ Bone mass remains constant until the age of around 50 years
  E ▷ Excluding the menopause, women still have a faster loss in bone mineral density than men

15 ▶ The following are true regarding osteoporosis:

  A ▷ Hypogonadism is the most common cause of osteoporosis in men
  B ▷ An increase in body weight makes osteoporotic fractures more common
  C ▷ Heparin increases the risk of osteoporotic fractures
  D ▷ It is more common in hyperthyroidism
  E ▷ It is more common in Cushing syndrome

## Sample questions relating to fat, carbohydrate and protein metabolism

### EXTENDED MATCHING QUESTIONS

#### Questions 1–9

■ *The list of options relates to lipoproteins. For each item below, choose the* **single** *best option from the list of options (A–H). Each option may be used once, more than once or not at all.*

OPTIONS

▷ A Chylomicron
▷ B Very-low-density lipoprotein
▷ C Low-density lipoprotein
▷ D High-density lipoprotein
▷ E Fatty acid–albumin
▷ F Free fatty acid
▷ G Vitamin E
▷ H Brown fat

1 ▶ Made of dietary triacylglycerols

2 ▶ Transports cholesterol from tissues to the liver

3 ▶ Made from endogenous triacylglycerols

4 ▶ Transports triacylglycerols from the liver to other tissues

5 ▶ Made from cholesterol and cholesteryl ester

6 ▶ Made from fatty acids

7 ▶ Made from cholesteryl ester only

**8 ▶** Transports triacylglycerols from the intestine to other tissues

**9 ▶** Transports cholesterol from the liver to other tissues

## MULTIPLE CHOICE QUESTIONS

**10 ▶** Regarding metabolism:

 **A** ▷ All reactions are reversible
 **B** ▷ All pathways run at the same speed
 **C** ▷ Triacylglycerols are broken down to free fatty acids
 **D** ▷ All substances are eventually converted to acetyl coenzyme A
 **E** ▷ Acetyl coenzyme A is hydrolysed

**11 ▶** Regarding the metabolism of carbohydrates:

 **A** ▷ They can be ingested as huge polymers
 **B** ▷ Disaccharides are a readily available glucose source
 **C** ▷ Sucrose produces a slow rise in blood sugar
 **D** ▷ Glucose polymers are slow to be digested
 **E** ▷ All dietary carbohydrate can be converted to glucose

**12 ▶** Regarding the metabolism of glucose:

 **A** ▷ Aerobic glucose metabolism yields more ATP than anaerobic metabolism
 **B** ▷ Under anaerobical conditions, glucose is converted into pyruvate
 **C** ▷ All tissues can consume glucose
 **D** ▷ Glucose is quickly replenished in the blood after it has been removed
 **E** ▷ Glucose is the only fuel that can be respired anaerobically

**13 ▶** Regarding the anaerobic metabolism of glucose:

 **A** ▷ The presence of lactate confirms anaerobic glucose metabolism
 **B** ▷ Lactate is a metabolic dead end
 **C** ▷ Lactate cannot be reduced back to pyruvate
 **D** ▷ The formation of lactate from pyruvate requires oxidised nicotinamide adenine dinucleotide ($NAD^+$)
 **E** ▷ Glucose can be formed from lactate

**14 ▶** Regarding the homeostasis of blood glucose:

 **A** ▷ In people without diabetes, the fasting blood glucose concentration can be as low as 3 mmol/l
 **B** ▷ In people without diabetes, the postprandial blood glucose concentration can be as high as 8 mmol/l
 **C** ▷ Pregnant women tolerate lower fasting blood glucose concentrations than nonpregnant women
 **D** ▷ Glucose only appears in the urine if the blood glucose concentration rises above 9 mmol/l
 **E** ▷ Hypoglycaemic coma can result from overconsumption of alcohol

**15 ▶** The following increase the breakdown of triacylglycerols:

 **A** ▷ Adrenaline
 **B** ▷ Diabetic coma
 **C** ▷ Glucagon
 **D** ▷ Insulin
 **E** ▷ Noradrenaline

**16 ▶** Regarding the plasma concentration of triacylglycerols:

 **A** ▷ It is lowered in exercise
 **B** ▷ It is lowered in stress
 **C** ▷ It is raised in people with diabetes
 **D** ▷ If elevated, this increases the risk of coronary heart disease
 **E** ▷ It is at its lowest in the normal fed state

**17 ▶** Regarding diabetic ketoacidosis:

 **A** ▷ It occurs predominantly in type 2 diabetes
 **B** ▷ It causes a hypoxic coma
 **C** ▷ It occurs in people with diabetes who have a concurrent illness
 **D** ▷ There is a decrease in the affinity of haemoglobin for $O_2$
 **E** ▷ Treatment is by rapid infusion of insulin

**18 ▶** The following are signs of diabetic ketoacidosis:

 **A** ▷ Hyperglycaemia
 **B** ▷ Glycosuria
 **C** ▷ Hyperkalaemia
 **D** ▷ Low partial pressure of $O_2$
 **E** ▷ High partial pressure of $CO_2$

19 ▶ The following are related to the development of diabetic ketoacidosis:

A ▷ Dehydration
B ▷ Hypoxia
C ▷ Low fatty acids
D ▷ Low kidney excretion of H$^+$
E ▷ Osmotic diuresis

20 ▶ Regarding gestational diabetes:

A ▷ All women have some insulin resistance in pregnancy
B ▷ Blood levels of insulin are high
C ▷ Blood levels of fatty acids are low
D ▷ It is diagnosed using a random blood sugar test
E ▷ It lasts for the duration of pregnancy only

21 ▶ The following elements form parts of proteins:

A ▷ Carbon
B ▷ Hydrogen
C ▷ Nitrogen
D ▷ Oxygen
E ▷ Silicon

22 ▶ The following increase protein breakdown:

A ▷ Exercise
B ▷ Growth
C ▷ High-protein diet
D ▷ Pregnancy
E ▷ Starvation

23 ▶ Regarding the urea cycle:

A ▷ It incorporates 1 mole of nitrogen into 1 mole of urea
B ▷ Its dysfunction causes brain oedema in newborn babies
C ▷ It produces energy
D ▷ It occurs in the liver
E ▷ Its product (urea) is nonsoluble

24 ▶ Regarding amino acids:

A ▷ They all enter the tricarboxylic acid cycle
B ▷ They can all be used to form glucose
C ▷ Some amino acids can produce both glucose and ketones
D ▷ Alanine and glutamine represent 70% of the amino acids released by muscle to produce glucose
E ▷ Tyrosine is ketogenic

25 ▶ The following are end products of the metabolism of phenylalanine by phenylalanine hydroxylase:

A ▷ Thyroxine
B ▷ Melanin
C ▷ Oxygen
D ▷ Water
E ▷ Phenylacetate

26 ▶ Regarding phenylketonuria:

A ▷ The accumulation of phenylalanine increases the uptake of other amino acids by the brain
B ▷ Affected people have mild mental restriction
C ▷ Screening involves the Guthrie test
D ▷ Screening should take place within 3 days of birth
E ▷ Treatment is with a special diet until the age of 5 years

27 ▶ Regarding the complex metabolism of the maternal and fetal unit:

A ▷ There is insulin resistance in maternal tissues throughout pregnancy
B ▷ Maternal insulin sensitivity is reduced by at least 50% in pregnancy
C ▷ Maternal anabolic activities are increased in the first trimester
D ▷ Fetal nutrient uptake is favoured throughout pregnancy
E ▷ The fetus oxidises ketone bodies and fatty acids

28 ▶ Regarding metabolism of glucose and fats in the newborn baby:

A ▷ Gluconeogenesis is inactive in the fetus
B ▷ The newborn baby activates the ketogenic pathway
C ▷ There is little lipogenic capacity
D ▷ Newborns have a low-fat diet
E ▷ Lipoprotein lipase activity increases in the newborn's heart

# Biophysics

# CHAPTER 10

# Biophysics

*Nazar N Amso and Neil Pugh*

## Introduction

Most obstetricians and gynaecologists use a wide range of equipment and instruments in their clinical practice, including ultrasound, X-rays and electronic instruments for monitoring the heart. However, not all practitioners fully appreciate the background principles on which these techniques are based. It is not so much the complex knowledge of physics and formulae that is required but rather a knowledge of how the principles of physics are applied in clinical practice. This is fundamental to a better understanding of the techniques as well as their safe, optimal and efficient use. In this chapter, each of the principal sections outlines the scientific foundations and uses of a procedure frequently used in our obstetric and gynaecological practice.

## Principles and use of electrocardiography

Electrocardiography is a commonly used noninvasive procedure for the recording of electrical changes in the heart. The printed record, called electrocardiogram (ECG or EKG), traces the electrical impulses that are generated during each cardiac cycle. The waves in a normal record are labelled P, Q, R, S and T. The test evaluates cardiac function and identifies any problems that might exist in the frequency and rhythm of the heart rate or in the size and position of the heart's chambers; the test also assesses whether there is any myocardial damage.

### RELATIONSHIP BETWEEN THE CARDIAC CYCLE AND ELECTROCARDIOGRAM

Electrical stimulation of the myocardium (depolarisation) is followed by restoration of the electrical potential of the myocardial cell (repolarisation). The electrical stimulation starts at the sinoatrial node, which acts as the natural cardiac pacemaker. The electrical signal then propagates through the internodal tracts of the atria to the atrioventricular node and subsequently activates the ventricles via the His–Purkinje system. This system con-

FIGURE 10.1 **His–Purkinje system**

*Adapted by permission from*: BMJ Publishing Group Ltd. Meek S, Morris F. ABC of clinical electrocardiography. Introduction. I – Leads, rate, rhythm, and cardiac axis. *Br Med J* 324:415–8.

sists of a bundle of fibres that divides into right and left branches. The left branch further divides into left anterior and posterior hemifascicles (Figure 10.1).

In an ECG, the P wave represents atrial depolarisation, while atrial repolarisation occurs during ventricular depolarisation and hence is not visualised. The QRS wave represents ventricular depolarisation, while the T wave represents ventricular repolarisation.

The ECG is recorded onto standard paper travelling at a rate of 25 mm/second. The paper is divided into large squares, each measuring 5 mm in width and representing 0.2 seconds. Each large square is divided into 25 small squares; a small square is 1 mm wide and represents 0.04 seconds.

## ELECTRODE PLACEMENT AND SKIN PREPARATION

ECG lead electrodes are placed either in a bipolar or in a unipolar arrangement. In the bipolar lead arrangement, the electrical activity at a single positive electrode is compared with that at a single negative electrode. In the unipolar lead arrangement, the electrical potential at a single positive electrode, the so-called exploring electrode, is compared with the average electrical activity at several other electrodes, which serve as the negative pole.

The limb leads (I, II, III) are bipolar leads, while the augmented voltage leads (aVR, aVL, aVF) are unipolar leads. These six leads explore the electrical activity of the heart in the frontal plane (the orientation of the heart seen when looking directly at the anterior chest; see Figure 10.2).

The chest leads (V1, V2, V3, V4, V5, V6) explore the electrical activity of the heart in the horizontal plane (Figure 10.2). The reference point for the chest leads is obtained by connecting the left-arm, right-arm and left-leg electrodes together. The position of the six chest electrodes for standard 12-lead electrocardiography is depicted in Figure 10.3.

In a standard 12-lead ECG:

- leads II, III and aVF 'view' the inferior surface of the heart
- leads V1 to V4 view the anterior surface of the heart
- leads I, aVL, V5 and V6 view the lateral surface of the heart
- leads V1 and aVR view the right atrium and the cavity of the left ventricle.

FIGURE 10.2 **Vertical and horizontal perspectives of the electrode leads**

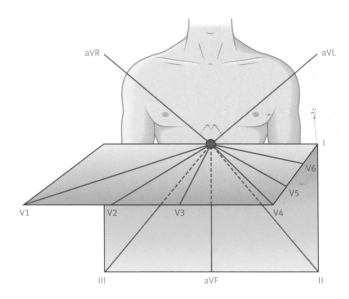

Red = frontal plane of the heart; green = horizontal plane of the heart.

*Adapted by permission from*: BMJ Publishing Group Ltd. Meek S, Morris F. ABC of clinical electrocardiography. Introduction. I – Leads, rate, rhythm, and cardiac axis. *Br Med J* 324:415–8.

FIGURE 10.3 **Position of the six chest electrodes for standard 12-lead electrocardiography**

*Adapted by permission from*: BMJ Publishing Group Ltd. Meek S, Morris F. ABC of clinical electrocardiography. Introduction. I – Leads, rate, rhythm, and cardiac axis. *Br Med J* 324:415–8.

The shape of the QRS complex in any lead depends on the orientation of that lead to the vector of depolarisation.

To obtain good electrical contact, the skin is cleaned and gel is applied before placing the electrodes. After removal of the electrodes at the end of the procedure, the skin should be thoroughly cleaned again to avoid skin irritation from the salty gel. No special precautions are required and no complications from this procedure have been observed.

### FEATURES OF A NORMAL ELECTROCARDIOGRAM

Normal sinus rhythm on an ECG has the following cardinal features:

- The heart rate is 60–99 beats/minute.
- The cardiac rhythm is regular except for minor variations with respiration.
- The P wave is upright in leads I and II.
- The normal duration of the PR interval is 0.12–20 seconds. This is the time required for the completion of atrial depolarisation, conduction through the atrioventricular node and His–Purkinje system and arrival at the ventricular myocardial cells.
- Each P wave is usually followed by a QRS complex.
- The normal duration of the QRS interval is 0.06–0.10 seconds. This represents the time required for ventricular cells to depolarise.
- Normal values for the QT interval are between 0.30 and 0.43 seconds (0.30–0.45 seconds for women). This is the time required for depolarisation and repolarisation of the ventricles.

Young healthy individuals, especially athletes, may also display various other rhythms, especially during sleep. For example, respiration may cause sinus arrhythmia, characterised by beat-to-beat variation in the RR interval, with the heart rate increasing during inspiration. This is a vagally mediated effect in response to the increased volume of blood that returns to the heart during inspiration. Other normal findings noted in healthy individuals include tall R waves, prominent U waves (reflecting repolarisation of the papillary muscles or His–Purkinje fibres), ST segment elevation, exaggerated sinus arrhythmia, sinus bradycardia and first-degree heart block.

## Principles and use of ultrasound

Diagnostic ultrasound uses the transmission of mechanical vibrations through matter to obtain some information about that matter. Ultrasound allows us to:

- determine the nature of a tissue (for example cystic or solid)
- assess the movement of tissues (such as fetal heart, bowel)
- measure blood flow (for example in the ovarian/ follicular circulation, fetal circulation)
- measure structures (such as follicular diameter, femur length).

Ultrasound has an advantage over other imaging modalities because it is noninvasive and does not use ionising radiation. For these reasons, ultrasound can be used as a screening test and repeated examinations can be made with relative safety. Therefore, ultrasound is ideally suited for use in obstetrics and gynaecology.

### THE SOUND WAVE AND ITS GENERATION

Sound is a pulsating pressure wave (that is, a mechanical disturbance of a medium) that passes through the medium at a fixed speed. Any sound wave can be defined by two main parameters, namely its amplitude, which is related to its acoustic power, and its frequency. Sound waves with frequencies above 20 kHz are termed ultrasound, with medical ultrasound operating in the low MHz range. Figure 10.4 shows the range of ultrasound frequencies used in the medical environment.

To produce ultrasound, there is the need to generate a pressure wave. This is achieved by incorporating a piezoelectric crystal within a transducer that is placed in contact with the tissue under investigation. The piezoelectric crystal converts electrical energy into mechanical energy and vice versa. When excited by a high-voltage current, the crystal oscillates at a given frequency, which is determined by the thickness of the crystal.

Two types of ultrasound can be produced, namely continuous-wave ultrasound and pulsed-wave ultrasound. For imaging purposes, pulsed-wave ultrasound is used. It consists of bursts or 'packets' of ultrasound that are sent out at a given frequency. The rate at which these bursts of ultrasound are sent out is known as the

FIGURE 10.4 **Typical range of ultrasound frequencies used in clinical practice**

TU = transvaginal ultrasound

FIGURE 10.5 **Temporal profile of pulsed-wave ultrasound**

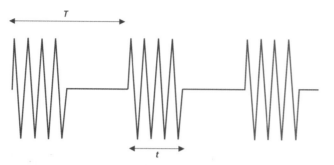

$T$ = pulse repetition period | $t$ = pulse length

pulse repetition frequency. Figure 10.5 shows the temporal profile of pulsed-wave ultrasound. The advantage of this type of ultrasound is that it is possible to obtain spatial information and therefore imaging is possible.

### INTERACTIONS OF ULTRASOUND WITH TISSUE

To build up an ultrasound image, the ultrasound pressure wave needs to interact with the tissue under investigation. The pressure wave then needs to return to the piezoelectric crystal to be converted from mechanical into electrical energy. There are three principal interactions with tissue:

- reflection
- scatter
- absorption.

Reflection occurs at interfaces between tissues with different characteristics. The tissue property that determines the degree of reflection is called the acoustic impedance ($Z$), which is related to the density ($\rho$) of the tissue and the velocity ($c$) of ultrasound in that particular tissue:

$$Z = \rho \times c$$

The greater the difference in acoustic impedance between two tissues, the greater the degree of reflection.

Scatter occurs when ultrasound interacts with a structure whose dimensions are similar to, or smaller than, the wavelength of the ultrasound wave. This is known as Rayleigh scattering and the resulting wave is scattered in all directions (360 degrees scattering). This type of interaction typically occurs when ultrasound interacts with very small structures such as blood cells or parenchyma. The intensity of the scattered wave depends primarily on the dimensions of the target tissue and the wavelength of the ultrasound wave. Generally, the intensity of the scatter increases very rapidly with the frequency of the ultrasound pressure wave, which puts an upper limit on the frequency of ultrasound that can be used in clinical practice.

Absorption is the conversion of mechanical (ultrasound) energy into heat or internal molecular energy. This can obviously have detrimental results in that the heating effect can produce unwanted bioeffects. In addition, energy is lost from the ultrasound beam, reducing the penetration of the beam. Absorption increases with frequency, which effectively puts an upper limit of 20 MHz on the frequency of ultrasound that can be used.

The echoes generated from the reflection at tissue boundaries and the scattering within tissues and organs give rise to the complex echo trains from which the diagnostic information is derived.

### REAL-TIME B-MODE (BRIGHTNESS MODE) ULTRASOUND SCANNING

Ultrasound scanning is a highly operator-dependent technique. To produce a B-mode ultrasound image, the ultrasound beam needs to be swept across the field of view (Figure 10.6 A). Typically, 200 effective ultrasound beams will be used to produce an image (Figure 10.6 B).

Figure 10.7 illustrates the main components of a typical B-mode ultrasound scanner. We will now discuss the role of these components in image formation.

The transducer houses the piezoelectric crystal and generates the ultrasound beam. Modern transducers tend to be broadband transducers with selectable frequencies. Transducers come in different shapes and sizes, depending on the frequencies used and the specific applications.

FIGURE 10.6  **Image acquisition with ultrasound**

**A** transducer sweeps a narrow
ultrasound beam across the area
to be imaged

**B** Resulting ultrasound image

Transducer

Ultrasound
beam

Field of
view limit

Direction of sweep

The power control allows adjustment of the amount of electric voltage that is applied to generate the ultrasound pulses.

The echoes received from the tissues are converted into electrical signals by the transducer. However, the received signal is much weaker than the transmitted signal and therefore a receiver amplifier boosts the returning signals to useful levels. As an analogy, the gain control acts like the volume control on a radio.

Owing to the attenuation of ultrasound pulses with depth, echoes from similar reflectors reduce in amplitude as the tissue depth increases. To ensure that echoes from similar reflectors at different depths are displayed at the same amplitude, it is necessary to compensate for attenuation. This is achieved using a technique called time-gain compensation, which essentially employs a series of amplifiers that can be adjusted to increase the image amplification at specific depths.

FIGURE 10.7 **Main operator-dependent components of a typical B-mode ultrasound scanner**

TGC = time-gain compensation

The scan converter controls the way in which the image is presented. It basically consists of computer memory elements that store grey-scale information and produces a digital image that is comprised of tiny picture elements (pixels). Each pixel has a unique address where the value of the echo amplitude is stored. This allows the appropriate shade of grey for each pixel to be displayed on the screen. In the scan converter, various parameters such as preprocessing and postprocessing curves can be altered, which can improve image quality.

Flat screens or conventional monitors are used to display the images.

### Limitations of real-time B-mode scanning

B-mode ultrasound scanning has several practical limitations including:

- inadequate spatial resolution
- inadequate penetration
- poor image quality (grey scale)
- low frame rate
- compromised field of view
- low line density.

Spatial resolution is the minimum distance between two reflectors or scattering surfaces that is necessary to be able to distinguish two separate echo signals. There are two main components to spatial resolution. Firstly, axial resolution, which is the minimum distance between two points that are located along the beam axis. The axial resolution is determined by the pulse length, which is shorter at higher frequencies. In fact, the axial resolution is equal to half the pulse length and this is why higher frequencies are used to give better axial resolution. The second component of spatial resolution is lateral resolution, which is the minimum distance between two points that are located at the same range or depth within the tissue (objects side by side in the image). The lateral resolution is determined by the beam width and is highly dependent on beam focusing. The spatial resolution also depends on the slice thickness, which is determined by the thickness of the transducer and is therefore inherent in the transducer's design.

Penetration is reduced by the attenuation of ultrasound. The main factors influencing penetration are absorption and scatter. As alluded to earlier, both absorption

FIGURE 10.8 **Doppler frequency shift**

An ultrasound wave is transmitted towards a blood vessel; the ultrasound echo reflected by the red blood cells moving through the vessel incurs a Doppler frequency shift that is proportional to the velocity of the blood flow. | $f_t$ = frequency of the transmitted ultrasound wave | $v$ = velocity of the red blood cells | $\theta$ = angle between the transmitted ultrasound wave and the direction of the blood flow and scatter increase with increasing frequencies. Hence, lower frequencies have to be used to achieve greater penetration. As a result, better penetration comes at the price of poorer resolution.

Image quality depends on several factors: the contrast resolution, which is influenced by the preprocessing and postprocessing carried out in the scan converter; the dynamic range (the range of echo strengths that can be handled by the amplifiers), which dictates how the echo train is converted to a grey scale; and the temporal resolution, which depends on the number of frames displayed per second (frame rate). All of these factors need to be optimised to obtain the best possible image quality.

Frame rate, line density (the number of scan lines in the image) and field of view (the size of the image displayed) are all interrelated. Ideally, one would like to have a fast frame rate, a high line density and a large field of view to obtain the best possible image. Unfortunately, the interrelation of theses factors means that something has to be compromised and, depending on the scan being performed, one has to decide which of the factors are the most important to optimise.

## DOPPLER ULTRASOUND

The wavelength recorded by an observer depends on the movement of the source and the observer relative to one another. This phenomenon can be used in medical ultrasound to give two pieces of useful information:

- the speed at which the target is moving
- the direction of the motion.

The difference in frequency between the returning echo and the transmitted ultrasound wave is known as the Doppler frequency shift; in medical ultrasound, it is particularly used to assess blood flow.

### Doppler equation

If the red blood cells are moving through a blood vessel at velocity $v$ and the angle of insonation between the red blood cells and the ultrasound beam is $\theta$ degrees (Figure 10.8), then the Doppler frequency shift ($f_d$) is given by the following equation:

$$f_d = \frac{2 f_t v \cos \theta}{c}$$

where $c$ is the velocity of ultrasound in soft tissue and $f_t$ is the frequency of the ultrasound wave transmitted by the ultrasound transducer.

### Doppler instrumentation

The simplest way to detect blood flow is by use of continuous-wave ultrasound. Instruments of this kind will give us no imaging capability and the devices therefore tend to be fairly basic, designed to assess the pulse or the fetal heart beat.

To get more information about the nature of blood flow, the Doppler information needs to be coupled with an imaging device. To this end, the main instrument now available is a colour flow scanner, which combines a B-mode real-time grey-scale imaging system with pulsed-wave Doppler and colour flow imaging. Colour flow images display direction and velocity information pictorially (Figure 10.9). Information on the direction of blood flow is colour-coded; generally, flow towards the transducer is red and flow away from the transducer is blue. Information on the velocity of red blood cells is also colour-coded, with dark hues representing low velocities and bright hues representing high velocities.

FIGURE 10.9  **Colour flow Doppler scan of a carotid artery**

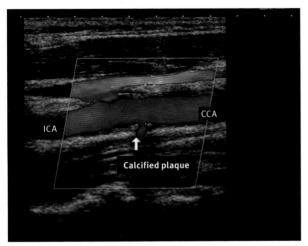

Red signifies flow towards the direction of the colour box; blue signifies flow away from the box; the hue of each colour represents the mean velocity. | CCA = common carotid artery | ICA = internal carotid artery

## SAFETY OF DIAGNOSTIC ULTRASOUND

Diagnostic ultrasound has been used for many years with no proven adverse effects, so why should we worry? Modern ultrasound equipment uses a broader range of ultrasound intensities than were ever used before; there is an increased use of Doppler imaging, which requires higher intensities than B-mode and M-mode ultrasound (M-mode stands for movement mode and is used exclusively in cardiac application); and in some circumstances there is the use of microbubble contrast agents. All of these factors in combination produce the potential for bioeffects. The following bioeffects have been variably reported in epidemiological studies:

- effects on isolated cells *in vitro*
- functional changes in multicellular organisms
- reduction in birthweight
- increase in childhood malignancies
- changes in neurological development
  - dyslexia
  - handedness
  - speech development.

The interactions of ultrasound with tissue can give rise to potentially harmful bioeffects, the most important of these being heating and mechanical effects.

### Heating

As stated earlier, absorption of ultrasound energy can lead to the heating of tissue. Heating is more likely to occur at sites in the body where the absorption is higher than in the surrounding tissue. For example, bone absorbs energy more strongly than soft tissue does and therefore the surrounding soft tissue can experience secondary heating as a result of conduction from the bone. This is particularly important as fetal bone matures, when large increases in absorption have been documented. Consequently, heating effects during routine fetal assessment need to be considered. Diagnostic ultrasound can produce temperature rises that are hazardous to sensitive organs and the developing embryo.

To this end, the thermal index has been developed in an attempt to account for the possibility of bioeffects resulting from heating. This index is an estimate of the rise in tissue temperature that might be possible under 'reasonable worst-case conditions' and is defined as the ratio of the acoustic power emitted to the power required to heat a particular target tissue by 1 degree C. As heating is tissue-specific, there are in fact three thermal indices: the thermal index in soft tissues (TIS), the thermal index in bone (TIB) and the thermal index in the cranium (TIC).

The responsibility for safety issues is with the operator. The operator should therefore continually monitor the thermal index and keep it as low as is consistent with achieving a diagnostic result. Regarding the safe use of ultrasound in obstetric investigations, the British Medical Ultrasound Society (BMUS) recommends monitoring of the TIS during scans carried out in the first 8 weeks following conception and monitoring of the TIB during subsequent scans.

### Cavitation

Since the early days of ultrasound, it has been known that ultrasound can lyse or otherwise damage cells in suspension. This effect is not a result of the thermal properties of ultrasound; instead, it is attributable to the presence of gas-filled cavities in tissue exposed to ultrasound waves. These cavities can either oscillate or collapse under the pressure of the ultrasound beam, producing either considerable shear forces or high pressures and temperatures that can damage cell membranes or produce highly reactive free radicals. This phenomenon is known as cavitation. Gas in the lung, in the intestine and in contrast agents increases the likelihood of cavitation and mechanical damage.

Once again, an index has been developed in an attempt to account for the possibility of bioeffects resulting from mechanical effects. This is known as the mechanical index and is related to the maximum negative pressure and frequency in an ultrasound field.

The importance of cavitation has been summed up by the European Federation of Societies for Ultrasound in Medicine and Biology (EFSUMB) as follows: 'biological effects of nonthermal origin have been reported in animals but, to date, no such effects have been demonstrated in humans, except when a microbubble contrast agent is present.'

### Guidelines and recommendations for the safe use of diagnostic ultrasound

There are a number of guidelines and recommendations for the safe use of diagnostic ultrasound and these change or are updated at regular intervals. A good review of the current guidelines and recommendations can always be found on the website of the BMUS [www.bmus.org]. The BMUS also provides recommended thermal and mechanical index values. The EFSUMB [www.efsumb.org] and the American Institute of Ultrasound in Medicine [www.aium.org] also publish their latest documents on their websites.

## Principles and use of X-rays, computed tomography and magnetic resonance imaging

### X-RAYS

X-radiation is a form of electromagnetic radiation. X-rays have a wavelength in the range of 10–0.01 nm, corresponding to frequencies in the range of $0.03–30 \times 10^{18}$ Hz and energies in the range of 120 eV to 120 keV. They are longer than gamma rays but shorter than ultraviolet rays. X-rays with energies below 12 keV are classified as soft X-rays and those above as hard X-rays, owing to their penetration abilities.

Radiography is considered to be a noninvasive medical test method that is primarily used for diagnostic purposes. It is the oldest and most frequently used form of medical imaging. As a result, the term X-ray is used to refer to a radiographic image produced using this method as well as to the method itself. X-rays are a form of ionising radiation and as such can be dangerous. X-rays were listed as a carcinogen by the US government in 2005.

The sievert (Sv) is the SI unit of measure of radiation and denotes the amount of energy delivered to a human body by gamma radiation or X-radiation (ionising radiation). The old-fashioned counterpart is the rem; 1 Sv is equivalent to 100 rem. Commonly, the radiation exposure from an X-ray is in the microsievert range, whereby 1 mrem equals 10 microsievert. The average person living in the USA receives approximately 3 mSv annually from background sources alone.

### Beam formation and detection

X-rays are produced by accelerating electrons, which are then made to collide with a metal target; the precise nature of the metal target depends on the type of application. In the X-ray tube, the electrons suddenly decelerate upon collision with the metal target and can knock out an electron from the inner shell of the metal atom. Electrons from higher energy levels then fill up the vacancy and X-ray photons are emitted as a result. The process is extremely inefficient and a considerable amount of energy and heat has to be wasted to produce a reasonable flux of X-rays.

X-rays were originally detected by use of a photographic plate and later by use of an X-ray film in a cassette. These devices are generally referred to as image receptors. Plates and films have been largely replaced in hospitals by computed and digital radiography, although film technology is still used in some countries and for industrial applications. Computed and digital technologies have several advantages: they do not require wet processing facilities on site; they do not require the use of silver, which is a nonrenewable resource; and the archiving and retrieval of digital images is considerably easier, with additional space-saving benefits.

### Use of X-rays in clinical practice

The body region to be imaged is positioned between the X-ray source and the image receptor, which captures a shadow image of internal body structures. X-rays may be blocked (attenuated) by dense tissues such as bone but pass more easily through soft tissues. On the X-ray, the areas where the image receptor is exposed to high X-ray energy will appear black. Soft tissue and bone will appear as shades of grey or white because some of the radiation energy is lost on its way from the source to the receptor.

X-rays are useful for identifying skeletal disease as well as chest, lung and abdominal pathologies. Their use in some cases, such as in the imaging of muscle or brain structures, is debatable and alternative imaging methods such as computed tomography (CT), magnetic resonance imaging (MRI) or ultrasound might be more appropriate.

Radiopaque contrast agents are used to highlight organs or vessels depending on the mode of their administration. They are often used in real-time procedures carried out with a so-called X-ray image intensifier resulting in a sequence of images that are projected on to a fluorescent screen or a television-like monitor. Such procedures include barium meal or enema, hysterosalpingography and uterine artery embolisation for the treatment of uterine fibroids.

In gynaecology, hysterosalpingography is frequently used to assess tubal patency in subfertile women (Figure 10.10). The procedure is usually performed in the first 10 days of the menstrual cycle to avoid inadvertent exposure of early pregnancy to radiation. There is no need for anaesthesia, although pain relief medications and antispasmodics are often given orally.

Hysterosalpingography has the following advantages:

- radiation does not persist after the procedure
- the procedure is minimally invasive
- complications are rare
- the procedure is relatively quick
- the procedure can provide valuable information on the appearance of the uterine cavity and the patency of the fallopian tube
- X-rays usually have no immediate adverse effects in the diagnostic range.

The effective radiation dose from hysterosalpingography is about 1 mSv, which is about the same as the amount received by the average person from background radiation in 4 months. The procedure carries the following risks:

- a very small risk of cancer from excessive exposure to radiation
- risk of flare-up of undiagnosed chronic pelvic infection or untreated sexually transmitted disease
- risk of inadvertent exposure of an unsuspected early pregnancy to X-ray
- small teratogenic risk associated with ovarian irradiation.

## DUAL ENERGY X-RAY ABSORPTIOMETRY

Bone density scanning is also called dual energy X-ray absorptiometry (DEXA) or bone densitometry. In this test, the machine sends two beams of low-dose X-rays (approximately one-tenth that of a standard chest X-ray) with distinct and differing energy levels through the

**FIGURE 10.10 Hysterosalpingogram showing an anterior view of the uterine fundus and patent tubes**

R = right side

**FIGURE 10.11 Dual energy X-ray absorptiometry scan of the lumbar spine**

L1–4 = lumbar vertebrae

FIGURE 10.12 **Bone densitometry machine**

FIGURE 10.13 **MRI scan of a fibroid uterus**

bones being examined. One beam is absorbed mainly by soft tissue and is subtracted from the total beam. The bone mineral density (BMD) can be calculated from the absorption of each beam by bone, although small and usually insignificant changes may be observed between scans owing to differences in positioning. The machine's special software calculates and displays the BMD measurements on the monitor. A DEXA image of the lumbar spine is shown in Figure 10.11.

DEXA is the most widely used BMD measurement technology. The test results are plotted as a graph and are also presented in the form of two scores: T score and Z score.

The T score is used to estimate an individual's risk of developing a fracture and compares the amount of bone in this individual with that in a young adult of the same gender with peak bone mass. A score above –1 is considered to be normal. A score between –1 and –2.5 is classified as osteopenia, the first stage of bone loss. A score below –2.5 is indicative of osteoporosis.

The Z score reflects the amount of bone in an individual compared with other individuals in the same age group and of the same size and gender. This is particularly relevant in children, where BMD is lower than in adults; hence, comparison with the reference data of adults would result in overdiagnosis of osteopenia in children.

When interpreting the results, the bone size should also be considered. DEXA tends to overestimate the BMD of taller subjects and underestimate the BMD of smaller subjects. This error is attributable to the way in which the BMD is calculated: the DEXA scanner divides the bone mineral content by the area scanned by the machine (a two-dimensional figure), whereas density is actually defined as mass divided by volume (a three-dimensional figure).

Two types of DEXA equipment are available. In central devices, the X-ray generator is positioned below a large, flat table and a detector, or imaging device, is suspended overhead (Figure 10.12). Central devices measure BMD in the hip and spine. Peripheral devices are much smaller; they measure BMD in the wrist, heel or fingers.

## COMPUTED TOMOGRAPHY

Ultrasound is usually the modality of first choice to assess female pelvic disease but CT is also used as part of the assessment of pelvic tumours and other abdominal disease. CT scanning uses X-rays and the principles of X-ray formation, detection and contrast outlined previously apply here as well. CT, however, produces transverse cross-sectional images of the body by reconstructing the attenuation of fine X-ray beams passed through the body. This gives images of higher contrast resolution than plain radiography does.

Recent software developments enable the reconstruction and display of three-dimensional images. These images are generated by stacking a series of two-dimensional planes on top of each other to generate a volumetric display of the area under examination. Advanced three-dimensional rendering techniques such as surface and volume rendering allow the construction of different three-dimensional models, with each anatomical structure being represented by a different colour. It is also possible to remove certain unwanted structures from the image through a process known as segmentation.

### MAGNETIC RESONANCE IMAGING

MRI is another imaging technique used to visualise the structure and function of the body. Unlike CT, MRI does not use ionising radiation. Instead, a powerful magnetic field is created to align the $H^+$ ions (protons) present in tissue $H_2O$ molecules. A radiofrequency pulse is then used to disrupt the alignment of these protons with the main magnetic field. Following the pulse, the protons drift back into alignment with the magnetic field, emitting a detectable radiofrequency signal as they do so. Contrast agents may be injected directly into the area being examined or intravenously to enhance the appearance of vessels, tumours or inflammatory tissue.

In clinical practice, MRI is used to differentiate pathological tissue such as brain or ovarian tumours from normal tissue (Figure 10.13). The spatial resolution (the ability to distinguish two structures that are very close to each other as separate) provided by MRI is comparable with that of CT, but its contrast resolution (the ability to distinguish between two similar but not identical tissues) is far better because modern MRI scanners include a complex library of pulse sequences that can be employed to characterise different tissues on the basis of their interaction with the pulse signal.

### Magnetic resonance imaging and pregnancy

No harmful effects of MRI have been demonstrated on the fetus, especially as no ionising radiation is used. However, as a precaution, MRI in pregnant women should be undertaken only where necessary, especially in the first trimester. Contrast agents, for example gadolinium-based compounds, are known to cross the placenta and their use during pregnancy is controversial. Nevertheless, on the basis of the available evidence, European Society of Radiology guidelines conclude that gadolinium-based contrast agents seem to be safe in pregnancy and that any gadolinium that reaches the fetus would rapidly be eliminated into urine. Gadolinium use should therefore be considered if the diagnostic study is important for the health of the mother and MRI also plays a role in the diagnosis and monitoring of congenital defects of the fetus.

### Interventional magnetic resonance imaging

In view of its safety record, MRI is well suited for interventional radiology, where the images produced by an MRI scanner are used to guide minimally invasive procedures. Such procedures, naturally, must be done in the absence of any ferromagnetic instruments. A subspecialty of interventional MRI is that of intraoperative MRI, where systems have been developed to allow imaging concurrent with the surgical procedure. More typical, however, is the temporary interruption of the surgical procedure so that MRI scans can be acquired to verify the success of the procedure or guide subsequent surgical work.

### Radiation therapy simulation

MRI is used to locate tumours within the body before the initiation of radiation therapy. The person to be treated is placed in a specific, reproducible, body position and scanned. The MRI system then computes the precise location, shape and orientation of the tumour mass, correcting for any spatial distortion inherent in the system. The person is then marked with triangulation points that will permit the delivery of precise, targeted radiation therapy.

### Magnetic-resonance-guided focused ultrasound

MRI is also used to guide ultrasound surgery, in which a high-energy ultrasound beam is focused on a small spot in a target tissue such as a uterine fibroid. The ultrasound beam heats the tissue to a temperature of more than 65 degrees C, destroying it completely. The three-dimensional view of the target tissue offered by MRI allows accurate focusing of the ultrasound energy as well as monitoring of the treatment cycle, resulting in precise ablation of the diseased tissue.

### Drawbacks of magnetic resonance imaging

Claustrophobia is one of the most common reasons for people to refuse to undergo an MRI examination. Traditionally, owing to the construction of the original machines, the person under investigation had to be placed in the centre of the magnet and, coupled with a somewhat lengthy examination time, the experience was often unpleasant. Modern scanners have short bores and faster scan times, so the procedure is better tolerated. Certain groups of people, such as children, obese individuals and pregnant women, are difficult to accommodate within the machine without special provisions. Acoustic noise associated with the operation of an MRI scanner can also exacerbate the discomfort associated with the procedure. Metal fragments in the eyes (welders), neurosurgical clips, pacing wires and other ferrous prostheses are contraindicated.

Guidance and safety notes on the use of MRI were first published by the American College of Radiology in 2002,[1] with an update published in 2007. [2] In the UK, the Medicines and Healthcare products Regulatory Agency published its *Safety Guidelines for Magnetic Resonance Imaging Equipment in Clinical Use* in December 2007. [3]

## Principles and use of electrosurgery

The use of thermal energy for therapy dates back many centuries. Hippocrates (460–370 BC) already recorded

the use of heat for incising suprapubic abscesses. With the advent of electricity in the early 1800s, electrically heated surgical instruments became available. Surgical diathermy machines were first introduced in the late 1920s.

A diathermy machine converts the mains low-frequency current (230 V, 50 Hz) into a high-frequency current in the radiofrequency range (between 200 kHz and 3.3 MHz) to obtain a desired surgical effect, such as cutting, coagulation (clotting of blood), vaporisation and/or destruction.

### INTERACTIONS OF ELECTRIC CURRENT WITH TISSUE

#### Low-frequency versus high-frequency currents

The effect of an electric current on tissues depends on the frequency of the current. A low-frequency current causes cyclic polarisation and depolarisation of cells owing to the transmembrane exchange of ions, resulting in neuromuscular stimulation. Depending on the actual frequency, this manifests as clonic or tetanic contraction.

By contrast, a high-frequency current changes direction so rapidly that ionic exchange at the cellular level does not happen because of the fixed time that such ions require to move through nerve tissue. Hence, no neuromuscular stimulation takes place. Nevertheless, the high energy delivered to tissue produces collision of intracellular ions and other materials, which manifests as heat.

FIGURE 10.14 **Impact of electrode size on current density**

**A** Two electrodes of equal size: the heating effect is the same beneath each electrode

**B** Unequal electrodes: the heating effect is greater under the smaller electrode

**C** Current density and thermal effects are highest when the electrode is pointed

FIGURE 10.15 **Electrosurgery electrodes**

Bipolar electrode used in hysteroscopic surgery (top); a grasping bipolar electrode used in laparoscopic surgery (bottom).

### Grounded versus isolated electrosurgery systems

Earthed (grounded) diathermy systems allow the current to return back to the unit via earth. If the return electrode is faulty or poorly applied, an alternative return pathway such as the treated person's skin is used, resulting in severe burns. By contrast, in an isolated system, minimal or no current flows to earth and the circuit through the human body is isolated. Hence, should there be a faulty connection or appliance, the current does not return to the machine and there is no risk of burns.

The return electrode, or patient plate, in grounded diathermy systems provides a safe return pathway for the passage of the current from the active electrode through the human body. As the current that passes through the tissues produces a greater current density and heat intensity under the smaller electrode (Figure 10.14), the surface area of the return electrode should be much larger than that of the active electrode. Generally, a minimum surface area of 69 cm² or 10 inch² is recommended to keep the temperature increase at very low levels.

### Monopolar versus bipolar electrosurgery

Surgical diathermy can be either monopolar or bipolar. During monopolar surgical diathermy, the electric current is transported through the human body and back to the generator. An electrode used in monopolar dia-

FIGURE 10.16 **Generator for monopolar and bipolar electrosurgery applications**

FIGURE 10.17 **Bipolar diathermy generator with autocoagulation capability**

FIGURE 10.18 **Modes of electrosurgical currents**

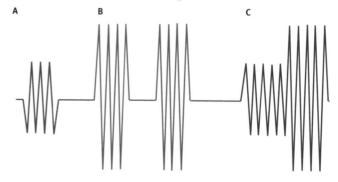

A Cutting mode | B Coagulation mode | C Blended mode

FIGURE 10.19  **Cutting effect**

FIGURE 10.20  **Desiccation effect**

**A** Desiccation accomplished by use of a low-voltage 'cutting' waveform with 100% duty cycle

**B** Desiccation accomplished by use of an intermittent high-voltage 'coagulation' waveform

thermy may be a blade, a ball, a needle tip or an open or closed loop. It is important to remember that the smaller the tip, the greater the heating effect will be because the current density will be concentrated at the smaller area (Figure 10.14). The monopolar electrode is connected to the diathermy machine (Figure 10.16), which in turn is connected to a return plate that is attached to another body part of the person undergoing the operation.

In bipolar diathermy, the current flows between the tips of a forceps' blades (Figure 10.15), which are separated by an insulating material. One blade acts as an active electrode and the other as a return. The tissue in between the blades acts as the conducting medium for the current. Many bipolar diathermy generators incorporate a facility for autocoagulation (Figure 10.17), where the degree of coagulation is sensed by the generator and the current is discontinued when the optimum effect has been achieved. Unlike monopolar diathermy, where cutting and coagulation modes are possible, bipolar diathermy only permits coagulation with no cutting. Several new bipolar electrodes are now available on the market.

### Tissue effects of various waveforms

Electrosurgical generators can produce current in several modes (Figure 10.18), with distinct tissue effects for each modality.

A cutting current is produced with a continuous unmodulated sinusoidal waveform, with a relatively low voltage needed to produce the desired tissue vaporisation effect (Figure 10.18 A). The tip of the electrode is held just above the target tissue. Electric arcs are formed between the cutting electrode and the tissue, generating points of extremely high temperatures that vaporise cells in such a way that a clean tissue cut is achieved (Figure 10.19). There is insufficient time for the heat to dissipate to adjacent tissue; hence there is less tissue trauma and cutting occurs without significant haemostasis.

A coagulation effect is produced with a higher voltage current than that used for cutting but the current is applied intermittently (Figure 10.18 B) and modulated with a duty cycle that is on for about 6% of the time, although this may vary depending on the desired effect. This modulation, or dampening, allows the tissue to cool between heating bursts. Thus, no vaporisation occurs but the current causes coagulation, a complex process that is

FIGURE 10.21 **Fulguration effect**

an important part of haemostasis. Higher voltage with longer modulation intervals results in greater coagulation or haemostatic effect.

Desiccation is the process of extreme drying, whereby tissues are coagulated while being heated to 70–100 degrees C. Soft coagulation uses a peak voltage of about 200 volts or less and the power output is precisely limited or minimal leading to minimal carbonisation, quick coagulation and as little sticking to the electrode as possible. Desiccation and soft coagulation both require contact by the active electrode with the tissue.

Monopolar or bipolar instruments can be used to desiccate tissues and the effect can be produced with either the cutting mode or the coagulation mode of the generator (Figure 10.20), although the cutting mode is the preferred option. A blended waveform combines bursts of low-voltage (cutting) and high-voltage (coagulation) currents (Figure 10.18 C) and produces cutting with coagulation effects.

Other variables can impact the tissue effect, namely the duration of application, the power setting and the precise type of active electrode. Too long an activation should be avoided as it may lead to adherence of the coagulum to the electrode and subsequent tearing of the coagulum from the vessels, resulting in inadequate

haemostasis. Modern generators may monitor the flow of current through the tissue to optimise the coagulation effect.

Fulguration (electrofulguration) or forced coagulation results when a high-powered current is used to produce a sparking effect to coagulate a large bleeding area or to char tissue without touching the tissue with the electrode (Figure 10.21). This effect produces deeper coagulation than can be achieved with soft coagulation and is used in specific circumstances only.

Argon-enhanced electrosurgery was introduced in the late 1980s. The inert, nonreactive argon gas wraps the electrosurgical current and concentrates and delivers the spark to the tissue in a beam-like fashion, creating a smoother, more malleable dry scab.

## SAFETY OF ELECTROSURGERY

In the past 15 years, considerable improvements in electrosurgical safety have been achieved. Modern generators produce efficient and effective cutting and coagulation currents, automatically measure tissue impedance and adjust the output, monitor and warn of any potentially dangerous low-frequency leaks of current from the human body to earth and warn of incomplete application of the return electrode. These features reduce the risk of adverse effects to people undergoing electrosurgery. Additionally, modern generators have two separate return plates and the resistance is constantly measured in each. If for any reason there is a difference in the resistance of the return plates, the system will automatically be turned off. It is also important that the diathermy machine displays the power output and that the surgeon uses the lowest effective power setting, for example 30 W. Higher outputs are required when using diathermy with glycine, such as in transcervical resection or rollerball ablation of the endometrium.

Hazards associated with the use of active monopolar electrodes also include direct coupling, insulation failure and capacitive coupling, each of which may cause severe injury.

Direct coupling occurs when the electrode is activated in close proximity or direct contact with another conductive instrument within the body. This risk is avoidable or greatly minimised through the adoption of strict safety rules during surgery.

Insulation failure occurs when the coating that covers the active electrode is compromised. This may result from repeated use or incorrect handling of instruments and may not be detected by the surgeon or theatre staff.

Capacitive coupling may occur between two conductors that are separated by an insulator. For example, if an insulated active electrode is inserted down a metal cannula, the electric current can be transferred from the active electrode through its insulation and into the conductive metal cannula, which can discharge electrical energy if it comes into contact with body structures.

The following practices are recommended to ensure the safe use of electrical surgical instruments:

- Check the instrument's isolation before surgery.
- Use the lowest possible power and voltage settings to achieve the desired effect.
- Activate the electrode only when necessary.
- Never activate the electrode when in close proximity or direct contact with a metal or conductive object.

Consideration should also be given to the following points:

- Bipolar instruments are safer than monopolar devices.
- An all-metal or all-plastic cannula system is the safest option.
- Active-electrode monitoring systems reduce the risk of capacitive coupling.

## Principles and use of lasers in endoscopic surgery

The term laser is an acronym for light amplification by stimulated emission of radiation. The laser device emits light photons (electromagnetic radiation) through a process called stimulated emission to vaporise, dissect and coagulate tissue. Laser beams additionally have a natural sterilisation effect as they evaporate bacteria, viruses and fungi and seal nerve endings, thus decreasing postoperative pain. Laser devices used in endoscopic surgery are either gas ($CO_2$ or argon ions) or solid-state lasers and are described as class 4 lasers with a capacity to cause fires, burns and retinal damage. Lasers can interact with tissues in four ways, namely photothermally (commonly employed in gynaecology), photochemically, photomechanically and photoablatively.

### CARBON DIOXIDE GAS LASERS

$CO_2$ gas lasers have a wavelength of 10 600 nm and are absorbed to a high degree by soft tissues that contain water. This enables precise tissue cutting and dissection with minimal lateral damage. The vaporisation capability of $CO_2$ lasers is useful for the removal of endometriotic implants, especially near the ureters. However, the beam has to be transmitted from the generator to the endoscope by a system of articulated arms and mirrors, which are expensive and difficult to clean, and is then sent through a semiflexible fibre that runs down the endoscopic operating channel. As $CO_2$ lasers are invisible to the human eye, an additional visible aiming laser is needed to assist with treatment. Overall, the depth of the $CO_2$ laser is very limited making it unsuitable for laparoscopic surgery.

### SOLID-STATE LASERS

Solid-state lasers are commonly made by 'doping' a crystalline solid host with ions that provide the required energy states. Examples include the neodymium-doped yttrium aluminium garnet (Nd:YAG) laser, which can produce high-energy beams in the infrared spectrum at 1064 nm and can be transmitted down a fibreoptic cable to the operating site. The Nd:YAG laser provides good cutting and haemostatic effects as well as being able to vaporise tissue. When the beam is transmitted down a bare quartz fibre, it penetrates deeply into tissues, a property that may be useful for hysteroscopic surgery but may be unsafe in laparoscopic procedures. In laparoscopic procedures, the beam should be focused at the tip (the focal spot size varies from approximately 0.1 mm to 0.4 mm) to limit the amount of unintended tissue damage to 0.2–1.0 mm.

Passage of the Nd:YAG beam through a crystal of potassium titanyl phosphate (KTP) results in doubling of the original frequency and a wavelength that is half the original, with beam characteristics that are somewhere between those of the $CO_2$ laser and the Nd:YAG laser. The KTP laser produces a visible beam at a wavelength of 532 nm, is easily transmitted down flexible fibreoptic cables and penetrates tissue for about 1–2 mm. The beam can vaporise, cut and coagulate tissue with a single, bare and reusable quartz fibre.

During the use of Nd:YAG and KTP lasers, staff must wear protective goggles and the person undergoing laser surgery must be provided with suitable protection to prevent inadvertent exposure and injury to the retina by the beam.

## Principles and use of radiotherapy

Radiation therapy or radiotherapy is the use of ionising radiation as a medical intervention, primarily for the treatment of cancer. The amount of radiation used is measured in gray (Gy). Use of radiotherapy for nonmalignant conditions is very limited because of concerns about the risk of radiation-induced cancers.

Radiotherapy acts by damaging cellular DNA. This damage may be caused by photons, electrons, protons, neutrons or ion beams and may occur either directly or indirectly. The indirect effect is the most common mechanism of action and results from the ionisation of $H_2O$ molecules, which generates $H^+$ and hydroxyl ($OH^-$) ions and free radicals ($H^\bullet$ and $OH^\bullet$) that damage the DNA. This can lead to the irreversible loss of the cells' reproductive integrity and their eventual death.

Radiotherapy also affects intracellular processes that are necessary for cellular growth, senescence and apoptosis and the intrinsic ability to repair damage. Cell survival curves depend on the dose of radiation, the position of the cell in the mitotic cycle, the $O_2$ tension, the intrinsic cellular radiosensitivity and the cellular environment. Tissue hypoxia increases resistance to the effects of radiation as $O_2$ makes the radiation damage to DNA permanent. Several strategies have been developed to increase tissue oxygenation and enhance the effectiveness of radiotherapy, including the practice of total dose fractionation (spreading the dose out over time). Details of logarithmic survival curves and information on how manipulation of the cellular environment alters these curves are provided in the literature.

When protons (positively charged particles) are used, their biological effects are the same as those of other particles. However, unlike photons (soft X-rays), protons release their energy at the point of impact within the tumour, with a rapid fall-off in dose in the healthy tissue beyond. Adverse effects are minimised and a higher dose can be used for treatment.

Radiotherapy may be used as primary therapy, in conjunction with either surgery, chemotherapy or endocrine therapy or in combination with one or more of these modalities.

When used as a primary therapeutic modality where there is survival benefit, it can be curative (resulting in the radical removal of disease) or palliative (where the aim of treatment is symptom control or the local control of disease).

When used as an adjuvant therapy, radiotherapy is usually given after the surgical removal of all detectable disease and its aim is to improve disease-specific and overall survival. Thus, adjuvant radiotherapy is essentially administered to minimise the risk of recurrence, rather than for the treatment of a proven disease, and a proportion of people who receive adjuvant therapy will already have been cured by their primary surgery.

When radiotherapy is given before the main treatment, it is described as neoadjuvant therapy and its aim is to reduce the size of the tumour so as to facilitate more-effective surgery.

If administered at the same time as other therapies, it is described as concomitant or concurrent therapy.

### DELIVERY OF RADIOTHERAPY

#### External-beam radiotherapy

Linear accelerator (linac) machines deliver two-dimensional beams from several (one to four) directions to the area being treated. In conventional techniques, the treatment is first simulated on a specially calibrated diagnostic X-ray machine known as the simulator, which has the same geometry as the linear accelerator employed during treatment. Treatment simulation is used for tumour localisation, treatment plan verification and treatment monitoring.

An enhancement of virtual simulation is three-dimensional conformal radiotherapy (CRT), which uses a variable number of beams with the profile of each radiation beam being shaped to fit the profile of the target. As the shape of the treatment volume matches the shape of the tumour, the relative toxicity of radiation to the surrounding normal tissues is reduced, allowing a higher dose of radiation to be delivered to the tumour than possible with conventional techniques.

Intensity-modulated radiation therapy (IMRT) is the next generation of three-dimensional CRT. In this form of high-precision radiation therapy, the intensity of each radiation beam can be modulated so that a given treatment field may be targeted by beams of variable intensity. This allows for greater control of the distribution of the dose within the target, thereby creating limitless possibilities to sculpt the radiation dose to the tumour itself.

Despite such advances, the limitations of radiotherapy include the inability to identify microscopic disease with accuracy, the difficulty of immobilising the treated person/tumour for the duration of a treatment session (with IMRT this is typically 15–30 minutes) and problems arising from tumour shrinkage with treatment.

The next challenge in radiation oncology is therefore to accommodate changes in the position of the treated person and/or movement or shrinkage of the tumour during treatment. Incorporating real-time imaging with real-time adjustment of the therapeutic beams, an approach commonly called four-dimensional CRT, allows 'online' imaging of the individual during treatment and real-time reconstruction of the actual daily delivered dose on the basis of the individual's and the tumour's changing anatomies. This approach results in adaptive radiotherapy – the modulation of prescription and delivery on the basis of the actual daily delivered dose as opposed to the planned dose.

### Internal-beam radiotherapy

Internally delivered radiotherapy may be in the form of:

- sealed-source radiotherapy
- unsealed-source radiotherapy.

Brachytherapy involves the use of sealed sources, which are placed directly into, or adjacent to, the volume of tissue to be irradiated. The advantage is that it allows the tumour to be treated at very short distances and the radiation passes through less healthy tissue. In addition, brachytherapy sources generally emit lower-energy radiation compared with external-beam radiotherapy. The proximity of the radiation source in brachytherapy allows the dose to be better localised to the tumour volume. The clinician can therefore treat the tumour with very high doses while the dose to the surrounding healthy tissue is minimised.

Brachytherapy is used to treat many gynaecological cancers including vaginal, cervical, ovarian and uterine cancer. The radioactive material, such as caesium-137 ($^{137}$Cs) or iridium-192 ($^{192}$Ir), is placed temporarily inside or near a tumour for a specific amount of time and then withdrawn. It may be administered at a low or high dose. Occasionally, radioactive seeds or pellets, such as iodine-125 ($^{125}$I) seeds, are placed in or near the tumour and are left there permanently. After several weeks or months, the radioactivity level of the implants eventually diminishes to nothing. The seeds then remain in the body with no lasting effect.

Radioisotope therapy is an unsealed form of radiotherapy. It is delivered by injection, for example intravenous infusion of a radioisotope substance to treat neuroblastoma, or by ingestion, for example ingestion of iodine-131 ($^{131}$I) to treat thyroid cancer or thyrotoxicosis.

Other examples of radioisotope therapy are the intravenous administration of hormone-bound lutetium-177 ($^{177}$Lu) and yttrium-90 ($^{90}$Y) to treat neuroendocrine tumours in what is called peptide receptor radionuclide therapy, and the injection of radioactive glass or resin microspheres into the hepatic artery to radioembolise liver tumours or liver metastases.

Further developments include the introduction of a monoclonal antibody against CD20 conjugated to a radioisotope molecule such as $^{131}$I or $^{90}$Y for the treatment of refractory non-Hodgkin lymphoma. This is referred to as radioimmunotherapy.

### SAFETY OF RADIOTHERAPY

Acute adverse effects of radiotherapy include:

- damage to epithelial surfaces (such as skin, oral and bowel mucosa)
- oedema and swelling of soft tissues as part of the inflammatory reaction, which may be ameliorated with steroids
- infertility caused by damage to the radiation-sensitive gonads
- generalised fatigue.

Medium-term and long-term adverse effects depend on the particular area being treated and may be minimal. These include:

- fibrosis and diffuse scarring of the irradiated tissue
- hair loss
- dryness as a result of damage to the salivary and tear glands or vaginal dryness as a result of damage to the cervical glands
- fatigue and lethargy
- cancer secondary to irradiation
- death.

Reirradiation may cause additional acute or intermediate adverse effects or exacerbation of already existing adverse effects and people undergoing reirradiation must be monitored closely.

## REFERENCES

1. KANAL E, BORGSTEDE JP, BARKOVICH AJ, BELL C, BRADLEY WG, FELMLEE JP, et al. American College of Radiology White Paper on MR Safety. *Am J Roentgenol* 2002;178:1335–47.

2. KANAL E, BARKOVICH AJ, BELL C, BORGSTEDE JP, BRADLEY WG JR, FROELICH JW, et al. ACR Guidance Document for Safe MR Practices. *Am J Roentgenol* 2007;188:1–27. [www.acr.org/SecondaryMainMenuCategories/quality_safety/MRSafety/safe_mr07.aspx].

3. Medicines and Healthcare Products Regulatory Agency. *Safety Guidelines for Magnetic Resonance Imaging Equipment in Clinical Use. Device Bulletin* DB2007(03). London: MHRA; 2007. [www.mhra.gov.uk/home/idcplg?LdcService=GET_FILE& dDocName=CON2033065&RevisionSelectionMethod= LatestReleased].

## FURTHER READING

### Electrocardiography

MORRIS F, BRADY W, CAMM J, editors. *ABC of Clinical Electrocardiography*. 2nd ed. London: BMJ Books; 2008.

### Ultrasound

KREMKAU F W. *Diagnostic Ultrasound: Principles and Instruments*. 7th ed. Philadelphia: Saunders/Elsevier; 2005.

CLAUDON M, COSGROVE D, ALBRECHT T, BOLONDI L, BOSIO M, CALLIADA F, et al. Guidelines and good clinical practice recommendations for contrast enhanced ultrasound (CEUS) – update 2008. *Ultraschall Med* 2008;29:28–44 [www.efsumb.org/mediafiles01/ceus-guidelines2008.pdf].

### X-ray, CT and MRI

DE WILDE J P, RIVERS A W, PRICE D L. A review of the current use of magnetic resonance imaging in pregnancy and safety implications for the fetus. *Prog Biophys Mol Biol* 2005;87:335–53.

### Electrosurgery

MANE S, PENKETH R. Hysteroscopy. In: Shaw R W, Soutter W P, Stanton S L, editors. *Gynaecology*. 3rd ed. London: Churchill Livingstone; 2003. p.37–53.

SMITH A R B, PARSONS J. Diathermy and lasers. In: Shaw R W, Soutter W P, Stanton S L, editors. *Gynaecology*. 3rd ed. London: Churchill Livingstone; 2003. p.67–77.

### Radiotherapy

BUCCI M, BEVAN A, ROACH M. Advances in radiation therapy: conventional to 3D, to IMRT, to 4D, and beyond. *CA Cancer J Clin* 2005;55:117–34 [http://caonline.amcancersoc.org/cgi/content/full/55/2/117].

POULIOT J, XIA P, AUBIN M, VERHEY L, BANI-HASHEMI A, GHELMANSARAI F, et al. Low-dose megavoltage cone-beam CT for dose-guided radiation therapy. *Int J Radiat Oncol Biol Phys* 2003;57 Suppl 1:S183–4.

# Sample questions relating to biophysics

## EXTENDED MATCHING QUESTIONS

### Questions 1–7

■ *This question relates to electrosurgery. For each item below, select the **single** best option from the list of options (A–F). Each option may be used once, more than once or not at all.*

OPTIONS

▷ **A** Argon-enhanced electrosurgery
▷ **B** Blended waveform
▷ **C** Coagulation current
▷ **D** Cutting current
▷ **E** Desiccation
▷ **F** Fulguration

1 ▶ Produced by a continuous unmodulated sinusoidal waveform with a relatively low voltage

2 ▶ Does not allow for haemostasis

3 ▶ Produced with a higher-voltage current than used for cutting

4 ▶ Applied intermittently and modulated with a duty cycle that is on for about 6% of the time

5 ▶ Alternates between low and high voltage

6 ▶ Causes coagulation by drying tissues

7 ▶ Used for deep coagulation

## MULTIPLE CHOICE QUESTIONS

8 ▶ Ultrasound can be used for the following:

A ▷ Fetal therapy
B ▷ To determine the nature of a tissue
C ▷ To assess the movement of tissues
D ▷ To measure blood flow
E ▷ To measure structures

9 ▶ The following are ultrasound interactions with tissues:

A ▷ Reflection
B ▷ Scatter
C ▷ Absorption
D ▷ Refraction
E ▷ Radiation

10 ▶ Regarding the detrimental effects of diagnostic ultrasound:

A ▷ It has proven harmful adverse effects
B ▷ The main safety issue concerns the heating of tissues
C ▷ Soft tissues are at greatest risk of heating
D ▷ Soft tissues experience secondary heating
E ▷ The thermal index is the same for all tissues

11 ▶ X-rays:

A ▷ are a form of electromagnetic radiation
B ▷ are shorter than gamma rays
C ▷ are measured in candela
D ▷ are very energy-inefficient to produce
E ▷ are formed by the acceleration of electrons

12 ▶ Regarding X-rays:

A ▷ They pass easily through soft tissues
B ▷ Structures that let most of the X-rays pass through appear white on film
C ▷ They can be used to produce real-time images
D ▷ They are used to embolise the uterine artery for the treatment of fibroids
E ▷ They are useful in imaging the brain

13 ▶ Hysterosalpingography:

A ▷ is usually performed in the second half of the menstrual cycle
B ▷ leaves no radiation after the procedure has ended
C ▷ involves an effective radiation dose that is equivalent to 1 month's background radiation
D ▷ can cause a flare-up of untreated sexually transmitted disease
E ▷ carries a small teratogenic risk owing to ovarian irradiation

**14 ▶** Regarding dual energy X-ray absorptiometry:

A ▷ It allows the calculation of bone mineral density

B ▷ It involves the firing of three different energy beams at bone

C ▷ The T score predicts the risk of developing a fracture

D ▷ A T score of −1 is normal

E ▷ It underestimates the bone mineral density of tall people

**15 ▶** Magnetic resonance imaging:

A ▷ provides high contrast between different soft tissues

B ▷ produces the same amount of ionising radiation as computed tomography

C ▷ affects all protons in the body

D ▷ works by emitting a radiofrequency pulse as protons move between magnetic fields

E ▷ is used to characterise pathological tissue

**16 ▶** Regarding magnetic resonance imaging:

A ▷ There are no harmful effects on the developing fetus

B ▷ Contrast agents do not cross the placenta

C ▷ It is contraindicated in people with metal fragments in the eyes

D ▷ It is contraindicated in claustrophobic people

E ▷ It is a very noisy procedure

**17 ▶** Regarding electrosurgery:

A ▷ The electric current during monopolar diathermy runs from the generator to the person being treated and back

B ▷ The electric current used in monopolar diathermy has a lower frequency than the current of the mains supply

C ▷ Low-frequency currents have no effect on cells

D ▷ High-frequency currents directly produce heat

E ▷ Bipolar diathermy does not allow cutting

**18 ▶** Regarding radiotherapy:

A ▷ The radiation used is measured in sievert

B ▷ Its use is widespread in malignant and nonmalignant conditions

C ▷ The process entails damaging malignant cell walls

D ▷ Tissue hypoxia decreases the resistance to radiation

E ▷ Using protons rather than X-rays decreases the adverse effects of radiotherapy

**19 ▶** Regarding radiotherapy:

A ▷ It can be used as primary or adjuvant therapy

B ▷ It is best used prior to surgery if used as an adjuvant

C ▷ It can be used prior to surgery to reduce the tumour size

D ▷ A linear accelerator uses only one two-dimensional beam

E ▷ With internal-beam radiotherapy, the dose of radiation to the tumour is increased while the dose to surrounding tissues is decreased

**20 ▶** The following are recognised medium- and long-term adverse effects of radiotherapy:

A ▷ Oedema

B ▷ Fatigue

C ▷ Fibrosis

D ▷ Hair loss

E ▷ Dryness due to gland damage

# Embryology

# CHAPTER 11

# Early embryology

*Ram Sharma*

## Overview

Human development begins when a sperm fertilises an ovum. By definition, an embryo consists of cells and tissues formed once mitosis of a zygote begins, thus even at the two-cell stage it is an embryo. These few cells multiply in number over an 8-week period into a fetus, by which time it will consist of many millions of cells. Table 11.1 summarises the major events of the prenatal stages of development. The critical phase during which there is potential for malformation is in the embryonic period, when the embryo is most vulnerable to environmental agents such as viruses and other teratogens.

## Gametogenesis

Gametogenesis is a process in which female and male germ cells (called oogenesis and spermatogenesis respectively) undergo cytoplasmic and chromosomal changes to form the definitive oocyte and the spermatozoon. There are, however, a number of differences between the two processes. Oogenesis is a cyclical event, while spermatogenesis begins at puberty and continues throughout adult life. The monthly female cycle consists of maturation of a single (usually) oocyte and is accompanied by changes in the hormone secretion. There are concurrent changes in the endometrium to prepare the uterus for pregnancy.

The primordial germ cells arise from the wall of the yolk sac during the second week of development. In the sixth week they migrate into the body of the embryo to occupy the gonadal ridges. The primordial germ cells undergo rapid mitotic divisions. However, the pattern of proliferation of these cells differs in the two sexes. In the female, the germ cells differentiate into oogonia and multiply rapidly in the embryonic ovary until the fifth month to reach up to 7 million in number. After this period, large numbers of oogonia undergo degeneration (atresia). In the male, primordial germ cells form spermatogonia, in contrast to female germ cells, which continue to proliferate from puberty throughout life.

Both oogenesis and spermatogenesis require two meiotic cell divisions, which reduce the number of chromosomes from diploid to haploid (covered in Chapters 29 and 30 on female and male reproductive physiology). Meiosis also allows random assortment of maternal and paternal chromosomes and redistribution of genetic information through the process of crossing over. Thus,

TABLE 11.1 **Stages of development before birth**

| Time period | Stage | Main events |
|---|---|---|
| Conception to week 2 | Pre-embryonic | Fertilised ovum undergoes mitosis, formation of morula; appearance of blastocyst; blastocyst implanted; germ layers develop |
| Week 2 to week 8 | Embryonic period | Germ layers and placenta develop; main body systems form |
| Week 9 to birth | Fetal period | Further growth and development of organs; locomotor system becomes functional |

reshuffling of genes adds to the genetic variability among the offspring.

### OOGENESIS

The process of oogenesis begins during the fetal period but is not completed until after puberty. During fetal life, the majority of oogonia proliferate by mitosis and differentiate into primary oocytes. At birth, most of the surviving primary oocytes enter the prophase of first meiotic division and remain suspended in the diplotene phase until puberty. This meiotic arrest is produced by secretion of oocyte maturation inhibitor (OMI), a small peptide produced by follicular cells surrounding the primary oocyte. A primary oocyte surrounded by a single layer of follicular cells is called a primary follicle.

As the primary oocyte grows during puberty, the follicular cells become stratified to produce a layer of granulosa cells. The primary oocyte becomes surrounded by a layer of glycoprotein secreted by the granulosa cells, and the ovarian connective tissue cells around the follicle condense to form theca folliculi; this layer then differentiates into an inner vascular and secretory layer, the theca interna, and an outer fibrous layer, the theca externa.

### SPERMATOGENESIS

Spermatogenesis is the process by which the primitive germ cells or spermatogonia are transformed into spermatozoa. Spermatogonia, which have formed in the fetal period, remain dormant in the seminiferous tubules of the testes until puberty, when they increase in number after several mitotic divisions.

## Fertilisation

The ovulated oocyte enters the abdominopelvic cavity and soon reaches the ampulla of the uterine tube, where it may be fertilised. Fertilisation takes place approximately 12–24 hours after ovulation. Fertilisation is a series of events that begins with penetration of a sperm into an oocyte and ends with a combination of maternal and paternal chromosomes at metaphase of the first mitotic division of the zygote. The several sequential events of fertilisation are:

- sperm activation and penetration of corona radiata
- attachment to zona and penetration of the zona pellucida
- fusion of the oocyte and sperm cell membranes
- completion of meiosis in the oocyte and formation of pronuclei
- formation of the zygote.

### SPERM ACTIVATION AND PENETRATION OF CORONA RADIATA

Before the sperm reach the distal uterine tube, they must undergo a process of capacitation, which makes them capable of penetrating the ovum. During this phase, the glycoprotein and cholesterol of the acrosomal membrane are removed by the secretions from the cervix and the uterine tube. When viable sperm come in contact with the corona radiata surrounding a secondary oocyte, they surround it, undergo an acrosomal reaction and release the enzyme hyaluronidase, which is needed to penetrate the corona radiata. The active movements of sperm also play an important role in penetration.

### ATTACHMENT TO AND PENETRATION OF THE ZONA PELLUCIDA

Once the path has been cleared through the cells of the corona radiata, a sperm binds to the zona pellucida and releases its acrosomal enzymes. The enzymes responsible for penetration include esterases, neuraminidase and acrosin. A spermatozoon binds to the zona pellucida and initiates a zona reaction, changing its physical properties to prevent attachment of any more sperm. The zona reaction is believed to result from a cortical reaction in which the cortical granules release their lysosomal enzymes into the space between the zona pellucida and oocyte cell membrane.

### FUSION OF THE OOCYTE AND SPERM CELL MEMBRANES

Once the sperm makes its way through the zona pellucida into the privitelline space, it comes in contact with the cell membrane of the oocyte, resulting in the fusion of the membranes of the sperm head and oocyte. After this fusion, the cell membranes of sperm and egg break down at the area of their contact.

## COMPLETION OF MEIOSIS IN THE OOCYTE AND FORMATION OF PRONUCLEI

Soon after entry of spermatozoa, the oocyte resumes second meiotic division, forming a mature oocyte and a second polar body. The chromosomes of the oocyte and sperm condense and enlarge to form pronuclei. As the pronuclei grow and approach each other, their haploid chromosomes become arranged on a spindle and split longitudinally to form chromatids.

## FORMATION OF THE ZYGOTE

When the male and female pronuclei meet, their membranes break down and the chromosomes mix to produce a single cell called a zygote. At this stage, the process of fertilisation is completed and the zygote prepares for its first mitotic division.

## The first week

A fertilised ovum has a diploid number of chromosomes and, once the second meiotic division has been completed, the stage of cleavage can begin. This consists of a series of rapid mitotic cell divisions in which the zygote divides over a period of about 3 days, resulting in the so-called 16-cell-stage embryo (Figures 11.1, 11.2). Each cell is known as a blastomere. After each cleavage division, while the number of cells increases, the size of each cell diminishes. The solid sphere of cells that forms is known as a morula (Figure 11.2 A). Each of these new daughter cells is, at this stage, pluripotential.

The morula soon shows signs of further differentiation. Cavities appear within the centre of the sphere of cells, forming a blastocyst, the cavity itself being the blastocoele (Figure 11.2 B, C). Once this stage has been reached, the outer layer of the blastocyst soon thins to single-cell thickness to become the trophoblast, enclosing the enlarging fluid-filled blastocyst cavity. The central

FIGURE 11.1 **Stages of pre-embryonic development during the first week**

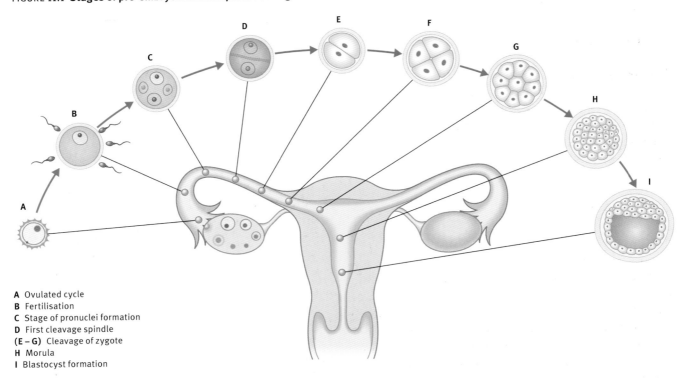

**A** Ovulated cycle
**B** Fertilisation
**C** Stage of pronuclei formation
**D** First cleavage spindle
**(E – G)** Cleavage of zygote
**H** Morula
**I** Blastocyst formation

*Reproduced with permission from: Embryology: An Illustrated Colour Text.* Mitchell B, Sharma R. London: Churchill Livingstone; 2009. Copyright Elsevier.

FIGURE 11.2 **Early stages of implantation**

**A** Morula at day 3

**B** Blastocyst at day 5

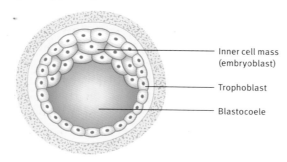

Inner cell mass (embryoblast)

Trophoblast

Blastocoele

**C** Blastocyst at day 6 making contact with uterine wall

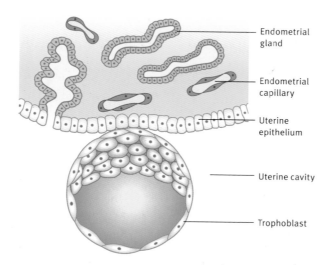

Endometrial gland

Endometrial capillary

Uterine epithelium

Uterine cavity

Trophoblast

FIGURE 11.3 **Implantation of blastocyst**

**A** Blastocyst at day 7 beginning to implant

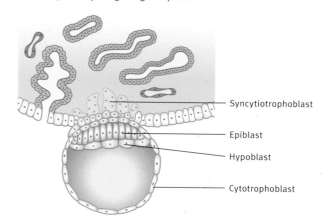

Syncytiotrophoblast

Epiblast

Hypoblast

Cytotrophoblast

**B** By day 8 the amniotic cavity appears

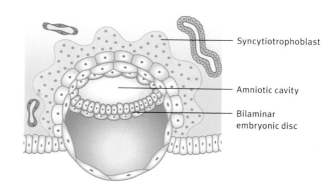

Syncytiotrophoblast

Amniotic cavity

Bilaminar embryonic disc

**C** By day 9 the syncytiotrophoblast invades the uterine glands and capillaries

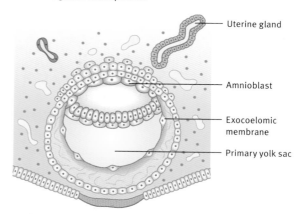

Uterine gland

Amnioblast

Exocoelomic membrane

Primary yolk sac

group of cells moves to one pole of the blastocyst (the embryonic pole) to form the inner cell mass from which the whole embryo itself will form. The trophoblast contributes to the fetal component of the placenta.

The process of morula and blastocyst formation occurs while the sphere of dividing cells is in transit along the uterine tube (Figure 11.1). The first mitotic division of cleavage will be completed by the time the two-cell stage embryo reaches the middle of the tube, at about 30 hours post-fertilisation. By 3 days the morula of 12–16 cells will have reached the junction of the uterine tube and the uterus. By 4–5 days the fully formed blastocyst reaches the uterine lumen in preparation for implantation, which occurs a day later (Figure 11.2).

## The second week – implantation and formation of bilaminar embryonic disc

At this stage the embryo is partly implanted in the endometrium. The implantation process initiates the decidual reaction or decidualisation in the uterine stroma, the cells of which contribute the maternal component of the placenta. The trophoblast begins to differentiate: its inner part becomes a single layer of cells, hence its name the cytotrophoblast (Figure 11.3 A). The outer layer is more extensive and is the invasive layer. It is a syncytium and, at this stage, although it has invaded the endometrium, it has not invaded endometrial blood vessels. It is known as the syncytiotrophoblast. By this stage, the inner cell mass of the blastocyst has differentiated into two layers: the epiblast and the hypoblast (Figure 11.3 A). These two layers are in contact and form a bilaminar embryonic disc (Figure 11.3 B). Within the epiblast a cavity develops, the amniotic cavity, which fills with amniotic fluid. Some epiblast cells become specialised as amnioblasts and they secrete the amniotic fluid. The exocoelomic membrane is derived from the hypoblast and lines the cavity that appears beneath the endoderm, the primary yolk sac (Figure 11.3 C). The fluid contained in this sac is the source of nutrition for the embryo before the placenta is fully formed and functional.

By 12 days there have been significant changes, particularly in the trophoblast. Small clefts, called lacunae, appear in the syncytiotrophoblast. These lacunae communicate with the maternal endometrial sinusoids, thereby deriving nutritional support for the developing embryo (Figure 11.4). Concurrent with this is the further development of the cytotrophoblast, which is thickest at the embryonic pole of the conceptus. Clefts appear between the exocoelomic membrane and the cytotrophoblast (Figure 11.4). These clefts merge to form the extra-embryonic coelom, which almost completely surrounds the embryo.

By day 13 the lacunae have enlarged substantially. The cytotrophoblast has begun to form primary chorionic villi, which are finger-like protrusions into the lacunae. The embryo proper consists of two layers, the epiblast and the hypoblast, still closely applied to each other. The two cavities continue to enlarge, with the amniotic cavity above the epiblast and the yolk sac below the hypoblast, now known as the secondary yolk sac because of the presence of the chorionic cavity. The embryo is connected to the cytotrophoblast by a connecting stalk of extra-embryonic mesoderm. This stalk is the forerunner of the umbilical cord. By this stage the uterine epithelium has reformed, thus completely engulfing the conceptus. The largest development of trophoblastic lacunae is on the deepest surface of the conceptus. By the end of the second week, the syncytiotrophoblast produces the hormone human chorionic gonadotrophin (hCG), which maintains the corpus luteum in the ovary, which in turn sustains the thickness of the endometrium. The hormone is secreted in the urine and thus its presence is an early indicator of pregnancy.

## The third week – further development of the embryo and formation of trilaminar disc

The embryo develops further by forming three germ layers, the process known as gastrulation. Two layers have already formed: the epiblast and the hypoblast. These two closely apposed layers take up the form of two elliptical plates and together are termed the bilaminar embryonic disc. From this point the epiblast becomes known as the ectoderm and the hypoblast as the endoderm.

The ectoderm gives rise to the third layer that comes to lie between the two original germ layers, the intra-embryonic mesoderm. As a useful generalisation, the ectoderm (the outer skin) forms the covering of the body (the epidermis) as well as the nervous system; the endo-

FIGURE 11.4 **Implanted blastocyst**

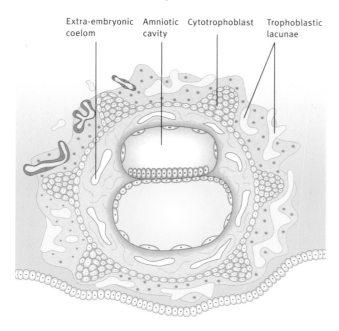

At day 12 cavities develop that coalesce to form the extra-embryonic coelom.

*Reproduced with permission from: Embryology: An Illustrated Colour Text.* Mitchell B, Sharma R. London: Churchill Livingstone; 2009. Copyright Elsevier.

FIGURE 11.5 **Germ layer derivatives**

derm (the inner skin) forms the lining of the gastrointestinal and respiratory systems; and the mesoderm (the middle skin) forms the skeletal, connective and muscle tissues of the body. The main tissue derivatives of germ layers are shown in Figure 11.5.

## Development of the ectoderm

### PRIMITIVE STREAK FORMATION

By the end of the second week of development there is a groove-like midline depression in the caudal end of the bilaminar embryonic disc. This marks the appearance of the primitive streak. By the beginning of week 3 the streak deepens. At the cephalic end of the streak the primitive node develops. Cells of the ectoderm layer migrate towards the streak and then detach from it, spreading out laterally beneath it. This migration forms a new germ layer, the intra-embryonic mesoderm. The new germ layer spreads out in all directions to lie between the ectoderm and the endoderm, except in two locations where the original two germ layers remain in contact: the prochordal plate, at the cephalic end of the disc, and the cloacal plate at the caudal end of the disc (Figure 11.6). The prochordal plate is

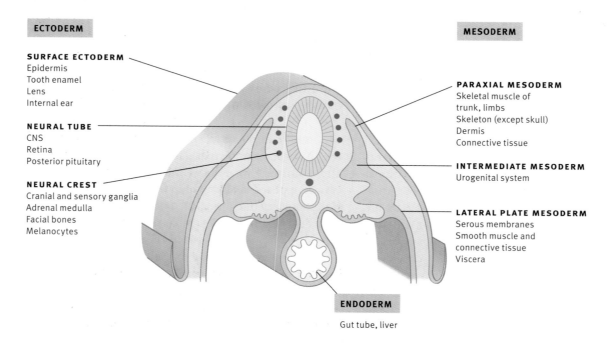

**ECTODERM**

**SURFACE ECTODERM**
Epidermis
Tooth enamel
Lens
Internal ear

**NEURAL TUBE**
CNS
Retina
Posterior pituitary

**NEURAL CREST**
Cranial and sensory ganglia
Adrenal medulla
Facial bones
Melanocytes

**MESODERM**

**PARAXIAL MESODERM**
Skeletal muscle of
trunk, limbs
Skeleton (except skull)
Dermis
Connective tissue

**INTERMEDIATE MESODERM**
Urogenital system

**LATERAL PLATE MESODERM**
Serous membranes
Smooth muscle and
connective tissue
Viscera

**ENDODERM**
Gut tube, liver

FIGURE 11.6  **Dorsal view of the embryonic disc showing the formation of the notochord**

By day 18 the notochord induces the overlying ectoderm to form the neural plate. Arrows indicate the migration of intra-embryonic mesoderm.

*Reproduced with permission from: Embryology: An Illustrated Colour Text.* Mitchell B, Sharma R. London: Churchill Livingstone; 2009. Copyright Elsevier.

soon replaced by the buccopharyngeal membrane, which forms a temporary seal for the future oral cavity. In week 4 this membrane breaks down to establish communication between the gut tube and the amniotic cavity. The cloacal plate is replaced by the cloacal membrane.

## NOTOCHORD FORMATION

Cells derived from the primitive node migrate cranially towards the buccopharyngeal membrane (Figure 11.6). This results in the appearance of the notochordal plate, which in turn folds in to form the solid cylinder of the notochord. The notochord thus comes to underlie the future neural tube (the future brain and spinal cord) and forms both a longitudinal axis for the embryo and the centres (nuclei pulposi) of the intervertebral discs of the vertebral column.

## NEURULATION

The process of the formation of the brain and spinal cord is known as neurulation. The ectoderm germ layer gives rise to neuroectoderm, which gives rise to most of the major components of the nervous system. At about 19 days, at the cranial end of the primitive streak, the under-lying mesoderm and notochord induce the ectoderm to form the neural plate (Figure 11.6), which rounds up to form the neural folds. The neural plate enlarges initially at the cranial end. At 20 days, the neural plate in the mid-region of the embryo remains narrowed, but it expands at the caudal end. The plate deepens to form the neural groove from which the neural tube forms. The cranial and caudal ends of the tube are open and are known as the anterior and posterior neuropores; these eventually close. At the edges of the neural tube, where the neuro-ectoderm is continuous with the surface ectoderm, the neural crests are formed. The neural crest cells detach themselves from the rest of the neural groove, before the tube forms, forming discrete aggregations of neural crest cells (Figure 11.7). They contribute to the formation of dorsal root, cranial, enteric and autonomic ganglia, connective tissues of the face and bones of the skull, the adrenal medulla, glial cells, Schwann cells, melanocytes, parts of the meninges and parts of the teeth.

## Further development of the mesoderm

As the number of mesodermal cells increases on either side of the notochord, by day 17 the layer becomes thickest

FIGURE 11.7 **Transverse sections of the embryo showing the origin and migration of neural crest cells between days 19 and 21**

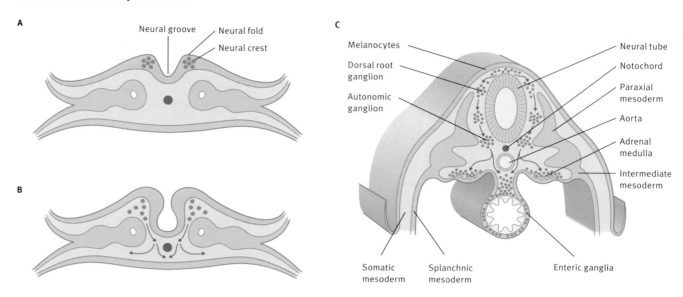

closest to the midline, which is known as the paraxial mesoderm. The parts further out are known as the intermediate and lateral plate mesoderm (Figure 11.7 C). At day 19, clefts begin to appear in the lateral plate. The mesoderm of the lateral plate is continuous with the extra-embryonic mesoderm covering the amniotic sac and the yolk sac (Figure 11.7 A, B). The mesoderm covering the amniotic sac is termed the parietal or somatic layer and that covering the yolk sac the visceral or splanchnic layer (Figure 11.7 B). The diverging limbs of the extra-embryonic mesoderm open into the extra-embryonic coelom. The clefts that appear within the lateral plate merge to form the intra-embryonic coelom, a cavity which is the forerunner of the serous cavities (the pericardial, pleural and peritoneal cavities). The intra-embryonic and extra-embryonic coeloms are therefore continuous.

Arising between the paraxial and lateral plate mesoderm is the intermediate mesoderm from which the urogenital system develops (Figure 11.7 C).

## Segmentation of the mesoderm

### PARAXIAL MESODERM

The paraxial mesoderm undergoes further differentiation in paired blocks of tissue in a craniocaudal direction on each side of the notochord, called somites. The first pair of somites forms at about 20 days and thereafter at a rate of about three per day until 42–44 pairs are formed, though not all persist into adulthood. The age of an embryo is related to the number of somite pairs present. From the beginning of the fourth week, the somites undergo further differentiation to form dermomyotomes (which form connective tissue and skeletal muscle) and sclerotomes (which form bone and cartilage) (Figure 11.8). Cells from the sclerotomes surround the notochord and spinal cord and give rise to the vertebral column.

### SOMITE DEVELOPMENT

In the fourth week, the medially placed mesenchymal cells of the somites migrate towards the notochord to form sclerotomes (mesenchyme is the loosely arranged embryonic connective tissue in the embryo). The ventro-

FIGURE 11.8 **Transverse sections of the embryo showing development of the somite**

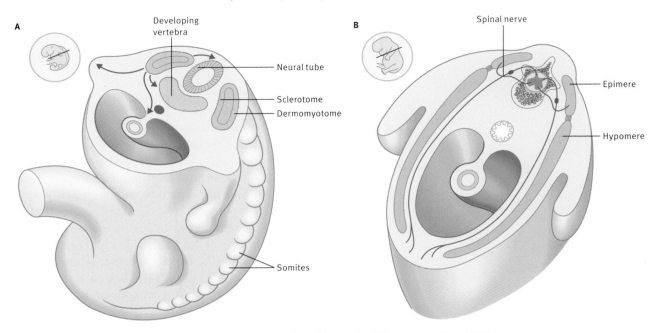

lateral cells of the somites become the myotomes, and those remaining become the dermatomes (Figure 11.8 A). The myotomes split into dorsal epimeres and ventral hypomeres. The dorsal epimeres give rise to epaxial muscles, the erector spinae muscles. The ventral hypomeres give rise to hypaxial muscles, which include muscles of the body wall (Figure 11.8 B). The ventrolateral parts of the somites in the regions of the future limb buds that remain after the sclerotomal portion has formed migrate to differentiate into limb musculature. The dermatomes form the dermis of the skin and, thus, these cells come to lie beneath the surface ectoderm, which forms the uppermost layer of the skin, the epidermis. It is important to appreciate that, as the myotomes and dermatomes migrate to their adult position, they bring with them their innervation, from the segment of origin of the developing spinal cord.

## LATERAL PLATE MESODERM

The two layers of the lateral plate mesoderm enclose the intra-embryonic coelom. The mesodermal cells of the lateral plate arrange themselves as thin layers, which become the serous membranes of the body: the pleura, pericardium and peritoneum. These two continuous layers differentiate therefore to become a lining for the future body wall, a covering for the future endodermal gut tube and the smooth muscle and connective tissue of the gut wall. The serous layer in contact with the future body wall is the parietal layer; the serous layer in contact with the endodermal gut tube is the visceral layer. Other names for these two layers are somatopleure and splanchnopleure (Figure 11.7 B, C).

## ENDODERM

The epithelial lining of the gastrointestinal tract is derived from the endoderm germ layer. The formation of the endodermal gut tube depends on the transverse and longitudinal folding of the embryo. In addition to the lining of the gastrointestinal and respiratory systems, the endoderm also gives rise to the parenchymal cells of the liver and pancreas and of the thyroid and parathyroids, as well as the lining of the urinary bladder.

FIGURE 11.9 **Formation of the lateral body folds between day 18 and day 21 in transverse sections of the embryo**

**A** Day 18

- Amniotic cavity
- Neural tube
- Notochord
- Yolk sac

**B** Day 21

**C** Day 24

- Peritoneal cavity
- Gut
- Anterior body wall

Arrows indicate the lateral folds. By day 24 lateral folding is complete.

*Reproduced with permission from: Embryology: An Illustrated Colour Text.* Mitchell B, Sharma R. London: Churchill Livingstone; 2009. Copyright Elsevier.

## The fourth week – folding of the embryo

Folding takes place in two directions: longitudinal (also referred to as cephalocaudal) and lateral (or transverse). Longitudinal folding occurs mainly as a consequence of the rapid enlargement of the cranial end of the neural tube to form the brain. Lateral folding is a consequence of the enlargement of the somites. The process of lateral folding is illustrated in Figure 11.9.

Longitudinal folding, which occurs between days 21 and 24, results in bending of the embryo so that the head and tail are brought closer together (Figure 11.10). The endoderm forms a tube-like structure with an initially wide communication with the yolk sac: this communication narrows as the longitudinal folding increases. The amniotic cavity pushes in at the cranial and caudal ends of the embryonic disc, thus increasing the degree of longitudinal folding at the head and tail folds. The amniotic cavity also pinches the connection of the yolk sac and gut to form the narrowed communication of the vitello-intestinal (or vitelline) duct (Figure 11.10). Later, this duct is lost.

The yolk sac plays a role in the early nutrition of the embryo but this is lost after the first month or so and a vestigial yolk sac lies freely in the chorionic cavity.

FIGURE 11.10 **The process of longitudinal folding by day 25 in a saggital section of an embryo**

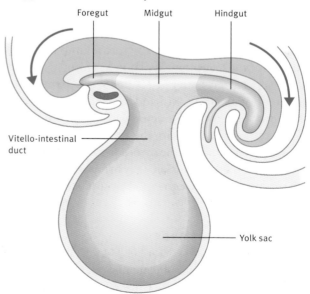

Foregut  Midgut  Hindgut

Vitello-intestinal duct

Yolk sac

Arrows indicate the formation of head and tail folds.

*Reproduced with permission from: Embryology: An Illustrated Colour Text.* Mitchell B, Sharma R. London: Churchill Livingstone; 2009. Copyright Elsevier.

# Development of the urogenital tract

*Vivek Nama*

## Development of the urogenital system

The urogenital system develops from the intermediate mesoderm. A longitudinal elevation of the intermediate mesoderm appears on either side of the aorta known as the urogenital ridge. The part that develops into the urinary system is known as the nephrogenic cord and the part that develops into the genital system is known as the gonadal ridge. The urinary system develops before the genital system (Box 12.1). The origins of the different parts of the fully formed urogenital system are listed in Table 12.1.

## Development of the kidney

Figure 12.1 shows the structures present early in embryonic development, at week 3. Three types of excretory organs are formed in a cranial to caudal sequence – the pronephros, mesonephros and metanephros – which are shown schematically in Figure 12.2.

The pronephros that appears at the beginning of week 4 of gestation is rudimentary and nonfunctional. It is seen as seven solid cell groups in the cervical region. All the elements of the pronephros disappear a week after their appearance. The pronephric ducts persist and are used by the mesonephros.

The mesonephros appears at week 4, becomes functional between weeks 6–10 and disappears by the end of week 10. The mesonephric ducts function as interim kidneys for 4 weeks (see Figure 12.4). They originate from the intermediate mesoderm between the upper thoracic and the upper lumbar segment (L3). They form excretory tubules that lengthen and acquire a tuft of capillaries. The tubules immediately adjacent to the vascular tuft differentiate into the Bowman's capsule and, laterally, the tubules open into the wolffian duct. The tubules then degenerate but the wolffian ducts persist and participate in the formation of the genital system in the male but disappear in the female.

The metanephros forms the permanent kidney that appears in week 5 and urine production starts by week 12. The excretory units develop from the metanephric mesoderm (metanephric blastema). The collecting ducts develop from the ureteric bud, which is an outgrowth of the mesonephric duct close to its entrance to the cloaca. This bud penetrates the metanephric mesoderm, the stalk of the ureteric bud forms the ureter and the expanded part forms the renal calyx. Each newly formed collecting tubule is covered at its distal end by a metanephric tis-

---

**BOX 12.1  Useful time points in the development of the urinary system and the gonads**

**URINARY SYSTEM**
- Pronephros – week 4, never functional
- Mesonephros – week 4, functions from weeks 6–10
- Metanephros – week 4, functions from week 12

**GONADS**
- Primordial germ cells develop in the endodermal yolk sac – week 4
- Germ cells migrate to mesodermal endothelium – week 5
- Gonads remain as indifferent – week 6
- Interstitial cells produce testosterone – week 8
- Secondary sex cords (cortical cords) – weeks 10–12
- Primordial follicles – week 16

**TABLE 12.1 Embryonic structures, adult derivatives and vestigial remnants in male and female**

| Male | Embryonic structure | Female |
|---|---|---|
| Testis | Indifferent gonad | Ovary |
| Seminiferous tubules | Cortex | Ovarian follicles |
| Rete testis | Medulla | Rete ovarii |
| Gubernaculum testis | Gubernaculums | Ovarian ligament and round ligament |
| Efferent ductules | Mesonephric tubules | Epoophoron, paroophoron |
| Duct of epididymis, also appendix of epididymis | Mesonephric duct (wolffian) | Duct of epoophoron, appendix vesiculosa |
| Ductus deferens | | Duct of Gartner |
| Ejaculatory duct and seminal vesicle | | No homologue |
| Ureter, renal pelvis, calyces, collecting tubules | | Ureter, renal pelvis, calyces, collecting tubules |
| Appendix of testes | Paramesonephric duct | Uterine tube, uterus, hydatid |
| Urinary bladder | Urogenital sinus | Urinary bladder |
| Urethra | | Urethra |
| Prostate gland | | Urethral and paraurethral glands |
| Prostatic utricle | | Vagina |
| Penis | Genital tubercle | Clitoris |
| Glans penis | | Glans clitoridis |
| Ventral aspect of penis | Urethral folds | Labia minora |
| Scrotum | Genital swellings | Labia majora |

*(handwritten annotations: "Trigone of bladder", "(Müllerian)", "Trigone of bladder")*

sue cap. The mesoderm adjacent to the collecting tubule develops into cells known as the metanephric vesicle. These vesicles differentiate later into the renal tubules and acquire a tuft of capillaries that later form glomeruli. Hence, the uriniferous tubule consists of the nephrons derived from the metanephric mass of intermediate mesoderm and a collecting tubule derived from the metanephric diverticulum. The glomerular integrity depends on signalling between the three major cell lineages: podocytes, and endothelial and mesangial cells. These tubules, together with their glomeruli, form nephrons. Hence, the kidney develops from two sources: metanephric mesoderm and the ureteric bud. In animal models, kidney formation is known to be controlled by the proteins RET (rearranged during transfection pro-tooncogene), GDNF (giant cell line-derived neutrophilic

**FIGURE 12.1 The intermediate mesoderm and the development of the urogenital organs in the early embryo (week 3)**

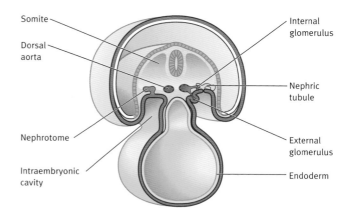

FIGURE 12.2 **Schematic representation of the three types of excretory organs formed in the human embryo**

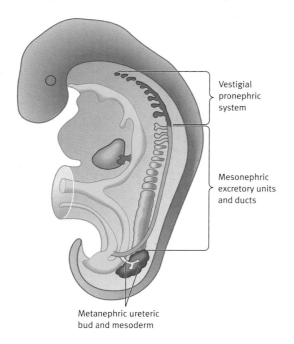

Vestigial pronephric system

Mesonephric excretory units and ducts

Metanephric ureteric bud and mesoderm

TABLE 12.2 **Development of the kidney and its regulators**

| Embryo | Adult derivatives |
|---|---|
| **PRONEPHROS** | Not functional and completely regresses, paramesonephric duct forms internal genitalia of the female |
| **MESONEPHROS** | Completely regresses but the mesonephric duct forms the internal male genital organs |
| **METANEPHROS** | |
| Ureteric bud | Collecting duct, minor calyx, major calyx, renal pelvis, ureter (regulated by WT1, GDNF9 glial cell line-derived neurotrophic factor, C-RET9 tyrosine kinase receptor) |
| Metanephric mesoderm | Renal glomerulus, renal capsule, proximal convoluted tubule, loop of Henle, distal convoluted tubule, connecting tubule (regulated by fibroblast growth factor 2, bone morphogenetic protein 7, GFRA1, WNT11) |

factor) and GFRA1 (GDNF family receptor alpha-1) (Table 12.2). Mutations in *RET* are found in both unilateral (20%) and bilateral (37%) renal agenesis.

## POSITION OF THE KIDNEY

The kidney develops in the pelvic region and later ascends to a more cranial position. The change in position is due to the differential growth of the lumbar and sacral regions. As the kidney ascends, it rotates by 90 degrees and derives its blood supply from the aorta, and the lower vessels disappear.

### Clinical correlates

- Wilms tumour occurs as a result of mutation in WT1, which regulates the mesoderm to respond to induction by the ureteric bud.

- Renal agenesis can occur if the ureteric bud fails to contact and/or induce the metanephric mesoderm. Unilateral renal agenesis occurs in one in 1000 infants. It is more common on the left side and in males. Unilateral renal agenesis is associated with a single umbilical artery. Bilateral renal agenesis is associated with oligohydramnios and characteristic facial appearance and occurs in one in 3000 births.

- Duplication of the ureter results from early splitting of the ureteric bud. Splitting may be partial or complete and metanephric tissue may be divided into two parts, each with its own renal pelvis and ureter. Partial division results in a divided kidney with a bifid ureter and complete division results in a double kidney with a bifid ureter.

- Accessory renal arteries occur from the persistence of embryonic vessels formed during the ascent of the kidney. About 25% of adult kidneys have two to four renal arteries. Accessory renal arteries usually arise from the aorta. Accessory arteries are about twice as common as accessory veins.

- Polycystic kidney disease is an autosomal that occurs because of the wide dilatation of the nephrons, particularly the loop of Henle. Gene mutations and faulty signalling have been implicated.

## Development of the bladder

During weeks 4 and 7 of development, the cloaca is divided into the urogenital sinus anteriorly and the anal canal posteriorly by the urogenital septum. The urogenital septum is a layer of mesoderm and its tip forms the perineal body. The urogenital sinus now develops into three parts. The cranial part forms the urinary bladder, which is continuous with the allantois. The narrower middle pelvic part forms the prostatic and membranous urethra in the male and the entire urethra in the female. The caudal, or phallic, part forms the genital organs (Figure 12.3). Later, the lumen of the allantois becomes obliterated to form the urachus (median umbilical ligament). During differentiation of the cloaca, caudal portions of the mesonephric ducts are absorbed into the wall of the urinary bladder. Consequently, the ureters outgrow the mesonephric ducts and enter the bladder separately. Since both mesonephric ducts and ureters originate in the mesoderm, the mucosa of the bladder (trigone) formed by the incorporation of the ureteric and ejaculatory ducts is mesodermal in origin.

## Development of the urethra

The epithelium of the urethra in both sexes originates in the endoderm; the surrounding connective and smooth muscle tissue is derived from the mesoderm. In males, the cranial part of the prostatic urethral epithelium forms numerous outgrowths that form the prostate. In females, the cranial part gives rise to the urethral and paraurethral glands.

### Clinical correlates

- When the lumen of the intraembryonic portion of the allantois persists, a urachal fistula drains urine into the umbilicus. If only a small area persists, then a urachal cyst is formed.

- Congenital megacystis is a pathologically large bladder and results from maldevelopment of the ureteric bud. It is usually associated with renal failure and pulmonary hypoplasia unless intrauterine treatment is performed.

FIGURE 12.3 **The bladder after week 5**

Gonad and remnants of mesonephros

Metanephros

Bladder

Phallus

Urogenital sinus

Rectum

- Exstrophy of the bladder is caused by a lack of mesodermal migration and incomplete closure of the inferior abdominal wall between the umbilicus and genital tubercle followed by rupture of the thin layer of ectoderm. It occurs in 10 in 40 000 births. The anomaly is characterised by protrusion of the posterior wall of the bladder. Complete exstrophy is associated with epispadias and wide separation of the pubic bones.

- Exstrophy of the cloaca occurs because of the failure of migration of mesoderm to the midline. The defect includes exstrophy of the bladder, spinal defects, imperforate anus and usually omphalocele.

## Development of the genital system

The genital system consists of gonads, gonadal ducts and external genitalia. All three components go through an indifferent stage, during which they may develop into either male or female.

### GONADS

Gonadal development begins at week 4 and starts as an area of thickened mesothelium on the medial side of the

## FIGURE 12.4  Transverse section of the embryo at week 6 showing the genital ridge and the mesonephros

The sex of the embryo is determined by its genotype. The sexual differentiation in the genital ducts and external genitalia is then determined by the type of gonad. The *SRY* (sex-determining region on Y) gene located on the short arm of chromosome Y (Yp11) determines the differentiation of the gonads. The SRY protein is the testis-determining factor; under its influence male development occurs and in its absence female development (Figure 12.5).

### The testis

If the embryo is genetically male, the primordial germ cells carry an XY sex chromosome complex. Under influence of the *SRY* gene on the Y chromosome, which encodes the testis-determining factor, the primitive sex cords continue to proliferate and penetrate deep into the medulla to form the testis or medullary cords. A layer of dense connective tissue appears which separates the cords from the surface epithelium and later forms the tunica albuginea (white covering). The enlarging testis becomes separated from the mesoderm and develops its own mesentry, the mesochorium. The cords of cells, now called seminiferous cords, develop into seminiferous tubules: tubuli seminiferi recti (straight seminiferous tubules) and rete testis. The Sertoli cells are derived from the surface epithelium of the gland and interstitial cells

mesonephros (Figure 12.4). The gonads appear initially as a pair of longitudinal ridges, the genital or gonadal ridges, and remain indifferent until week 7. Finger-like epithelial cords, the gonadal cords, grow into the underlying mesenchyme, dividing the ridge into the external cortex and the internal medulla. Primordial germ cells from the yolk sac migrate by amoeboid movement along the dorsal mesentery, invading the genital ridges in week 6. If they fail to reach the ridges, the gonads do not develop and there is a lack of the inductive influence of these cells on the development of the gonad into ovary or testis.

## FIGURE 12.5  Events in the differentiation of the gonadal ridge based on the genotype and hormones produced

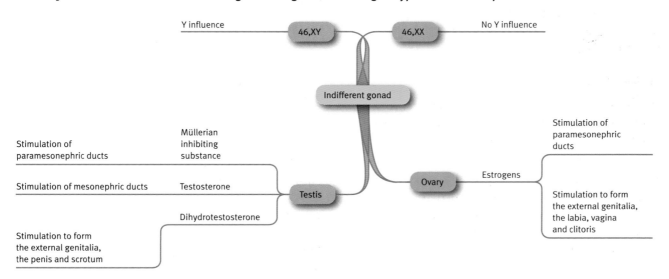

of Leydig from the mesenchyme of the gonadal ridge. By week 8, Leydig cells begin production of testosterone and are able to influence sexual differentiation of the genital ducts and external genitalia. The seminiferous tubules canalise at puberty, which in turn enter the ductuli efferentes (excretory mesonephric tubules), which link the rete testis and the mesonephric duct, which becomes the ductus deferens (mesonephric duct) (Figure 12.6).

### The ovary

In embryos with XX chromosomes, the sex cords dissociate into irregular cell clusters. The germ cells in the medullary part of the ovary are replaced by vascular stroma but the surface epithelium continues to multiply, forming cords of cells. During multiplication, the primordial germ cells are incorporated into the cords. At month 4, these cords split into isolated cell clusters surrounding the primitive germ cells. Later, the germ cells develop into oogonia and the epithelial cells surrounding the oogonia form follicular cells (Figure 12.7).

### GENITAL DUCTS

There are two pairs of genital ducts: wolffian (mesonephric) ducts and müllerian (paramesonephric) ducts.

### In the male embryo

The mesonephric ducts under the influence of testosterone form the epididymis, ductus deferens and ejaculatory duct. As the mesonephros regresses, the tubules divide into epigenital and paragenital tubules. The epigenital tubules join the rete testis and form the efferent ductules, whereas the paragenital tubules do not join the rete testis and form the paradidymis. The mesonephric ducts below the paradidymis elongate and convolute to form the epididymis. The seminal vesicle grows as an outbudding from the tail of epididymis and the region beyond the seminal vesicle is called the ejaculatory duct. The paramesonephric ducts degenerate in the male to form the appendix testis (Figure 12.8).

### In the female embryo

The paramesonephric ducts arise as a longitudinal invagination of the mesothelium on the lateral surface of the urogenital ridge. Cranially, the duct opens into the abdominal cavity and caudally it merges with the paramesonephric duct of the opposite side to form the uterovaginal primordium. The caudal tip then projects into the posterior wall of the urogenital sinus causing a small swelling known as the müllerian tubercle. As the ducts fuse in the midline, they take a sheet of peritoneum with them, which forms the broad ligament of the uterus. The fused paramesonephric ducts give rise to the corpus and cervix and the surrounding layer of mesenchyme forms the myometrium. The mesonephric ducts open into the urogenital hiatus on either side of the müllerian tubercle. The female may retain some parts of the excretory tubules known as epoophoron and paraoophoron. Small cranial portions of the mesonephric duct persist in the epoophoron. If the caudal part persists, then it may develop into a cyst in the uterus or the vagina known as a Gartner's cyst (Figure 12.9).

### EXTERNAL GENITALIA

### Indifferent stage

At week 3, the mesenchyme around the cloacal membrane becomes slightly elevated to form the cloacal fold. The folds cranial to the cloacal membrane unite to form the genital tubercle and caudally they are divided into urethral folds anteriorly and anal folds posteriorly. As the urorectal septum fuses with the cloacal membrane, it divides the cloacal membrane into a dorsal anal membrane and a ventral urogenital membrane. On either side of the urethral fold, another pair of swellings becomes more apparent, known as genital swellings. The genital swellings will form the scrotal swellings in the male and the labia majora in the female (Figure 12.10).

### In the male embryo

In the presence of androgens secreted by the testis, the genital tubercle elongates and is now called the phallus. As the phallus elongates it pulls the urethral folds forward so that they form the lateral walls of the urethral

FIGURE 12.6 **The embryonic testis**

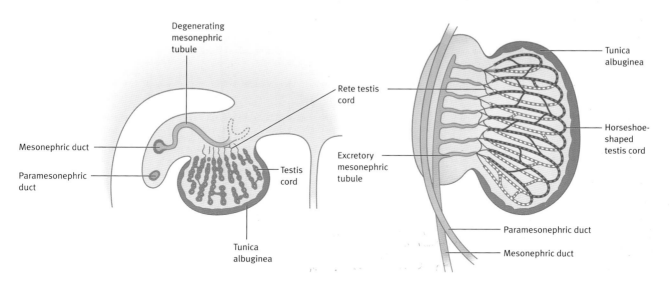

**A** Transverse section at week 8

**B** Sagittal section at month 4

FIGURE 12.7 **The embryonic ovary**

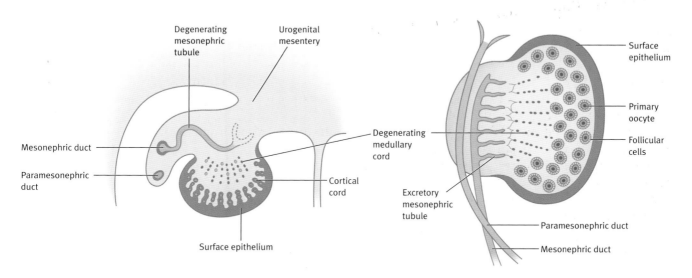

**A** Transverse section at week 7

**B** Sagittal section at month 5

groove. The epithelial lining of the groove originates in the endoderm and forms the urethral plate, which extends from the phallic portion of the urogenital sinus. The two urethral folds close over the urethral plate to form the penile urethra. Ectodermal cells penetrating inward and joining the urethra from the tip of the glans form the external urethral meatus. The corpora cavernosa and corpus spongiosum develop from mesenchyme in the phallus. The labioscrotal swellings fuse to form the scrotum (Figure 12.11).

FIGURE 12.8 **The male genital ducts**

**A** At month 4

Epigenital tubule

Rete testis

Testis cord

Tunica albuginea

Paragenital tubule

Mesonephric duct

Paramesonephric tubercle

**B** After descent of the testis

Seminal vesicle

Uticulus prostaticus

Mesonephric duct

Appendix epididymis

Appendix testis

Excretory mesonephric tubule

Testis cord

Rete testis

Epididymis

Paradidymis

FIGURE 12.9 **The female genital ducts**

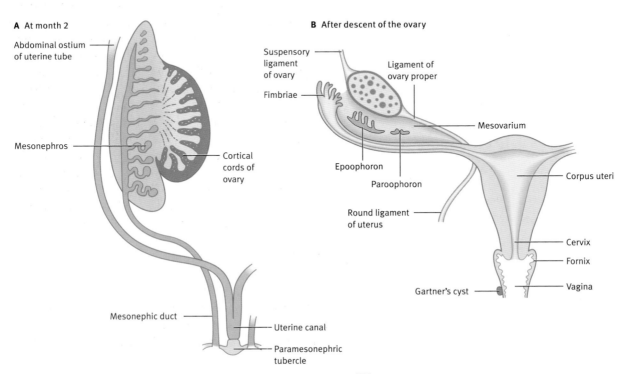

**A** At month 2

Abdominal ostium of uterine tube

Mesonephros

Cortical cords of ovary

Mesonephic duct

Uterine canal

Paramesonephric tubercle

**B** After descent of the ovary

Suspensory ligament of ovary

Ligament of ovary proper

Fimbriae

Mesovarium

Epoophoron

Paroophoron

Corpus uteri

Round ligament of uterus

Cervix

Fornix

Gartner's cyst

Vagina

### FIGURE 12.10  Indifferent stages of external genitalia

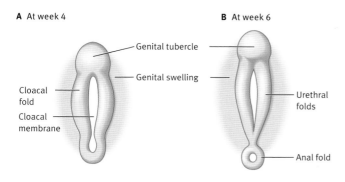

**A** At week 4

**B** At week 6

Genital tubercle

Genital swelling

Cloacal fold

Cloacal membrane

Urethral folds

Anal fold

### FIGURE 12.11  Male external genitalia

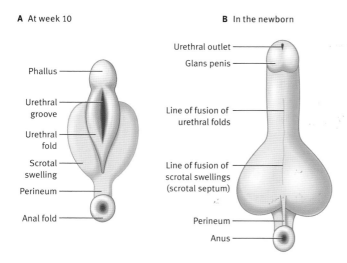

**A** At week 10

**B** In the newborn

Phallus

Urethral groove

Urethral fold

Scrotal swelling

Perineum

Anal fold

Urethral outlet

Glans penis

Line of fusion of urethral folds

Line of fusion of scrotal swellings (scrotal septum)

Perineum

Anus

### FIGURE 12.12  Female external genitalia

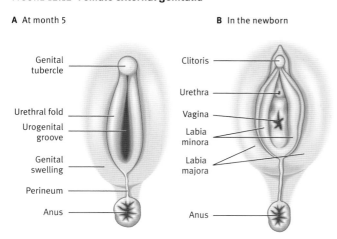

**A** At month 5

**B** In the newborn

Genital tubercle

Urethral fold

Urogenital groove

Genital swelling

Perineum

Anus

Clitoris

Urethra

Vagina

Labia minora

Labia majora

Anus

## Clinical correlates

- Androgen insensitivity syndrome occurs in one in 20 000 births and is phenotypically female but genotypically male. The external genitalia are female but end in a blind pouch. The uterus and uterine tubes are absent or rudimentary. It results from a defect in the androgen receptor mechanism.

- Hypospadias occurs as a result of failure of the fusion of the urethral folds near the glans or at the shaft or near the base of the penis. It is the most common anomaly of the penis and occurs in one in 300 male infants. Hypospadias is said to occur because of inadequate production of androgens by the fetal testes.

- Epispadias is the result of the genital tubercle developing in the region of the urorectal septum instead of the cranial end of the cloacal membrane. This places the urethra on the dorsum of the penis. It occurs in one in 30 000 male infants and is often associated with exstrophy of the bladder.

### In the female embryo

As the paramesonephric ducts reach the urogenital sinus, two solid evaginations grow out of the pelvic part of the urogenital sinus. These evaginations are known as the sinovaginal bulbs, which proliferate and form a solid vaginal plate. Proliferation of the cranial end of the plate continues until it reaches the cervix. The lower part of the paramesonephric ducts are absorbed into the sinovaginal bulbs. Hence, the vaginal fornices develop from the paramesonephric ducts. Later, the vaginal plate acquires a lumen by the breakdown of the central cells to form the vagina. In the presence of estrogens, the genital tubercle elongates only slightly to form the clitoris and the urethral folds develop into the labia minora. The genital swellings enlarge and form the labia majora and the urogenital groove forms the vestibule (Figure 12.12).

### DESCENT OF GONADS

The urogenital mesentery attaches the testis and mesonephros to the posterior abdominal wall. With the degeneration of the mesonephros, the attachment serves as a mesentery for the gonad. Caudally it becomes ligamentous (caudal genital ligament). The gubernaculum is a band of mesenchyme extending from the tip of the testis and ending in the anterior abdominal wall. As the fetus grows and the testis passes through the inguinal canal, the lower part of the gubernaculum develops from the scrotal floor and joins the intra-abdominal part. The testis reaches the inguinal canal by week 12, migrates through the inguinal canal by week 28 and reaches the scrotum by week 33. As the testis descends, the peritoneum covering the testis is called a processus vaginalis (vaginal process), which later forms the tunica vaginalis. The communication between the abdominal cavity and the tunica vaginalis is obliterated at birth. The transversalis fascia (transverse fascia) forms the internal spermatic fascia, the internal abdominal oblique muscle forms the cremasteric fascia and muscle and the external oblique forms the external spermatic fascia.

The descent of the ovary is considerably less and settles below the rim of the true pelvis. The cranial genital ligament forms the suspensory ligament of the ovary whereas the caudal genital ligament forms the ligament of the ovary proper and the round ligament of the uterus.

## Clinical correlates

- Absence of vagina and uterus occurs in one in 4000–5000 female births. The failure of the sinovaginal bulbs to develop and form the vaginal plate leads to absent vagina. It is usually associated with an absent uterus as the sinovaginal plates are induced by the paramesonephric ducts fusion and migration to the urogenital sinus.

- Vaginal atresia is failure of canalisation of the vaginal plate, which results in vaginal atresia. This leads to formation of the transverse vaginal septum usually located at the junction of the middle and superior thirds of the vagina.

- Cryptorchidism or undescended testes occur in 30% of premature infants and 3–4% of infants born at term. In most cases, the testes descend into the scrotum by the end of the first year; if they remain within the abdominal wall, by the end of 1 year sterility is common. Deficient production of androgen by the fetal testes plays a role in its causation.

### SUGGESTED FURTHER READING

KEITH L, MOORE T V N P, editors. *The Developing Embryo.* 7th ed. Philadelphia: Saunders; 2003.

QUAGGIN S E, KREIDBERG J A. Development of the renal glomerulus: good neighbors and good fences. *Development* 2008;135:609–20.

THOMAS W, SADLER J L, LELAND J, editors. *Langman's Medical Embryology.* 10th ed. Philadelphia: Lippincott Williams & Wilkins; 2006.

# Development and congenital anomalies of the gastrointestinal tract

*Rohan D'Souza*

## Development of the digestive system

During week 4 of development, the embryo folds cephalo-caudally and laterally, incorporating a portion of the endoderm-lined yolk sac cavity to form the primitive gut: the yolk sac and the allantois remain outside the embryo (Figure 13.1). This gut system extends from the buccopharyngeal membrane to the cloacal membrane and is divided into the pharyngeal gut, foregut, midgut and hindgut, the derivatives of which are shown in Table 13.1. The relative contributions of the three germ layers of the primitive gut are outlined in Table 13.2 while the arterial supply is outlined in Table 13.3.

### FOREGUT

#### Development of the oesophagus

In week 4, a respiratory diverticulum (lung bud) appears in the ventral wall of the foregut just beneath the pharyngeal gut. This diverticulum gradually gets partitioned from the dorsal part of the foregut by the tracheoesopha-

FIGURE 13.1 **Sagittal sections showing the cephalocaudal folding of the embryo and the formation of the primitive gut**

**A** Presomite embryo

**B** Embryo at 22 days

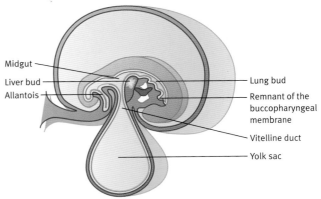

TABLE 13.1 **Derivatives of the primitive gut**

| Pharyngeal gut | Pharynx and related glands |
|---|---|
| Foregut | Oesophagus |
| | Trachea and lung buds |
| | Stomach |
| | Duodenum proximal to the entrance of the bile duct |
| | Liver, biliary apparatus and pancreas |
| Midgut | Duodenum distal to the opening of the bile duct |
| | Small intestine |
| | Caecum and appendix |
| | Ascending colon and two-thirds of the transverse colon |
| Hindgut | Distal third of the transverse colon, descending colon and sigmoid colon |
| | Rectum and the superior part of the anal canal |
| | Epithelium of the urinary bladder and most of the urethra |

TABLE 13.2 **Contributions of the germ layers in the development of the gut**

| Germ layer | Derived components |
|---|---|
| Endoderm | Epithelium of the digestive system |
| | Parenchyma of the derivates of the gut |
| Splanchnic mesoderm | Connective tissue |
| | Muscular components |
| | Peritoneal components |
| Ectoderm | Distal part of the anal canal |

TABLE 13.3 **Arterial supply of the primitive gut**

| Portion of primitive gut | Arterial supply |
|---|---|
| Foregut | Branches of the coeliac trunk |
| Midgut | Branches of the superior mesenteric artery |
| Hindgut | Branches of the inferior mesenteric artery |

geal septum. Thus, the foregut divides into a ventral respiratory primordium and a dorsal oesophagus. The oesophagus rapidly lengthens as the heart and lungs descend. The characteristics of the muscle coat of the oesophagus are outlined in Table 13.4.

### Development of the stomach

The stomach appears as a fusiform dilation of the foregut during week 4. It subsequently rotates around a longitudinal and an anteroposterior axis (Figure 13.2). The effects of this rotation have been summarised in Table 13.5.

During rotation, the original posterior wall (now on the left) grows faster than the anterior portion (now on the right), forming the greater and lesser curvatures respectively. The stomach thus assumes its final position, its axis running from above left to below right.

### Mesenteries of the stomach

The stomach is suspended from the dorsal wall and ventral body wall by mesenteries, known as the dorsal and ventral mesogastrium respectively. Its rotation and disproportionate growth alter the position of these mesenteries.

The dorsal mesogastrium is pulled to the left, creating a space behind the stomach called the omental bursa (lesser peritoneal sac). It continues to grow down, forming a double-layered sac – the greater omentum (Figure 13.3). The two leaves of the greater omentum later fuse with each other and with the mesentery of the transverse colon.

The ventral mesogastrium is pulled to the right, forming the lesser omentum (which passes from the liver to the lesser curvature of the stomach) and the falciform ligament (which extends from the liver to the ventral abdominal wall). On its way from the umbilical cord to the liver, the umbilical vein passes in the free border of the falciform ligament (Figure 13.4).

TABLE 13.4 **Characteristics of the oesophageal muscle coat**

| Portion of oesophagus | Muscle type | Nerve supply |
|---|---|---|
| Upper two-thirds | Striated | Vagus nerve |
| Lower two-thirds | Smooth | Splanchnic plexus |

TABLE 13.5 **Rotation al changes during development of the stomach**

| Rotational change | Effects |
|---|---|
| 90° clockwise rotation around its longitudinal axis | The original left side now faces anterior and the original right side faces posterior |
| | The left vagus nerve consequently innervates the anterior wall and the right innervates the posterior wall |
| Anteroposterior rotation | The cephalic and caudal ends of the stomach no longer lie in the midline |
| | The caudal or pyloric part moves to the right and upward and the cephalic or cardiac portion moves to the left and slightly downward |

### Development of the duodenum

The duodenum also develops early in week 4. Since it develops from both the terminal part of the foregut and the proximal part of the midgut, it is supplied by branches of both the coeliac artery and the superior mesenteric artery. The junction of these two parts is just distal to the origin of the bile duct. As the stomach rotates, the duodenum takes on the form of a C-shaped loop, rotates to the right and becomes retroperitoneal. The region of the duodenal cap, however, retains its mesentery and remains intraperitoneal. During weeks 5–6, proliferation of epithelial cells results in temporary obliteration of the lumen of the duodenum, but this is recanalised by the end of the embryonic period.

FIGURE 13.2 **Schematic representation of the rotation of the stomach on its anteroposterior axis**

A Stomach prior to rotation

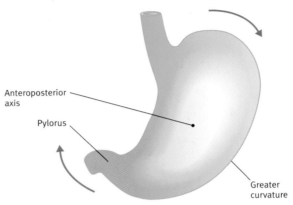

B Final position of the stomach after rotation

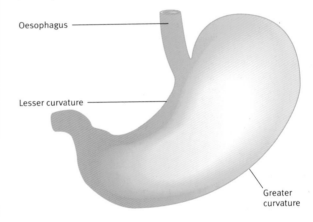

### Development of the liver and biliary apparatus

Rapidly proliferating cells at the distal end of the foregut result in the formation of a ventral outgrowth early in week 4. This is the hepatic diverticulum (liver bud), which then penetrates the septum transversum and goes on to form the liver and the biliary apparatus (Figure 13.5). The bile duct is formed when the connection between the hepatic diverticulum and the foregut (duodenum) subsequently narrows. The bile duct develops a small ventral outgrowth that then goes on to form the gallbladder and the cystic duct.

The surface mesoderm of the liver differentiates into visceral peritoneum, except on the cranial surface, where the liver remains in contact with the rest of the original

FIGURE 13.3 **The formation of the omental bursa and the greater omentum**

A Transverse section at 4 weeks, showing the formation of the omental bursa and lesser omentum

B Sagittal section at 4 months, showing the final position of the omental bursa and the greater omentum

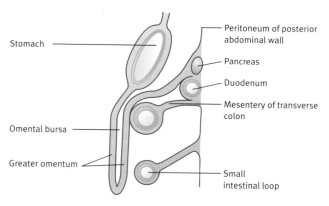

septum transversum. This portion of the septum, which comprises densely packed mesoderm, forms the central tendon of the diaphragm, and the surface of the liver that is in contact with the future diaphragm forms the bare area of the liver. This area is never covered by peritoneum. The liver grows rapidly and, by week 9, accounts for approximately 10% of the body weight. Initially, the right and left lobes are approximately the same size, but the right lobe soon becomes larger.

Haematopoiesis begins during week 6, giving the liver a bright red appearance. Bile formation by hepatic cells begins during week 12. When the cystic duct joins the hepatic duct to form the bile duct, bile enters the gastrointestinal tract and its contents take on a dark green colour. This entrance of the bile duct is initially anterior but, because of positional changes of the duodenum, it moves posteriorly and finally comes to lie behind the duodenum. The origin of various hepatic cells is outlined in Table 13.6.

### Development of the pancreas

Two separate buds, the ventral and dorsal pancreatic buds, originate from the endodermal lining of the duodenum and grow rapidly between the layers of the dorsal mesentery. These go on to form the pancreas. The larger dorsal pancreatic bud appears first and develops cranial to the ventral pancreatic bud, which in turn develops near the entry of the bile duct into the duodenum. Rotation of the duodenum causes the ventral bud to move dorsally and finally to lie immediately below and behind the dorsal bud. Subsequently, the parenchyma and the duct systems of the two buds fuse and the main pancreatic duct enters the

FIGURE 13.4 **The effect of rotation of the stomach on the position of the mesenteries**

A Embryo at week 5

B Embryo at week 11

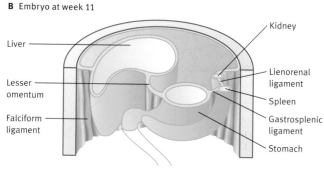

TABLE 13.6  **Origin of hepatic cells and sinusoids**

| Origin | Cell type |
|--------|-----------|
| Mesoderm of the septum transversum | Haematopoetic cells |
| | Kupffer cells |
| | Connective tissue cells |
| Liver cords | Parenchyma (liver cells) lining the biliary ducts |
| Intermingling of epithelial liver cords with vitelline and umbilical veins | Hepatic sinusoids |

duodenum along with the bile duct at the major papilla. The accessory pancreatic duct (when present) enters the duodenum at the minor papilla. Figure 13.6 and Table 13.7 provide more details.

The main pancreatic duct, together with the bile duct, enters the duodenum at the site of the major papilla; while the accessory duct (when present) enters at the site of the minor papilla, which is located approximately 2 cm cranial to the major papilla. In 10% of cases, the duct system fails to fuse and the original double system persists.

The origin of various cell-types in the pancreas is outlined in Table 13.8. Insulin secretion begins at approximately month 5.

### Development of the spleen

The spleen is derived from a mass of mesenchymal cells located between the layers of the dorsal mesogastrium. It begins to develop during week 5. In the fetus, the spleen is lobulated and functions as a haemopoietic centre. The splenic lobules normally disappear before birth, but the potential for blood cell formation is retained even in adult life. The splenic artery is the largest branch of the coeliac trunk.

## MIDGUT

The portion of the gut that is supplied by the superior mesenteric artery undergoes rapid elongation and forms the primary loop. Its derivatives are outlined in Table 13.9. At its apex, it remains in open connection with the yolk sac by way of the vitelline duct.

FIGURE 13.5  **Sagittal sections showing the penetration of the septum transversum by the rapidly proliferating cells of the hepatic diverticulum (liver bud) and the subsequent development of the liver and the biliary apparatus**

A  Embryo at day 25

B  Embryo at day 36

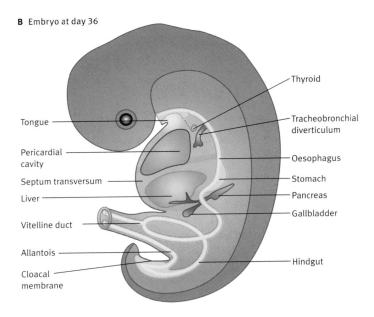

FIGURE 13.6 **Development of the pancreas**

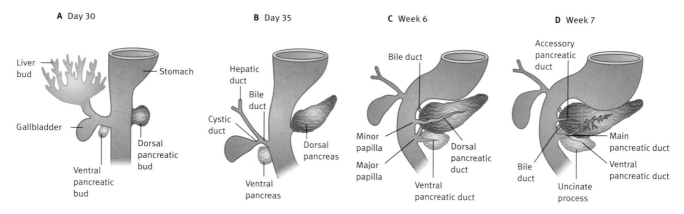

A Day 30     B Day 35     C Week 6     D Week 7

TABLE 13.7 **Origin of parenchyma and duct system of the pancreas**

| Origin | Final structure |
| --- | --- |
| Ventral pancreatic bud | Uncinate process and inferior part of head of pancreas |
| Dorsal pancreatic bud | Entire pancreas except for the above |
| Ventral pancreatic duct and the distal part of dorsal pancreatic duct | Main pancreatic duct (of Wirsung) |
| Proximal part of dorsal pancreatic duct (if and when it persists) | Accessory pancreatic duct (of Santorini) |

TABLE 13.8 **Origin of pancreatic cells and connective tissue**

| Origin | Cell/tissue |
| --- | --- |
| Parenchymatous pancreatic tissue | Pancreatic islets (of Langerhans) |
| | Glucagon- and somatostatin-secreting cells |
| Splanchnic mesoderm surrounding the pancreatic buds | Connective tissue |

### Physiological umbilical herniation and subsequent retraction of herniated loops

The primary loop, and especially its cephalic limb, elongates rapidly. As a result of this, as well as the rapid growth and expansion of the liver, the abdominal cavity temporarily becomes too small to contain all the intestinal loops. During week 6 of development, the loops therefore enter the extraembryonic cavity in the umbilical cord. This is known as physiological umbilical herniation.

During week 10, regression of the mesonephric kidney, reduced growth of the liver and expansion of the abdominal cavity cause these herniated intestinal loops to return to the abdominal cavity. The first part to re-enter the cavity is the proximal part of the jejunum, which comes to lie on the left side. The loops that enter later settle more and more to the right.

### Rotation of the midgut

The primary intestinal loop rotates around an axis formed by the superior mesenteric artery, by approximately 270 degrees in the anti-clockwise direction. This rotation occurs during herniation (about 90 degrees) as well as during return of the intestinal loops into the abdominal cavity (remaining 180 degrees).

### Caecum and appendix

The caecal bud, which appears at about week 6 as a small conical dilation of the caudal limb of the primary intesti-

TABLE 13.9 **Derivatives of the midgut**

| Part of the midgut | Derivatives |
|---|---|
| Cephalic limb of the primary loop | Distal part of the duodenum |
| | Jejunum |
| | Part of the ileum |
| Caudal limb of the primary loop | Lower part of the ileum |
| | Caecum and appendix |
| | Ascending colon |
| | Proximal two-thirds of the transverse colon |

nal loop, is the last part of the gut to re-enter the abdominal cavity. At first it lies in the right upper quadrant below the right lobe of the liver. Later it descends into the right iliac fossa and during this process its distal end forms a narrow diverticulum, the appendix. The appendix grows rapidly in length and at birth it is a relatively long tube arising from the distal end of the caecum. After birth, as a result of unequal growth of the caecal wall, it comes to lie medially, although it may sometimes lie posterior to the caecum and colon.

### Fixation of the intestines

The enlarged colon presses the duodenum and pancreas against the posterior abdominal wall resulting in the absorption of most of the duodenal mesentery. Similarly, when the ascending and descending colon obtain their definitive positions, their mesenteries press against the peritoneum of the posterior abdominal wall and are eventually absorbed. The following structures therefore become retroperitoneal:

- duodenum (except for the first 2.5 cm)
- ascending colon
- descending colon.

The following structures, however, retain their free mesenteries:

- other derivatives of the midgut loop (the jejunum and ileum)
- lower end of the caecum and the appendix

- transverse colon (although its mesentery fuses with the posterior wall of the greater omentum)
- sigmoid colon.

The line of attachment of the fan-shaped mesentery of the small intestine passes from the duodenojejunal junction inferolaterally to the ileocaecal junction.

### HINDGUT

#### Partitioning of the cloaca

The cloaca is the expanded terminal part of the hindgut. It is an endoderm-lined chamber that is in contact with the surface ectoderm at the cloacal membrane. This membrane is composed of endoderm of the cloaca on the inside and ectoderm of the proctodeum (anal pit) on the outside. As illustrated in Figure 13.7, at week 5, the allantois enters the anterior portion of the cloaca (the future urogenital sinus), while the hindgut enters the posterior portion (the future anorectal canal). A layer of mesoderm, the urorectal septum, separates the region between the allantois and hindgut. By week 6, the urorectal septum moves closer to the cloacal membrane, although the two never make contact. At the end of week 7, breakdown of the cloacal membrane creates the anal opening for the hindgut and a ventral opening for the urogenital sinus. The tip of the urorectal septum forms the perineal body. Proliferation of the ectoderm of the proctodeum closes the lowermost region of the anal canal but this region recanalises during week 9.

#### Anal canal

The superior two-thirds of the anal canal originates in the endoderm of the hindgut, while the inferior one-third originates in the ectoderm of the proctodeum. The junction between these regions is delineated by the pectinate line (also called the anocutaneous line or simply the 'white line'), just below the anal columns. The differences in blood supply, nerve supply and venous and lymphatic drainage of the superior and inferior parts of the anal canal are clinically important and are outlined in Table 13.10. The other layers of the wall of the anal canal are derived from the splanchnic mesoderm.

**179**

FIGURE 13.7 **Partitioning of the cloaca**

**A** Week 5

Allantois
Cloaca
Cloacal membrane
Urorectal septum
Hindgut

**B** Week 6

Primitive urogenital sinus

**C** Week 7

Urogenital membrane
Perineum
Anal membrane
Urinary bladder
Anorectal canal

## Congenital anomalies of the gut

### ABNORMALITIES OF THE FOREGUT

#### Oesophageal atresia

Oesophageal atresia occurs in about one in 3000–4500 live births. When associated with a tracheo-oesophageal fistula (85–90%), it occurs as a result of posterior deviation of the tracheo-oesophageal septum. When it occurs as an isolated abnormality, the cause is failure of recanalisation of the oesophagus during week 8 of development. This may be associated with anorectal atresia and anomalies of the urogenital system.

Oesophageal atresia manifests as polyhydramnios in fetal life and excessive drooling and regurgitation after birth. Diagnosis is suspected when there is an inability to pass a catheter through the oesophagus and confirmed on radiography when the nasogastric tube is arrested in the proximal oesophageal pouch. This abnormality can be corrected surgically.

#### Congenital hiatal hernia

Congenital hiatal hernia results from the failure of the oesophagus to elongate sufficiently as the neck and thorax develop. The stomach therefore gets pulled into the oesophageal hiatus through the diaphragm. This condition generally manifests in middle age.

#### Congenital hypertrophic pyloric stenosis

Congenital hypertrophic pyloric stenosis occurs in one in 150 males and one in 750 females. There is a marked muscular thickening of the circular muscles and, to a lesser degree, the longitudinal muscles in the pylorus. Its cause

TABLE 13.10 **Distinctive features of the two parts of the anal canal**

| Feature | Superior two-thirds | Inferior one-third |
| --- | --- | --- |
| Origin | Endoderm (hindgut) | Ectoderm (proctodeum) |
| Length | 25 mm | 13 mm |
| Epithelium | Columnar | Stratified squamous |
| Arterial supply | Superior rectal artery (continuation of the artery of the hindgut, the inferior mesenteric artery) | Inferior rectal arteries, branches of the internal pudendal artery |
| Venous drainage | Superior rectal vein, a tributary of the inferior mesenteric vein | Inferior rectal vein, a tributary of the internal pudendal vein that drains into the internal iliac vein |
| Lymphatic drainage | Inferior mesenteric lymph nodes | Superficial inguinal lymph nodes |
| Nerve supply | Autonomic nervous system (hence 'painless carcinomas') | Inferior rectal nerve (hence 'painful carcinomas') |

TABLE 13.11 **Frequencies of atresias and stenoses of the gut**

| Type of anomaly | Percentage |
|---|---|
| Loss of a region of the bowel | 50 |
| Fibrous cord remnant | 20 |
| Narrowing of lumen with a thin diaphragm separating the larger and smaller pieces of bowel | 20 |
| Stenoses | 5 |
| Multiple atresias | 5 |

is unknown, but genetic factors may be involved: there is a high rate of concordance in monozygotic twins.

Neonates present with projectile vomiting and marked distension of the stomach. Management is essentially surgical (pyloromyotomy).

### Duodenal stenosis and atresia

The frequencies of occurrence of atresias and stenoses of the gut are shown in Table 13.11.

Duodenal stenosis results when there is incomplete recanalisation of the duodenum. This generally involves the horizontal (third) and/or fourth parts of the duodenum.

Duodenal atresia results when the duodenal lumen fails to recanalise. This almost always occurs at the junction of the bile and pancreatic ducts, but rarely in the third part of the duodenum. Duodenal atresia shows autosomal recessive inheritance and may be associated with other anorectal and cardiovascular abnormalities or annular pancreas. One-third of affected infants have Down syndrome.

Duodenal atresia presents as polyhydramnios in fetal life and bilious vomiting and distension of the epigastrium after birth. Diagnosis is made on X-ray (double bubble sign) or ultrasound.

## ABNORMALITIES OF THE HEPATOBILIARY APPARATUS

### Liver abnormalities

Major liver anomalies are rare, but minor variations of liver lobulation, accessory hepatic ducts and a duplicated gall-

bladder are common. These are of surgical importance.

### Extrahepatic biliary atresia

Extrahepatic biliary atresia occurs in one in 10 000–15 000 live births. It results from infections, immunological reactions or the failure of the remodelling process at the hepatic hilum. It commonly occurs at or just above the porta hepatis, a deep transverse fissure on the visceral surface of the liver.

The main signs are pathological jaundice after birth and clay-coloured stools. Surgical correction is by Kasai hepatoportoenterostomy or liver transplant.

### Intrahepatic biliary atresia or hypoplasia

Intrahepatic biliary atresia occurs in one in 100 000 live births. It may be caused by fetal infections. It can be lethal or may run an extended benign course.

### Annular pancreas

Migration of the left portion of the ventral bud of the pancreas in the opposite direction results in the formation of a ring (annulus) around the pancreas. Annular pancreas may be associated with Down syndrome, intestinal atresia, imperforate anus, pancreatitis and malrotation of the gut. Males are affected more frequently. Although uncommon, an annular pancreas can result in serious duodenal obstruction, especially when inflamed.

### Accessory pancreatic tissue

Accessory pancreatic tissue is extrapancreatic tissue that shows all the histological characteristics of the pancreas. The tissue lies most frequently in the mucosa of the stomach or in a Meckel diverticulum.

### Accessory spleens

Accessory spleens are seen in approximately 10% of people. They are usually isolated but may be attached to the spleen by thin bands.

## ABNORMALITIES OF THE ANTERIOR ABDOMINAL WALL

### Omphalocele (exomphalos)

Omphalocele occurs in one in 5000 live births. It is a central abdominal wall defect and refers to the herniation of abdominal viscera, which may include liver, bowel, spleen or gallbladder, covered in amnion, through an enlarged umbilical ring. It results from the failure of the bowel to return to the body cavity from its physiological herniation during weeks 6–10. Omphalocele is associated with chromosomal abnormalities (50%), cardiac malformations (50%), neural tube defects (40%) and high mortality rates (25%).

Surgical repair is required. Infants with very large omphalocele suffer from pulmonary and thoracic hypoplasia and a delayed closure is recommended.

### Gastroschisis

Gastroschisis occurs in one in 10 000 live births, but the frequency is increasing, especially among young mothers and probably related to cocaine use. Its occurrence is more common in males.

Gastroschisis is herniation of abdominal contents, not covered by peritoneum/amnion, through the body wall. This herniation occurs lateral to the umbilicus, usually on the right, through a region weakened by regression of the right umbilical vein. Since it is not associated with chromosomal abnormalities or severe defects, the prognosis is generally excellent. However, a volvulus, resulting in a compromised blood supply, may damage large regions of the intestine and lead to fetal death.

### Congenital umbilical hernia

Congenital umbilical hernia is herniation of abdominal contents through an imperfectly closed umbilicus. There is a defect in the linea alba, the fibrous band between the rectus muscles. The protruding mass is generally omentum and/or small bowel and is covered by subcutaneous tissue and skin. The condition presents as an umbilical swelling that becomes prominent during crying or coughing.

Surgery is not performed unless it persists beyond 3–5 years.

## GUT ROTATION DEFECTS

### Abnormal/incomplete rotation of the gut and its effects

Rotation by 90 degrees results in the colon and caecum returning first to the abdominal cavity and being situated to the left, while the small bowel returns to the right. The caecum lies just inferior to the pylorus of the stomach and is fixed to the posterolateral abdominal wall by peritoneal bands that pass over the duodenum. The peritoneal bands and the twisting of the intestines results in duodenal obstruction. Infants may present with bilious vomiting. The diagnosis is confirmed by a simple contrast study.

In cases where there is malrotation of the gut, the intestine remains improperly positioned and improperly fixed. This may lead to a catastrophic twisting of the gut (midgut volvulus), wherein the superior mesenteric vessels can be obstructed resulting in infarction and gangrene of the intestine.

Rotation sometimes occurs by 90 degrees in the clockwise direction. This reversed rotation results in the duodenum lying anterior to the superior mesenteric artery and the transverse colon lying posterior to it. The transverse colon may be obstructed by pressure from the superior mesenteric artery.

## OTHER ABNORMALITIES OF THE MIDGUT

### Meckel diverticulum

A Meckel diverticulum occurs in 2–4% of the population. It is the most common anomaly of the digestive tract and is three to five times more prevalent in males. There is a persistence of a small portion of the vitelline duct, forming an outpocketing of the ileum. In the adult, it lies approximately 40–60 cm from the ileocaecal valve on the antimesenteric border of the ileum.

Inflammation (diverticulitis) mimics appendicitis. The wall may contain small patches of gastric and pancreatic tissues. The ectopic gastric mucosa often secretes acid, producing ulceration and bleeding. Variations, in the form of vitelline cysts and fistulae are also described, which could present with features of a volvulus or faecal discharge at the umbilicus, respectively.

## Duplications of intestinal loops and cysts

Duplications may occur anywhere along the length of the gut but are most frequently found in the region of the ileum. The duplicated segment lies on the mesenteric side. Thirty-three percent are associated with other defects, such as intestinal atresias, imperforate anus, gastroschisis and omphalocele. Symptoms usually occur early in life. The duplicated intestine often contains ectopic gastric mucosa, which may result in local peptic ulceration and lower gastrointestinal bleeding.

## Gut atresias and stenoses

Gut atresias and stenoses occur in one in 1500 live births. They may occur anywhere along the intestine, although most occur in the duodenum and fewest occur in the colon. Atresias in the upper duodenum are usually due to a lack of recanalisation, while those distal to this region are usually caused by deficient blood supply to the gut.

Apple-peel atresia accounts for 10% of atresias. Here, the intestine is short and the atresia is in the proximal jejunum, with the portion distal to the lesion coiled around a mesenteric remnant. Babies with this defect have low birth weight and other abnormalities.

## Subhepatic caecum and appendix

Subhepatic caecum and appendix occurs in 6% of fetuses and is more common in males. The caecum adheres to the inferior surface of the liver where it returns to the abdomen and is drawn superiorly as the liver diminishes in size. This malposition can pose difficulty in the diagnosis of appendicitis and during appendicectomy.

## ABNORMALITIES OF THE MESENTERIES

### Mobile caecum

Mobile caecum occurs in 10% of the population. A failure of the ascending colon to fuse to the posterior abdominal wall results in the persistence of a portion of mesocolon. In the most extreme form, the long mesentery allows abnormal movements of the gut or even a volvulus of the caecum and colon. In unusual cases, it may herniate into the right inguinal canal.

### Retrocolic hernia

A retrocolic hernia is an entrapment of portions of the small intestine behind the mesocolon. It is generally asymptomatic and often is only discovered at autopsy.

## ANOMALIES OF THE HINDGUT

### Low anomalies

Rectoanal atresias and fistulae occur in one in 5000 live births. They are caused by abnormalities in formation of the cloaca, generally due to ectopic positioning of the anal opening and not due to defects in the urorectal septum.

Imperforate anus occurs in one in 5000 live births and is more common in males. There is no anal opening. This defect occurs because of a lack of recanalisation of the lower portion of the anal canal. It requires surgical correction.

Anal stenosis is seen when the anus is in the normal position but the anus and anal canal are narrow. It is probably caused by a slight dorsal deviation of the urorectal septum as it grows caudally to fuse with the cloacal membrane.

Membranous atresia of the anus is seen when the anus is in the normal position but a thin layer of tissue separates the anal canal from the exterior. It results from the failure of the anal membrane to perforate at the end of week 8.

Congenital megacolon (aganglionic megacolon or Hirschsprung disease) occurs in one in 5000 live births and males are four times more likely to be affected. Congenital megacolon accounts for 33% of all neonatal obstructions. It is a dominantly inherited, multigenic disorder with incomplete penetrance and variable expressivity. There is an absence of parasympathetic ganglia in the bowel wall. This occurs because neural crest cells fail to migrate into the wall of the colon during weeks 5–6. Of the genes so far identified, the *RET* proto-oncogene is the major susceptibility gene, accounting for most cases. In most cases the rectum is involved and in 3% the entire colon is affected.

### High anomalies

Anorectal agenesis, with or without fistula, is the most common type of anorectal anomaly. The rectum ends blindly, superior to the puborectalis muscle, often with a fistula to the bladder, urethra or vestibule of the vagina. This is the result of incomplete separation of the cloaca by the urorectal septum. The main symptom is the passage of meconium or flatus in urine or in the vestibule of the vagina. Children with high malformations tend to have poorer outcome, with higher rates of faecal incontinence.

Rectal atresia is seen when the rectum and anus are separated; sometimes the two segments of bowel are connected by a fibrous cord. This may be caused by abnormal recanalisation or deficient blood supply.

## FURTHER READING

Bates M D, Balistreri W F. Development and function of the liver and biliary system. In: Behrman R E, Kliegman R M, Jenson H B, editors. *Nelson Textbook of Paediatrics*. 17th ed. Philadelphia: WB Saunders; 2004. p.1304–8.

Gosche J R, Vick L, Boulanger S C, Islam S. Midgut abnormalities. *Surg Clin North Am* 2006;86:285–99.

Lau S T, Caty M G. Hindgut abnormalities. *Surg Clin North Am* 2006;86:301–16.

Ledbetter D J. Gastroschisis and omphalocele. *Surg Clin North Am* 2006;86:249–60.

Magnuson D K, Parry R L, Chwals W J. Selected abdominal gastrointestinal anomalies. In: Martin R J, Fanaroff A A, Walsh M C, editors. *Fanaroff and Martin's Neonatal-perinatal Medicine. Diseases of the Fetus and Infant*. 8th ed. Philadelphia: Mosby; 2006. p.1381–402.

Moore K L, Persaud T V N. The gastrointestinal system. In: *The Developing Human: Clinically Oriented Embryology*. 8th ed. Philadelphia: W B Saunders; 2008. p.211–42.

Naik-Mathuria B, Olutoye O O. Foregut abnormalities. *Surg Clin North Am* 2006;86:261–84.

Nievelstein R A J, Van derWerff J F A, Verbeek F J, Vermeij-Keers C. Normal and abnormal development of the anorectum in human embryos. *Teratology* 1998;57:70–8.

Orenstein S, Peters J, Khan S, Yaussef N, Hussain S Z. Congenital anomalies. Esophageal atresia and tracheoesophageal fistula and function of the esophagus. In: Behrman R E, Kliegman R M, Jenson H B, editors. *Nelson Textbook of Paediatrics*. 18th ed. Philadelphia: W B Saunders; 2007. chap.316.

Sadler T W. The gastrointestinal system. In: *Langman's Medical Embryology*. 10th ed. Baltimore: Lippincott Williams & Wilkins; 2006. p.203–27.

# CHAPTER 14

# Development of the heart and the fetal circulation

*Rohan D'Souza*

## Development of the heart

The cardiovascular system is the first major system to function in the embryo. The primordial heart and vascular system appears in the middle of week 3, to satisfy the nutritional and oxygen requirements of the developing embryo.

## The cardiogenic field

Cardiac progenitor cells lie in the epiblast, immediately lateral to the primitive streak (Figure 14.1). They migrate through the streak and then proceed towards the cranium, coming to lie in the splanchnic layer of the lateral plate mesoderm. They are then induced to form cardiac myoblasts. Blood islands also appear in this mesoderm, where they form blood cells and vessels by the process of vasculogenesis. With time, the islands unite and form a horseshoe-shaped endothelial-lined tube surrounded by

FIGURE 14.1 **Embryo at day 18 showing the cardiogenic field and the formation of the pericardial cavity**

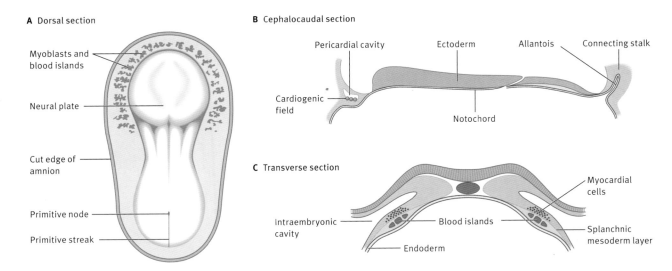

**A** Dorsal section

Myoblasts and blood islands

Neural plate

Cut edge of amnion

Primitive node

Primitive streak

**B** Cephalocaudal section

Pericardial cavity

Ectoderm

Allantois

Connecting stalk

Cardiogenic field

Notochord

**C** Transverse section

Intraembryonic cavity

Blood islands

Myocardial cells

Splanchnic mesoderm layer

Endoderm

Myoblasts and blood islands can be seen in the splanchnic mesoderm in front of the neural plate and on each side of the embryo. Note the position of the pericardial cavity and the cardiogenic field in (**B**).

FIGURE 14.2 **Cephalocaudal sections through an embryo**

A Day 20

B Day 22

The effects of the rapid growth of the brain on the positioning of the heart can be seen. The cardiogenic field moves from in front of the buccopharyngeal membrane to the thorax.

myoblasts. This region is known as the cardiogenic field. The intraembryonic cavity over it later develops into the pericardial cavity.

### THE HEART TUBE

The embryo folds both cephalocaudally and laterally (Figures 14.2 and 14.3). As a result of cephalocaudal folding, as well as the rapid growth of the brain, the cardiogenic area moves caudally to the thorax. As a result of the lateral folding of the embryo, the caudal regions of the

paired cardiac primordia merge except at their caudal-most ends. The heart now becomes a continuous tube consisting of an inner endothelial lining (the future endocardium), which is separated from an outer muscular layer (the future myocardium) by a gelatinous connective tissue called cardiac jelly (Figures 14.3 and 14.4 A). The pericardium is formed from mesothelial cells that arise from the external surface of the sinus venosus. This outer layer is responsible for formation of the coronary arteries, including their endothelial lining and smooth muscle.

FIGURE 14.3 **Transverse sections through an embryo**

A Day 17    B Day 18    C Day 22

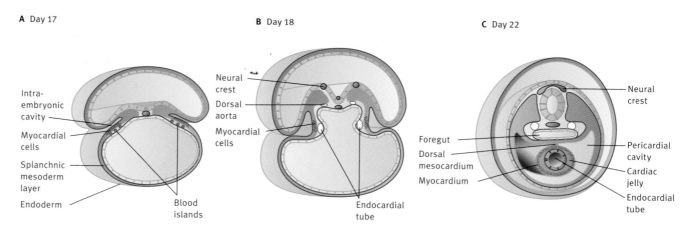

The effect of the lateral folding of the embryo and the merging of the paired cardiac primordial to form the endocardial tube can be seen.

FIGURE 14.4 **Ventral views of the developing heart**

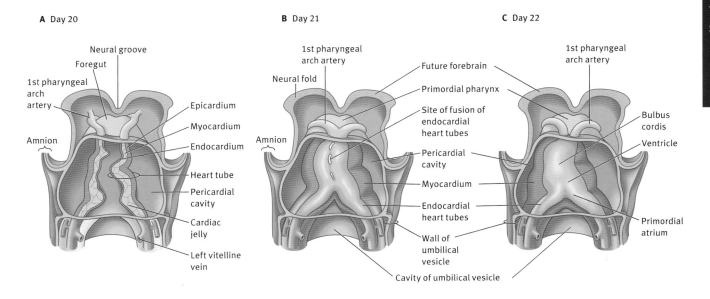

**A** Day 20

**B** Day 21

**C** Day 22

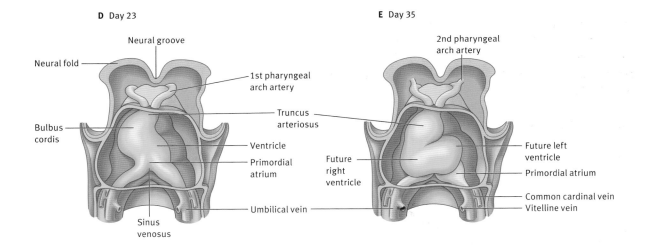

**D** Day 23

**E** Day 35

Fusion of the two heart tubes begins at the cranial ends of the heart tubes and extends caudally. A single tubular heart is formed as a result of the fusion of heart tubes. The heart elongates, forming regional segments and begins to fold on itself. This folding is completed by day 28 to form an S-shaped heart.

FIGURE 14.5 **Partitioning of the atrioventricular canal**

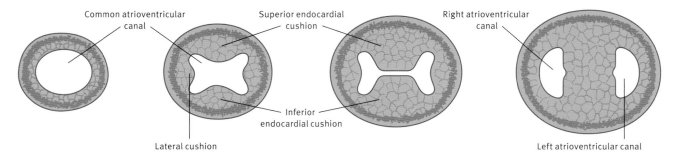

Endocardial cushions grow into the common atrioventricular canal (day 23) and result in the formation of the atrioventricular septum and the atrioventricular canals by day 35.

## THE CARDIAC LOOP

The tubular heart elongates and develops alternate dilatations and constrictions (Figure 14.4). The primordial heart is composed of four chambers – the bulbus cordis (conotruncus), ventricle, atrium and sinus venosus. The cranial part of the bulbus cordis is the truncus arteriosus and is continuous cranially with the aortic sac. The sinus venosus receives the umbilical, vitelline and common cardinal veins from the chorion, umbilical vesicle and embryo, respectively. Because the bulbus cordis and ventricle grow faster than other regions, the heart bends upon itself forming a U-shaped loop: the cardiac loop or the bulboventricular loop. This is completed by day 28. The developing heart bulges more and more into the pericardial cavity. Eventually, it is suspended in the cavity, remaining attached only at the cranial and caudal ends by blood vessels.

## PARTITIONING OF THE PRIMORDIAL HEART

The partitioning of the various chambers of the primordial heart begins simultaneously around the middle of week 4 and is largely completed by the end of week 8.

### *Partitioning of the atrioventricular canal*

In week 4 of development, endocardial cushions form on the dorsal and ventral walls of the atrioventricular canal. They approach each other and fuse, dividing the common atrioventricular canal in to right and left atrioventricular canals (Figure 14.5). These canals partially separate the primordial atrium from the primordial ventricle.

### *Partitioning of the atrium*

The partitioning of the atrium occurs between day 27 and day 37 (week 4 to week 6) (Figure 14.6). A thin crescent-shaped membrane, the septum primum, grows from the roof of the primordial atrium towards the endocardial cushions, partially dividing the primordial atrium into right and left halves. This septum primum bears a large opening called the foramen primum (ostium primum), which serves as a shunt, enabling oxygenated blood to pass from the right to left atrium. As the septum primum fuses with the endocardial cushions, the foramen primum becomes progressively smaller and then disappears. Before this can happen, however, perforations appear in the central part of the septum primum, which subsequently coalesce to form a new opening, the foramen secundum (ostium secundum). Thus, although the foramen primum closes, shunting of blood from the right to the left atrium continues via the foramen secundum. Now, a thick crescentic muscular fold grows from the ventrocranial wall of the right atrium, just adjacent to the septum primum. As this grows downwards, the upper part of the septum primum disappears, thus forming a flap-like valve between the two, called the foramen ovale (oval foramen). Owing to the flap-like mechanism, the oval foramen allows only unidirectional flow of blood from the right atrium to the left during fetal life.

FIGURE 14.6  **Partitioning of the atrium**

A  Coronal section through an embryo at day 30

Septum primum
Foramen primum
Endocardial cushion
Atrioventricular canal

B  Right lateral section through an embryo at day 30

Interventricular foramen

C  Coronal section through an embryo at day 33

Septum secundum
Foramen secundum
Septum primum
Endocardial cushion
Interventricular foramen

D  Right lateral section through an embryo at day 33

Endocardial cushions fused

E  Coronal section through an embryo at day 37

Venous valves
Septum primum
Septum secundum

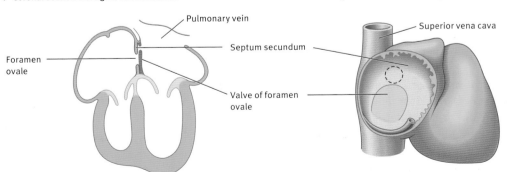

F  Coronal section through a newborn heart

Pulmonary vein
Septum secundum
Foramen ovale
Valve of foramen ovale

G  Right lateral section through a newborn heart

Superior vena cava

**A** and **B** show the formation of septum primum and foramen primum; note the development of perforations in the septum primum as the foramen primum begins to shrink. **C** and **D** show the formation of foramen secundum by the coalescence of perforations within the septum primum; note the formation of septum secundum as a growth from the ventrocranial wall of the right atrium. **E** shows the further growth of the septum secundum and the obliteration of the upper part of the septum primum, allowing unidirectional flow of blood from the right to left atrium. **F** and **G** show the foramen ovale and its flap-like valve formed by the lower part of the septum primum.

FIGURE 14.7 **Partitioning of the sinus venosus**

**A** Dorsal view at approximately day 26

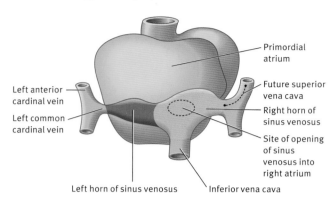

FIGURE 14.8 **Development of the left atrium**

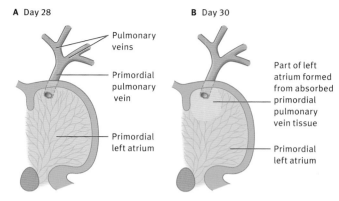

**A** Day 28      **B** Day 30

**B** Dorsal view in week 8

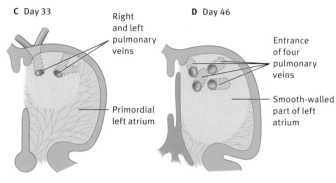

**C** Day 33      **D** Day 46

Red = fully oxgenated blood | blue = deoxygenated blood |
purple = mixed blood

FIGURE 14.9 **Closure of the interventricular foramen**

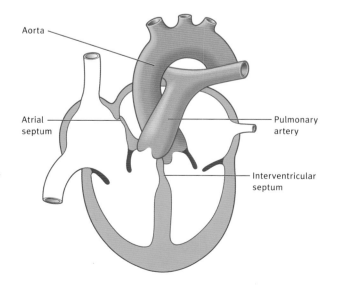

### Partitioning of the sinus venosus

Partitioning of the sinus venosus occurs between week
4 and week 10 (Figure 14.7). Initially, the sinus venosus
opens into the centre of the dorsal wall of the primordial
atrium and its right and left horns are approximately of
the same size. During weeks 4–5, left-to-right shunts in
the venous system cause the right sinus horn to enlarge
progressively. The left sinus horn rapidly loses its importance as the right umbilical vein and the left vitelline vein
obliterates during week 5. At week 10, the left common
cardinal vein also obliterates and now all that remains
of the left sinus horn is the oblique vein of the left atrium
and the coronary sinus. The enlarged right horn begins
to receive all blood from the cranial and caudal regions

FIGURE 14.10 **Partitioning of the bulbus cordis and truncus arteriosus**

**A** Ventral view through an embryo at week 5

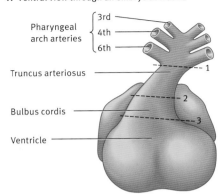

Pharyngeal arch arteries
- 3rd
- 4th
- 6th

Truncus arteriosus — 1

Bulbus cordis — 2 — 3

Ventricle

**B** Transverse section through an week 5

1

Truncal ridge

2

Bulbar ridges

3

**C** Coronal section through an embryo at week 5

Left atrioventricular canal

**D** Ventral views though an embryo at week 6

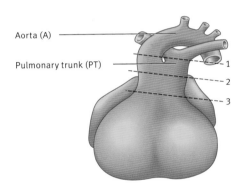

Aorta (A)

Pulmonary trunk (PT)

— 1
— 2
— 3

**E** Transverse section though an embryo at week 6

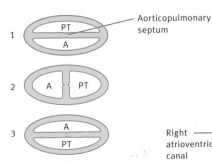

1     PT     Aorticopulmonary septum
       A

2    A    PT

3     A
      PT

**F** Coronal section though an embryo at week 6

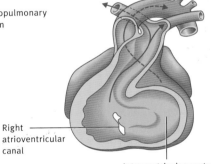

Right atrioventricular canal

Interventricular septum

**G** Spiral form of the aorticopulmonary septum

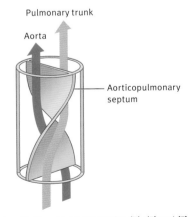

Pulmonary trunk

Aorta

Aorticopulmonary septum

**H** Aorta and pulmonary trunk twisting around each other

Ascending aorta

Pulmonary trunk

Left pulmonary artery

Aorticopulmonary septum

(A–C) show the truncal and bulbar ridges at 5 weeks. (D), (E) and (F) show the aorticopulmonary septum at 6 weeks. (G) and (H) show the final position of the ascending aorta and pulmonary trunk at the end of 8 weeks, twisting around each other as they leave the heart.

FIGURE 14.11 **Schematic coronal section through a ventricle, showing the formation of atrioventricular valves**

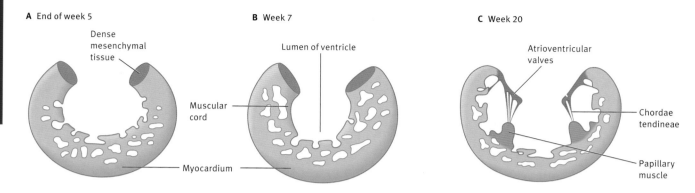

**A** End of week 5

Dense mesenchymal tissue

Myocardium

**B** Week 7

Lumen of ventricle

Muscular cord

**C** Week 20

Atrioventricular valves

Chordae tendineae

Papillary muscle

The atrioventricular orifice is surrounded by local proliferations of mesenchymal tissue. The tissue on the ventricular surface of these proliferations thins and forms valves, which remain attached to the ventricular wall by muscular cords. The muscular tissue in the cords degenerates by week 20 and is replaced by dense connective tissue forming chordae tendineae, which now connect valves with the papillary muscles.

of the body via the superior and inferior vena cava and gets incorporated into the wall of the right atrium forming the smooth-walled part of the right atrium, the sinus venarum. The remainder of the right atrial wall has a rough trabeculated appearance. The smooth and rough parts are demarcated internally by a vertical ridge, the crista terminalis, and externally by a shallow groove, the sulcus terminalis.

Most of the wall of the left atrium is formed by incorporation of the primordial pulmonary vein and is therefore smooth (Figure 14.8).

### Partitioning of the ventricles

A muscular septum arises in the floor of the primordial ventricle, near its apex. This interventricular septum contains a crescent-shaped interventricular foramen, which permits communication between the two ventricles, until week 7. After the closure of this foramen, the pulmonary trunk communicates with the right ventricle and the aorta with the left ventricle (Figure 14.9).

### Partitioning of the bulbus cordis and truncus arteriosus

During week 5, mesenchymal cells in the walls of the bulbus cordis proliferate actively and form bulbar ridges. Similar ridges that are continuous with the bulbar ridges form in the truncus arteriosus. The bulbar and truncal ridges (conotruncal ridges) then undergo 180-degrees

spiralling, resulting in the formation of a spiral aorticopulmonary septum when the ridges fuse. This septum divides the bulbus cordis and the truncus arteriosus into two distinct channels, the ascending aorta and pulmonary trunk. Because of the spiralling of the aorticopulmonary septum, the pulmonary trunk twists around the ascending aorta (Figure 14.10).

## Formation of the cardiac valves

### ATRIOVENTRICULAR VALVES

After the fusion of the atrioventricular endocardial cushions, each atrioventricular orifice is surrounded by proliferations of mesenchymal tissue. The bloodstream hollows out and thins these tissue proliferations on the ventricular surface resulting in the formation of valves. These valves remain attached to the ventricular wall by muscular cords. Over time, the muscular tissue in the cords degenerates and is replaced by dense connective tissue. The valves then consist of connective tissue covered by endocardium. They are connected to thick trabeculae in the wall of the ventricle, the papillary muscles, by means of chordae tendineae (Figure 14.11). In this manner, two valve leaflets (mitral valve) form in the left atrioventricular canal, and three valve leaflets (tricuspid valve) form on the right side.

FIGURE 14.12  **Formation of the semilunar valves**

Longitudinal sections through the semilunar valves illustrate successive stages in the hollowing (shown by arrows) and thinning of the valve swellings to form valve cusps.

## SEMILUNAR VALVES

At the time of partitioning of the truncus arteriosus, three swellings of subendocardial tissue develop around the orifices of the aorta and pulmonary trunk. These swellings are hollowed out and reshaped to form three thin-walled cusps, the future semilunar valves (Figure 14.12).

## The conducting system of the heart

In the early stages of development, the function of pacemaker is assumed by the atrium and later by the sinus venosus. As the sinus venosus is incorporated into the right atrium, pacemaker tissue comes to lie near the opening of the superior vena cava resulting in the formation of the sinoatrial node by week 5. The atrioventricular node and bundle (bundle of His) are derived from cells in the left wall of the sinus venosus and the atrioventricular canal. Fibres from the atrioventricular bundle pass from the atrium into the ventricle, split into right and left bundle branches and are distributed throughout the ventricular myocardium (Figure 14.13). Innervation of the sinoatrial node, atrioventricular node and atrioventricular bundle occurs later.

## Congenital heart defects

Abnormalities of the cardiovascular system account for 1% of malformations among liveborn infants and almost 10% among stillborn babies, making up the largest category of human birth defects. Some cause very little disability and their impact may only become apparent at birth. Some others are incompatible with extrauterine life.

### FACTORS LINKED WITH CONGENITAL HEART DEFECTS

The following factors are linked with congenital heart defects.

### *Genetic and chromosomal factors*

It is estimated that 8% of cardiac malformations are due to genetic factors. Congenital heart defects are associated with a number of genetic syndromes such as DiGeorge, Goldenhar and Down syndromes. Of those children with chromosomal abnormalities, 33% have a congenital heart

FIGURE 14.13  **The conducting system of the heart at week 20**

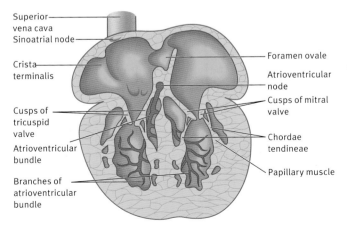

defect, with an incidence of nearly 100% in children with trisomy 18. Of newborns with congenital heart defect, 6–10% have an unbalanced chromosomal abnormality.

### Environmental factors

A small proportion (2%) of congenital heart defects are due to environmental agents. Classic examples of cardiovascular teratogens include alcohol, the rubella virus and drugs such as thalidomide and isotretinoin (vitamin A). Maternal insulin-dependent diabetes and hypertension have also been linked to congenital heart defect.

### Multifactorial inheritance

In most cases, the causes of congenital heart defects are unknown and are believed to occur as a result of a complex interplay between a number of factors, genetic and environmental.

### POSITIONAL ANOMALIES

Occasionally, the heart is found to lie on the wrong side of the thorax or even outside the thoracic cavity. While the former condition may not be clinically relevant, the latter may be associated with significant perinatal morbidity and mortality.

### Dextrocardia

With dextrocardia, the heart lies on the right side of the thorax instead of the left. It is the most frequent positional anomaly of the heart and is caused when the heart loops to the left instead of the right. Dextrocardia may coincide with situs inversus, where there is a complete reversal of symmetry in all organs, or heterotaxy, where the position of some organs is randomly reversed. Generally these conditions are associated with normal physiology, although there is a slight risk of heart defects.

### Ectopia cordis

With ectopia cordis, the heart is in an abnormal location, most commonly partly or completely exposed on the surface of the thorax. It is also sometimes found to protrude through the diaphragm, into the abdomen. The thoracic

form results from faulty development of the sternum and pericardium. Death from infection, cardiac failure or hypoxemia occurs in most cases during the first few days of life. Surgical correction is required and the clinical outcome has now improved, with some surviving to adulthood.

### ENDOCARDIAL CUSHIONS AND HEART DEFECTS

Because of their key location, abnormalities in endocardial cushion formation contribute towards many cardiac malformations. Since neural crest cells, which contribute to the development of the head and neck, also populate the conotruncal cushions, abnormalities of these cells often produce both heart and craniofacial defects in the same individual.

### Atrial septal defects

Atrial septal defects occur in 6.4 in 10 000 births. There is a two in one prevalence in girl versus boy infants. The most common form of atrial septal defect is a patent foramen ovale, which may be present in up to 25% of the population. It is generally not clinically significant unless forced open because of other cardiac defects. There are four clinically significant types of atrial septal defect.

Foramen secundum atrial septal defect is characterised by a large opening between the atria. It is caused either by excessive cell death and resorption of the septum primum or by inadequate development of the septum secundum. It is generally tolerated well in childhood; symptoms of pulmonary hypertension usually appear after the third decade of life.

Endocardial cushion defects with foramen primum atrial septal defect include a group of abnormalities resulting from a common developmental defect: deficiency of the endocardial cushions and the atrioventricular septum. Here, the septum primum does not fuse with the endocardial cushions.

Sinus venosus atrial septal defect is the rarest type of atrial septal defect. It results from incomplete incorporation of the sinus venosus into the right atrium or abnormal development of the septum secundum. It is commonly associated with partial anomalous pulmonary venous connections.

Common atrium (cor triloculare biventriculare) is the most serious abnormality in this group. It represents

FIGURE 14.14 **Abnormalities of the conotruncal region**

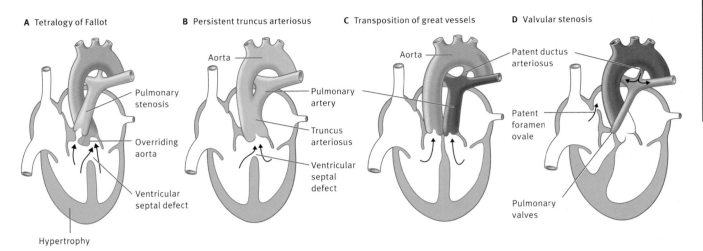

**A** Tetralogy of Fallot    **B** Persistent truncus arteriosus    **C** Transposition of great vessels    **D** Valvular stenosis

Red = fully oxgenated blood  |  blue = deoxygenated blood  |  purple = mixed blood

the combination of all the above atrial septal defects and refers to the complete absence of the atrial septum.

### Ventricular septal defect

Ventricular septal defect is the most common type of congenital heart defect, accounting for approximately 25% of defects. It occurs more commonly in boys than in girls. It may be found as an isolated lesion or associated with abnormalities in partitioning of the conotruncal region. Dyspnoea, pulmonary hypertension and cardiac failure are known to occur depending on the size of the defect and associated conditions. The following subtypes have been identified.

Membranous ventricular septal defect is the most common type of ventricular septal defect (12 in 10 000 births) resulting from failure of development of the membranous part of the interventricular septum. About 30–50% of these defects close within the first year of life. Muscular ventricular septal defect is less common and may appear anywhere in the muscular part of the interventricular septum. Sometimes there are multiple small defects, producing what is sometimes called the 'Swiss cheese ventricular septal defect'.

Single ventricle (cor triloculare biatriatum) is a complete absence of the interventricular septum. It is an extremely rare anomaly resulting in a three-chambered heart, where both aorta and pulmonary trunk arise from the common ventricle.

Atrioventricular septal defect is a failure of fusion of the endocardial cushions and results in a large defect in the centre of the heart. Although rare, it occurs in approximately 20% of people with Down syndrome.

### ABNORMALITIES OF THE CONOTRUNCAL REGION

Four of the most common abnormalities of the conotruncal region are discussed below and illustrated in Figure 14.14.

### Tetralogy of Fallot

Tetralogy of Fallot is the most frequently occurring abnormality of the conotruncal region. It occurs in 9.6 in 10 000 births and is not fatal. It is an anterior displacement of the conotruncal septum that results in unequal division of the conus and produces four cardiovascular alterations: pulmonary stenosis (obstruction of right ventricular outflow), ventricular septal defect, dextroposition of aorta (overriding or straddling aorta) and right ventricular hypertrophy. Cyanosis may not be present at birth but it is an obvious sign of this condition. Primary surgical repair in early infancy is the treatment of choice.

### Persistent truncus arteriosus

Persistent truncus arteriosus occurs in 0.8 in 10 000 births. The truncal ridges and aorticopulmonary septum fail to develop normally. It can result in the failure of division of the truncus arteriosus into aorta and pulmonary trunk, such that the undivided truncus overrides both ventricles and receives blood from both sides. It can also result in a ventricular septal defect, because the ridges participate in the development of the interventricular septum.

### Transposition of the great vessels

Transposition of the great vessels occurs in 4.8 in 10 000 births. It is the most common cause of cyanotic heart disease in newborn infants. The conotruncal septum runs straight down, instead of following a spiral course. This results in the aorta originating from the right ventricle and the pulmonary artery originating from the left ventricle. This condition may be associated with a membranous ventricular septal defect or an open ductus arteriosus. Death would ensue within a few months if not surgically corrected.

### Valvular stenosis

Valvular stenosis of the pulmonary artery and aorta occurs in 3–4 in 10 000 births. It is caused by fusion of the semilunar valves. Stenosis could occur over a variable distance and could be either a mild narrowing or complete atresia. In valvular stenosis of the pulmonary artery, the trunk of the pulmonary artery is narrow or even atretic. Here, the patent oval foramen forms the only outlet for blood from the right side of the heart, while the patent ductus arteriosus is the only access route to the pulmonary circulation. In aortic valvular stenosis, the size of the aorta is usually normal. However, in aortic valvular atresia, the aorta, left ventricle and left atrium are markedly underdeveloped. Here the patent ductus arteriosus delivers blood into the aorta.

### Tricuspid atresia

Tricuspid atresia is the absence or fusion of the tricuspid valves and results in obliteration of the right atrioventricular orifice. It is associated with a patent foramen ovale, a ventricular septal defect, an underdeveloped right ventricle and a hypertrophied left ventricle.

### ABNORMALITIES OF THE CONDUCTING SYSTEM

Abnormalities of the conducting system are the most common cause of sudden infant death syndrome in developed countries, accounting for 40–50% of infant deaths in the first year. No mechanism has been identified, although there is a suggestion that they have an abnormality in the autonomic nervous system.

## Fetal circulation

The umbilical vein carries blood from the placenta to the fetus. Figure 14.15 illustrates the passage of blood from the umbilical vein through the fetal heart to the umbilical arteries. The blood in the umbilical vein is nutrient-rich and 80% saturated with oxygen and it loses its high oxygen content as a result of mixing with deoxygenated blood at various places (Table 14.1) This is discussed in greater detail in chapter 32.

Most of this blood bypasses the liver and flows directly through the ductus venosus into the right atrium at the junction with the inferior vena cava. A smaller amount enters the liver sinusoids and mixes with blood from the portal circulation. The flow of umbilical blood through

TABLE 14.1 **Mixing of oxygenated and deoxygenated blood, as shown in Figure 14.15**

| Label | Site | Source of deoxygenated blood |
|---|---|---|
| I | Liver | Blood returning from the portal system |
| II | Inferior vena cava | Blood returning from lower extremities, pelvis and kidneys |
| III | Right atrium | Blood returning from the head and upper extremities |
| IV | Left atrium | Blood returning from lungs |
| V | Junction of ductus arteriosus and descending aorta | Blood from the proximal aorta |

FIGURE 14.15 **Fetal circulation *in utero***

Ductus arteriosus

Pulmonary vein

Superior vena cava

Pulmonary vein

Crista dividens

*Foramen ovale*

Inferior vena cava

*Ductus venosus*

Pulmonary artery

Descending aorta

Portal vein

Inferior vena cava

Umbilical vein

Umbilical arteries

Red = fully oxygenated blood  |  blue = deoxygenated blood  |  red/blue = mixed blood  |  *Shunts in italics*

the sinusoids is said to be regulated by a sphincter mechanism in the ductus venosus close to the entrance of the umbilical vein. This sphincter supposedly closes when a uterine contraction renders the venous return too high, thereby preventing sudden overloading of the heart.

In the inferior vena cava, placental blood mixes with deoxygenated blood returning from the lower limbs. It then enters the right atrium, from where most of the blood is guided through the oval foramen to the left atrium. A small amount remains in the right atrium where it mixes with deoxygenated blood returning from the head and arms via the superior vena cava. Blood in

the left atrium mixes with a small amount of deoxygenated blood returning from the lungs through the pulmonary veins.

Blood from the left atrium enters the left ventricle and ascending aorta. The coronary and carotid arteries are the first branches of the ascending aorta, ensuring that the heart and the brain are supplied with well-oxygenated blood.

Blood from the superior vena cava flows into the right ventricle and the pulmonary trunk. Since resistance in the pulmonary vessels is high during intrauterine life, most of this blood passes through the ductus arteriosus

FIGURE 14.16 **Circulatory changes at birth**

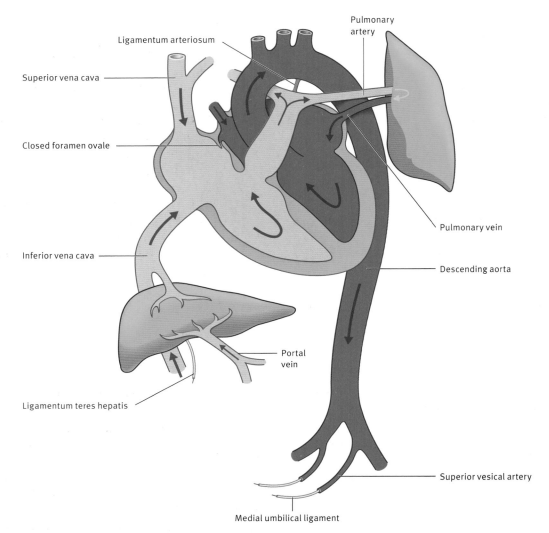

Labels (clockwise): Pulmonary artery; Ligamentum arteriosum; Superior vena cava; Closed foramen ovale; Inferior vena cava; Pulmonary vein; Descending aorta; Portal vein; Ligamentum teres hepatis; Superior vesical artery; Medial umbilical ligament

in to the descending aorta, where it mixes with blood from the proximal aorta.

Blood from the descending aorta flows toward the placenta by way of the two umbilical arteries. The oxygen saturation in the umbilical arteries is about 58%.

## Circulatory changes at birth

Cessation of placental blood flow and the beginning of respiration bring about profound changes in the vascular system: compare Figures 14.15 and 14.16.

## CLOSURE OF THE UMBILICAL ARTERIES

Thermal and mechanical stimuli along with a change in oxygen tension bring about contraction of the smooth muscle in the walls of the umbilical arteries. Functional closure of the arteries occurs a few minutes after birth, although actual obliteration of the lumen by fibrous proliferation could take 2–3 months. The proximal portions of the arteries remain open as the superior vesical arteries, while the distal portions form the medial umbilical ligaments.

## CLOSURE OF THE UMBILICAL VEIN AND DUCTUS VENOSUS

The umbilical vein and ductus venosus close shortly after the umbilical arteries. After obliteration, the umbilical vein forms the ligamentum teres hepatis (round ligament of the liver) in the lower margin of the falciform ligament while the ductus venosus forms the ligamentum venosum, which courses from the ligamentum teres hepatis to the inferior vena cava.

## CLOSURE OF THE DUCTUS ARTERIOSUS

Closure of the ductus arteriosus is mediated by bradykinin, a substance released from the lungs during initial inflation. Immediately after birth, its muscular wall contracts, but complete anatomical obliteration by proliferation of the intima is thought to take 1–3 months.

When the ductus arteriosus closes, there is a rapid increase in the amount of blood flowing through the lung vessels. This increases pressure in the left atrium. The obliterated ductus arteriosus forms the ligamentum arteriosum.

## CLOSURE OF THE OVAL FORAMEN

There already is increased pressure in the left atrium as a result of closure of the ductus arteriosus and reduced pressure in the right atrium as a result of interruption of placental blood flow. Now, when the first breath is taken, the septum primum presses against the septum secundum, resulting in functional closure of the oval foramen.

This closure is reversible during the first days of life and when the baby cries a right-to-left shunt is created, accounting for cyanotic periods in the newborn. Constant apposition gradually leads to fusion of the two septa at about 1 year of age.

### FURTHER READING

Bruyer H J, Kargas S A, Levy J M. The causes and underlying developmental mechanisms of congenital cardiovascular malformation: a critical review. *Am J Med Genet* 1987;3:411–31.

Clark E B. Cardiac embryology: its relevance to congenital heart disease. *Am J Dis Child* 1986;140:41–4.

Fishman M C, Chien K R. Fashioning the vertebrate heart: earliest embryonic decisions. *Development* 1997;124:2099–117.

Hirakow R. Development of the cardiac blood vessels in staged human embryos. *Acta Anat* 1983;115:220–30.

Moore, K L, Persaud, T V N. The cardiovascular system. In: *The Developing Human: Clinically Oriented Embryology.* 8th ed. Philadelphia: W B Saunders; 2008. p. 285–337.

Noden D M. Origins and assembly of avian embryonic blood vessels. *Ann N Y Acad Sci* 1990;588:236–49.

Sadler T W. Cardiovascular system. In: *Langman's Medical Embryology.* 11th edn. Baltimore: Lippincott Williams & Wilkins; 2010. p. 165–200.

Skandalakis J E, Gray S W. *Embryology for Surgeons: The Embryological Basis for the Treatment of Congenital Anomalies.* 2nd edn. Baltimore: Williams & Wilkins; 1994.

Waldo K, Miyagawa-Tomita S, Kumiski D, Kirby M L. Cardiac neural crest cells provide new insight into septation of the cardiac outflow tract: aortic sac to ventricular septal closure. *Dev Biol* 1998;196:129–44.

## Sample questions relating to early embryology

### EXTENDED MATCHING QUESTIONS

#### Questions 1–4

■ *For each item below, choose the **single** correct primary cell layer from which it is derived from the list of options (A–G). Each option may be used once, more than once or not at all.*

OPTIONS

▷ **A** Endoderm
▷ **B** Intermediate mesoderm
▷ **C** Lateral mesoderm
▷ **D** Neural crest
▷ **E** Neuroectoderm
▷ **F** Paraxial mesoderm
▷ **G** Surface ectoderm

1 ▶ Epithelial lining of the anal canal

2 ▶ Epithelial lining of the bladder

3 ▶ Gonads

4 ▶ Urethral epithelia

### MULTIPLE CHOICE QUESTIONS

5 ▶ Regarding fertilisation and implantation:

**A** ▷ Fertilisation occurs in the fimbrial end of the fallopian tube
**B** ▷ Capacitation is necessary prior to fertilisation
**C** ▷ The acrosome enzymes allow the spermatozoon to penetrate the zona pellucida
**D** ▷ Fertilisation begins the resumption of the second mitotic division
**E** ▷ The embryo implants during the proliferative phase of the endometrium

6 ▶ Regarding implantation and placentation:

**A** ▷ Implantation usually occurs on day 4 after fertilisation
**B** ▷ Cells for the syncytiotrophoblast are derived from the inner cell mass
**C** ▷ By day 12, the uteroplacental circulation has formed
**D** ▷ The decidual reaction occurs only at the site of implantation
**E** ▷ Beta human chorionic gonadotrophin is produced by the cytotrophoblast

7 ▶ Regarding the amnion and chorion:

**A** ▷ The amniotic cavity begins to develop on day 9
**B** ▷ The amniotic cavity is formed between cells of the hypoblast
**C** ▷ The trophoblast lines the blastocyst cavity
**D** ▷ The chorion begins to form in the extraembryonic mesoderm
**E** ▷ By week 2, the embryo is connected to the cytotrophoblast by a connecting stalk of extraembryonic mesoderm

8 ▶ Regarding neural development:

**A** ▷ The primitive streak starts to form by the end of the second week
**B** ▷ The primitive pit represents the caudal end of the fetus
**C** ▷ Cells that displace the hypoblast form the mesoderm
**D** ▷ The notochord is the basis of the formation of the skeleton
**E** ▷ The neural plate derives from the ectoderm

9 ▶ Regarding fertilisation:

**A** ▷ The process usually takes place within 24 hours of ovulation
**B** ▷ Capacitation is aided by secretions of the uterine wall
**C** ▷ The acrosome reaction occurs when the spermatozoon comes into contact with the zona pellucida
**D** ▷ Pronuclei are formed by condensation of the chromosome of the gametes
**E** ▷ A zygote is formed when the male and female pronuclei meet

**10 ▶** Regarding blastocyst formation:

**A** ▷ Cleavage begins after completion of the second meiotic division
**B** ▷ Cleavage occurs by mitosis
**C** ▷ After 3 days, there are 32 cells
**D** ▷ The morula is a solid sphere of cells
**E** ▷ A blastomere forms when there is a cavity in the morula

**11 ▶** Regarding the first week of development:

**A** ▷ The blastocoele is a cavity within the blastocyst
**B** ▷ The wall surrounding the blastocoele is two cells thick
**C** ▷ The cells surrounding the blastocoele becomes the trophoblast
**D** ▷ The blastocyst enters the lumen of the uterus on day 6
**E** ▷ The inner cell mass is formed from the cells on the outer surface of the blastocoele

**12 ▶** Regarding week 2 of development:

**A** ▷ Fertilisation initiates the decidual reaction
**B** ▷ Cells of the decidual reaction form part of the placenta
**C** ▷ The syncytiotrophoblast is invasive
**D** ▷ The primary yolk sac is the source of nutrition for early embryos
**E** ▷ Hypoblast cells adapt to produce amniotic fluid

**13 ▶** Regarding week 2 of development:

**A** ▷ Maternal sinusoids are small veins
**B** ▷ Maternal sinusoids connect the lacunae in the cytotrophoblast
**C** ▷ Primary chorionic villi are formed from the cytotrophoblast
**D** ▷ The umbilical cord is a stalk of epiblast
**E** ▷ Uterine epithelium eventually reforms to cover the conceptus

**14 ▶** Regarding week 3 of development:

**A** ▷ The bilaminar disc is made up of the epiblast and hypoblast
**B** ▷ The formation of the early gut is called gastrulation
**C** ▷ The hypoblast becomes the ectoderm
**D** ▷ The middle layer is formed from the hypoblast
**E** ▷ The mesoderm forms muscles

**15 ▶** Regarding week 3 of development:

**A** ▷ The cloacal plate is made of two germ cell layers
**B** ▷ The gut is continuous with the amniotic cavity from week 4
**C** ▷ Cells for neurulation are derived from the endoderm
**D** ▷ The neural plate enlarges to fill most of the caudal end of the bilaminar disc
**E** ▷ The neural fold forms the spinal cord

**16 ▶** The neural crest cells form:

**A** ▷ the dorsal root
**B** ▷ sympathetic ganglia
**C** ▷ adrenal cortex
**D** ▷ glial cells
**E** ▷ melanocytes

**17 ▶** Regarding mesoderm segmentation:

**A** ▷ Somites are formed from the paraxial mesoderm
**B** ▷ Forty pairs of somites are formed in total
**C** ▷ Dermomyotomes form connective tissue
**D** ▷ Sclerotomes form skeletal muscles
**E** ▷ Somites carry with them the innervations from the spinal cord

## Sample questions relating to development of the urogynaecological tract

### EXTENDED MATCHING QUESTIONS

#### Questions 1–6

■ *These questions relate to the embryological development of the female urogenital tract. For each item below, select the **single** best option from the list of options (A–H). Each option may be used once, more than once or not at all.*

OPTIONS

▷ **A** Gonads
▷ **B** Labioscrotal swelling
▷ **C** Mesonephric ducts
▷ **D** Mesonephric tubules
▷ **E** Paramesonephric ducts
▷ **F** Phallus
▷ **G** Urogenital folds
▷ **H** Urogenital sinus

1 ▶ Forms the fallopian tubes

2 ▶ Forms the ducts of Gartner

3 ▶ Forms the epoophoron

4 ▶ Forms the paraoophoron

5 ▶ Forms the lower two-thirds of the vagina

6 ▶ Forms the clitoris

#### Questions 7–11

■ *These questions relate to the abnormal development of the urogenital tract. For each item below, select the **single** best option from the list of options (A–G). Each option may be used once, more than once or not at all.*

OPTIONS

▷ **A** Female pseudohermaphrodite
▷ **B** Hypospadias
▷ **C** Male pseudohermaphrodite
▷ **D** Pseudohermaphroditism
▷ **E** Androgen insensitivity syndrome
▷ **F** True hermaphrodite
▷ **G** Turner syndrome

7 ▶ Have gonads that are both ovary and testicle

8 ▶ Is caused by deficiency of androgen receptors

9 ▶ The most common abnormality of the penis

10 ▶ Is usually due to congenital adrenal hyperplasia

11 ▶ Has gonads and external genitalia of different sexes

#### Questions 12–15

■ *These questions relate to the congenital kidney abnormalities. For each item below, select the **single** best option from the list of options (A–F). Each option may be used once, more than once or not at all.*

OPTIONS

▷ **A** Autosomal recessive polycystic kidney disease
▷ **B** Duplication of the ureters
▷ **C** Dysplastic kidneys
▷ **D** Horseshoe kidney
▷ **E** Pelvic kidney
▷ **F** Renal agenesis

12 ▶ Is caused by the kidneys being in close proximity as they move up through the abdomen

13 ▶ Is caused by early splitting of the ureteric bud

14 ▶ Is caused by failure of the ureteric bud to induce the metanephros

15 ▶ Forms cysts in the collecting ducts and causes renal failure in the young

## Questions 16–20

■ *These questions relate to gonadogenesis. For each item below, select the **single** best option from the list of options (A–H). Each option may be used once, more than once or not at all.*

OPTIONS

▷ **A** Gonads
▷ **B** Labioscrotal swelling
▷ **C** Mesonephric ducts
▷ **D** Mesonephric tubules
▷ **E** Paramesonephric ducts
▷ **F** Phallus
▷ **G** Urogenital folds
▷ **H** Urogenital sinus

16 ▶ Forms the seminiferous tubules

17 ▶ Forms the rete testis

18 ▶ Forms the testicular appendix

19 ▶ Forms the seminal vesicles

20 ▶ Forms the ventral aspect of the penis

## MULTIPLE CHOICE QUESTIONS

21 ▶ During the development of the urinary system from the nephrogenic cord of the urogenital ridge:

   **A** ▷ There are three types of kidneys during embryonic life
   **B** ▷ The kidneys develop from the intermediate mesoderm
   **C** ▷ The mesonephros appears during week 5 of development
   **D** ▷ The mesonephric tubules are involved in renal corpuscle formation
   **E** ▷ The mesonephros has stopped functioning by week 9

22 ▶ During the development of the urinary system from the nephrogenic cord of the urogenital ridge:

   **A** ▷ The ureteric buds form from intermediate mesoderm
   **B** ▷ Expansion of the ureteric bud forms the renal pelvis
   **C** ▷ The metanephric blastema forms the collecting ducts
   **D** ▷ The proximal and distal convoluted tubules meet at week 10
   **E** ▷ Urine production starts during week 12

23 ▶ During development of the metanephros:

   **A** ▷ The metanephros starts off as a pelvic organ
   **B** ▷ The metanephric mesoderm forms the minor calyces
   **C** ▷ The metanephric vesicles differentiate into the renal tubules
   **D** ▷ The metanephric vesicles form glomeruli
   **E** ▷ All nephrons are formed by 20 weeks

24 ▶ During development of the bladder from the urogenital sinus:

   **A** ▷ The urogenital septum is derived from mesoderm
   **B** ▷ The cranial part of the urogenital septum forms the bladder
   **C** ▷ The middle part forms the whole urethra in males
   **D** ▷ The caudal part forms the prostate in males
   **E** ▷ The mucosa is mesodermal in origin

25 ▶ During development of the bladder from the urogenital sinus:

   **A** ▷ The cloaca is divided by the endodermal urorectal septum
   **B** ▷ The allantois persists into adult life as the urachus
   **C** ▷ The bladder is lined with mesodermal epithelium
   **D** ▷ In females, the urogenital sinus becomes the vaginal vestibule
   **E** ▷ Urethral epithelium is endodermal in origin

26 ▶ During the development of the urethra:

   **A** ▷ The epithelium is derived from the endoderm
   **B** ▷ The smooth muscle is derived from mesoderm
   **C** ▷ In males, the urethral epithelium gives rise to paraurethral glands
   **D** ▷ Urachal fistulas drain urine into the vagina
   **E** ▷ The base of the bladder is exposed in bladder exstrophy

**27 ▶ Regarding gonadogenesis:**

A ▷ Gonadal development begins in week 4
B ▷ The gonads are undifferentiated until week 8
C ▷ The gonadal ridges form laterally to the mesonephros
D ▷ The sex-determining region is located on the long arm of chromosome Y
E ▷ The gonadal cords divide the gonadal ridges

**28 ▶ Regarding gonadogenesis:**

A ▷ The seminiferous cords develop in the rete testis
B ▷ Sertoli cells are formed from the mesenchyme of the gonadal ridge
C ▷ The seminiferous tubules are patent from week 12
D ▷ In the ovary, the medullary sex cords degenerate
E ▷ The primordial germ cells originate from the intermediate mesoderm

**29 ▶ During the process of external genital development:**

A ▷ The genital tubercle forms from the cloacal folds
B ▷ In males, the external urethral meatus is derived from the same epithelium as the rest of the urethral lining
C ▷ The corpora cavernosa develops from mesenchyme in the phallus
D ▷ The vaginal fornices develop from the paramesonephric ducts
E ▷ The urethral folds meet to form the clitoris

**30 ▶ The following pairs of structures are derived from the same embryonic structure:**

A ▷ The epoophoron and the gubernaculum
B ▷ The efferent ductules and the paraoophoron
C ▷ The ductus deferens and the duct of Gartner
D ▷ The appendix of the testis and the uterus
E ▷ The ventral aspect of the penis and the labia majora

**31 ▶ During the development of the male genital tract:**

A ▷ Sertoli cells begin to form in the mesonephric duct
B ▷ Sertoli cells form testis cords that become the seminiferous tubules
C ▷ The vas deferens is formed by the mesonephric ducts
D ▷ Leydig cells produce testosterone
E ▷ The prostate develops independently from the urethra

**32 ▶ In the male embryo, the mesonephric ducts form:**

A ▷ appendix of testes
B ▷ ductus deferens
C ▷ efferent ductules
D ▷ ejaculatory duct
E ▷ epididymis

**33 ▶ The following structures form a layer of the covering of the testis:**

A ▷ Gubernaculum
B ▷ Processus vaginalis
C ▷ Transversalis fascia
D ▷ Internal abdominal oblique muscle
E ▷ External abdominal oblique muscle

**34 ▶ During the development of the female genital tract:**

A ▷ The primitive sex cords form clusters
B ▷ The oogonia enter and are inhibited at the first mitotic stage
C ▷ The mesonephric ducts form the fallopian tubes, uterus and upper one-third of the vagina
D ▷ The lower part of the vagina is formed by the vaginal plate
E ▷ The epoophoron and paroophoron are remnants of the mesonephric and paramesonephric ducts respectively

**35 ▶ In the female embryo, the mesonephric ducts form:**

A ▷ appendix vesiculosa
B ▷ duct of epoophoron
C ▷ duct of Gartner
D ▷ epoophoron
E ▷ paroophoron

# Sample questions relating to development of the gastrointestinal tract and heart

## EXTENDED MATCHING QUESTIONS

OPTIONS

### Questions 1–8

■ *These questions relate to atrial septal defects. For each item below, select the **single** best option from the list of options (A–I). Each option may be used once, more than once or not at all.*

OPTIONS

▷ **A** Common atrium (cor triloculare biventriculare)
▷ **B** Endocardial cushion defects with foramen primum atrial septal defect
▷ **C** Ostium secundum atrial septal defect
▷ **D** Premature closure of the oval foramen
▷ **E** Sinus venosus atrial septal defect
▷ **F** Atrioventricular septal defect
▷ **G** Membranous atrial septal defect
▷ **H** Muscular atrial septal defect
▷ **I** Single ventricle (cor triloculare biatriatum)

1 ▶ Is associated with partial anomalous pulmonary venous connections

2 ▶ Causes pulmonary hypertension in adult life

3 ▶ Is caused by failure of the septum primum to fuse with the endocardial cushions

4 ▶ Is characterised by a large opening between the left and right atria

5 ▶ Is the complete absence of the atrial septum

6 ▶ Is the most serious abnormality

7 ▶ Is the rarest atrial septal defect

8 ▶ Results from the failure of development of both the septum primum and secundum

### Questions 9–15

■ *These questions relate to ventricular septal defects. For each item below, select the **single** best option from the list of options (A–I). Each option may be used once, more than once or not at all.*

OPTIONS

▷ **A** Atrioventricular septal defect
▷ **B** Membranous ventricular septal defect
▷ **C** Muscular ventricular septal defect
▷ **D** Single ventricle (cor triloculare biatriatum)
▷ **E** Common atrium (cor triloculare biventriculare)
▷ **F** Endocardial cushion defects with foramen primum ventricular septal defect
▷ **G** Foramen secundum ventricular septal defect
▷ **H** Premature closure of the oval foramen
▷ **I** Sinus venosus ventricular septal defect

9 ▶ Closes in up to 50% of cases in the first year of life

10 ▶ Forms a three-chambered heart

11 ▶ Results from failure of fusion of the endocardial cushions

12 ▶ Is the most common ventricular septal defect

13 ▶ Occurs in 20% of Down syndrome neonates

14 ▶ Is extremely rare

15 ▶ When multiple, is known as the 'Swiss cheese' ventricular septal defect

**Questions 16–22**

- *These questions relate to the fetal circulation. For each item below, select the **single** best option from the list of options (A–L). Each option may be used once, more than once or not at all.*

OPTIONS

▷ **A** Ascending aorta
▷ **B** Descending aorta
▷ **C** Ductus arteriosus
▷ **D** Ductus venosus
▷ **E** Inferior vena cava
▷ **F** Left atrium
▷ **G** Left ventricle
▷ **H** Pulmonary trunk
▷ **I** Right atrium
▷ **J** Right ventricle
▷ **K** Umbilical arteries
▷ **L** Umbilical vein

**16** ▶ Allows blood to bypass the liver

**17** ▶ Carries blood 80% saturated with oxygen

**18** ▶ Carries blood from the fetus to the placenta

**19** ▶ Carries blood from the placenta to the fetus

**20** ▶ Connects the right ventricle to the descending aorta

**21** ▶ Contains the highest level of oxygenated blood in the heart

**22** ▶ Is closed by a sphincter during a uterine contraction

## MULTIPLE CHOICE QUESTIONS

**23** ▶ Regarding the development of the fetal heart:

    **A** ▷ The primordial heart and vascular system appears in the middle of week 3
    **B** ▷ The cardiac jelly separates the myoblasts from the endothelial tube
    **C** ▷ The endocardium is formed by the endothelial lining in the cardiac loop
    **D** ▷ The pericardium is formed from the outermost myoblasts
    **E** ▷ The coronary arteries are formed from the mesothelial cells covering the myocardium

**24** ▶ Regarding the process of cardiac looping:

    **A** ▷ The truncus arteriosus connects to the aortic sac
    **B** ▷ The sinus venosus receives the umbilical blood supply
    **C** ▷ The ventricle and bulbus cordis are the fastest growing parts of the fetal heart
    **D** ▷ Is completed by day 35
    **E** ▷ The heart is in contact with the pericardium until week 8

**25** ▶ Regarding cardiac partitioning:

    **A** ▷ The atria are separated from the ventricles first
    **B** ▷ The septum primum separates the atria into two
    **C** ▷ The foramen primum remains patent
    **D** ▷ The foramen ovale forms in the septum primum
    **E** ▷ The foramen secundum forms around the foramen ovale

**26** ▶ During partitioning of the sinus venosus:

    **A** ▷ There are left and right sinus horns
    **B** ▷ The left sinus horn becomes obliterated
    **C** ▷ The right sinus horn receives all blood from the entire body
    **D** ▷ The right sinus horn becomes the right atrium
    **E** ▷ The sulcus terminalis is the internal wall of the sinus venosus

**27** ▶ During partitioning of the heart:

    **A** ▷ The interventricular septum grows as a continuation of the septum primum
    **B** ▷ The interventricular septum closes in week 9
    **C** ▷ Bulbar ridges form during week 5
    **D** ▷ The bulbus cordis and truncus arteriosus form the descending aorta
    **E** ▷ The bulbus cordis and truncus arteriosus form the pulmonary trunk

**28** ▶ Regarding the formation of heart valves:

    **A** ▷ The atrioventricular valves are formed by hollowing of the ventricle by the bloodstream
    **B** ▷ The valves are formed from the thick muscular wall
    **C** ▷ The valves are covered in endocardium
    **D** ▷ The semilunar valves form from four swellings around the aorta and pulmonary trunk
    **E** ▷ The semilunar valves form by rotation of the great vessels

29 ▶ Congenital heart defects:

A ▷ are the most common birth defects

B ▷ account for 10% of malformations in live births

C ▷ account for 10% of malformations in stillbirths

D ▷ are genetic in 20% of cases

E ▷ affect one-third of children with chromosomal abnormalities

30 ▶ Regarding congenital heart defects:

A ▷ Almost all children with Edwards syndrome (trisomy 18) have a heart defect

B ▷ They are not associated with DiGeorge syndrome

C ▷ 5% are due to environmental factors

D ▷ Gestational diet-controlled diabetes increases the incidence of congenital heart effects

E ▷ Isotretinoin (vitamin A) is a known cardiovascular teratogen

31 ▶ Regarding cardiac anomalies:

A ▷ In dextrocardia, the heart lies on the right side of the thorax

B ▷ Dextrocardia is associated with situs inversus

C ▷ Ectopia cordis is the most frequent cardiac positional anomaly

D ▷ In ectopia cordis, the heart is exposed on the surface of the thorax

E ▷ Ectopia cordis is due to abnormal cardiac development

32 ▶ Regarding atrial septal defect:

A ▷ Incidence is about six in 10 000

B ▷ Incidence in males is equal to that in females

C ▷ Patent foramen ovale is the most common type

D ▷ Patent foramen ovale occurs in 10% of neonates

E ▷ Foramen secundum atrial septal defect often leads to pulmonary hypertension after the third decade of life

33 ▶ Tetralogy of Fallot:

A ▷ is the most common abnormality of the conotruncal region

B ▷ is usually fatal

C ▷ causes a ventricular septal defect

D ▷ causes left ventricular hypertrophy

E ▷ causes right ventricular outflow obstruction

34 ▶ Regarding the conducting system of the heart:

A ▷ The atrium is the initial pacemaker of the heart

B ▷ The sinoatrial node is formed in week 6 of life

C ▷ The bundle of His forms in the ventricle and passes up towards the atrioventricular node

D ▷ Nerve supply to the heart develops before the conducting system

E ▷ 50% of sudden infant deaths are due to abnormalities of the conducting system

35 ▶ Mixing of oxygenated and deoxygenated fetal blood takes place in:

A ▷ the inferior vena cava

B ▷ the left atrium

C ▷ the liver

D ▷ the right atrium

E ▷ the superior vena cava

36 ▶ During the formation of the stomach:

A ▷ The stomach rotates 90° anticlockwise around its longitudinal axis

B ▷ The left side rotates to face anteriorly

C ▷ The posterior wall grows faster than the anterior wall

D ▷ The ventral mesogastrium forms the lesser omentum

E ▷ The caudal mesogastrium forms the greater omentum

37 ▶ During the development of the liver and biliary apparatus:

A ▷ The bile duct arises from the duodenum

B ▷ The bile duct originally enters the duodenum posteriorly

C ▷ The gallbladder and cystic duct develop from the same outgrowth

D ▷ Bile formation begins during week 10

E ▷ Hepatic sinusoids are made up of, amongst others, umbilical veins

38 ▶ During the development of the liver:

A ▷ The septum transversum provides mesodermal cells for the liver parenchyma

B ▷ The septum transversum provides mesodermal cells for connective tissue

C ▷ The entire surface of the liver differentiates into visceral peritoneum

D ▷ The central tendon of the diaphragm is formed from the embryological liver

E ▷ Haematopoiesis begins during week 6

**39** ▶ During development of the midgut:

 A ▷ The superior mesenteric artery supplies the entire midgut

 B ▷ The vitelline duct is an open connection between the midgut and the yolk sac

 C ▷ The midgut forms the proximal one-third of the transverse colon

 D ▷ The primary loop of bowel rotates around an axis by 270°

 E ▷ The primary intestinal loop rotation occurs during the bowel herniation time only

**40** ▶ During development of the midgut:

 A ▷ The midgut enters the umbilical cord in week 8

 B ▷ Herniated bowel begins to return to the abdomen by week 12

 C ▷ On returning to the abdomen, the caecum lies below the liver

 D ▷ The appendix is relatively large in the neonate

 E ▷ The pancreas becomes retroperitoneal by being pressed by the colon to the posterior abdominal wall

**41** ▶ During development of the hindgut:

 A ▷ The hindgut is supplied by the middle mesenteric artery

 B ▷ The cloaca is lined with mesoderm

 C ▷ The urorectal septum is made of mesoderm

 D ▷ The urorectal septum comes into contact with the cloacal membrane

 E ▷ The tip of the urorectal septum forms the perineal body

**42** ▶ Regarding the development of the anal canal:

 A ▷ The junction between the superior and inferior anal canal is marked by the pectinate line

 B ▷ Above the pectinate line, the epithelium is stratified squamous

 C ▷ Below the pectinate line, the epithelium is keratinised

 D ▷ The lymphatic drainage is the same for the entire anal canal

 E ▷ Carcinomas from the upper two-thirds are painful

**43** ▶ The inferior two-thirds of the anal canal:

 A ▷ are derived from endoderm

 B ▷ are 13 mm long

 C ▷ receive blood from arteries originating from the inferior mesenteric artery

 D ▷ drain to the superficial inguinal nodes

 E ▷ have a nerve supply from the autonomic nervous system

**44** ▶ Regarding omphalocele:

 A ▷ Incidence is one in 10 000 births

 B ▷ Omphalocele is caused by failure of the bowel to return to the abdomen

 C ▷ Diagnosis can be from week 9 onwards

 D ▷ The viscera are uncovered

 E ▷ Mortality rate is 25%

**45** ▶ Gastroschisis:

 A ▷ occurs in one in 10 000 births

 B ▷ occurs in older mothers

 C ▷ is equally spread between male and female fetuses

 D ▷ herniation occurs through a weakness due to regression of the right umbilical vein

 E ▷ is associated with chromosomal abnormalities

# Endocrinology

CHAPTER 15

# Placental structure and function

*Desmond Holden*

## Introduction

The placenta anchors the developing pregnancy within the uterus, is responsible for nutrient and waste exchange, is important in preventing the mother from recognising and rejecting paternally derived antigens, has important endocrine functions that equip the mother to survive childbirth and is involved in the signalling to initiate labour. This highly evolved organ has also been implicated in the aetiology of miscarriage, fetal growth restriction, pre-eclampsia and abruption. In this chapter, the mechanisms by which some of these functions are accomplished will be discussed. Definitions of terms are shown in Table 15.1.

## The early conceptus

The fertilised egg is moved along the fallopian tube by cilial and muscular action. The first cleavage division takes place in the ampulla, within 30 hours of fertilisation, with subsequent divisions every 12 hours to the 16-cell stage. The daughter cells (blastomeres) remain totipotent until this stage is reached. This redundancy allows preimplantation diagnosis in the field of assisted conception by the removal of a single cell. These early divisions are directed by maternally derived proteins and RNA. The embryo enters the uterus at the eight-cell stage. Differences in the development of the early embryo in different species are shown in Table 15.2.

TABLE 15.1 **Terminology of pregnancy**

| Term | Definition |
|------|-----------|
| Morula | The conceptus up until approximately 16-cell stage, prior to fluid collection and development of the inner cell mass |
| Blastocyst | The next stage of development from the morula, with fluid separating inner cell mass from outer cells, which become trophoblast |
| Blastomere | Individual cells of the blastocyst |
| Zona pellucida | Glycoprotein layer surrounding the oocyte, which persists to the morula/blastocyst stage, allowing growth in cell number without loss of cells prior to trophoblast invasion of the decidua |
| Trophoblast | Derived from the outer cell layer of the blastocyst, forms cytotrophoblast (retain single nucleus per cell) and syncytiotrophoblast, a true syncytium. The trophoblast is the key placental cell for synthesis, invasion and anchoring the pregnancy in the uterus |
| Decidua | Specialised modulation of the uterine endometrium, with species-specific alteration of blood vessels, connective tissue and leucocyte content |
| Haemochorial placenta | Maternal blood in direct contact with the chorionic (syncytio)trophoblast |

TABLE 15.2 **Comparison of mouse, sheep and human early pregnancies**

| Species | Cleavage to 4 cells | Transcriptionally active stage | Conceptus enters uterus | Formation of blastocyst | Time of attachment | Time to luteal regression if not pregnant | Pregnancy duration |
|---|---|---|---|---|---|---|---|
| **INVASIVE** | | | | | | | |
| Mouse | 1.5–2 | 2 cell | 3 | 3 | 4.5 | 10–12 | 19–20 |
| Human | 2 | 4–8 cell | 3.5 | 4.5 | 7–9 | 12–14 | 270–290 |
| **NON-INVASIVE** | | | | | | | |
| Sheep | 4 | 8 cell | 2–3 | 6–7 | 16 | 16–18 | 144–152 |

Values are time in days unless otherwise stated.

The development of the conceptus from the eight-cell stage to the time of implantation is shown in Figure 15.1. From the 16-cell morula stage, subcellular differentiation of organelles occurs with a greater concentration seen at the apex compared with the basal pole. The apical surface develops numerous microvilli. The outer cells of the morula (which are destined to become the trophoblast and placenta) develop tight intercellular junctions (gap junctions and desmosomes). Fluid collects in this outer layer, separating it from the cells that will become the inner cell mass (and ultimately the fetus). At this stage the morula becomes much more metabolically active, with increased protein synthesis and increased oxygen consumption. The energy fuelling these processes is derived from pyruvate rather than glucose metabolism.

In the preimplantation phase, new trophoblast develops from the base of the inner cell mass (polar trophoblast). This is the blastocyst stage of development. It is at this morula–blastocyst stage that one of the two X chromosomes of a female embryo becomes deactivated and condensed as a Barr body.

## Implantation

Placental attachment to the maternal uterine wall is fundamental to successful human reproduction. Inadequate invasion of the decidua by the trophoblast is associated with various pregnancy complications, while excessive invasion compromises the health of the mother and, therefore, the infant.

The characteristics of trophoblast cells are:

- paternal X chromosome inactivation
- unmethylated DNA
- ability to form multinucleated cells
- variable expression of major histocompatibility complex (MHC) class 1 antigens; no MHC class 2 antigen expression.

The functions of the trophoblast cells are:

- attachment of the placenta to the uterine wall
- transport of nutrients, oxygen and maternal immunoglobulins to the fetus
- elimination of fetal waste products
- synthesis and secretion of proteins and hormones
- barrier between maternal and fetal circulations
- contact site between maternal immune system and conceptus.

Implantation can be thought of in three phases.

### APPOSITION

Initially at the site of contact between the polar trophoblast and the endometrium, but subsequently more widely, the endometrium increases mitotic activity and undergoes localised changes in stromal cell morphology and intercellular matrix composition. There is also an influx of cells associated with host defence, including natural killer (NK) cells. This process is called decidualisation. The endometrium develops pinopodes, which remove fluid from the uterine cavity (by pinocytosis) and allow closer apposition between the blastocyst and the decidua.

## FIGURE 15.1 Development of the conceptus from the eight-cell stage to the time of implantation

### A  Eight-cell stage

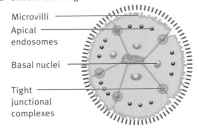

- 2nd polar body
- Zona pellucida
- Blastomere

### B  Sixteen-cell stage

- Microvilli
- Apical endosomes
- Basal nuclei
- Tight junctional complexes

### C  Morula

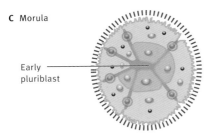

- Early pluriblast

### D  Blastocyst

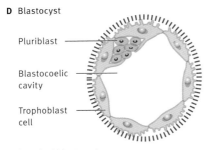

- Pluriblast
- Blastocoelic cavity
- Trophoblast cell

### E  Attached blastocyst

- Primary decidua
- Uterine epithelium
- Pinopodes
- Trophoblast

## ADHESION

Adhesion is accompanied by destruction of the zona pellucida, allowing contact between maternal and trophoblast cells. Within a few hours of attachment, the surface epithelium adjacent to the trophoblast becomes eroded. This, and the destruction of the zona pellucida, is accomplished by a variety of metalloproteases and by the expression of adhesion molecules on the trophoblast cell membrane that are specific for ligands on the forming decidua.

## PENETRATION

The production of metalloproteases by trophoblast allows the digestion of the extracellular matrix. This facilitates trophoblast invasion into the uterine decidua and makes a variety of lipids, proteins, nucleotides and sugars available as metabolic substrates and fuel. Trophoblast cells can actively transport small molecules across their cell membranes and are able to transport large molecules and cellular fragments by pinocytosis and phagocytosis. This early nutrition is independent of any placental circulation. Trophoblast cells contain microfilaments as part of their internal cytoskeleton. These allow the trophoblast cells to squeeze between endometrial cells and the blastocyst to thereby invade the underlying stroma so deeply that the surface epithelium becomes restored over it (interstitial implantation).

The biochemical signalling involved in these processes is incompletely understood. There may be considerable biochemical redundancy in this control as well, because transgenic mice with genes inactivated for each of the supposed key control cytokines (so called 'knockout mice') are still able to reproduce successfully. The peptide hormone vascular endothelial growth factor (VEGF) is

From the eight-cell stage, the conceptus becomes compacted with maximum contact between adjacent cell membranes. After cell division and differentiation, the cells become wedge-shaped and develop tight intercellular junctions that prevent intercellular diffusion. The nuclei become basally located and the polarised cells develop microvilli centrally and at their outer (zonal) ends. Further cell division to 16–32 cells leads to early division into an outer layer (destined to be trophoblast) and an inner, pluriblast layer. By the 64-cell stage (blastocyst), fluid has accumulated within the blastocoelic cavity, facilitated by tight intercellular junctions. The pluriblast is eccentric and will form the inner cell mass. After attachment, the zona pellucida is lost and the trophoblast is starting to penetrate the uterine epithelium.

FIGURE 15.2 **Formation of the intervillous space and primary stem villi**

Anatomy of the developing placenta

The trophoblast differentiates into two layers: an inner layer of cytotrophoblast, where the cells remain recognisably individual, and an outer syncytiotrophoblast layer, where cellular walls are largely lost (Figure 15.2). Before implantation is complete (11–12 days), lacunae form in the polar syncytiotrophoblast. These trophoblast-lined lacunae will eventually be the intervillous space, allowing circulation of maternal blood in the placental bed. By 13 days after conception, some cells from the trophoblast shell will invade deeply through the decidua and into the myometrium, providing a supportive or attaching function. Also by the end of week 2, primary villous stems are formed. These comprise an outer layer of syncytiotrophoblast cells with a core of cytotrophoblast, which itself has a core of extraembryonic mesoderm (Figure 15.2).

Differentiation of the extraembryonic mesoderm allows vascularisation of the stem villus, which then becomes continuous with the vessels of the body stalk (which will become the umbilical vessels) during week 3 (Figure 15.3). The primary villous stems give rise to syncytiotrophoblast buds, again with a cytotrophoblast and mesodermal core, which become primary villi. Those primary villi adjacent to the uterine cavity regress to form the chorion laeve (nonplacental part of the chorion). The villi on the decidual side of the conceptus (chorion frondosum) undergo further growth and branching as secondary and tertiary villi, filling the intervillous space to form the definitive placenta. It is from the tertiary villi that the true placental villi arise. The elaboration of villi centred on a single primary stem villus is called a placental lobule, of which the placenta has approximately 200. This process is complete by 8–10 weeks of gestation. There is no relation between placental lobules, or groups of lob-

FIGURE 15.3 **Formation of tertiary stem villi, which provide the architecture of the placenta**

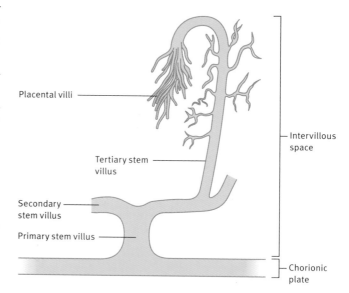

**FIGURE 15.4  Types of placentation and relationships between fetal trophoblast cells and maternal blood**

**A** Epitheliochorial placentation

**B** Endotheliochorial placentation

**C** Haemochorial placentation

Fetal vascular endothelium

FB

Trophoblast cells

Uterine epithelium

Maternal vascular smooth muscle

MB

Maternal vascular endothelium

Cytotrophoblast

Syncytiotrophoblast

Maternal blood in intervillous space

MB

FB = fetal blood  |  MB = maternal blood

ules, and the cotyledons (or lobes) seen when examining the maternal surface of the term placenta.

By 12 weeks, the placenta has reached its definitive form and subsequently enlarges laterally. The placenta exceeds the weight of the fetus until about 17 weeks and typically weighs about one-sixth of the fetus at term.

**THE CHORIONIC VILLUS**

Several different patterns of placental function (Figure 15.4) have developed in different mammalian species and these can be classified on the basis of the cell types intervening between maternal and fetal blood cells. In epitheliochorial placentation, the trophoblast cells attach to the surface epithelium of the uterus (no invasion). Endotheliochorial placentation sees trophoblast invasion of the uterine epithelium but no invasion of maternal blood vessels. Haemochorial placentation shows the greatest invasion, with maternal blood vessels invaded by trophoblast cells, which become bathed in maternal blood. Species with epitheliochorial placentation increase maternal blood flow to the placental bed through decidual angiogenesis (an increased number of similar-sized vessels). This contrasts with human (haemochorial) pregnancy where an increase in blood flow through the placental bed is achieved through trophoblast invasion of the spiral arteries of the decidua and outer myometrium.

In the nonpregnant state, the spiral artery is a muscular high-resistance vessel. In pregnancy, trophoblast invasion converts the spiral artery to a wider bore capaci-

tance vessel, allowing blood flow through the uterus to increase 10–15-fold. The mechanism by which trophoblast cells invade decidual spiral arteries and replace the vascular endothelium is only just beginning to be understood. It seems likely that trophoblast cells recognise vascular smooth muscle and endothelial cells through specific adhesion molecule expression. This recognition can induce an intracellular sequence of events that alters trophoblast motility, induces apoptosis in the vascular myocytes and endothelial cells and causes the functional and histological changes in spiral arteries (reduced muscular wall and endothelial lining replaced by trophoblast cells) that are the characteristics of haemochorial placentation.

Two observations about placental architecture in pre-eclampsia have remained constant despite the growing understanding of placental development. Placental villi are less developed in placentas taken from pre-eclamptic pregnancies, with fewer branches and less complex vascular loops than placentas associated with normal pregnancy outcome. The second observation is that change in spiral artery architecture is less evident or patchy when the placental bed is examined histologically at placental bed biopsy (Figure 15.5).

## Immunology of pregnancy tolerance

While there are advantages of close contact between the trophoblast of placental villi and maternal blood (nutri-

FIGURE 15.5 **Differences in placental architecture for a normal pregnancy and a pre-eclamptic pregnancy**

**A** Normal pregnancy       **B** Pre-eclamptic pregnancy

Placental villus
Spiral artery
Vascular loops
Syncytiotrophoblast
Decidua
Myometrium
Maternal vascular smooth muscle
Maternal vascular endothelium

In **A** the placental villus contains an elaborate fetal vasculature and the spiral artery wall has been replaced by the endovascular syncytiotrophoblast; in **B** the fetal villous vessels are less branched and the spiral artery has remained as a narrow, high-resistance vessel with reduced replacement by the endovascular trophoblast. | MB = maternal blood

■ Uterine NK cells are similar to a minor (10%) fraction of blood NK cells, but have phenotypic differences, including unusual adhesion molecule expression and poor cytotoxicity.

■ The origin of decidual NK cells, as discrete lineage, or differentiated from circulating NK cells, is unclear.

■ Decidual NK cells produce a range of soluble products including angiogenic cytokines (angiopoietin-2 and vascular endothelial growth factor), immunoregulatory cytokines and chemokines and lytic enzymes.

■ The reduced cytotoxicity of decidual NK cells may relate to a lack of intracellular cytoskeletal and lytic granule organisation.

■ Diagnostic tests on NK cells in peripheral blood of women with reproductive failure give no information about decidual NK cell function.

■ Possible roles for decidual NK cells include maintenance of mucosa and blood vessel stability, modification of spiral arteries in the decidua and regulation of trophoblast invasion of the decidua and its structures.

tion and waste elimination) as seen in the haemochorial placenta, the disadvantage is that the circulations are no longer separated by an epithelial barrier. Trophoblastic cells in human pregnancy are therefore exposed to potential allogenic immune responses by the mother.

Advances have been made in understanding the immune reactions of pregnancy by focusing on the relationship between trophoblast – the outermost layer of fetal cells – and the cells with which they are in contact. These are the cells of the uterus that undergo highly specialised differentiation during decidualisation. The most obvious features include enlargement of the uterine stromal cells and the presence of a distinct lymphocyte population of uterine NK cells. The presence of NK cells is seen widely in all species with a decidual response to invasive placentation. Similar cells are not seen in other tissues. The roles and characteristics of uterine NK cells are as follows:

■ CD56$^{hi}$CD16$^-$ uterine NK cells represent 70% of leukocytes at the implantation site and increase in number in the late luteal phase of the menstrual cycle and in early pregnancy.

The relationship between the decidual response in the uterus and invasion has been argued both to permit and to control the degree of invasion. Both roles may occur, allowing the balance of sufficient placental invasion without excess. Uncontrolled trophoblast cell invasion is seen where the decidua is deficient or absent (for example, in tubal ectopic pregnancy or implantation on scar tissue within the uterus). Trophoblast cells implanted at distant ectopic sites (in animal experiments and in *in vitro* cell culture) show inherent invasive growth. Overinvasion of the fetal–maternal interface compromises the mother's health, resulting in haemorrhage in the absence of medical intervention.

At the opposite end of the spectrum, the decidua may prevent adequate invasion into the spiral arteries. This shift of fetal–maternal interface in favour of the mother is associated with reduced blood supply to the placental bed and a growth restricted, hypoxic fetus. Pre-eclampsia has a high maternal and fetal mortality and yet has an incidence of 5–10% in first-time mothers. That natural selection has not removed this complication may be a trade in human reproduction: balancing human trophoblasts' highly invasive tendencies against the consequent risk of maternal haemorrhage, death and subsequent compromise of neonatal survival. Exactly how the degree of trophoblast invasion is controlled is not yet understood, although there is evidence that apoptosis in invasive trophoblast may be a limiting and controlling factor.

## PLACENTA–UTERUS IMMUNE INTERACTION

A mother does not biologically reject her pregnancy but would reject a tissue graft from a genotypically dissimilar donor. The rejection of an allograft (for example, renal or heart transplant) is through powerful antibody and T-cell-mediated responses to allogeneic MHC molecules expressed by the vascularised graft. However, the fetus is not in contact with the mother's immune system but is shielded by the trophoblast of the placental interface. Trophoblast cells never express MHC class 2 molecules and are thereby unable to present antigen to maternal CD4+ T-cells. In humans, the placental trophoblast encounters the maternal immune system in two locations: (i) the villous syncytiotrophoblast is bathed by maternal blood; and (ii) the extravillous cytotrophoblast interacts with uterine tissue.

The syncytiotrophoblast expresses no MHC antigens, which is consistent with the concept that the placenta is immunologically neutral. This theory also fits with the observation that while fetal cells that enter the maternal circulation provoke an immune reaction (for example, rhesus isoimmunisation and haemolytic disease of the newborn), no such systemic T- or B-cell immune response to trophoblast cells has been described.

The second area of contact is between the decidua and the invasive, anchoring, extravillous cytotrophoblast. Unlike the syncytiotrophoblast, the extravillous trophoblast expresses unusual combinations of cell surface human leucocyte antigen (HLA) C, G and E molecules, but does not express polymorphic HLA-A and HLA-B, the molecules that are important in initiating allograft rejection. Polymorphic HLA-C is expressed but does not lead to allograft rejection. There are a number of hypotheses to explain this.[1] One difference from allograft rejection is that CD8+ regulatory T cell populations present in the uterus in pregnancy are specific for a carcinoembryonic antigen-like ligand, rather than being MHC restricted. Another mechanism by which the placenta might alter the local immune environment is that trophoblast HLA-G binds with highly avidity leukocyte immunoglobulin-like receptors on myelomonocytic cells. Increased expression of these receptors is associated with graft tolerance, possibly through reduced MHC class 2 pathways, and may be important in the decidua where macrophages and dendritic cells expressing MHC class 2 are found.

## UTERINE NATURAL KILLER CELL RECOGNITION BY TROPHOBLAST CELLS

Uterine, but not peripheral, NK cells express an array of receptors for trophoblast MHC class 1 antigens. One of the C-type lectins (CD94-NKG2A) binds HLA-E and reduces NK cell cytotoxicity. All NK cells also express a killer cell immunoglobulin-like receptor family antigen, KIR2DL4, that can bind HLA-G, the effect of which is the upregulation of proinflammatory and proangiogenic cytokines. This may be a mechanism by which the placenta can enhance its blood supply, while soluble HLA-G entering the systemic circulation might interact with blood NK cells and contribute to the systemic vascular and inflammatory changes of pregnancy.

The polymorphic HLA-C expressed by trophoblast also interacts with NK cell KIR ligands, of which there are both activating (KIR2DS) and inhibitory (KIR2DL) receptor types. Hence, there are two polymorphic gene systems, maternal KIRs and fetal HLA-C antigens, at this site of the maternal–fetal interface. Decidual invasion by the trophoblast therefore has the potential to vary in different pregnancies, as some ligand–receptor interactions are likely to favour trophoblast invasion while others may prevent adequate placentation.

## The placenta and maternal–fetal exchange

The placenta acts as a barrier between the maternal and fetal circulations. Simple diffusional exchange between the circulations is only significant for low-molecular-weight substances (such as gases, sodium, urea and water) and for nonpolar molecules (such as unconjugated steroids and fatty acids). This simple diffusion changes with gestation as the anatomy of the terminal villus changes. In early pregnancy, the terminal villi are large (diameter

150–200 micrometres) and the fetal vessels are located centrally, beneath 10 micrometres of syncytiotrophoblast, so metabolites need to diffuse relatively far to access the fetal circulation. As pregnancy progresses, the villi are smaller (40 micrometres diameter) and the vessels are more eccentric, giving a 90% reduction in diffusional distance. While the diffusion rate of most molecules is inversely proportional to this distance, oxygen is highly soluble and its diffusion is dependent more on blood flow than thickness of the intervening barrier.

### OXYGEN AND CARBON DIOXIDE

Oxygen consumption in pregnancy is proportional to the growing conceptus. Cardiac output and blood flow through the uterus and placental bed increase and ventilation increases, reducing carbon dioxide and bicarbonate concentrations in maternal plasma. Concentration gradients promote oxygen and carbon dioxide diffusion into and out of the fetus, respectively. Fetal oxygen carriage, however, is approximately equal to that of maternal blood. This is due to the greater intrinsic affinity for oxygen and reduced binding for 2,3-diphosphoglycerate with embryonic and fetal haemoglobin. Oxygen transfer to the fetus is also promoted by fetal blood in the placenta increasing in pH, which favours the uptake of oxygen by haemoglobin, while the reduction in maternal blood pH as it picks up carbon dioxide favours maternal haemoglobin giving up oxygen (double Bohr effect).

### GLUCOSE AND CARBOHYDRATE

As gestation progresses, maternal tissues become relatively less sensitive to insulin. This can allow latent diabetes to appear, but also allows more of the plasma glucose to be taken up by the fetal–placental unit and relatively less to be taken up by maternal tissues. Placental uptake of glucose is by facilitated diffusion in which specific carriers use concentration gradients to drive the uptake of D-glucose. The maximum rate of transfer for this transport is 0.6 mmol/minute/g placenta. This transport only becomes saturated at 20 mmol/l glucose. The placenta metabolises considerable amounts of glucose to lactate and this is available to the fetus as fuel at about one-third the availability of glucose. The rate of fetal use of glucose is largely related to fetal insulin production.

### AMINO ACIDS AND UREA

Deamination of amino acids by the maternal liver is reduced in pregnancy and the maternal excretion of resultant urea also falls. This makes more ingested and absorbed amino acids available to the placenta and fetus. Some amino acids are synthesised within the trophoblast cells (for example, acidic nonessential amino acids and neutral straight-chained amino acids). There are also a number of active transport systems for different groups of amino acids (neutral branched-chain and basic amino acids) in the placenta, which are used as building blocks for the placenta itself and for the dependent fetus. These concentrate amino acids within the trophoblast to five times the maternal plasma concentration. The urea generated by fetal amino acid metabolism diffuses passively back across the placenta into the maternal circulation, which has a reduced urea concentration.

### WATER AND ELECTROLYTES

Exchange of water between mother and fetus occurs at two main sites: the placenta and the remainder of the non-placental chorion. The amnion and chorion are freely permeable to water and either diffusion or hydrostatic forces must account for transfer. A large difference in hydrostatic pressure between maternal and fetal circulations within the placenta does not occur and it is likely that the necessary flux of water from fetus to mother is accomplished across small and intermittent hydrostatic gradients. Isotope studies have shown that sodium trafficking across the placenta occurs as co-transport for various active transport molecules and also by paracellular diffusion.

Fetal blood contains iron at between two and three times the concentration of maternal blood. This iron is delivered by active transport across the placenta and an intratrophoblast ferritin-binding stage has been described. Calcium and phosphate are transferred to the fetus against a concentration gradient by an active transport system that is sensitive to metabolic and competitive inhibitors.

### AMNIOTIC FLUID

The volume of amniotic fluid increases during pregnancy from about 15 ml at 8 weeks to 450 ml at 20 weeks, after which net production declines to zero by 34 weeks (approximate volume 750 ml). The composition of amniotic fluid suggests that it is initially a transudate. Towards term, the total solute concentration in amniotic fluid falls but the concentrations of urea, creatinine and uric acid rise. Amniotic fluid is in a dynamic state, with complete exchange of its water occurring approximately every 3 hours.

## PLACENTAL MEMBRANES

The amnion arises as an epithelial layer between the ectodermal disc of the inner cell mass and the trophoblast (chorion). The amnion has five layers: cuboidal epithelium (with prominent intracellular canals and vacuoles), basement membrane, compact layer, fibroblast layer and spongy layer of mucoid reticular tissue (remnant of extraembryonic coelom). The amniotic cavity lies between the amnion and the ectodermal disc.

The chorion has four layers: fibroblasts, reticular layer, basement membrane and trophoblast layer. The trophoblast layer is 2–10 cells thick, lies immediately adjacent to the deciduas and is continuous with placental trophoblast. Obliterated chorionic villi have been described.

Neither the amnion nor the chorion has blood vessels, lymphatics or nerves.

# Hormonal control of placental synthesis

## HUMAN CHORIONIC GONADOTROPHIN

For a pregnancy to survive, it is necessary that the corpus luteum does not involute during the first trimester. In humans, human chorionic gonadotrophin (hCG) is secreted by the syncytiotrophoblast from as early as 6–7 days post-fertilisation. It consists of two amino acid chains (alpha and beta) linked by non-covalent bonds and has a relative molecular weight of 38 400 kDa. Both chains have attached carbohydrate residues. hCG is chemically and functionally similar to pituitary luteinising hormone (LH), with the alpha subunit being similar to all glycoprotein hormones: LH, follicle-stimulating hormone (FSH), thyroid-stimulating hormone. The beta subunit of hCG is similar to LH but with an additional 30 amino acids at the carboxy terminus. Immunoassays

directed at this beta-subunit terminus are therefore specific for hCG and the basis for urinary pregnancy tests. The levels of hCG in maternal serum and urine rise rapidly in early pregnancy, peak at about 12 weeks of gestation and then decline. hCG binds to LH receptors in the corpus luteum. That hCG is the luteotrophic hormone of human pregnancy is suggested by observations that the corpus luteum does not involute in women who are not pregnant but are given parenteral hCG injections, and by the observation in animal studies that antibodies directed at hCG that prevent binding at the LH receptor site cause involution of the corpus luteum and abortion.

## PROGESTERONE

hCG maintains the progestogenic activity of the corpus luteum, but within 2 weeks of fertilisation the conceptus is also synthesising all the steroid hormones required for pregnancy. Although the corpus luteum remains active throughout pregnancy, it is not essential after about 6 weeks and contributes only a small amount to the total pregnancy production of progesterone. In blighted ovum pregnancies, where no embryo forms, and in choriocarcinoma or hydatidiform moles, progesterone production by the conceptus is unaffected. This observation and immunocytochemical studies of the trophoblast *in vitro* have localised production of progesterone to the trophoblast itself. This synthesis uses maternal cholesterol and appears autonomous to the placenta (with no external control identified). The peak concentration of progesterone in human pregnancy is at term when it is ten-fold greater than the luteal phase of the ovarian cycle. The main maternal urinary excretion product is pregnanediol.

## ESTROGEN

The main estrogen in pregnancy is not the ovarian-cycle steroid 17-estradiol but the less potent estriol. The synthesis of this steroid is severely reduced in molar and choriocarcinoma pregnancies and production requires the presence of a fetus (unlike the production of progesterone). Estriol synthesis occurs in the placenta but uses dehydroepiandrosterone (DHEA), derived from the fetal adrenal cortex, as a substrate. DHEA is hydroxylated to 16-hydroxy DHEA in the fetal liver and this product undergoes aromatisation of the A-ring in the trophoblast to form estriol. Deficiency of fetal adrenal activity (congenital adrenal hyperplasia and anencephaly) is associated with low estriol levels. In fetal blood, 16-hydroxy DHEA circulates as a sulphate conjugate and a placental sulphatase is essential for estriol synthesis. This sulphination of the steroid in the fetus and desulphination in the placenta is important as sulphination creates a steroid that is water soluble and inactive. This allows the fetus to be less exposed to the biological effects of a steroid that in the mother is bioactive and important in a range of pregnancy adaptations. Maternal estriol concentration rises to 100 times the nonpregnant estrogen concentration at term. Estrone and estradiol are also synthesised by the placenta, but in smaller amounts than estriol and from maternal precursors.

### HUMAN PLACENTAL LACTOGEN

As the trophoblast makes less hCG towards the end of the first trimester of pregnancy, it synthesises human placental lactogen, a 21 600 kDa single-peptide protein with 191 amino acids, two disulphide bridges and a plasma half-life of 15 minutes. It is chemically and functionally similar to prolactin and pituitary growth hormone but less biologically active. Its plasma concentration plateaus after 35 weeks and, while it may have a role in modifying carbohydrate metabolism, pregnancies lacking any human placental lactogen appear to progress normally.

## Abnormal placentation

### MULTIPLE PREGNANCY

One of the functions of the zona pellucida is to prevent the blastomeres of the early conceptus from falling apart during early cleavage. If the conceptus does become divided into two distinct groups of cells at this stage, monozygotic twins result. If this division occurs early, then two completely separated pregnancies occur with implantations that may be separated within the uterus or may be coincidentally close to each other. In either case, the placentas are anatomically and functionally separate from each other. If division into two pregnancies occurs after 9 days from conception, then there will be either two distinct fetuses in a single amniotic sac with a single placenta (monoamniotic twins) or, if later still, then conjoined fetuses will result. If cleavage occurs between 4 and 8 days after conception, monochorionic diamniotic twins will result: two fetuses in two amniotic sacs but with a single chorion and a single placenta. In this placental arrangement, while most placental cotyledons will drain oxygenated blood to the umbilical vein of the same cord which has supplied it with deoxygenated blood, some cotyledons drain to the other cord and twin and one twin can become a net donor of blood to its sibling (the recipient). This is called twin-to-twin transfusion, with the recipient becoming hypervolaemic, with excessive amniotic fluid, a hyperdynamic circulation and a high haemoglobin concentration. Its donor becomes anaemic, oliguric and growth restricted (twin-to-twin transfusion syndrome).

### MOLAR PREGNANCY

The chromosome complement within the developing trophoblast can have profound effects on the phenotype of the developing placenta. Clinically, this effect is seen most commonly with molar pregnancy. Molar, or hydatidiform molar, pregnancies are classified as partial or complete on the basis of their chromosome complement and the presence or absence of fetal tissue. A complete molar pregnancy occurs with fertilisation of an oocyte where the maternally derived chromosomes are lost and the paternally derived chromosomes are duplicated. There are 46 chromosomes in each cell, but they comprise 23 chromosomes from a single spermatozoon, duplicated to 46. As there are no maternally derived chromosomes, no fetal tissue forms. In a partial mole, there are 69 chromosomes in each cell, two sets paternally derived and one set from the oocyte. In this case, fetal tissue does form. In both situations, the trophoblast is more invasive than normal and secretes more pregnancy hormones per gestational stage than a normal conceptus.

### UNIPARENTAL DISOMY

Uniparental disomy results in an imbalance between paternally and maternally derived chromosomes in the conceptus, with effects on placental structure and function. It occurs when conception produces a 46-chromosome complement, but one pair is formed by loss of the maternal or paternal chromosome and duplication of the remaining one; hence, 22 chromosomes are derived from one parent and 24 from the other. The best-characterised example of this relates to chromosome 15. Loss of maternal chromosome 15, with duplication of the paternal chromosome, is a rare cause of Angelman syndrome, while the reverse of this situation, with maternal disomy for chromosome 15, gives rise to Prader–Willi syndrome.

## REFERENCE

1.  Moffat A, Loke C. Immunology of placentation in eutherian mammals. *Nature Rev Immunol* 2006;324:584–94.

## FURTHER READING

Huppertz B, Peeters L L H. Vascular biology in implantation and placentation. *Angiogenesis* 2005;8:157–67.

Johnson M, Everitt B. *Essential Reproduction*. Oxford: Blackwell Science; 2000.

Rezende-Filhoe J, Castro P, Pereira Leite S, Barbosa Montenegro CA, de Lourdes de Almeida Lima M. Pre-eclampsia: an overview in placentation, endothelial dysfunction and flow-mediated vasodilatation. *Ultrasound Rev Obstet Gynecol* 2005;5:242–53.

# Hypothalamus and pituitary gland

*Gul Bano*

## Anatomy of the hypothalamo–pituitary region

The hypothalamus is bounded anteriorly by the optic chiasm, laterally by the subthalamus and internal capsule and posteriorly by the mammillary bodies. Dorsally, it is delineated from the thalamus by the hypothalamic sulcus. The pituitary stalk descends from its central region, which is termed the median eminence. This region stands out because of its dense vascularity, which is formed by the primary plexus of the hypophysial portal system. The long portal veins run along the ventral surface of the pituitary stalk.

The pituitary gland or hypophysis weighs roughly 0.5 g in adult life and measures approximately 10–15 mm in each dimension. It protrudes from the bottom of the hypothalamus at the base of the brain, rests in a small bony cavity (the sella turcica) in the sphenoid bone and is covered by a dural fold called the diaphragma sellae. The pituitary gland is in close proximity to the optic chiasm, the cavernous sinus and the floor of the third ventricle. It is heavier in women than in men and becomes larger during pregnancy.

The pituitary gland is composed of two main lobes: the anterior pituitary or adenohypophysis and the posterior pituitary or neurohypophysis. The adenohypophysis in turn can be subdivided into the pars distalis (anterior lobe) and the pars tuberalis. The neurohypophysis is composed of the pars nervosa, the pituitary stalk (also known as the infundibular stalk or infundibulum) and the median eminence. The pituitary stalk connects the pituitary and the hypothalamus, enabling hypothalamic releasing factors to stimulate the release of pituitary hormones.

The blood supply to the hypothalamo–pituitary axis is complex (Figure 16.1). The hypothalamus receives its blood supply from the circle of Willis, whereas the neurohypophysis and adenohypophysis receive blood from the inferior and superior hypophysial arteries, respectively. The capillary plexus of the inferior hypophysial artery drains into the dural sinus, although some of these capillaries in the neural stalk form short portal veins that drain into the anterior pituitary gland. The major portion of the circulation arises from the long portal veins. These are formed from the capillary network of the superior hypophysial arteries that supply the nerve endings of the neurosecretory cells in the median eminence. Here, the portal veins form a secondary capillary network into which the hormones of the anterior pituitary are secreted. The venous channels from the anterior pituitary gland drain into the cavernous sinuses and from there into the superior and inferior petrosal sinuses and into the jugular vein.

## Histology of the hypothalamo–pituitary region

There are three types of hypothalamic neurosecretory cells. Magnocellular neurons secrete arginine vasopressin (AVP) or oxytocin. The cell bodies, which are located in the supraoptic or paraventricular hypothalamic nucleus, project their neuronal processes via the pituitary stalk into the posterior neural lobe and neurohormone is released from the nerve endings into the blood.

Hypophysiotrophic neurons are located in nuclear groups, including the paraventricular nucleus and the arcuate nucleus, in the medial basal hypothalamus. The

FIGURE 16.1 **Blood supply to, and venous drainage from, the hypothalamo–pituitary axis**

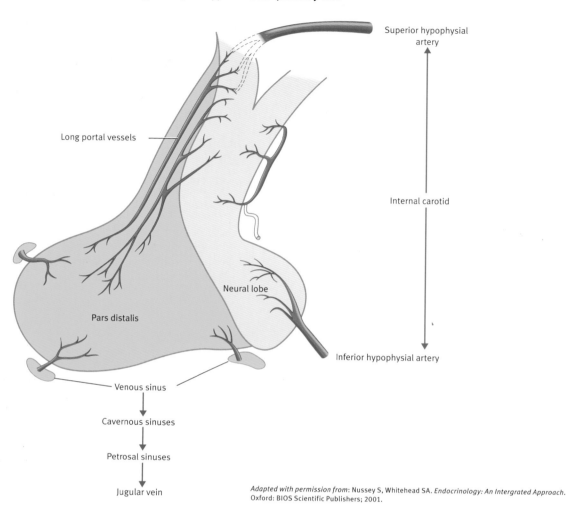

Adapted with permission from: Nussey S, Whitehead SA. *Endocrinology: An Intergrated Approach.* Oxford: BIOS Scientific Publishers; 2001.

hypophysiotrophic neuropeptides are released into a specialised blood supply called the hypothalamic–hypophysial portal system and regulate the secretion of hormones from the pituitary. Hypophysiotrophic neuropeptides include thyrotrophin-releasing hormone (TRH), corticotrophin-releasing hormone (CRH), somatostatin, growth-hormone releasing hormone (GHRH), gonadotrophin-releasing hormone (GnRH) and dopamine.

Projection neurons are found in the paraventricular and arcuate nuclei and in the lateral hypothalamic area. These neurons project to autonomic preganglionic neurons in the brain stem and spinal cord.

Microscopic examination of the conventionally stained adenohypophysis reveals three distinctive cell types termed acidophils, basophils and chromophobes. This pattern of staining reflects the chemical character of intracellular hormone-laden granules within the pituitary cells.

The neurohypophysis is an extension of the hypothalamus and is composed of bundles of axons from hypothalamic neurosecretory neurons intermixed with glial cells.

## Embryology of the hypothalamo–pituitary region

The anterior lobe of the pituitary gland develops from an evagination of ectodermal cells of the oropharynx in the primitive gut and is recognisable at weeks 4–5 of gestation. This evagination, known as the Rathke pouch, is eventually pinched off from the oral cavity and becomes separated from it by the sphenoid bone of the skull. The lumen of the pouch is reduced to a small cleft, while the upper portion of the pouch surrounds the neural stalk and forms the pars tuberalis. This, together with the anterior lobe, is called the adenohypophysis. When cells from the Rathke pouch are left behind and form tumours, these are called craniopharyngiomas.

The posterior lobe develops from neural crest cells as a downward evagination of the floor of the third ventricle of the brain. The lumen of this pouch closes as the sides fuse to form the neural stalk, while the upper portion of the pouch forms a recess in the floor of the third ventricle known as the median eminence.

The neural stalk together with the median eminence forms the infundibular stalk and this, together with the posterior lobe, is collectively termed the neurohypophysis. The cleft-like remnant of the Rathke pouch demarcates the boundary between the anterior and posterior lobes of the pituitary gland.

The hypothalamo–pituitary axis is established by week 20 of gestation.

## Physiology of the hypothalamus and pituitary gland

Functions of the hypothalamus include the control of the autonomic nervous system and the regulation of body temperature, hunger and thirst; it also has a role in memory, behaviour and emotional responses. In this chapter, we restrict discussion to the regulation of the endocrine system.

### ANTERIOR PITUITARY GLAND

The anterior pituitary gland is regulated by three interacting elements: hypothalamic input (releasing and inhibitory factors), feedback effects of circulating hormones and paracrine and autocrine secretions of the pituitary gland itself. From a clinical perspective, the anterior pituitary gland synthesises and secretes six major hormones: growth hormone (GH, also called somatotrophin), thyroid-stimulating hormone (TSH, also called thyrotrophin), adrenocorticotrophin (ACTH), follicle-stimulating hormone (FSH), luteinising hormone (LH) and prolactin.

The physiological control of TSH and ACTH is described in chapter 17.

### Growth hormone

GH is synthesised and secreted by cells called somatotrophs in the anterior pituitary gland. It is a single-chain polypeptide containing 191 amino acids. GH shares structural homologies with prolactin and human chorionic somatomammotrophin (also called human placental lactogen), the latter being a GH variant synthesised exclusively in the placenta.

GH predominantly affects growth, metabolism, cell differentiation and lactation. The effects of GH on protein metabolism include increases in amino acid uptake and protein synthesis and a decrease in the oxidation of proteins. GH enhances the metabolism of fats by stimulating triglyceride breakdown and oxidation in adipocytes. In carbohydrate metabolism, GH is one of the hormones that maintain blood glucose levels within the normal range. It suppresses insulin-mediated glucose uptake in peripheral tissues and insulin-mediated glucose synthesis in the liver. Somewhat paradoxically, GH stimulates insulin secretion and GH administration can therefore lead to hyperinsulinaemia.

GH exerts its effects directly and indirectly through the family of insulin-like growth factors (IGFs). The IGF family consists of three members (insulin, IGF-I and IGF-II) that share common structural similarities. Insulin, IGF-I and IGF-II have metabolic functions, but they also have important roles in cellular proliferation and differentiation (mediated by the IGF-I receptor). IGF-II is a major fetal growth factor. IGF-I is more important for postnatal growth. Insulin also plays a role in fetal growth. A reflection of this role is the development of fetal macrosomia in pregnancies associated with maternal diabetes.

Mean daily GH secretion is high in childhood with a peak at puberty. Secretion falls during adulthood. In the adult human, approximately five pulses of GH are secreted during a 24-hour period with a larger peak

FIGURE 16.2 **Actions and regulation of growth hormone and prolactin**

GH = growth hormone | GHRH = growth-hormone-releasing hormone |
IGF = insulin-like growth factor | MB = mamillary bodies |
OC = optic chiasm | PRF = prolactin-releasing factor |
TRH = thyrotrophin-releasing hormone | + = stimulatory effects |
− = inhibitory effects

Adapted with permission from: Nussey S, Whitehead SA. *Endocrinology: An Intergrated Approach.*
Oxford: BIOS Scientific Publishers; 2001.

occurring at the onset of sleep at night. The half-life of GH in the circulation is about 20 minutes.

Synthesis and secretion of GH are controlled by two hypothalamic neurohormones: GHRH, which stimulates GH secretion, and somatostatin, which inhibits GH secretion (Figure 16.2). Ghrelin also causes GH release.

GHRH is released from nerve terminals in the median eminence and transported to the anterior pituitary gland via the hypophysial portal capillaries. Somatostatin is a 14-amino-acid peptide that is synthesised in hypothalamic neurons mainly located in the anterior periventricular nuclei.

Factors affecting GHRH and somatostatin secretion include sleep, exercise, stress and blood glucose levels. In addition, IGF-I provides negative feedback to the pituitary gland and hypothalamus. Finally, estradiol acts to increase the sensitivity of tissues to GH.

### Prolactin

Prolactin is a single-chain protein made up of 199 amino acids with three disulphide bridges. It shares strong structural homologies with GH and the cell surface receptors of prolactin and GH are also similar.

FIGURE 16.3  **Actions and regulation of gonadotrophins**

FSH = follicle-stimulating hormone  |  G = G-protein-linked receptor  |  GnRH = gonadotrophin-releasing hormone  |  LH = luteinising hormone

*Adapted with permission from:* Nussey S, Whitehead SA. *Endocrinology: An Intergrated Approach.* Oxford: BIOS Scientific Publishers; 2001.

In animals, prolactin has a plethora of actions but in humans it is mainly involved in preparation of the female breast for lactation. Other roles are poorly understood, although there is widespread tissue expression of prolactin receptors. It is also notable that men have the same circulating concentrations of prolactin as nonlactating women. Prolactin has effects on the hypothalamo–pituitary–gonadal axis, it can inhibit pulsatile secretion of GnRH from the hypothalamus and it can alter the activity of certain steroidogenic enzymes.

Prolactin secretion is regulated by a dual hypothalamic inhibitory and stimulatory system. In addition, it can regulate its own secretion through a short feedback loop (Figure 16.2). The control of prolactin release by the hypothalamus is unique in that the predominant hypothalamic influence is inhibitory, whereas it is stimulatory for all other hormones. Thus, damage to the hypothalamic control causes increased prolactin levels.

Dopamine, released into the hypophysial portal veins from nerve terminals in the hypothalamus, is the main neurohormone inhibiting prolactin secretion. Somatostatin also has an inhibitory effect. Stimulatory factors include TRH, other releasing factors, pregnancy, lactation (suckling), estrogen, opioids, dopamine $D_2$ receptor antagonists, sleep and stress.

### Gonadotrophins

The gonadotrophins, such as FSH, LH and human chorionic gonadotrophin, are glycoproteins (molecular weights approximately 30 000 Dalton) made up of a gonadotrophin-specific alpha subunit and a beta subunit that confers biological specificity to each hormone. LH and FSH are secreted from cells called gonadotrophs in the anterior pituitary gland (Figure 16.3). Their receptors are typical G-protein-linked proteins. Receptor activation by gonadotrophin binding stimulates adenylate cyclase, resulting in a rise in cyclic adenosine monophosphate (cAMP) levels.

LH and FSH are important regulators of steroidogenesis in the gonads. In the testis, LH acts on the interstitial or Leydig cells, whereas FSH acts on the Sertoli cells. In the ovary, each hormone acts on more than one cell type. There are numerous isoforms of circulating LH and FSH and biological potency depends on the degree and sites of glycosylation and the electrical charge of the molecule. Thus, different assays of LH and FSH concentrations may not always give a true index of biological activity.

### POSTERIOR PITUITARY GLAND

AVP and oxytocin are small peptides with strong structural homologies. They consist of nine amino acids arranged in a ring structure with a short 'tail'. AVP is mainly synthesised in the supraoptic nuclei and to a lesser extent the paraventricular nuclei, whereas the reverse is true for oxytocin. The hormones synthesised in the large (or magnocellular) neurosecretory cells of these nuclei are transferred to the posterior pituitary gland, whereas those synthesised in the smaller (or parvocellular) neurons control the hormone secretions of the anterior pituitary gland.

Like all other peptide and protein hormones, AVP and oxytocin are synthesised as large prohormones. Once packaged into secretory granules, the AVP and oxytocin prohormones pass by axonal flow to the nerve terminals (Herring bodies) in the neurohypophysis. During this passage, the prohormones are cleaved into the biologically active AVP or oxytocin molecules and a larger polypeptide fragment. Neurophysin II is the product cleaved from the AVP prohormone, neurophysin I that cleaved from the oxytocin prohormone. Both neurophysins are cosecreted with the active hormones upon electrical activation of the neurosecretory cells.

### Arginine vasopressin

AVP derives its name from the first action ascribed to it nearly 100 years ago: an increase in systemic blood pressure (it is a pressor agent). The actions of AVP on water balance in the kidney (where it is effective in very low concentrations) gave rise to an alternative name, antidiuretic hormone, and the two names tend to be used interchangeably. AVP has three known receptors and acts in concert with aldosterone and atrial natriuretic peptide to control blood volume and pressure. However, this chapter will consider exclusively the actions of AVP.

In the kidney, AVP acts on the G-protein linked $V_2$ receptors on the capillary (basal) side of the distal convoluted and collecting ducts and stimulates the synthesis of cAMP (Figure 16.4). cAMP activates a kinase on the luminal (apical) side of the ducts, which initiates a series of events culminating in the insertion of water channels, known as aquaporins, into the luminal membrane. Water passes into the collecting-duct cells and, by osmosis, across the basal membrane into the interstitial fluid and hence back into the circulation. There is also an osmotic gradient (set up by the countercurrent activity of the loop of Henle) from the cortex to the medulla of the kidney. Thus, as the collecting ducts pass through the cortex to the medulla, increasing amounts of solute-free water (also termed free water) can be reabsorbed by the osmotic gradient. This is governed by the aquaporins and hence AVP.

Increased osmolality of the extracellular fluids stimulates AVP release (Figure 16.4). Changes in osmolality are detected by osmoreceptors. Osmotically sensitive cells were first described in the hypothalamus but it is now known that there are additional osmoreceptors in the circumventricular organs and in systemic viscera. These are not only important in regulating AVP secretion but also in stimulating thirst. As a result, AVP induces an

FIGURE 16.4 **Actions and regulation of arginine vasopressin**

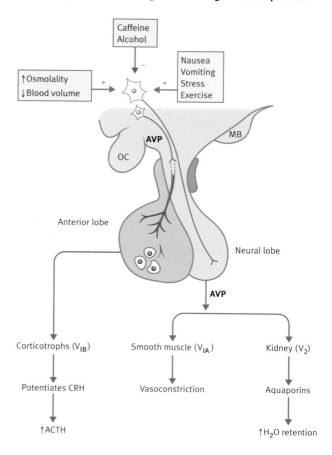

$\downarrow$ = decrease | $\uparrow$ = increase | ACTH = adrenocorticotrophin | AVP = arginine vasopressin | CRH = corticotrophin-releasing hormone | $V_{1A}$, $V_{1B}$ and $V_2$ = AVP receptor subtypes | + = stimulatory effects | − = inhibitory effects

*Adapted with permission from*: Nussey S, Whitehead SA. *Endocrinology: An Intergrated Approach.* Oxford: BIOS Scientific Publishers; 2001.

increase in water retention and a reduction in serum osmolality.

Another potent stimulus to AVP secretion is a reduction in effective blood volume; in fact, AVP secretion is stimulated by a volume reduction of just 5–10%. This is controlled by so-called stretch receptors that detect changes in blood volume or pressure. These include the baroreceptors and other receptors in the cardiovascular system. Thus, for example after a haemorrhage, AVP secretion will be stimulated and water will be retained to increase blood volume. The reverse occurs in response to an increase in blood volume or pressure.

Other stimulants of AVP secretion include emotional stress, pain and a variety of drugs. Nausea and vomiting are also extremely potent stimulators of AVP release. The effects of these stimuli can be important in situations such as the postoperative state, affecting water balance. By contrast, alcohol is a potent inhibitor of AVP release (as little as 30–90 ml of whisky is sufficient) resulting in inappropriate dehydration and some of the symptoms associated with a hangover. The preventative measure is to drink a restorative volume of water after excess ethanol consumption.

Apart from its primary role in water conservation, AVP is also important in maintaining blood pressure after a haemorrhage as a result of its vasopressive effects on arteriolar smooth muscle. Acting on smooth muscle cells, it induces vasoconstriction via $Ca^{2+}$ and phospholipase-C-generated second messengers.

The final established role of AVP is to potentiate the action of CRH on the pituitary corticotrophs.

### Oxytocin

The major action of oxytocin is in lactation, when, through a neuroendocrine reflex, it initiates the let-down of milk by inducing contractions of the myoepithelial cells surrounding the alveoli of the mammary gland. In animals, there is evidence that oxytocin has a major role in parturition but in humans there is much less evidence to support this role. Oxytocin does, however, have a contributing role in that it induces powerful contractions of the uterine muscle. Thus, synthetic oxytocin is widely used therapeutically in obstetrics, not only to induce labour but also to reduce postpartum bleeding.

Oxytocin can have stimulatory effects at the AVP $V_2$ receptor in the kidney. There is no naturally occurring disease associated with excess oxytocin secretion but in obstetric situations, when given in high doses as an intravenous infusion with 5% dextrose, it can cause water retention and iatrogenic hyponatraemia. (For more information on oxytocin, see Chapter 6.)

## Hypothalamic and pituitary control of puberty

Puberty is defined as the stage of physical maturation in which an individual becomes physiologically capable of sexual reproduction. It is associated with marked endocrine changes, including an increase in growth rate, skeletal changes (such as increase in hip width in girls), increase in fat and muscle and profound psychological changes.

### PHYSIOLOGY OF PUBERTY

The onset of puberty is characterised by an increase in the secretions of LH and FSH, which in turn is driven by GnRH release from neurons that are diffusely situated in the arcuate nucleus and other nuclei of the hypothalamus. Before the onset of puberty, both LH and FSH are secreted in very small amounts (with low concentrations in peripheral blood) and there is no apparent stimulation of the gonads. However, as puberty approaches, the amplitudes of LH and FSH pulsatile secretions (and hence the mean secretion rates) increase and the nocturnal rise in LH secretion is amplified. It is notable that this nocturnal rhythm is specific to puberty as it disappears in adulthood. The gonad itself does not seem necessary for the changes to occur and thus it must be concluded that the brain is in some way programmed to produce more GnRH and hence LH and FSH.

The increasing circulating concentrations of LH and FSH stimulate pubertal development of the gonads and thus an increase in the output of sex steroids. These, together with adrenal androgens, induce the physical changes that occur at this time (Figure 16.5).

In boys, the earliest sign of increasing LH and FSH secretions is an increase in testicular size (a volume increase of more than 4 ml or a length increase of more than 2.5 cm). In girls, thelarche (breast development) is a sensitive indicator of LH- and FSH-stimulated ovarian steroid secretions. Before the menarche, however, estradiol secretion fluctuates widely, probably reflecting waves of follicular development in which the follicles fail to reach the ovulatory stage. Estrogen stimulates growth of the uterus but menarche does not occur until the estrogens have stimulated sufficient uterine growth such that their withdrawal causes the first menstruation. The onset of menstruation is such a milestone in the development of girls that primary amenorrhoea can be relied upon to indicate underlying pathology. The growth of axillary and pubic hair in both sexes is a consequence of increased concentrations not only of gonadal steroids (gonadarche) but also of adrenal steroids (adrenarche).

FIGURE 16.5  **Tanner stages of puberty**

**FEMALE**

| STAGE | BREAST DEVELOPMENT |
|---|---|
| 1 | Prepubertal; no breast tissue |
| 2 | Areolar enlargement with breast bud |
| 3 | Enlargement of breast and areola, which arise as a single mound |
| 4 | Projection of areola above breast as a secondary mound |
| 5 | Adult; papilla projects out of areola, which is part of breast contour |

**MALE**

| STAGE | GENITAL DEVELOPMENT |
|---|---|
| 1 | Prepubertal |
| 2 | Testes enlarge (4 ml); scrotum enlarges, reddens and develops coarser skin |
| 3 | Penis enlarges, initially in length; continued growth of testes and scrotum |
| 4 | Penis grows in length and breadth; continued growth of testes and scrotum, which becomes pigmented |
| 5 | Testes, scrotum and penis adult size |

**BOTH SEXES**

| STAGE | PUBIC HAIR DEVELOPMENT |
|---|---|
| 1 | None |
| 2 | Few darker hairs along labia or at base of penis |
| 3 | Curly pigmented hairs across pubes |
| 4 | Small adult configuration |
| 5 | Adult configuration with spread onto inner thighs |

*Adapted with permission from: Nussey S, Whitehead SA. Endocrinology: An Intergrated Approach. Oxford: BIOS Scientific Publishers; 2001.*

## PRECOCIOUS PUBERTY

The changes during puberty normally follow a reliable pattern that is sometimes called consonance. If these changes happen early (before the age of 8 years in girls and before the age of 9 years in boys), puberty is considered to be precocious. When the normal pattern is not followed, this is termed precocious sexual development (or pseudoprecocious puberty). Precocious puberty is gonadotrophin-dependent and idiopathic in 90% of girls.

## DELAYED PUBERTY

Delayed puberty is defined as an increase in testicular

TABLE 16.1 **Causes of delayed puberty**

| Cause | Frequency |
|---|---|
| **CONSTITUTIONAL DELAY** | Common (~90%) |
| **HYPOGONADOTROPHIC HYPOGONADISM** | Rare (~10%) |
| GnRH deficiency[a] | |
| Gonadotrophin deficiency[b] | |
| **HYPERGONADOTROPHIC HYPOGONADISM** | Rare (~10%) |
| Sex chromosome abnormality[c] | |
| Gonadal dysgenesis with normal karyotype | |
| Gonadal damage[d] | |
| Loss-of-function mutation in the beta subunit of LH[e] | |
| Loss-of-function mutation in gonadotrophin receptors (resistant ovary syndrome) | |

[a] May be isolated or associated with other features, for example anosmia (Kallmann syndrome), cognitive impairment or dysmorphic features (Prader–Willi syndrome) | [b] may be isolated (fertile eunuch syndrome resulting from LH deficiency) or more commonly associated with any form of hypopituitarism | [c] for example Klinefelter syndrome (47,XXY) in boys, Turner syndrome (45,X) in girls | [d] may be viral (for example mumps orchitis), iatrogenic (surgical, chemotherapy or radiotherapy) or autoimmune (often associated with Addison's disease) | [e] reduced LH bioactivity but elevated concentrations of LH in immunoassay | GnRH = gonadotrophin-releasing hormone | LH = luteinising hormone

volume of less than 4 ml by the age of 14 years in boys and no breast development by the age of 13.5 years in girls. Boys are much more likely than girls to have idiopathic delay (termed constitutional delay). Constitutional delay affects both growth and puberty and, by definition, the investigations are normal. The causes of delayed puberty are given in Table 16.1.

### AMENORRHOEA

Primary amenorrhoea is usually defined as no menarche by the age of 16 years. Secondary amenorrhoea is defined as absence of menstruation for at least 3 months in a previously menstruating girl or woman of reproductive age. Primary amenorrhoea can be a feature of delayed puberty.

From a clinical point of view, considerable diagnostic accuracy can be gained from defining the presence of breast development and a uterus. Thus, when a uterus is present and there is no breast development, the cause is probably a failure of the whole hypothalamo–pituitary–ovarian axis (for example Kallmann syndrome) or ovarian failure (for example Turner syndrome). If a uterus is present and the breasts have developed, this indicates that the failure of the axis has occurred after breast development. If breasts have developed and a uterus is absent, the likely cause is androgen insensitivity or congenital absence of the uterus.

From an endocrine point of view, the causes can be defined by considering the serum concentrations of the gonadotrophins LH and FSH. High gonadotrophin concentrations indicate a problem in the ovary, whereas low levels indicate hypothalamo–pituitary dysfunction.

## Diseases of the hypothalamus and pituitary gland

Endocrine disease of the hypothalamus or pituitary is characterised by a loss of hormone action. Excess pituitary hormone secretion is usually caused by a tumour and generally involves oversecretion of a single hormone. The vast majority of pituitary tumours are benign adenomas and these may compress the optic chiasm. Rare carcinomas may invade locally and may either compress or destroy the adjacent parts of the pituitary.

When end-organ diseases such as those of the thyroid gland, ovary or adrenal gland arise, these are termed primary disorders. Secondary disorders arise when function is affected by defective pituitary hormone secretion. Tertiary disorders result from hypothalamic dysfunction that produces both pituitary and target-organ hypofunction.

### ACROMEGALY

Acromegaly is a very rare disease (annual incidence approximately three/million). The syndrome results from a chronic exposure to GH leading to the classic clinical features outlined in Table 16.2. High exposure to GH before fusion of the epiphyseal plates produces gigantism. It is attributable to a pituitary adenoma in 95% of the total incidence. These adenomas are often

TABLE 16.2 **Clinical features of acromegaly**

| Body system | Symptoms (prevalence among those with acromegaly) | Signs (prevalence among those with acromegaly) |
|---|---|---|
| Skeletal | Arthralgia/arthritis (85%) Carpal tunnel syndrome (50%) | Enlarged hands and feet (100%) Jaw protrusion (90%) Dental malocclusion (80%) Osteoarthritis (30%) |
| Skin | Excessive sweating (85%) | Greasy skin, skin tags (60%) |
| Cardiovascular | Angina (5–10%) | Hypertension (50%) Cardiomyopathy (5%) |
| Respiratory | Diurnal drowsiness (30%) | Obstructive sleep apnoea (30%) |
| Metabolic | Polydipsia and polyuria (5%) | Neuropathy (50%) Retinopathy (15%) |
| Renal | Renal colic (20%) | Renal stones (20%) |
| Other endocrine | Menstrual irregularity (50%) Impotence (40%) | Hypogonadism (40%) |

over 1 cm in diameter when the diagnosis is established. Around 15% of GH-secreting tumours also hypersecrete prolactin. More rarely, acromegaly may be caused by hypothalamic tumours such as glioma and hamartoma and even less often by peripheral tumours such as adenocarcinoma of the pancreas.

In acromegaly caused by a pituitary tumour, the secretion of GH remains pulsatile but the duration, amplitude and number of secretory episodes are elevated. The characteristic nocturnal surge is absent and there are abnormal responses to suppression and stimulation of GH secretion.

Most of the deleterious effects of GH hypersecretion are caused by its stimulation of excessive amounts of IGF-I. IGF-I leads to the proliferation of bone, cartilage and soft tissue and an increase in the size of other organs. Clinical features of GH excess usually begin in the third or fourth decade of life and progress insidiously. The duration of symptoms before diagnosis is usually 5–10 years. The mean age at diagnosis is 42 years and the incidence is the same in both sexes.

Soft-tissue proliferation is one of the early manifestations, leading to enlarged hands and feet and exaggerated facial features (the most common clinical symptom).

Local symptoms of pituitary mass effect, that is, expansion of the tumour and compression of neighbouring structures, include headache and visual impairment (usually bitemporal hemianopia with loss of peripheral vision). Hypopituitarism may lead to the additional clinical features of hypothyroidism, hypogonadism and hypoadrenalism. The musculoskeletal abnormalities are generally not reversible but myalgias and arthralgias frequently decrease. There is an increase in the rates of mortality from cardiovascular and cerebrovascular atherosclerosis (36–62%), respiratory disease (0–25%) and malignancies (9–25%). Death rates tend to be higher when diabetes or hypertension is associated.

The best test to confirm a diagnosis of acromegaly is the oral glucose tolerance test. Glucose (75 g orally) is administered after an overnight fast. Healthy people usually respond with suppression of the serum GH concentration to less than 2 mU/l. In acromegaly, there is failure to suppress GH levels after a glucose load; in fact, GH levels may be increased (a paradoxical increase). TRH or GnRH stimulation will increase GH levels in 70–80% of people with acromegaly; this is not the case in healthy people.

Formal assessment of visual fields should be performed and the imaging modality of choice is magnetic resonance imaging (MRI).

Treatments for acromegaly include medical and surgical approaches and radiotherapy. Surgery may be curative, especially when the tumours are smaller than 10 mm in diameter. After radiotherapy, panhypopituitarism occurs in 15–20% of people treated, with a lag time of a few years.

## GROWTH HORMONE DEFICIENCY

GH deficiency in childhood is usually detected rapidly as a result of the effects on growth velocity. The causes of adult GH deficiency include any damage to the hypothalamo–pituitary axis.

The laboratory diagnosis of adult GH deficiency requires a stimulation test to confirm the diagnosis. The insulin tolerance test is the diagnostic test of choice, provided adequate hypoglycaemia is achieved and the person under investigation is not subject to seizures and does not have ischaemic heart disease. A peak GH response of less than 9 mu/l is indicative of GH deficiency.

## HYPERPROLACTINAEMIA

Serum prolactin concentrations can be elevated for a number of reasons (Table 16.3).

### Prolactinoma

Prolactinomas are benign, clonally expanded tumours and the clinical presentation is different in men and women. Women tend to have smaller tumours that come to light earlier because these tumours have a predilection for causing galactorrhoea or amenorrhoea owing to the inhibitory effects of excess prolactin on the pituitary gland and ovaries. Men tend to have larger tumours that come to light late, perhaps because men are reluctant to discuss gradually deteriorating gonadal and sexual function.

In the treatment of prolactinoma, surgery and radiotherapy may be used as in all pituitary tumours. However, dopamine agonist drugs (including cabergoline or bromocriptine) are recommended as first-line treatment for prolactinomas, even in the presence of visual field defects. These drugs lower serum concentrations of prolactin and shrink the tumours. In people who cannot tolerate these drugs or in whom the drugs fail to shrink the tumour

TABLE 16.3 **Causes of hyperprolactinaemia**

| Cause | Frequency |
|---|---|
| Drugs, such as neuroleptic agents (e.g. phenotiazine) or dopamine D$_2$ receptor antagonists used as antiemetics (e.g. metoclopramide)<br><br>Primary hypothyroidism | Common (~90%) |
| Macroprolactinaemia<br><br>Stalk syndrome [a]<br><br>Pituitary tumour (micro- or macroprolactinoma) [b] | Uncommon (~10%) |
| Renal failure | Rare (<1%) |

[a] Interference in the supply of dopamine to the normal lactotrophs; usually associated with moderately elevated circulating concentrations of prolactin (<3000 mu/l) | [b] usually associated with markedly elevated circulating concentrations of prolactin (>5000 mu/l)

sufficiently, surgery and/or radiotherapy may be used. In pituitary apoplexy associated with mass effects, such as visual loss, surgical intervention may be recommended to decompress the optic chiasm.

## NONFUNCTIONING PITUITARY ADENOMA

These tumours cause problems because of their size and location. The clinical features are headache, visual field defects, cranial nerve palsies and those of hypothyroidism, hypogonadism, hypoadrenalism and GH deficiency detailed elsewhere.

Investigation requires assessment of pituitary function, visual field assessment and use of MRI as the imaging modality of choice.

Treatment usually comprises surgery with or without radiotherapy.

## CRANIOPHARYNGIOMAS AND RATHKE CLEFT CYSTS

Craniopharyngiomas cause symptoms in three different ways:

- by increasing the intracranial pressure
- by disrupting the function of the pituitary gland resulting in hypopituitarism and diabetes insipidus
- by damaging the optic nerve.

Craniopharyngiomas are nearly always cystic, sometimes lobulated and filled with oily green fluid that has a characteristic appearance on MRI. They may also calcify and appear as suprasellar calcification on a plain skull X-ray. Craniopharyngiomas are usually picked up in people under the age of 20 years.

The usual treatment for craniopharyngiomas is surgery, with postoperative radiotherapy recommended for any residual tumour. Medical treatment involves the replacement of missing hormones.

Rathke cleft cysts are rare benign lesions requiring surgical treatment when they become symptomatic. Transsphenoidal surgery is the recommended therapy.

### DIABETES INSIPIDUS

Central diabetes insipidus is characterised by decreased secretion of AVP. This results in polyuria and polydipsia because the ability to concentrate urine is diminished. Reduced or absent AVP secretion can result from a defect in one or more sites involving the hypothalamic osmoreceptors, the supraoptic or paraventricular nuclei or the supraopticohypophysial tract. Lesions of the posterior pituitary rarely cause permanent diabetes insipidus because AVP is produced in the hypothalamus and can still be secreted into the circulation.

Nephrogenic diabetes insipidus is characterised by a decrease in the ability to concentrate urine owing to a resistance to AVP action in the kidney. It can be observed in chronic renal insufficiency, lithium toxicity, hypercalcaemia, hypokalaemia and tubulointerstitial disease.

There are also rare forms of hereditary nephrogenic diabetes insipidus. One potential cause is an X-linked genetic defect that results in failure of the AVP $V_2$ receptor in the kidney to function correctly. More rarely, a mutation in the gene encoding aquaporin-2 can cause a break in the kidney water channel, which results in the kidney being unable to absorb water. This mutation is inherited in an autosomal recessive manner.

The diagnosis of diabetes insipidus is usually made clinically and laboratory tests provide confirmation. Most people with diabetes insipidus can drink enough fluid to replace their urine losses if the thirst mechanism is intact. The synthetic AVP analogue desmopressin may be used twice a day as a subcutaneous, nasal or oral preparation to control symptoms. It is important to avoid

hyponatraemia through overuse of desmopressin.

## Pituitary diseases in pregnancy

### PROLACTINOMA

Excess levels of prolactin directly inhibit pulsatile GnRH secretion, resulting in anovulation/amenorrhoea and infertility. Correction of hyperprolactinaemia with dopamine agonists restores ovulation in approximately 90% of women with prolactinoma.

There are two key issues in a woman with a prolactinoma who becomes pregnant. The first is the effect of a dopamine agonist on early fetal development before the pregnancy is discovered. In principle, fetal exposure to dopamine agonists should be limited. Bromocriptine seems to be safe in pregnancy and available data suggest that cabergoline is also safe, although the evidence regarding cabergoline safety is based on a small number of pregnancies. Data on the safety of pergolide and quinagolide during pregnancy are too limited to recommend the use of these agents. The reported heart valve damage seen with high-dose cabergoline has not been demonstrated with cabergoline at the doses used to treat hyperprolactinaemia, nor with bromocriptine or quinagolide (a non-ergot-based dopamine agonist).

The second issue is the effect of pregnancy on the prolactinoma. Pregnancy stimulates normal lactotrophs and causes enlargement of the normal pituitary. This does not necessarily mean that the adenomatous pituitary gland may enlarge. Prolactinomas that enlarge and become symptomatic during pregnancy are uncommon. Symptoms suggestive of prolactinoma growth are headache and visual field changes. The risk of clinically significant enlargement for women with a microprolactinoma is 1–2%. The risk of enlargement for a woman with untreated macroprolactinoma is about 20%. A macroprolactinoma that has been previously treated with surgery, radiation or both has a 2–5% risk of clinically significant enlargement. Shrinkage of a prolactinoma with a dopamine agonist is associated with a reduced chance of symptomatic growth during pregnancy once treatment is discontinued.

Reinitiation of medical treatment is recommended for pregnant women with prolactinomas that become symptomatic. The symptoms tend to regress quickly. Transsphenoidal surgery or delivery is an alternative if the tumour does not respond to medical treatment or if further visual deterioration occurs. Careful follow-up with monthly visual field examinations is important in pregnant women with a known macroadenoma. MRI is performed on women who develop symptoms of tumour enlargement, visual field defects or both.

Breastfeeding has not been associated with any growth of an underlying prolactinoma. Resolution of hyperprolactinaemia and regression of the prolactinoma have been reported following the pregnancy. Idiopathic hyperprolactinaemia is even more likely to resolve following pregnancy.

### SHEEHAN SYNDROME

Severe haemorrhage, shock or hypotension at delivery may lead to postpartum pituitary necrosis or Sheehan syndrome. The syndrome is now fortunately uncommon owing to improved obstetric practice. The pathogenesis of Sheehan syndrome is still not completely clear. During pregnancy, there is an approximately 50% increase in the volume of the pituitary gland. A sudden fall in blood pressure after an event such as a postpartum haemorrhage causes ischaemia of the gland, cellular damage and oedema. In turn, the oedema results in swelling of the pituitary gland, further restricting the normal blood flow to the gland. Usually, only anterior pituitary function is affected because the posterior pituitary and hypothalamus are supplied by the inferior hypophysial artery and the circle of Willis, which makes them less vulnerable to ischaemic necrosis. Some women with Sheehan syndrome have an impairment of AVP secretion that may lead to partial or overt diabetes insipidus.

The clinical presentation of women with Sheehan syndrome is highly variable. Following destruction of 95–99% of the anterior pituitary gland, the disease is characterised by postpartum failure of lactation, secondary amenorrhoea, loss of axillary and pubic hair, genital and breast atrophy, increasing signs of secondary hypothyroidism and adrenocortical insufficiency. Less extensive pituitary destruction (50–95%) is associated with an atypical form of the disease with loss of one or more hormones. The pattern of loss of trophic hormones is unpredictable but the invariable result is hypothyroidism (owing to impaired TSH secretion) and hypoadrenalism (owing to impaired ACTH secretion). In some instances, gonadotrophin secretion may be preserved and a subsequent pregnancy is possible. Spontaneous recovery from hypopituitarism caused by postpartum haemorrhage has also been reported.

## Premature ovarian failure

Menopause is defined by the last menstrual period and marks the end of a woman's reproductive phase. The average age of menopause is reported to be approximately 51 years. Ovarian failure is diagnosed when sex steroid deficiency, elevated gonadotrophins and amenorrhoea occur. Premature ovarian failure (POF) is diagnosed statistically when ovarian failure occurs at an age that is more than two standard deviations below the mean age at menopause estimated for a reference population or, more arbitrarily, below the age of 40 years.

POF can occur before or after the onset of menarche and affects 1% of women under the age of 40 years and 0.1% under the age of 30 years. The prevalence of POF varies by ethnicity, with women of oriental origin having a lower risk and black women having a higher risk than white women. POF is diagnosed in 10–28% of women with primary amenorrhoea and in 4–18% of those with secondary amenorrhoea.

POF results from either a dysfunction or a depletion of the ovarian follicles. In contrast to normal menopause, 50% of the women with POF have intermittent ovarian function up to 15 years after the onset of POF. Pregnancies have been documented in those diagnosed with POF even in the absence of follicles on ovarian biopsy.

### CAUSES OF PREMATURE OVARIAN FAILURE

In the majority of women with POF, no aetiological factor can be identified. A small initial follicle pool and/or inappropriate luteinisation of graafian follicles have been suggested as causes of spontaneous POF. Other potential causes include:

- chromosomal and genetic abnormalities involving the X chromosome or autosomes

- autoimmune ovarian damage with positive antiovarian antibodies
- iatrogenic disease following pelvic surgery, radiotherapy or chemotherapy
- environmental factors such as viral infections or toxins, for which no clear mechanism is known.

## CLINICAL PRESENTATION

The clinical presentation of POF is variable. Rarely, POF presents as primary amenorrhoea with variable degrees of development of secondary sexual characters. More commonly, POF presents as secondary amenorrhoea. Some women present with symptoms of estrogen deficiency or menstrual disturbance, others present as part of a work-up for infertility and some as part of a syndromic condition, which can be genetic or autoimmune. Women with chromosomal defects commonly present with primary amenorrhoea and absent secondary sex characteristics. Those with mosaicism may have some functioning gonadal tissue. Various degrees of sexual development and transient menstruation may therefore be present.

There are no specific warning signs of approaching POF. Approximately 50% of women with POF have a history of oligomenorrhoea or dysfunctional uterine bleeding, which has been termed prodromal POF. In 25% of affected women, acute onset of amenorrhoea has been associated with pregnancy and delivery or with discontinuation of the oral contraceptive pill. Vasomotor symptoms are only present in women with secondary amenorrhoea and may become apparent while the woman is still having regular periods, suggesting prodromal POF.

In general, women with POF have normal fertility before the disorder starts to develop. A decline in fertility owing to resistant ovaries or an increase in the level of FSH may be a sign of developing POF.

Women with POF are at high risk of developing a variety of health problems and therefore have nearly twice the age-specific mortality risk. Sex steroid deficiency in young women with POF occurs for longer periods than it does in naturally menopausal women. This results in a significantly increased risk of osteoporosis, which is particularly high in those who have developed POF before achieving peak adult bone mass. Two-thirds of women with normal karyotype and POF have a bone mineral density one standard deviation below the mean for women of a similar age despite having taken standard hormonal therapy. This translates to a 2.6-fold increased risk of hip fracture.

The risk of cardiovascular disease in women with POF is also significantly increased. A significantly increased mortality owing to coronary heart disease, stroke, cancer and other causes has been documented (age-adjusted odds ratio of death: 1.29, 3.07, 1.83 and 2.14, respectively).

## AUTOIMMUNE PREMATURE OVARIAN FAILURE

Autoimmune mechanisms may be involved in the pathogenesis of POF in up to 30% of affected women. Autoimmune oophoritis is an important cause (10–30%) of reversible POF. It could be mediated either humorally or cellularly. Antibodies against steroidogenic enzymes (for example 3-hydroxy steroid dehydrogenase), gonadotrophins and their receptors, the corpus luteum, the zona pellucida and the oocyte have been indentified but their specificity for the disease is unknown.

Autoimmune lymphocytic oophoritis is commonly associated with an increased activity of peripheral T lymphocytes and may be isolated or associated with other endocrine or nonendocrine disorders, such as Addison's disease, diabetes mellitus, myasthenia gravis, systemic lupus erythematosus, rheumatoid arthritis and autoimmune hypothyroidism. Lymphocytic infiltration may also be present in the ovarian hilum, with an accumulation of lymphocytes around neural tissue. Forty percent of women with POF can be positive for at least one organ-specific autoantibody, the most common being antithyroid antibodies (found in about 20% of women with POF).

POF accounts for 25% of young women presenting with amenorrhoea. Some 5–30% of women with POF have another affected female relative. In these women, the mode of inheritance could be X-linked or autosomal, dominant or recessive. The causal mutation tends to be unknown.

Chromosomal and genetic abnormalities associated with POF include Turner syndrome (45,X), triple X syndrome, fragile X syndrome and fragile X premutation. Other causes include Swyer syndrome (pure gonadal dysgenesis with an XY chromosomal constitution), blepharophimosis, Perrault syndrome, Down syndrome and infections such as oophoritis following mumps, malaria, varicella and *Shigella* infections.

## DIAGNOSIS

The diagnosis of POF is based on the finding of elevated serum FSH concentrations (40 iu/l) on at least two occasions separated by a few weeks. The reason for two samples is that the natural history of POF can be very variable. In many women, the condition follows an unpredictable course of relapse and remission, often given the label fluctuating ovarian function. A pregnancy rate of approximately 1–5% has been reported in women with POF.

Ovarian biopsy adds little to the investigative process because the small samples obtained are not predictive of the natural history of the condition. Pelvic ultrasound is not predictive but may help to define those who may be candidates for oocyte preservation. An autoimmune screen for thyroid and adrenal autoantibodies may be helpful for future surveillance of other autoimmune problems.

A good family history can help to identify other affected members in as many as 30% of women with POF. Genetic screening is increasingly being used in women with a family history of POF but it can also be used in sporadic POF with a high index of suspicion of a genetic disorder. For example, fragile X premutations occur in 15% of women with POF who have a positive family history of POF and in 3% of sporadic presentations. Karyotype and fragile X premutation screening should be considered in persons with a family history or unusually young onset.

## MANAGEMENT

Management of POF will not be discussed in detail but has three main components: medical treatment, fertility advice and psychological support. The major medical issues are quality of life and bone protection. These issues can be addressed by prescribing hormone replacement therapy. Options for addressing infertility include oocyte donation and adoption. Psychological treatment requires personal and emotional support to deal with the impact of the diagnosis on a woman's health and relationships. Long-term follow-up is essential to monitor hormone replacement therapy and to allow surveillance for any emerging associated autoimmune pathology.

# CHAPTER 17

# Adrenal and thyroid glands and the pancreas

*Gul Bano*

## Adrenal gland

### PHYSIOLOGY OF THE ADRENAL CORTEX

#### Steroid synthesis

The adrenal cortex secretes three classes of steroid hormones:

- glucocorticoids – mainly cortisol, secreted by the zona fasciculata
- androgens – mainly dehydroepiandrosterone (DHEA), secreted by the zona reticularis
- mineralocorticoids – mainly aldosterone, secreted by the zona glomerulosa.

Details on the adrenocortical synthesis of steroid hormones are provided in Chapter 6.

#### Control of hormone synthesis

##### Glucocorticoids and androgens

The synthesis of glucocorticoids and androgens is regulated by the hypothalamo–pituitary axis (Figure 17.1).

Cells in the paraventricular nucleus of the hypothalamus secrete corticotrophin-releasing hormone (CRH). Released from nerve terminals in the median eminence, this 41-amino-acid peptide is transported in the hypophysial portal capillaries to the anterior pituitary corticotrophs to stimulate both the synthesis and the release of adrenocorticotrophin (ACTH).

ACTH is derived from a large precursor molecule, pro-opiomelanocortin (POMC), which is cleaved by the action of specific peptidase enzymes. Cleavage of the prohormone POMC can give rise to a number of hormones, including opioid peptides and melanocyte-stimulating hormone, but the main product of POMC cleavage in the corticotroph cells is ACTH. (In the brain, other products predominate.)

The main role of ACTH is to stimulate the synthesis and release of glucocorticoids and androgens from the adrenal cortex via a G-protein-coupled receptor. The immediate actions of ACTH in terms of steroid synthesis are:

- increase in the activity of cholesterol esterase
- transport of cholesterol into the mitochondria
- binding of cholesterol to the cholesterol side chain cleavage enzyme (CYP11A1).

This all leads to the induction of steroidogenic enzymes and to specific structural changes such as hypervascularisation, cellular hypertrophy and hyperplasia.

The action of CRH on pituitary corticotrophs is potentiated by stress and trauma and by arginine vasopressin (AVP), formally known as antidiuretic hormone. AVP is secreted by parvocellular (small) neurosecretory cells into the hypophysial portal capillaries and by magnocellular (large) neurosecretory cells into the general circulation (see Chapter 16).

The production of glucocorticoids is controlled by a classic negative feedback loop in which neurons in the hypothalamus detect circulating concentrations of glu-

FIGURE 17.1 **Hypothalamo–pituitary–adrenal axis and control of cortisol secretion**

ACTH = adrenocorticotrophin | AVP = arginine vasopressin | CRH = corticotrophin-releasing hormone | MB = mamillary bodies | OC = optic chiasm | PVN = paraventricular nucleus | SO = supraoptic nucleus | MB = mamillary bodies | OC = optic chiasm | + = stimulatory effects | – = inhibitory effects |

*Adapted with permission from*: Nussey S, Whitehead SA. *Endocrinology: An Intergrated Approach.* Oxford: BIOS Scientific Publishers; 2001.

cocorticoids and consequently stimulate or inhibit the release of CRH and AVP from the parvocellular neurons (Figure 17.1). The secretion of AVP by the magnocellular neurons is controlled by different stimuli, namely serum osmolality and blood volume.

In normal situations, CRH, ACTH and cortisol secretory rates demonstrate a circadian rhythm, with a peak in the early morning and a nadir in the evening. The negative feedback effect of cortisol on the anterior pituitary and the hypothalamus helps to control these increases and to regulate plasma cortisol concentrations.

As ACTH also stimulates the release of androgens by the adrenal gland, the secretion of these hormones parallels that of cortisol.

It should be noted that CRH is also produced in the placenta along with the binding protein CRH-BP. In this organ, CRH/CRH-BP are thought to play a role in the initiation of parturition. CRH synthesis and CRH receptors have also been identified in immune cells, where CRH has both anti-inflammatory and proinflammatory effects.

### Mineralocorticoids

The secretion of aldosterone is regulated by a number of factors, the most important of which involve the renin–angiotensin system and changes in the plasma $K^+$ concentration (Figure 17.2).

Renin, secreted by the granular cells (also called juxtaglomerular cells) of the afferent arterioles at the juxtaglomerular apparatus, is an enzyme that converts angiotensinogen (produced in the liver) to angiotensin I. In the lung, angiotensin-converting enzyme (ACE) converts angiotensin I to angiotensin II, a potent vasoconstrictor and stimulator of aldosterone release by the adrenal gland.

### *Actions of adrenocortical steroids*

### Glucocorticoids

Cortisol has many effects on the body:

- It stimulates gluconeogenesis, the overall result being an increase in serum glucose concentrations.
- It has a catabolic effect, decreasing protein stores in the body.
- It has clinically significant anti-inflammatory effects (for which it is used extensively therapeutically).
- It can adversely affect immunity (eosinophil and lymphocyte counts in the blood decrease with atrophy of lymphoid tissue).

### Adrenal androgens

The adrenal cortex continually secretes several male sex hormones, including DHEA and its sulphate (DHEAS), androstenedione and 11-hydroxyandrostenedione, as well as small quantities of the female sex hormones progesterone and estrogen. All have weak effects, but in boys they probably have a role in the early develop-

FIGURE 17.2  **Control of aldosterone secretion**

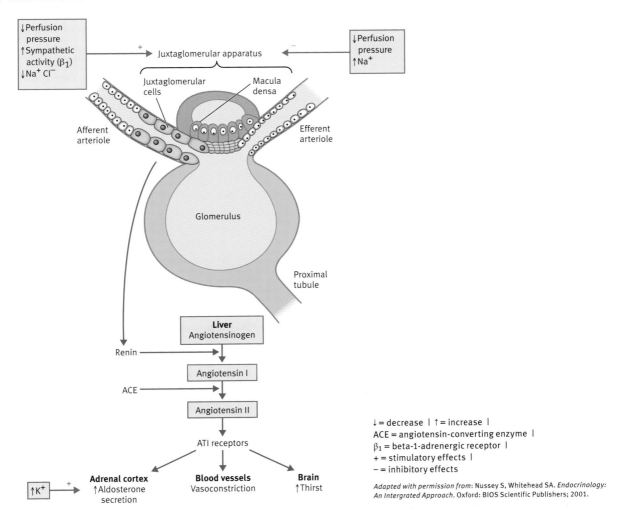

↓ = decrease  |  ↑ = increase  |
ACE = angiotensin-converting enzyme  |
$\beta_1$ = beta-1-adrenergic receptor  |
+ = stimulatory effects  |
− = inhibitory effects

*Adapted with permission from:* Nussey S, Whitehead SA. *Endocrinology: An Intergrated Approach.* Oxford: BIOS Scientific Publishers; 2001.

ment of the male sex organs and in girls they have an important role during puberty and menarche. Most androgenic effects result from extra-adrenal conversion of the androgens to testosterone (see Chapter 6).

### Mineralocorticoids

Aldosterone accounts for 90% of mineralocorticoid activity. This hormone promotes $Na^+$ reabsorption and $K^+$ excretion by the renal tubular epithelial cells of the collecting and distal tubules. As $Na^+$ is reabsorbed, $H_2O$ follows passively, leading to an increase in the extracellular fluid volume with little change in the plasma $Na^+$ concentration. Persistently elevated extracellular fluid

volumes cause hypertension. Without aldosterone, the kidney loses excessive amounts of $Na^+$ and consequently $H_2O$, leading to fluid depletion.

### Steroid transport and metabolism

Cortisol binds to proteins in the blood, mainly cortisol-binding globulin (also called transcortin). More than 90% of cortisol is transported in the blood in this bound form. Only 50% of aldosterone is bound to protein in the blood.

All adrenocortical steroids are degraded in the liver and conjugated predominantly to glucuronides, with lower amounts of sulphates formed. About 75% of these degradation products are excreted in the urine and the rest is excreted in the stool by means of bile.

## PHYSIOLOGY OF THE ADRENAL MEDULLA

### Catecholamine synthesis and secretion

The adrenal medulla constitutes less that 20% of the adrenal gland and the cells are polygonal and arranged in cords. The medulla receives blood either directly from the medullary arterioles or from the cortical venules, which are rich in cortisol and drain centripetally to the medullary venules. Epinephrine and smaller amounts of norepinephrine are synthesised by, and secreted from, the chromaffin cells of the medulla, in response to stimulation of preganglionic (cholinergic) sympathetic nerves that originate in the thoracolumbar lateral grey matter of the spinal cord. Chromaffin cells are so named because of their affinity for chromium salts, which leads to characteristic staining. As modified postganglionic nerve cells, they are classic neurosecretory cells (that is, neurons releasing hormones into the general circulation).

Like melatonin and thyroid hormones, the catecholamines are synthesised from tyrosine but, in contrast to thyroid hormones, they are made from single tyrosine molecules. These in turn are either synthesised from phenylalanine or imported from the circulation. The rate-limiting step in the synthesis of catecholamines is that catalysed by tyrosine hydroxylase, converting tyrosine to 3,4-dihydroxyphenylalanine (DOPA). The enzyme aromatic-L-amino-acid decarboxylase converts DOPA to dopamine. Hydroxylation of dopamine by dopamine β-hydroxylase leads to the formation of norepinephrine. In some adrenal medullary cells, the synthetic process stops at norepinephrine, but in most cells (particularly those at the corticomedullary junction) norepinephrine is converted to epinephrine by phenylethanolamine N-methyltransferase.

The output of the adrenal gland is controlled from nerve cells within the posterior hypothalamus, which can ultimately stimulate acetylcholine release from preganglionic nerve terminals. This induces depolarisation of the chromaffin cells and exocytosis of the catecholamine-containing granules following a transient rise in intracellular $Ca^{2+}$ concentration. Once secreted, catecholamines have a very short half-life in the circulation (approximately 1–2 minutes).

### Actions and metabolism of catecholamines

Catecholamines act on their target tissues through typical G-protein-linked membrane receptors. These receptors are classified as alpha-adrenergic or beta-adrenergic receptors on the basis of the physiological and pharmacological effects induced by hormone binding.

The physiological effects of the catecholamines are manifold and summarised in Table 17.1. They have been characterised as preparing us for 'fight or flight', with overall actions comprising an increase in heart rate and stroke volume, an increase in blood pressure, a dilatation of the bronchi, the mobilisation of glucose and the stimulation of lipolysis. These actions are mediated by beta-adrenergic receptors. Blood flow to the splanchnic bed is reduced by vasoconstriction of arterioles. This effect is mediated by alpha-adrenergic receptors and helps to divert blood flow to skeletal muscles.

While most catecholamines released from sympathetic nerves are taken back up into the presynaptic terminal (termed uptake 1), catecholamines released into the circulation are taken up by non-neuronal tissues (uptake 2) and are rapidly converted to deaminated products by monoamine oxidase (MAO) or to O-methylated products by catechol O-methyltransferase. The latter enzyme also catalyses the m-O-methylation of the products of MAO action (metanephrine, normetanephrine, epinephrine and vanillylmandelic acid). These may then be conjugated with glucuronide or sulphate and excreted in the urine.

## DISEASES OF THE ADRENAL GLAND

### Cushing syndrome

The term Cushing syndrome is used for an excess of glucocorticoids, however produced. The term Cushing's disease is used when the excess of glucocorticoids is attributable to an ACTH-secreting pituitary tumour. When Cushing syndrome is caused by ectopic ACTH secretion (for example secretion by a lung tumour), the clinical features may not be typical of classic disease and include hypokalaemia and metabolic alkalosis.

The clinical features of Cushing syndrome are given in Table 17.2 and the causes in Table 17.3. When the cause

TABLE 17.1 **Effects of catecholamines**

| Body system | Effect | Mediator of the effect |
|---|---|---|
| Cardiovascular | Increase in heart rate and force | $\beta_1$-receptors |
| | Increase in venous return | $\alpha$-receptors |
| | Increase in peripheral resistance | $\alpha$-receptors, especially those in the subcutaneous, mucosal, splanchnic and renal vascular beds |
| Autonomic nervous | Smooth muscle relaxation | $\beta_2$-receptors |
| | Smooth muscle contraction | $\alpha$-receptors |
| | Modulation of fluid and electrolyte transport in the gut, kidney and gall bladder | $\alpha$-receptors |
| Fuel metabolism | Glycogenolysis, lipolysis | $\beta$-receptors |
| | Increase in diet-induced and nonshivering thermogenesis | $\beta$-receptors |
| Fluid and electrolyte balance | Decrease in $Na^+$ excretion and glomerular filtration | Direct effects on the kidney |
| | Increase in aldosterone production resulting in enhanced $Na^+$ retention in the distal tubule | $\beta$-receptor-mediated effects on renin secretion |
| | Increase in serum $K^+$ levels | $\alpha$-receptor-mediated effects on the liver |
| | Decrease in serum $K^+$ levels | $\beta_2$-receptor-mediated effects on muscle |
| Endocrine | Modulation of the renin–angiotensin–aldosterone system | $\beta_1$-receptors |
| | Increase in the secretion of glucagon and insulin | $\beta_2$-receptors |
| | Inhibition of the carbachol-stimulated synthesis of catecholamines | $\alpha_2$-receptors |

*Adapted with permission from: Nussey S, Whitehead SA. Endocrinology: An Intergrated Approach. Oxford: BIOS Scientific Publishers; 2001.*

is a pituitary tumour, clinical features associated with the loss of other pituitary hormones may also be apparent. These include hypothyroidism, hypogonadism and growth hormone deficiency.

**Diagnosis**

Screening tests for Cushing syndrome include:

- measurement of 24-hour urinary levels of free cortisol
- measurement of midnight levels of salivary cortisol
- low-dose dexamethasone suppression test.

The latter may be combined with the CRH test to differentiate between pseudo-Cushing caused by obesity, alcoholism or depression, pituitary Cushing due to ACTH excess and Cushing syndrome caused by primary adre-

nal disease or ectopic ACTH production (Table 17.4).

When investigating solid lesions of the adrenal gland, unenhanced or delayed contrast-enhanced computed tomography (CT) may help in distinguishing benign from malignant lesions by their attenuation. Benign lesions tend to have decreased attenuation because of an increased fat content. Magnetic resonance imaging (MRI) is also useful and its main benefit over CT is its improved ability, with gadolinium enhancement or with chemical shift imaging, to help in differentiating benign from malignant lesions.

Ultrasonography is often the first imaging study performed in children who are suspected to have an ACTH-secreting adrenocortical tumour. It can differentiate cystic from solid adrenal masses and is useful to assess for vascular involvement and liver metastases. Radioiso-

TABLE 17.2 **Clinical features of Cushing syndrome**

| Overall frequency | Clinical feature (prevalence among those with Cushing syndrome) |
|---|---|
| Common | Moon face (with plethora) (100%) |
| | Weight gain, central obesity (100%) |
| | Hypertension (80%) |
| | Mental changes (80%) |
| | Impaired glucose tolerance/diabetes mellitus (70%) |
| | Hypogonadism [a] (70%) |
| | Hirsutism in women (70%) |
| | Purple striae (60%) |
| | Acne (60%) |
| | Osteopenia/osteoporosis (50%) |
| | Easy bruising (50%) |
| | Proximal myopathy (50%) |
| Less common | Poor wound healing (30%) |
| | Polycythaemia (10%) |
| | Renal stones (10%) |
| | Headache (10%) |
| | Exophthalmos (10%) |

[a] Menstrual irregularity/infertility in women, loss of libido in men

*Adapted with permission from*: Nussey S, Whitehead SA. *Endocrinology: An Intergrated Approach.* Oxford: BIOS Scientific Publishers; 2001.

tope scanning is now rarely used.

For lesions of the pituitary gland, MRI is the imaging modality of choice. Visual field examination most often reveals bitemporal hemianopia if a large pituitary tumour is present.

**Treatment**

The definitive treatment for Cushing syndrome is surgery. This includes transphenoidal surgery for pituitary disease and adrenalectomy (either laparoscopic or conventional) for adrenal disease.

Medical management includes supportive treatment for hypokalaemia with $K^+$-sparing diuretics and $K^+$ supplements.

TABLE 17.3 **Causes of Cushing syndrome**

| Overall frequency | Cause |
|---|---|
| Common (~99%) | Exogenous therapeutic glucocorticoids |
| Uncommon (<1%) | Anterior pituitary adenoma |
| | Ectopic ACTH production |
| | Adrenal adenoma |
| Rare (<0.01%) | Adrenal carcinoma |
| | Ectopic CRH production |
| | Alcoholism |
| | Bilateral multinodular hyperplasia |

ACTH = adrenocorticotrophin | CRH = corticotrophin-releasing hormone

*Adapted with permission from:* Nussey S, Whitehead SA. *Endocrinology: An Intergrated Approach.* Oxford: BIOS Scientific Publishers; 2001.

### Primary aldosteronism

An excess of mineralocorticoid steroids results in $Na^+$ retention in the kidney with loss of $K^+$. $Na^+$ retention promotes $H_2O$ retention and expansion in the extracellular volume, resulting in hypertension and a suppression of renin production. This condition is also called Conn syndrome. It accounts for up to 2% of the total incidence of hypertension in the general population. The causes include:

- adrenal adenoma (accounting for 80% of the total incidence)
  - solitary adenoma (65–70%)
  - multiple adenomas (13%)
  - microadenomatosis (6%)
- adrenal gland hyperplasia (20%)
- adrenal carcinoma (less than 1%).

**Diagnosis**

The diagnosis is made from the classic biochemical findings of hypokalaemia and metabolic alkalosis associated with hyperaldosteronism.

**Treatment**

In 75–90% of people with a solitary aldosterone-producing tumour, surgical adrenalectomy corrects hypertension and hypokalaemia. Surgery should be avoided in bilateral

TABLE 17.4 **Combined dexamethasone and corticotrophin-releasing hormone test**

| Condition | Cortisol level at baseline | ACTH level at baseline | Cortisol and ACTH levels after dex administration | Cortisol and ACTH levels after CRH administration | Ratio of ACTH precursors to ACTH |
|---|---|---|---|---|---|
| Pseudo-Cushing | Normal or high | Normal or high | Both suppressed | No response | Normal |
| Pituitary Cushing | High or normal | High | Incomplete suppression | Increase by ≥40% in both | Normal |
| Adrenal adenoma | High | Normal or low | No suppression | No change | Normal |
| Ectopic ACTH secretion | High | High | No suppression | No change | High |

ACTH = adrenocorticotrophin  |  CRH = corticotrophin-releasing hormone  |  dex = dexamethasone

hyperplasia. As a result, it is important to distinguish the two and, as with Cushing syndrome, CT or MRI scans are the best modalities to localise a tumour or establish bilateral adrenal hyperplasia. If hyperplasia is present, the aldosterone antagonist spironolactone is used to correct hypokalaemia and treat hypertension.

### Phaeochromocytoma

A phaeochromocytoma is a rare catecholamine-secreting tumour of the sympathetic nervous system. The majority (90%) of such tumours arise from adrenal sites, whereas 10% occur elsewhere in the sympathetic chain. Tumours that arise outside the adrenal gland are termed extra-adrenal phaeochromocytomas or paragangliomas.

Most tumours release both epinephrine and norepinephrine but large and extra-adrenal tumours produce almost entirely norepinephrine. Excessive catecholamine secretion from phaeochromocytomas may precipitate life-threatening hypertension or cardiac arrhythmias.

### Diagnosis

The diagnosis of phaeochromocytoma is made using assays of 24-hour urinary metanephrines and catecholamines. Localisation of the lesion is usually made with the help of CT or MRI scanning.

It is important to note the family history because, although phaeochromocytomas may occur sporadically, a number of germline mutations have been identified to be responsible for familial forms of phaeochromocytoma.

TABLE 17.5 **Causes of hypoadrenalism**

| Overall frequency | Type of hypoadrenalism | Cause |
|---|---|---|
| Common (>99%) | Primary hypoadrenalism (Addison's disease) | Abrupt cessation of exogenous sources of glucocorticoids |
| Rare (<1%) | Primary hypoadrenalism (Addison's disease) | Autoimmunity |
| | | Infection (e.g. tuberculosis or fungal infections) |
| | | Haemorrhage |
| | | Metastases |
| | | Drugs (e.g. etomidate, ketoconazole, metyrapone) |
| | Secondary hypoadrenalism | Any pituitary disease causing hypopituitarism |
| | Tertiary hypoadrenalism | Any hypothalamic disease causing hypopituitarism |

Adapted with permission from: Nussey S, Whitehead SA. *Endocrinology: An Intergrated Approach.* Oxford: BIOS Scientific Publishers; 2001.

### Treatment

The only form of curative therapy is complete surgical removal of the tumour after initial medical treatment. Preoperative medical treatment is required to reduce the risk of acute catecholamine release in response to anaesthetic drugs and surgical handling. The usual preoperative treatment is initially with alpha-adrenergic blockade followed by a combination of alpha-adrenergic and beta-adrenergic blockade.

### *Hypoadrenalism*

This condition can occur as a result of primary adrenal insufficiency (also termed Addison's disease) but it can also be secondary to pituitary damage and results in deficient production of hormones by the adrenal cortex. The causes are summarised in Table 17.5.

In autoimmune Addison's disease, the autoimmune destruction of the adrenal glands may be isolated or part of multiorgan involvement. There are two types of autoimmune polyendocrinopathy. Autoimmune polyendocrinopathy syndrome (APS) type 1 is also known as autoimmune polyendocrinopathy, candidiasis and ectodermal dystrophy (APECED) syndrome. APS type 1 occurs in association with autoimmune hypopara-thyroidism, chronic mucocutaneous candidiasis and other organ-specific autoimmune disorders. It is a monogenic autoimmune disorder and has autosomal recessive inheritance.

APS type 2 (Schmidt syndrome) is the association of autoimmune Addison's disease with autoimmune thyroid disease and/or type 1 diabetes. APS type 2 has a predilection for women in middle age and the average age of onset is between 35 and 40 years. The genetic basis of isolated autoimmune Addison's disease and APS type 2 is not clearly understood. Other autoimmune disorders can be associated with APS type 2 and these include primary gonadal failure, pernicious anaemia, vitiligo and alopecia. Antibodies to the adrenal cortex mediate autoimmune destruction of the adrenal glands.

The clinical features of Addison's disease are given in Table 17.6. High concentrations of ACTH result in buccal pigmentation and pigmentation of scars and palmar creases.

### Diagnosis

The diagnosis of hypoadrenalism may be suspected from evidence in routine biochemical tests of hyponatraemia, hyperkalaemia and hypercalcaemia. Biochemical confirmation may be made using a tetracosactrin test. Tetracosactrin is a peptide identical to the 24 amino-terminal amino acids of ACTH. ACTH and cortisol are measured in peripheral venous blood before a single injection of 250 micrograms of peptide and cortisol is assayed again 30 minutes thereafter. If the cortisol response is impaired and the baseline ACTH level is high, the diagnosis is primary adrenal failure. If the baseline ACTH level is low, the diagnosis is secondary adrenal failure. Stimulation of the adrenal gland in primary disease will not result in the release of cortisol. In secondary insufficiency, the atrophic adrenal glands still produce some cortisol when exposed to ACTH and the serum cortisol level rises to more than 1000 nmol/l.

Imaging studies can be useful in helping to elucidate the cause of hypoadrenalism. Both CT and MRI demonstrate a reduced adrenal gland size in people with autoimmune destruction and an enlarged adrenal gland in people with infection such as tuberculosis. MRI is superior to CT in differentiating adrenal masses but MRI cannot distinguish a tumour from an inflammatory process.

TABLE 17.6 **Clinical features of Addison's disease**

| Overall frequency | Clinical feature (prevalence among those with Addison's disease) |
|---|---|
| Common | Weakness (100%) |
| | Weight loss (95%) |
| | Pigmentation (95%) |
| | Anorexia (95%) |
| | Nausea (95%) |
| Less common | Abdominal pain (30%) |
| | Postural hypotension (25%) |
| | Vitiligo (20%) |
| | Salt craving (15%) |
| | Aches and pains (10%) |
| | Hypoglycaemia (in adults <1%) |

*Adapted with permission from*: Nussey S, Whitehead SA. *Endocrinology: An Intergrated Approach*. Oxford: BIOS Scientific Publishers; 2001.

## Treatment

Treatment of acute adrenal insufficiency requires immediate intravenous administration of 100 mg hydrocortisone followed by administration of 100–200 mg hydrocortisone over 24 hours as well as continuous infusion of large volumes of physiological saline solution, all under close monitoring. Individuals with adrenal insufficiency who require long-term replacement usually receive two or three daily doses of hydrocortisone. An extra dose of hydrocortisone may be required before strenuous exercise and doses are usually doubled for intercurrent illness.

The standard mineralocorticoid replacement is fludrocortisone acetate at 100–150 micrograms/day. The dose of fludrocortisone acetate is titrated individually on the basis of the clinical examination (mainly the body weight and arterial blood pressure) and the levels of plasma renin activity.

In women, the adrenal cortex is the primary source of androgen in the form of DHEA and DHEAS. Although the physiological role of these androgens in women has not been fully elucidated, their replacement is being increasingly considered in the treatment of adrenal insufficiency.

## Thyroid gland

### PHYSIOLOGY OF THE THYROID GLAND

The thyroid gland synthesises and secretes three hormones:

- follicular cells produce thyroxine ($T_4$) and triiodothyronine ($T_3$)
- C cells produce calcitonin.

The discussions in this chapter focus on the hormones produced by the follicular cells (referred to as thyroid hormones). For further information on calcitonin see Chapter 8.

### *Synthesis of thyroid hormones*

#### Iodine uptake

Iodine is an indispensable component of the follicular cell hormones $T_3$ and $T_4$. Ingested iodine is absorbed through the small intestine and transported in the plasma to the thyroid, where it is concentrated. Iodide uptake by thyroid cells is dependent on membrane ATPase. The protein responsible for iodide transport is the $Na^+$–iodide symporter. Passive transport occurs across the apical plasma membrane. The $Na^+$–iodide symporter is sensitive to iodine availability and stimulation by thyroid-stimulating hormone (TSH, also called thyrotrophin).

#### Formation of iodotyrosines and iodothyronines

After concentrating iodide, the thyroid rapidly oxidises it and binds it to tyrosyl residues in the protein thyroglobulin, followed by coupling of iodotyrosines to form $T_4$ and $T_3$. The process requires the presence of iodide, a peroxidase (thyroid peroxidase), a supply of hydrogen peroxide ($H_2O_2$) and thyroglobulin (the iodine acceptor). This process occurs at the apical plasma membrane–follicle lumen boundary. The final step in hormone synthesis is the coupling of two iodotyrosyl residues to form iodothyronine:

- two diiodotyrosines form $T_4$
- one diiodotyrosine and one monoiodotyrosine form $T_3$.

#### Hormone storage and secretion

Iodination and hormone formation of thyroglobulin results in mature hormone-containing ($T_4$ and $T_3$) molecules. These are stored in the follicular lumen, where they make up the bulk of the thyroid-follicle colloid content. When stimulated by TSH, colloid is taken up into follicular cells and lysosomal enzymes release $T_3$ and $T_4$ from thyroglobulin.

Estimates of average normal secretion for euthyroid humans are about 100 micrograms/day of $T_4$ and 20 micrograms/day of $T_3$. The thyroid may also convert some $T_4$ to reverse $T_3$.

### *Control of thyroid hormone synthesis*

TSH, released from the anterior pituitary gland, is a complex glycoprotein with a molecular weight of about 30 000 Dalton. TSH acts on G-protein-coupled transmembrane receptors on the surface of thyroid follicle cells, thereby increasing cyclic adenosine monophosphate (cAMP) and phosphatidylinositol concentrations. TSH stimulates the expression of the $Na^+$–iodide symporter, thyroid peroxidase and thyroglobulin and the generation of $H_2O_2$. TSH

### Transport and metabolism of thyroid hormones

Thyroid hormones circulate bound to plasma proteins. Approximately 70% are bound to T$_4$-binding globulin, with the rest being bound to transthyretin and albumin. Only 0.1% of T4 and 1% of T3 are unbound or free. Peripheral tissues can regulate local T$_3$ levels by increasing or decreasing T$_3$ synthesis. T$_4$ is converted to T$_3$ by deiodination. There are three main forms of deiodinase.

### Effects of thyroid hormones

Thyroid hormones have effects on virtually every cell in the body, as reflected by the wide range of clinical manifestations caused by their lack or excess. Many actions of thyroid hormones are mediated by nuclear receptors that have a preferential affinity for T$_3$. Like all steroid hormone receptors, T$_3$ receptors are members of a family of nuclear transcription factors that, in combination with other transcription factors, regulate gene expression in target cells. Unlike some steroid receptors (such as those for sex steroids and glucocorticoids), thyroid hormone receptors exist in the nucleus, not the cytoplasm, and may remain bound to DNA in the absence of hormone binding.

Thyroid hormones were once considered to be lipid-soluble and able to readily cross cell membranes. It is now recognised that there are transport mechanisms in the membrane. Once inside the nucleus, T$_3$ binds to its receptor. This dimerises with another T$_3$ receptor (to form a homodimer) or with a different receptor, notably the retinoic acid receptor, to form a heterodimer. The dimers then interact with DNA.

In most tissues (exceptions include the brain, spleen and testis), thyroid hormones stimulate the metabolic rate by increasing the number and size of mitochondria, stimulating the synthesis of enzymes in the respiratory chain and increasing membrane Na$^+$,K$^+$-ATPase concentration and membrane Na$^+$ and K$^+$ permeability. As much as 15–40% of a cell's resting energy expenditure is used to maintain its electrochemical gradient (pumping Na$^+$ out in exchange for K$^+$). Increasing the Na$^+$,K$^+$-ATPase activity therefore increases the resting metabolic rate.

---

FIGURE 17.3 **Control of thyroid hormone secretion**

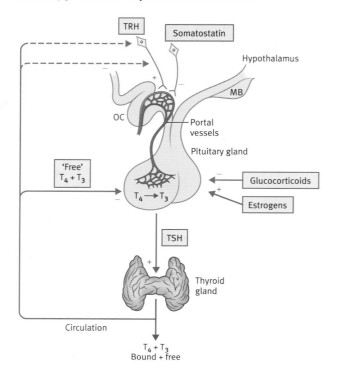

IL-1β = interleukin-1 beta | T$_3$ = triiodothyronine | T$_4$ = thyroxine | TRH = TSH-releasing hormone | TSH = thyroid-stimulating hormone | MB = mamillary bodies | OC = optic chiasm | + = stimulatory effects | − = inhibitory effects

*Adapted with permission from*: Nussey S, Whitehead SA. *Endocrinology: An Intergrated Approach.* Oxford: BIOS Scientific Publishers; 2001.

also increases the formation of T$_3$ relative to T$_4$, alters the priority of iodination and hormonogenesis among tyrosyls and promotes the rapid internalisation of thyroglobulin by thyrocytes.

TSH forms part of a negative feedback loop and its release is inhibited by increased T$_3$ and T$_4$ serum concentrations, by somatostatin and glucocorticoids and by chronic illness (Figure 17.3). The hypothalamic tripeptide thyrotrophin-releasing hormone (TRH) stimulates the release of TSH from the thyrotrophs in the anterior pituitary and upregulates transcription of the gene encoding TSH. T$_3$ receptors present in the pituitary and hypothalamus inhibit TSH release and transcription of the gene encoding the TRH prohormone. T$_3$ excess also inhibits TSH release. This negative feedback system helps to maintain serum T$_3$ concentrations.

TABLE 17.7 **Causes of hyperthyroidism**

| Cause (prevalence among those with hyperthyroidism) | Overall frequency |
|---|---|
| Graves disease[a] (80%) | Common |
| Toxic multinodular goitre (15%) | |
| Toxic adenoma ('hot' nodule) (2%) | Uncommon |
| Thyroiditis (1%) | |
| Thyrotoxicosis factitia[b] (<1%) | Rare |
| TSH-secreting pituitary tumour[c] (<0.01%) | |
| Thyroid follicular carcinoma (<0.01%) | |
| Trophoblastic tumour[d] (<0.001%) | |

[a] Autoimmune disease with stimulating antibodies to the TSH receptor | [b] excess T$_4$ ingestion to achieve weight loss and other perceived benefits associated with hyperthyroidism | [c] must be distinguished biochemically from thyroid hormone resistance, where TSH secretion is increased because of a loss of negative-feedback effects | [d] associated with increased concentrations of human chorionic gonadotrophin, which can stimulate the TSH receptor | TSH = thyroid-stimulating hormone

*Adapted with permission from:* Nussey S, Whitehead SA. *Endocrinology: An Intergrated Approach.* Oxford: BIOS Scientific Publishers; 2001.

## DISEASES OF THE THYROID GLAND

### *Hyperthyroidism*

This is defined as overactivity of the thyroid gland leading to excessive synthesis of thyroid hormones and accelerated metabolism in the peripheral tissues. The terms hyperthyroidism and thyrotoxicosis are frequently used interchangeably but the former refers to hyperfunction of the thyroid gland, while the latter refers to any state characterised by thyroid hormone excess, including ingestion of excess amounts of thyroid hormone and thyroiditis.

Hyperthyroidism is a common disorder that affects approximately 3% of women and 0.5% of men. The causes are given in Table 17.7 and it is noteworthy that they tend to be different at different ages. In young people aged 50 years or less, Graves disease is almost always the cause, whereas in elderly people toxic nodular goitre is a more common cause. The signs and symptoms of hyperthyroidism are summarised in Table 17.8.

#### Graves disease
Graves disease is an autoimmune disease that is characterised by hyperthyroidism attributable to circulating autoantibodies. In some people, Graves disease represents part of a more extensive autoimmune polyglandular syndrome.

TABLE 17.8 **Clinical features of excess thyroid hormone**

| Symptom (prevalence among those with excess thyroid hormone) | Sign (prevalence among those with excess thyroid hormone) | Overall frequency |
|---|---|---|
| Anxiety and irritability (>90%) | Tachycardia (100%) | Common |
| Palpitations (90%) | Goitre (100%) | |
| Increased perspiration and heat intolerance (90%) | Tremor (95%) | |
| Fatigability (80%) | Warm moist skin (95%) | |
| Weakness (70%) | | |
| Increased appetite and weight loss (85%) | | |
| Dyspnoea (65%) | Atrial fibrillation (10%) | Less common |
| Increased bowel frequency (30%) | 'Liver palms' (5%) | |
| Oligomenorrhoea (25%) | Heart failure (5%) | |
| Anorexia (10%) | Onycholysis (<5%) | |
| Weight gain (<5%) | | |

*Adapted with permission from:* Nussey S, Whitehead SA. *Endocrinology: An Intergrated Approach.* Oxford: BIOS Scientific Publishers; 2001.

In Graves disease, B- and T-lymphocyte-mediated autoimmunity is known to be directed at four thyroid antigens: thyroglobulin, thyroid peroxidase, the $Na^+$–iodide symporter and the TSH receptor. The TSH receptor itself is the primary autoantigen of Graves disease and is responsible for the manifestation of hyperthyroidism. The thyroid gland is under continuous stimulation by circulating autoantibodies against the TSH receptor and pituitary TSH secretion is suppressed because of the increased production of thyroid hormones. Antibodies to the $Na^+$–iodide symporter, thyroglobulin and thyroid peroxidase seem to have little role in the aetiology of hyperthyroidism in Graves disease and act as markers of autoimmune disease against the thyroid.

Graves disease is the most common cause of hyperthyroidism and affects more women than men, with hyperthyroidism due to Graves disease having a female-to-male ratio of 7–8 to 1.

Most of the clinical features of Graves disease are related to the hyperthyroid state. Clinical features that are virtually unique to Graves disease and not associated with other causes of hyperthyroidism include ophthalmopathy and dermopathy. The thyroid gland is diffusely enlarged and smooth. A bruit may be heard as a result of increased vascularity. Very rarely gynaecomastia may be present.

### Goitre

Goitre is a nonspecific term describing diffuse or nodular enlargement of the thyroid gland. The development of a goitre is independent of thyroid function. The thyroid gland becomes more nodular with increasing age. In multinodular goitre, nodules typically vary in size and most multinodular goitres are asymptomatic. Multinodular goitre can be toxic or nontoxic. Toxic multinodular goitre occurs when multiple sites of autonomous nodule hyperfunction develop, resulting in thyrotoxicosis.

### Diagnosis of hyperthyroidism

Assays have been developed to measure the serum concentrations of total $T_4$ and $T_3$, free thyroid hormone and TSH. Assays for TRH are not used. In hyperthyroidism, the concentrations of total and free $T_4$ and $T_3$ are elevated and the TSH level is suppressed as a result of negative feedback at the hypothalamus and pituitary gland.

Subclinical hyperthyroidism has been defined as the presence of free $T_4$ or $T_3$ levels within the reference range, with suppressed TSH. Subclinical hyperthyroidism can also be seen when only the levels of free $T_3$ are elevated, a syndrome known as $T_3$ toxicosis. This may be associated with toxic multinodular goitre or the ingestion of $T_3$.

Ultrasound, CT and MRI demonstrate the anatomy, size and presence of nodules within the gland. Radioactive isotope scanning and measurements of isotope uptake are useful in differentiating the causes of hyperthyroidism. In Graves disease, the uptake of radioactive iodine is increased and diffusely distributed within the entire gland. In thyroiditis and hyperthyroidism caused by excess iodine ingestion, there is poor radioactive uptake. In multinodular goitre, isotope uptake serves to define the functional characteristics of the gland and shows multifocal areas of varying activity.

### Treatment of hyperthyroidism

Treatment of hyperthyroidism involves alleviation of symptoms and correction of the thyrotoxic state. Correction of the high thyroid hormone levels can be achieved with antithyroid drugs, radioactive iodine or surgery, each of which has advantages and disadvantages. Factors to consider in determining the therapeutic modality include the age of the person to be treated, the size of the goitre and the presence of coexisting medical conditions that affect anaesthetic and operative risks.

Two types of drugs are used to inhibit thyroid hormone synthesis and release, namely thioamides and iodine (see also Table 17.9). Thioamides (such as carbimazole and propylthiouracil) inhibit thyroid hormone synthesis by competing with the tyrosyl residues of thyroglobulin for oxidised iodine, thereby inhibiting thyroid peroxidase. Propylthiouracil tends to be prescribed to pregnant and lactating women because it binds to plasma proteins and crosses the placenta or enters the breast milk in smaller amounts. It also has the added advantage of reducing the hepatic conversion of the less active $T_4$ to $T_3$.

Iodine is the fastest-acting antithyroid agent, reducing thyroid hormone synthesis within 3 days through a presumed autoregulatory mechanism.

Perchlorate also reduces thyroid hormone synthesis but this agent is no longer used routinely because it is relatively toxic with adverse effects on bone marrow.

Destruction of thyroid tissue is the alternative to drug therapy. This can be done surgically or using radioactive isotopes of iodine. Treatment with 131-iodine ($^{131}I$) is

TABLE 17.9  **Pharmacological treatment of hyperthyroidism**

| Drug | Indication | Advantages | Disadvantages/adverse effects |
|---|---|---|---|
| Thiocarbamides (e.g. carbimazole, propylthiouracil) | People with mild thyroid disease and small goitre<br><br>People with eye disease or cardiorespiratory disease<br><br>Pregnant women<br><br>Children | Cheap<br><br>Effective | Rash<br><br>Pruritus<br><br>Neutropenia<br><br>Hepatitis<br><br>Pneumonitis |
| Beta-adrenoreceptor-blocking drugs (e.g. propranolol) | Symptomatic relief (especially from cardiac symptoms)<br><br>Hyperthyroid storm | Propranolol inhibits conversion of $T_4$ to $T_3$ in the liver | Asthma<br><br>Heart failure |
| Glucocorticoids (e.g. prednisolone) | Hyperthyroid storm | Prednisolone inhibits conversion of $T_4$ to $T_3$ in the liver | Iatrogenic Cushing syndrome |
| Iodine (e.g. Lugol's solution) | Hyperthyroid storm<br><br>Before surgery to reduce blood flow | Rapid inhibition of thyroid hormone synthesis (Wolff–Chaikoff effect) | Becomes ineffective with time |
| Perchlorate | Iodine-induced hyperthyroidism | Discharge of iodide excess from thyroid gland | Rash<br><br>Gastric upset<br><br>Lymphadenopathy<br><br>Agranulocytosis<br><br>Aplastic anaemia |
| Lithium | Second-line alternative to thiocarbamides | Inhibits $T_4$ and $T_3$ release | Lithium toxicity (tremor, ataxia, coma)<br><br>Polydipsia<br><br>Polyuria |

*Adapted with permission from*: Nussey S, Whitehead SA. *Endocrinology: An Intergrated Approach*. Oxford: BIOS Scientific Publishers; 2001.

safe; many clinicians now use a fixed dose of isotope and aim to produce hypothyroidism. Once hypothyroidism is induced, the person can be treated with oral $T_4$, which is cheap, effective and easy to monitor. [131]I is also used to treat euthyroid goitres (so as to avoid surgery) and such treatment usually reduces the volume of the thyroid gland. It is contraindicated in children, pregnant women and women who are breastfeeding. Women of childbearing age should wait for at least 4 months after [131]I therapy before becoming pregnant.

Thyroid surgery is usually restricted to large and unsightly goitres that are not treatable medically or with radioactive iodine.

### Hypothyroidism

Hypothyroidism is a common endocrine disorder that results from deficiency of thyroid hormone. The causes are given in Table 17.10 and the signs and symptoms in Table 17.11. Worldwide, iodine deficiency remains the foremost cause of hypothyroidism. In areas of adequate iodine intake, autoimmune thyroid disease (Hashimoto thyroiditis) is the most common cause of hypothyroidism. The prevalence of antibodies is higher in women and increases with age. Unlike Graves disease, T-cell-mediated actions in Hashimoto thyroiditis result in thyroid gland destruction rather than stimulation.

### Chronic autoimmune thyroiditis (Hashimoto thyroiditis)

Hashimoto thyroiditis is similar to Graves disease in that it has an autoimmune aetiology and occurs with about the same incidence and with the same sex bias, peak age of presentation and family history of thyroid disease or related autoimmune diseases. It differs in being associated with cell-mediated destruction of the gland. When a goitre is present, it is the result of diffuse lymphocytic infiltration (which gives it a number of alternative names such as chronic lymphocytic thyroiditis), together with TSH-stimulated hyperplasia of surviving thyroid tissue owing to loss of feedback inhibition from the thyroid hormones.

Other features of Hashimoto thyroiditis are antibodies against thyroid peroxidase and thyroglobulin. Some people are affected by a period of hyperthyroidism, which is termed hashitoxicosis, but the degree of hyperthyroidism is usually milder than that in Graves disease.

### Diagnosis of primary hypothyroidism

In primary hypothyroidism caused by decreased function of the thyroid gland itself, the total and free concentrations of $T_4$ and $T_3$ are low and the levels of TSH are elevated as a result of negative feedback at the hypothalamus and pituitary gland.

Subclinical hypothyroidism has been defined as a free $T_4$ or free $T_3$ level within the reference range with an elevated thyrotrophin.

The presence of thyroid autoantibodies (antimicrosomal or antithyroid peroxidase antibodies) and antithyroglobulin is typical for autoimmune hypothyroidism. The occurrence of antithyroid peroxidase antibodies has been associated with a higher risk of infertility and miscarriage.

### Diagnosis of secondary hypothyroidism

Hypothyroidism can also arise because of a loss of TSH secretion from either pituitary or hypothalamic dysfunction (secondary and tertiary hypothyroidism, respectively). In these situations, TSH concentrations do not increase in appropriate relation to the low $T_4$ and $T_3$ concentrations. The absolute levels of TSH may be in the normal or even slightly elevated range but they are inappropriately low for the severity of the hypothyroid state. Hence, when secondary or tertiary hypothyroidism is suspected, measurement of serum TSH alone is inad-

TABLE 17.10  **Causes of hypothyroidism** [a]

| Type of hypothyroidism | Overall frequency | Cause |
|---|---|---|
| Primary hypothyroidism | Common (95%) | Hashimoto's disease [b] |
| | | Primary (atrophic) hypothyroidism [c] |
| | | Radioiodine therapy [d] |
| | | Surgery of the thyroid gland |
| | Uncommon (5%) | Thyroiditis (nonlymphocytic) |
| | | Genetic defect resulting in impaired $T_4$ synthesis |
| | | Antithyroid drugs |
| | Rare (<1%) | Loss-of-function mutation in the gene encoding the TSH receptor |
| | | Thyroid hormone resistance |
| Secondary (pituitary) hypothyroidism | 1% | Hypopituitarism caused by a tumour, surgery or radiotherapy |
| | | Impaired TSH synthesis |
| Tertiary (hypothalamic) hypothyroidism | <1% | Hypothalamic damage caused by a tumour, radiotherapy or trauma |

[a] In most Western countries, iodine deficiency is not a cause of hypothyroidism; it is a major cause in iodine-deficient areas  |  [b] autoimmune thyroid destruction  |  [c] probably end-stage Hashimoto disease  |  [d] destroys thyroid tissue

Adapted with permission from: Nussey S, Whitehead SA. *Endocrinology: An Intergrated Approach*. Oxford: BIOS Scientific Publishers; 2001.

equate; the level of free $T_4$ should also be determined.

### Treatment of hypothyroidism

The hypothyroidism treatment of choice is levothyroxine (synthetic $T_4$). It is chemically stable and $T_4$ is converted to $T_3$ in peripheral tissues. Measurement of TSH should be made after 6 weeks and the dose should be adjusted in increments of 25–50 micrograms.

Treatment with $T_4$ is also recommended in people with subclinical hypothyroidism who are positive for antithyroid microsomal antibodies.

Once the appropriate dose is established, it tends to remain constant except in pregnancy, when there is a need to increase the dose by at least 50 micrograms/day to maintain normal TSH concentration.

### *Altered thyroid function in nonthyroidal illness*

A number of changes can occur in the hypothalamo–pituitary–thyroid axis of people who are severely ill with a nonthyroidal disease. Most commonly, serum concentrations of TSH are normal or decreased, total $T_4$ levels are decreased and total $T_3$ levels are markedly decreased. This can be confused with secondary hypothyroidism. However, the primary abnormality is the decreased peripheral production of $T_3$ from $T_4$. There may be an increase in the level of reverse $T_3$, the magnitude of which correlates with the severity of illness. During recovery, some people have transient elevations in serum TSH concentrations (up to 20 mu/l).

Thyroid function should not be evaluated in a critically ill person unless thyroid dysfunction is strongly suspected. If so, screening with TSH measurement alone is insufficient.

### THYROID DISORDERS AND PREGNANCY

### *Changes in normal pregnancy*

During pregnancy, maternal thyroid function is modulated by three factors:

- increase in the concentration of human chorionic gonadotrophin (hCG), which stimulates the thyroid gland
- increase in urinary iodide excretion, resulting in a fall in plasma iodine concentrations
- increase in $T_4$-binding globulin during the first trimester, resulting in increased binding of $T_4$.

TABLE 17.11  **Clinical features of hypothyroidism**

| Overall frequency | Symptoms (prevalence among those with hypothyroidism) | Signs (prevalence among those with hypothyroidism) |
|---|---|---|
| Common | Fatigue (90%) | Dry, scaly skin (90%) |
| | Cold intolerance (80%) | Puffy eyes (90%) |
| | Depression (70%) | Hair loss or dryness (70%) |
| | Poor concentration (65%) | Coarse, brittle thinning hair (60%) |
| | Musculoskeletal aches and pains (25%) | Bradycardia (40%) |
| | Carpal tunnel syndrome (15%) | |
| Rare | Constipation | Anaemia |
| | Hoarse voice | Oedema |
| | Menorrhagia | Cerebellar signs [a] |
| | | Deafness [a] |
| | | Psychosis [a] |

[a] Cerebellar ataxia, deafness and myxoedema madness are commonly cited as signs of hypothyroidism but in clinical practice these signs are unusual and only seen in very severe disease

These factors are responsible for the increased demand for thyroid hormones during pregnancy. Women with hypothyroidism therefore require an increased dosage of levothyroxine during pregnancy to maintain the euthyroid state.

There is a structural similarity between hCG and TSH. Therefore, hCG possesses an intrinsic, weak thyroid-stimulating activity. In addition, homology exists between the TSH and luteinising hormone/hCG receptors. As a result, TSH levels fall predictably during the first trimester, mirroring in a reciprocal fashion the concomitant rise in hCG. The overall effect is a degree of thyroid stimulation and TSH suppression. Despite hCG-mediated stimulation of the thyroid gland, serum concentrations of free $T_4$ generally remain within, or slightly above, the normal range during the first trimester. The stimulatory effects of hCG are normally confined to the first half of gestation. In certain pathological conditions, including hyperemesis gravidarum and trophoblastic tumours, hCG concentrations may increase into a range sufficient to induce biochemical hyperthyroidism.

The maternal plasma concentration of inorganic iodine decreases as a result of increased glomerular filtration during pregnancy. The thyroid gland compensates by enlarging and increasing the plasma clearance of iodine to produce sufficient thyroid hormone so as to maintain the euthyroid state. This mechanism is responsible for an increase in thyroid size in pregnancy, particularly in iodine-deficient areas.

Serum concentrations of $T_4$-binding globulin increase in pregnancy owing to the effects of estrogen. As a result, the serum concentrations of total $T_3$ and $T_4$ are elevated between weeks 6 and 12 of gestation, stabilising by midgestation. The concentrations of free thyroid hormone remain within the normal range for nonpregnant women, although they tend to decrease by 10–15% in late pregnancy. During the first trimester, serum TSH values decrease slightly in response to elevations in hCG and its intrinsic thyroid-stimulating activity. During the remainder of a normal pregnancy, serum TSH values increase but remain well within the normal range.

There is evidence of maternal transfer of thyroid hormone to the fetus and there are fetal consequences of maternal hypothyroidism. The maternal thyroid provides all thyroid hormone necessary for fetal development until the fetal thyroid is able to produce sufficient amounts of endogenous hormone. Fetal TSH and $T_4$ are first detectable at week 10 of gestation. In a fetus at risk for thyroid dysfunction, surveillance with ultrasound may be performed, directed at detecting the presence of fetal goitre. This is of clinical relevance as fetal goitre may result in local airway compromise during delivery.

### Gestational hypothyroidism

The causes, symptoms and signs of maternal hypothyroidism are the same as those in any woman of reproductive age. The requirement for thyroid hormone replacement therapy is increased during pregnancy. If untreated, hypothyroidism worsens during pregnancy and there is increased risk of fetal loss and psychoneurological deficit in the fetus. There is no evidence for an increased risk of birth defects associated with a history of maternal hypothyroidism.

Women diagnosed with hypothyroidism in pregnancy should immediately be given full replacement doses of $T_4$ regardless of the degree of thyroid dysfunction. This will minimise further fetal exposure to the hypothyroid environment. Therapy should be titrated rapidly in young pregnant women with no other comorbid conditions. For women on thyroid hormone replacement therapy before conception, the dose of thyroid hormone commonly has to be increased by up to 50% during pregnancy. Such women will require close follow-up during pregnancy to maintain optimal thyroid hormone concentrations.

In women who have no previous history of hypothyroidism and in whom the diagnosis is made during pregnancy, thyroid hormone therapy may be discontinued during the postpartum period, with reassessment of thyroid function 5–6 weeks later. Recovery may be delayed because normal thyroid function may remain suppressed for a number of weeks after prolonged thyroid hormone therapy. Most will remain hypothyroid and will ultimately require chronic replacement therapy.

### Neonatal hypothyroidism

Neonatal hypothyroidism has a number of causes, including thyroid dysgenesis and thyroid hormone resistance. Prompt identification and treatment of newborn infants with congenital hypothyroidism is vital to ensure their appropriate neuropsychological development. Identification through screening programmes, with immediate institution of replacement therapy, leads to a normal IQ at 5–7 years of age. If left untreated, neonatal and early childhood hypothyroidism results in profound mental and developmental restriction.

### Gestational hyperthyroidism

Although menstrual irregularity is frequent in women with mild to moderate hyperthyroidism, fertility does not seem to be impaired. The effects of gestational hyperthyroidism include:

- effects on the mother (premature labour, pre-eclampsia, heart failure)
- effects on the fetus (neonatal mortality, low birth weight).

Mild to moderate thyrotoxicosis is not a contraindication to the continuation of pregnancy and pregnancy does not make thyrotoxicosis more difficult to control. Indeed, hyperthyroidism may be more easily controlled during pregnancy, although relapses tend to occur postpartum.

Treatment of hyperthyroidism during pregnancy is similar to that in nonpregnant individuals but limited to antithyroid drugs or surgery because radioactive iodine is contraindicated. Antithyroid drugs include the thioamides (propylthiouracil and carbimazole). Pregnant women tolerate mild degrees of hyperthyroidism without great difficulty and the goal of antithyroid therapy during pregnancy is to maintain the level of free $T_4$ at, or slightly above, the upper limit of the normal range.

Thioamides are transferred into the breast milk of women receiving these drugs but, overall, breastfeeding seems to be safe in mothers taking thioamides. Beta-blockers are not recommended for long-term treatment of thyrotoxicosis during pregnancy.

### Fetal thyrotoxicosis

Fetal thyrotoxicosis is usually caused by the placental transfer of thyroid-stimulating immunoglobulins. Maternal thyroid-stimulating antibodies may be present even when the maternal thyroid has been ablated or when the mother is in remission, as the antibodies can persist. Thus, the possibility of fetal thyrotoxicosis should be considered in all pregnant women with a history of Graves disease regardless of the current thyroid status.

The diagnosis is suggested by clinical features such as persistent fetal tachycardia, growth failure or increased fetal activity. There may be elevated concentrations of maternal thyroid-stimulating immunoglobulins and ultrasonography may detect the presence of a goitre in a thyrotoxic fetus. Fetal thyrotoxicosis is associated with increased fetal morbidity and mortality, so early diagnosis is crucial.

Antithyroid drug therapy directed specifically towards the fetus should be used and close monitoring is mandatory. After delivery, the baby should continue to be treated for thyrotoxicosis, which is usually self-limited.

### Thyroid nodules and their management in pregnancy

A solitary thyroid nodule during pregnancy is evaluated by ultrasound scan and fine-needle aspiration cytology. An ultrasound scan provides information about the size of the nodule and whether the nodule is solid or cystic. It is also useful in identifying the presence of diffuse thyroid disease and in revealing the presence of previously undetected, nonpalpable nodules. Fine-needle aspiration cytological assessment is indicated in:

- women with nodules that are larger than 1 cm in diameter
- women with enlarging nodules
- women who have nodules associated with palpable cervical lymph nodes.

If the biopsy specimen is adequate and does not reveal suspect cells, TSH suppression with $T_4$ may be instituted for the duration of the pregnancy. If the biopsy is suggestive of malignancy, surgery is indicated.

The diagnosis of thyroid carcinoma during pregnancy is not an absolute indication for termination of the pregnancy. Pregnancy does not have a direct effect on the natural history of thyroid carcinoma. Treatment options for thyroid carcinoma during pregnancy are more limited than in the nonpregnant state as radioactive iodine is contraindicated. Thyroid surgery remains the main option.

### Postpartum thyroiditis

This is defined as the occurrence of a period of transient thyrotoxicosis followed by transient hypothyroidism with return of the euthyroid state by 1 year postpartum. The thyrotoxicosis always predates hypothyroidism and occurs between 2 and 6 months postpartum. The hypothyroid phase can occur at any time between 3 and 12 months following delivery. Women who express antithyroid peroxidase or antithyroglobulin antibodies in the first trimester of pregnancy have a 33–50% risk of developing postpartum thyroiditis. The higher the thyroid antibody titre is, the more likely is the development of postpartum thyroiditis. Spontaneous recovery occurs in 90% of women with postpartum thyroiditis but the risk of recurrence after subsequent pregnancies is as high as 25%. In fact, there is an increased risk of developing permanent hypothyroidism, particularly in those with high titres of antithyroid peroxidase antibodies, so follow-up is recommended.

The signs and symptoms of postpartum thyroiditis are often subtle. Many of them, such as fatigue, irritability and fluctuations in weight, are common in the postpartum period. A painless small goitre is palpable in half the women with postpartum thyroiditis.

The laboratory diagnosis of thyrotoxicosis in postpartum thyroiditis is based on high levels of free $T_4$ with suppression of TSH on thyroid function tests. In contrast to Graves disease, the uptake of radioisotopes such as technetium in postpartum thyroiditis is low. Like primary hypothyroidism, the subsequent hypothyroid phase is diagnosed by an increased serum TSH concentration and a decreased serum $T_4$ concentration.

## Endocrine pancreas

### PHYSIOLOGY OF THE ENDOCRINE PANCREAS

The pancreas has both digestive and hormonal functions. The enzymes secreted by the exocrine tissue in the pancreas help to break down carbohydrates, fats, proteins and acids in the duodenum. The exocrine tissue also secretes bicarbonate to neutralise stomach acid in the duodenum. The hormones secreted by the endocrine tissue in the pancreas include insulin, glucagon, somatostatin, gastrin, vasoactive intestinal peptide (VIP) and pancreatic polypeptide.

### Insulin

Insulin is a protein with a molecular weight of about 6000 Dalton and is composed of two chains held together by disulphide bonds. The insulin mRNA is translated into a single-chain precursor protein called preproinsulin. Removal of the precursor's signal peptide during insertion into the endoplasmic reticulum generates proinsulin. Proinsulin consists of three domains: an amino-terminal B chain, a carboxy-terminal A chain and a connecting peptide in the middle known as the C peptide. Within the endoplasmic reticulum, proinsulin is exposed to several specific endopeptidases that excise the C peptide, thereby generating the mature form of insulin. When the beta cell is appropriately stimulated, insulin is secreted from the cell by exocytosis and diffuses into islet capillary blood.

Insulin is secreted after an oral glucose load. The early insulin response to glucose (at 30 minutes) is due to neuronal stimulation, whereas the late response (at 120 minutes) is primarily due to elevated blood concentrations of glucose. Glucose is transported into the beta cell by facilitated diffusion via a glucose transporter. This leads to membrane depolarisation and an influx of extracellular $Ca^{2+}$. The resulting increase in intracellular $Ca^{2+}$ is thought to be one of the primary triggers for exocytosis of insulin-containing secretory granules. Increased levels of glucose within beta cells also seem to activate $Ca^{2+}$-independent pathways that participate in insulin secretion.

The receptor for insulin is a tyrosine kinase that is embedded in the plasma membrane. It is composed of two alpha subunits and two beta subunits, which are linked by disulphide bonds.

The major targets for the anabolic actions of insulin are:

- liver
- adipose tissue
- muscle.

In the liver, insulin promotes glycogen synthesis by stimulating glycogen synthetase and inhibiting glycogen phosphorylase. Insulin induces the rapid uptake of glucose in muscle and fat tissue and as a consequence muscle converts glucose to glycogen.

In adipose tissue, glucose is converted to fatty acids for storage as triglyceride. Insulin also stimulates the uptake of amino acids into muscle. At the same time, insulin suppresses the mobilisation of fuels by inhibiting the breakdown of glycogen in the liver, the release of amino acids from muscle and the release of free fatty acids from adipose tissue. This partly explains weight loss in people with diabetes despite normal or increased appetite.

## Glucagon

Glucagon is a linear peptide of 29 amino acids that is initially synthesised as proglucagon, which is proteolytically processed within alpha cells of the pancreatic islets to yield glucagon. It is secreted in response to hypoglycaemia. Other stimuli of glucagon secretion include elevated serum concentrations of amino acids and exercise. Glucagon secretion is inhibited by high levels of blood glucose, either as a direct effect of glucose on the alpha cells or as a result of insulin secretion by the beta cells. Glucagon secretion is also inhibited by somatostatin.

Glucagon has counter-regulatory actions to insulin, promoting the mobilisation of fuels, particularly glucose. Its primary action is on the liver, where it stimulates the breakdown of glycogen to glucose and the production of glucose from amino acids (gluconeogenesis). In addition, it stimulates the release of free fatty acids from adipose tissue. Glucagon is both a hyperglycaemic and a ketogenic hormone. By and large, it is the molar ratio of insulin to glucagon in the portal blood that governs the metabolic state of the liver.

## Somatostatin

Somatostatin is secreted by a broad range of tissues, including the pancreas, the gastrointestinal tract and regions of the central nervous system outside the hypothalamus. Two forms of somatostatin are synthesised, termed somatostatin 14 and somatostatin 28 in reflection of the length of their amino acid chains. Both forms of somatostatin are generated by proteolytic cleavage of prosomatostatin. Somatostatin 14 is the predominant form produced in the nervous system, whereas the intestine secretes mostly somatostatin 28. The two forms have different biological potencies. Somatostatin 28 is nearly ten times more potent than somatostatin 14 in inhibiting the secretion of growth hormone but less potent than somatostatin 14 in inhibiting the release of glucagon.

Five somatostatin receptors have been identified, all members of the G-protein-coupled receptor superfamily. Four of the five receptors do not differentiate between somatostatin 14 and somatostatin 28.

Somatostatin acts by both endocrine and paracrine pathways to affect its target cells and inhibit the secretion of many other hormones, including growth hormone, from the pituitary gland.

In the pancreas, somatostatin seems to act primarily in a paracrine manner to inhibit the secretion of both insulin and glucagon. It also suppresses pancreatic exocrine secretions by inhibiting the cholecystokinin-stimulated secretion of enzymes and the secretin-stimulated secretion of bicarbonate.

In the gastrointestinal tract, somatostatin inhibits the secretion of many of the other gastrointestinal hormones. Moreover, somatostatin suppresses the secretion of gastric acid and pepsin, lowers the rate of gastric emptying and reduces smooth muscle contractions and blood flow within the intestine. These activities seem to have the overall effect of decreasing the rate of nutrient absorption.

## Vasoactive intestinal peptide

VIP is a peptide hormone that contains 28 amino acids and is produced in many areas of the human body, including the gut, the pancreas and the suprachiasmatic nuclei of the hypothalamus in the brain. In the digestive system, the roles of VIP are stimulation of $H_2O$ and electrolyte secretion, dilatation of peripheral blood vessels, stimulation of pancreatic bicarbonate secretion and inhibition of the gastrin-stimulated secretion of gastric acid.

VIP acts via two known VIP-specific receptors, termed VPAC1 and VPAC2.

## Gastrin

Gastrin is a linear peptide synthesised as a preprohormone that is cleaved to form a family of peptides. The predominant circulating form is gastrin-34 (big gastrin) but biological activity is present even in the smallest peptide (gastrin-14 or minigastrin). In fact, full bioactivity is preserved in the five carboxy-terminal amino acids of gastrin, known as pentagastrin.

Gastrin is synthesised in G cells, which are located in gastric pits found primarily in the antrum of the stomach. The hormone binds receptors that are found predominantly on parietal and enterochromaffin-like cells. These receptors also bind cholecystokinin and are known as gastrin/cholecystokinin type B receptors. They belong to the family of G-protein-coupled receptors.

Gastrin is a major physiological regulator of gastric acid secretion and has a growth-promoting influence on the gastric mucosa. The primary stimulus for the secretion of gastrin is the presence of certain foodstuffs (especially peptides, certain amino acids and $Ca^{2+}$) in the gastric lumen. Secretion of this hormone is inhibited when the lumenal pH of the stomach becomes very low.

## ENDOCRINE DISEASES OF THE PANCREAS

### Diabetes mellitus

The term diabetes mellitus describes a group of metabolic diseases that are characterised by hyperglycaemia resulting from defects in insulin secretion, insulin action or both. Diabetes mellitus is diagnosed on the basis of symptom history plus fulfilment of one of the following criteria:

- a random venous plasma glucose concentration of at least 11.1 mmol/l
- a fasting plasma glucose concentration of at least 7.0 mmol/l
- a plasma glucose concentration of at least 11.1 mmol/l 2 hours after administration of 75 g anhydrous glucose in an oral glucose tolerance test (OGTT).

In the absence of symptoms, the diagnosis should not be made on the basis of a single glucose estimation. At least one additional glucose test result on another day with a value in the diabetic range is essential, with the blood sample taken either randomly, after fasting or 2 hours after a glucose load. The diagnosis should never be based solely on the finding of glycosuria, a reading of capillary blood glucose or a reading of glycated haemoglobin ($HbA_{1c}$).

A normal fasting blood glucose reading is generally defined as a level below 6 mmol/l. Impaired fasting glucose is defined by values between 6.0 mmol/l and 7.0 mmol/l. Impaired glucose tolerance is recognised with serum glucose values between 7.8 mmol/l and 11.1 mmol/l 2 hours after administration of 75 g of oral glucose.

### Type 1 diabetes

Type 1 diabetes mellitus is considered to be a T-lymphocyte dependent autoimmune disease that is characterised by infiltration and destruction of the beta cells in the islets of Langerhans. Studies in twins have clearly established a major genetic element to type 1 diabetes. However, in fewer than half of instances where one twin of an identical pair has the disease, the other will develop it as well.

Currently, autoimmunity is considered to be the major factor in the pathophysiology of type 1 diabetes. The prevalence is increased in people with other autoimmune diseases, such as Graves disease, Hashimoto thyroiditis and Addison's disease. Approximately 85% of people with type 1 diabetes have circulating islet cell antibodies and the majority will have detectable anti-insulin antibodies before receiving insulin therapy. Most islet cell antibodies are directed against glutamic acid decarboxylase within pancreatic beta cells.

Environmental factors that have been hypothesised to induce an attack on beta cell function include viruses (for example mumps virus, rubella virus, Coxsackie B4 virus), toxic chemicals, cytotoxins and exposure to cow's milk in infancy.

Type 1 diabetes mellitus is predominantly a disease of white populations. It tends to develop after the age of 20 years. Overall, it occurs with equal frequency in men and women and there are increases in incidence around puberty and before starting school.

People with type 1 diabetes mellitus require insulin therapy to control hyperglycaemia. The goal of insulin treatment is to keep blood glucose levels at normal or near-normal levels. Careful control of blood glucose levels can help to prevent both the short-term effects of poorly controlled blood glucose, such as diabetic ketoacidosis, and the long-term effects, such as complications of the eye, kidney and cardiovascular system.

### Type 2 diabetes

Type 2 diabetes mellitus is characterised by:

- hyperglycaemia
- insulin resistance
- relative impairment of insulin secretion.

It is a common disorder with a prevalence that rises markedly with increasing degrees of obesity. For type 2 diabetes mellitus to develop, both insulin deficiency and defects of insulin resistance must coexist. All overweight individuals have insulin resistance but only those with an inability to increase beta cell production of insulin develop diabetes. About 90% of people who develop type 2 diabetes mellitus are obese. Relative insulin deficiency owing to damaged beta cells also results in a lack of glucagon suppression and this further contributes to hyperglycaemia. People with type 2 diabetes mellitus retain the ability to secrete some endogenous insulin and generally do not develop diabetic ketoacidosis.

Type 2 diabetes is often accompanied by other clinical features, such as hypertension and a dyslipidaemia including high serum levels of low-density lipoprotein (LDL) cholesterol and low serum levels of high-density lipoprotein (HDL) cholesterol. This constellation of clinical conditions is referred to as metabolic syndrome and is associated with an increased risk of cardiovascular disease.

### Treatment of diabetes mellitus

Diabetes is associated with serious complications that are generally divided into:

- microvascular complications (including retinopathy, nephropathy and neuropathy)
- macrovascular complications (including atherosclerotic disease of the coronary, carotid and femoral arteries).

Since the complications of diabetes are, by and large, related to the duration of the disease and the degree of blood sugar control, much effort is made to control blood glucose. A sensible approach to diet, control of body weight and exercise is therefore important in all forms of the disease. It is also important to manage dyslipidaemia and blood pressure.

Dietary modification is fundamental to the long-term treatment of all forms of diabetes mellitus. The generally recommended diet, the so-called healthy eating diet, contains more than 55% of carbohydrate, 10–15% of protein and less than 30% of fat (of which less than 10% saturates). In general, no further dietary modification is required other than to reduce sources of simple sugars (less than 25 g/day of added sucrose) and replace them with complex carbohydrates.

Glycaemic control is judged by measurement of the $HbA_{1c}$ level. An optimal $HbA_{1c}$ value for a person with diabetes lies between 6.5% and 7.0%. The majority of people with type 2 diabetes have inadequate glycaemic control. Monotherapy will fail by the end of 9 years in 75%. To achieve ideal glycaemic control in type 2 diabetes, early aggressive combination therapy is recommended, not allowing the $HbA_{1c}$ level to go above 7.8%.

Pharmacotherapy includes the use of:

- biguanides
- thiazolidinediones
- sulphonylureas
- incretins
- insulin.

The biguanide metformin reduces the release of hepatic glucose and is considered to be a first-line therapy in overweight and nonoverweight people. It reduces cardiovascular outcomes in obese individuals but can cause gastrointestinal adverse effects.

The primary mode of action of the thiazolidinediones is to improve insulin sensitivity in muscle and adipose tissue. These agents can be used as monotherapy or in combination therapy but they may be associated with modest weight gain.

Sulphonylureas work by increasing the insulin secretion from pancreatic islet cells. They are effective hypoglycaemic agents but are associated with weight gain and accelerated beta cell exhaustion.

Incretins are gut-derived factors that increase glucose-stimulated insulin secretion. There are two incretin hormones: glucagon-like peptide 1 (GLP-1) produced in the ileum and colon and gastric inhibitory peptide produced in the jejunum. GLP-1 action can be enhanced by the use of the oral dipeptidylpeptidase-4 inhibitor sitagliptin. A GLP-1 analogue called exenatide may be used by injection.

The three broad classes of insulin are defined by their duration of action (short-acting, intermediate-acting and long-acting). Most newly diagnosed persons with type 1 diabetes can be started on a total daily insulin dose of 0.2–0.4 units/kg. The majority will ultimately require 0.6–0.7 units/kg daily. Adolescents often need more, especially during puberty. About one in three people diagnosed with type 2 diabetes will require insulin at some stage.

There are two schemes for insulin treatment:

- Approximately one-half of the total dose should be given as a basal insulin. This can be either as once-per-day long-acting insulin or as twice-per-day intermediate-acting insulin (isophane). Long-acting insulin can be given either at bedtime or in the morning.
- The remainder of the total daily insulin requirement is given as short-acting or rapid-acting insulin before meals (sliding scale insulin therapy). The premeal dose is determined before each individual meal, taking into account the carbohydrate content of the meal, the blood glucose level and the activity level.

The treatment targets for diabetes are widely accepted and include a fasting blood sugar level below 7 mmol/l, an $HbA_{1c}$ value of no more than 6.5%, a systolic blood pressure below 130 mmHg, a diastolic blood pressure below 80 mmHg, a total cholesterol level below 4 mmol/l, an HDL cholesterol level above 1 mmol/l, an LDL cholesterol level below 2 mmol/l and a triglyceride level below 1.5 mmol/l.

### Endocrine tumours of the pancreas

The cells in pancreatic endocrine neoplasms are termed amine precursor uptake and decarboxylation (APUD) cells because they have a high amine content, are capable of amine precursor uptake and contain an amino acid decarboxylase. Most pancreatic endocrine neoplasms discovered clinically are functional apudomas and are named after the predominant secreted hormone. Thus, the following apudomas exist:

- insulinoma
- gastrinoma (also termed Zollinger–Ellison syndrome)
- glucagonoma
- VIPoma (Verner–Morrison syndrome)
- somatostatinoma.

The clinical features in people with functional pancreatic endocrine neoplasms reflect the physiological derangements related to the normal action of the hormonal product that the tumours overproduce.

By contrast, people with nonfunctional pancreatic endocrine neoplasms typically present later in the course of their disease, when their tumours begin to cause symptoms related to mass effect.

To a large part, investigation of pancreatic endocrine neoplasms consists of demonstrating that the concentrations of circulating hormone are inappropriate to the clinical situation.

### Treatment

Endocrine tumours of the pancreas usually grow slowly and have a relatively low metastatic potential. Definitive treatment is surgical removal. Medical treatment with somatostatin analogues may control symptoms in tumours that express somatostatin receptors. Proton pump inhibitors have a major role in providing symptomatic relief in the case of gastrinomas. Embolisation or radiofrequency ablation may be useful for hepatic metastases.

## ENDOCRINE PANCREAS AND PREGNANCY

### Glucose metabolism during pregnancy

Pregnancy changes both basal and postprandial glucose metabolism as early as by the end of the first trimester. In the nonpregnant state, the liver is the predominant source of endogenous glucose production. Normal pregnancy (especially late pregnancy) is associated with reduced levels of fasting plasma glucose and increased levels of fasting insulin, presumably because of an increase in glucose uptake by the fetal and placental unit. Despite these changes, maternal hepatic glucose production is increased suggesting reduced hepatic insulin sensitivity or the presence of hepatic insulin resistance to increase glucose availability to the fetus in the fasted state. Postprandial glucose values are slightly elevated in association with maternal postprandial hyperinsulinaemia, especially in the second and third trimester.

The physiological factors responsible for the decrease of insulin sensitivity or the development of insulin resistance in pregnancy are not fully known. The metabolic effects of several hormones (including human placental lactogen, progesterone, prolactin and cortisol) and cytokines (including tumour necrosis factor alpha [TNF-α]) have been implicated; their levels are elevated in the maternal circulation during pregnancy. An increase in TNF-α concentration is associated with decreased insulin sensitivity in a number of conditions, including obesity, ageing and sepsis.

In normal pregnancy, there are progressive increases in insulin concentration with advancing gestation. These increases are more pronounced in lean women than in obese women because lean women tend to begin their pregnancies with better insulin sensitivity. Lean women have a greater total decrease in insulin sensitivity than obese women with normal glucose tolerance.

Increased insulin secretion during pregnancy represents compensation for progressive insulin resistance. However, insulin secretion increases by as much as 50% early in the second trimester before insulin resistance of pregnancy becomes manifest. Pregnancy may therefore exert a primary effect to increase insulin secretion independent of the presence of insulin resistance.

## Lipid metabolism during pregnancy

Significant alterations during pregnancy also occur in lipid metabolism. Women who are not obese gain approximately 3.5 kg of fat during normal pregnancy but there is a wide variation both within and between various ethnic and racial groups. Subcutaneous fat mass, primarily centrally distributed, significantly increases in early gestation. There is an increase in both preperitoneal and subcutaneous fat regions by the late third trimester of pregnancy. The increases in visceral fat may relate to the decreases in insulin sensitivity in late gestation.

Lipid metabolism differs between lean and obese women with normal glucose metabolism.

Total triglyceride concentrations increase two- to four-fold and total cholesterol concentrations increase by 25–50% during normal human pregnancy. There is a 50% increase in LDL cholesterol and a 30% increase in HDL cholesterol by midgestation, followed by a slight decrease in HDL cholesterol at term. There is also an increase in the concentration of free fatty acids in late pregnancy.

## Fetal endocrine pancreas

The fetal pancreas appears during the fourth week of fetal life. The alpha cells, which contain glucagon, and the delta cells, which contain somatostatin, develop before differentiation of the beta cells. Human pancreatic insulin and glucagon concentrations increase with advancing fetal age and are higher than the concentrations found in the adult pancreas. In maternal diabetes mellitus, fetal islet cells undergo hypertrophy such that the rate of insulin secretion increases.

## Diabetes in pregnancy

Abnormal maternal glucose regulation occurs in 3–10% of pregnancies. The prevalence of diabetes mellitus among women of childbearing age is increasing worldwide. This increase is attributable to more sedentary lifestyles, changes in diet, continued immigration from high-risk populations and an epidemic of childhood and adolescent obesity. Gestational diabetes mellitus (GDM) accounts for 90% of the total incidence of diabetes in pregnancy.

### Gestational diabetes mellitus
The term GDM refers to carbohydrate intolerance that is first identified during pregnancy. GDM is characterised as follows:

- Women with GDM have increased fasting glucose concentrations. In obese women with GDM, the fasting insulin concentration also rises and is greater than in women without GDM. The increase in circulating glucose concentrations despite increased insulin concentrations suggests an imbalance between the requirements for tissue insulin needed for the regulation of the glucose metabolism and the ability of the pancreatic beta cells to meet those requirements.
- There is an increase in insulin resistance from the time before conception through early pregnancy (weeks 12–14 of gestation), particularly in women with reduced insulin sensitivity before conception.
- There is failure to suppress the hepatic production of free fatty acids.

In GDM, insulin signalling changes do not only occur at the postreceptor level, as seen in a normal pregnancy; tyrosine phosphorylation of the insulin-receptor beta subunit is also impaired. This defect is not found in either pregnant or nonpregnant women with normal glucose tolerance and results in a 25% decrease in glucose transport activity. These receptor defects may contribute in part to the pathogenesis of GDM and the increased risk of type 2 diabetes later in life.

In addition to the previously mentioned changes, women with GDM also have a decreased serum concentration of adiponectin and this change correlates with decreased insulin sensitivity and impaired glucose disposal. Adiponectin is a hormone that is secreted from adipose tissue and serum concentrations are negatively associated with obesity, hyperinsulinaemia and insulin resistance. Adiponectin and TNF-α produce opposing effects on insulin signalling (adiponectin increases insulin sensitivity whereas TNF-α reduces it).

GDM results from inadequate insulin secretion that arises in women with chronic insulin resistance and is therefore related to type 2 diabetes. The range of beta cell defects in GDM could be similar to the spectrum of beta cell defects that lead to diabetes in nonpregnant people. Women with GDM have a 30–70% decrease in beta cell function relative to women who maintain normal glucose tolerance during pregnancy. As women with GDM tend to have chronic insulin resistance, most beta cell dysfunction in GDM occurs against a background of insulin resistance. Insulin secretion increases in pregnant women with GDM but not to the required extent. GDM therefore represents the detection during pregnancy of chronic metabolic abnormalities that antedate pregnancy but are detected when pregnancy leads to the first evaluation of glucose tolerance in otherwise healthy young women. The risk of type 2 diabetes after GDM ranges from 20% to 50%.

In addition to having abnormalities in their glucose metabolism, women with GDM, like those with pregestational type 2 diabetes, have higher triglyceride and decreased HDL concentrations than pregnant women with normal glucose tolerance.

### Screening and diagnosis of gestational diabetes mellitus

GDM is found in 1–4% of evaluated pregnancies. It poses many challenges to screening and diagnosis. The difficulty in diagnosing GDM arises as a result of the fact that there is more than one diagnostic test and no agreed gold-standard. In addition, there are several threshold criteria for the tests that are currently used and there is no agreement on criteria that best identify women at risk of poor outcomes.

Screening for GDM can be accomplished in many ways. Generally, methods of screening comprise risk factor assessment and laboratory glucose measurement.

Factors often evaluated in risk assessment include:

- maternal age
- ethnicity
- obesity
- gestational weight gain
- suspected macrosomia
- polyhydramnios
- glycosuria.

In addition, the family history of diabetes is taken as well as the history of previous GDM, delivery of a macrosomic infant, stillbirth, neonatal death and congenital anomaly. Risk factor screening may also be used to identify a subset of women who are at low risk of GDM and in whom laboratory testing can be avoided.

Risk assessment for GDM should be undertaken at the first prenatal visit. Laboratory testing is usually undertaken at weeks 24–28 of gestation. A fasting plasma glucose level above 7.0 mmol/l or a casual plasma glucose level above 11.1 mmol/l is indicative of diabetes. If confirmed on a subsequent day, there is no need for any glucose challenge.

In the absence of this degree of hyperglycaemia, evaluation for GDM in women with average or high-risk characteristics should follow one of two approaches:

- The one-step approach involves a diagnostic OGTT without prior plasma or serum glucose screening. This strategy may be cost-effective in high-risk individuals or populations.
- The two-step approach involves initial screening for hyperglycaemia by measurement of plasma or serum glucose concentrations 1 hour after a 50-g oral glucose load (glucose challenge test) followed by performance of a diagnostic OGTT on the subset of women who exceed the glucose threshold value on the glucose challenge test.

When the two-step approach is employed, a glucose threshold value of 7.8 mmol/l identifies approximately 80% of women with GDM and the yield is further increased to 90% by using a cutoff level of 7.2 mmol/l.

With either approach, the diagnosis of GDM is based on an OGTT. A glucose load of either 100 g or 75 g can be used but the 75 g OGTT is not as well validated for the detection of at-risk infants or mothers as the 100 g OGTT.

### Maternal morbidity associated with diabetes during pregnancy

Women with diabetic microvascular complications at the start of pregnancy may experience a deterioration in their symptoms that may in part result from the rapid induction of glycaemic control in early pregnancy. As a result, current management recommendations include baseline ophthalmology referral for pregnant women with diabetes with follow-up according to the degree of retinopathy. Women with underlying nephropathy can have varying degrees of deterioration of renal function during a pregnancy. The degree of proteinuria also increases but generally pregnancy does not cause progression to end-stage renal disease. Chronic hypertension complicates approximately one in ten pregnancies in women with diabetes and pre-eclampsia is also more frequent among women with diabetes.

Women with GDM are at increased risk for the development of diabetes (usually type 2 diabetes) after pregnancy. Obesity and other factors that promote insulin resistance seem to enhance the risk of type 2 diabetes after GDM.

### Fetal morbidity associated with diabetes during pregnancy

There is a strong association between the degree of glycaemic control before pregnancy and the rate of miscarriage. Women with long-standing (more than 10 years) and poorly controlled (HbA$_{1c}$ exceeding 11%) diabetes have been shown to have a miscarriage rate of up to 44%.

Major birth defects occur in 1–2% of the general population. In women with overt diabetes and suboptimal glycaemic control before conception, the likelihood of a structural anomaly is increased four- to eight-fold. Two-thirds of anomalies involve the cardiovascular and central nervous systems. Periconceptional glycaemic control is the main determinant of abnormal fetal development in women with diabetes. Since birth defects occur during the critical 3–6 weeks after conception, nutritional and metabolic intervention must be initiated well before pregnancy begins.

If the maternal pancreatic insulin response is inadequate, maternal, and subsequently fetal, hyperglycaemia results. This typically manifests as recurrent postprandial hyperglycaemic episodes. These postprandial episodes lead to accelerated fetal growth and are accompanied by episodic fetal hyperinsulinaemia. Fetal hyperinsuli-

naemia promotes excess nutrient storage, resulting in macrosomia.

Macrosomia occurs in 15–45% of pregnant women with diabetes, a four-fold increase compared with the frequency in normoglycaemic pregnant women. Maternal obesity, common in type 2 diabetes, seems to significantly accelerate the risk of infants being large for gestational age. The macrosomic fetus in diabetic pregnancy develops a unique pattern of overgrowth, involving central deposition of subcutaneous fat in the abdominal and interscapular areas. The rates of neonatal morbidity among newborns with macrosomia are excessive.

The energy expenditure associated with the conversion of excess glucose into fat causes depletion in fetal O$_2$ levels. These episodes of fetal hypoxia are accompanied by surges in adrenal catecholamines, which in turn cause hypertension, cardiac remodelling and hypertrophy, stimulation of erythropoietin, red cell hyperplasia and increased haematocrit. Polycythaemia (haematocrit above 65%) occurs in 5–10% of newborns whose mothers have diabetes. This finding seems to be related to the level of glycaemic control and is mediated by decreased fetal O$_2$ tension. High haematocrit values in the newborn baby lead to vascular sludging, poor circulation and postnatal hyperbilirubinaemia.

While most fetuses of mothers with diabetes exhibit growth acceleration, growth restriction occurs with significant frequency in pregnancies in women with pre-existing type 1 diabetes. The most important predictor of fetal growth restriction is underlying maternal vascular disease. Pregnant women with diabetes-associated retinal or renal vasculopathies and/or chronic hypertension are most at risk of delivering a growth-restricted baby.

Infants of mothers with diabetes have five-fold higher rates of severe hypoglycaemia and a two-fold increase in neonatal jaundice. Birth injuries are also more common among infants of mothers with diabetes.

Excessive body fat stores, stimulated by excessive glucose delivery during diabetic pregnancy, often extend into childhood and adult life. Glucose intolerance and increased serum insulin levels are more frequent in children of mothers with diabetes than in children of healthy controls. By the age of 10–16 years, children of mothers with diabetes during pregnancy have a 19.3% rate of impaired glucose intolerance. Development of childhood metabolic syndrome includes childhood obesity, hypertension, dyslipidaemia and glucose intolerance. Fetuses of women with diabetes that are born large for gestational age seem to be at the greatest risk. Markers of islet-cell-directed autoimmunity, if present, are associated with an increase in the risk of type 1 diabetes.

### Prepregnancy counselling for women with diabetes

For women with pre-existing diabetes, prepregnancy counselling is a major way of achieving a reduction in diabetes-associated neonatal morbidity. A thorough assessment of cardiovascular, renal and ophthalmological status is required. A regimen of frequent and regular monitoring of both preprandial and postprandial capillary glucose levels is required with the aim of keeping fasting plasma glucose levels at 5.0–5.5 mmol/l, 1-hour postprandial plasma glucose levels below 7.8 mmol/l and 2-hour postprandial plasma glucose levels below 6.7 mmol/l. The $HbA_{1c}$ level should ideally be within the reference range for at least 3 months before conception.

Women with diabetes should be advised to take a vitamin supplement containing at least 1.0 mg/day of folic acid for at least 3 months before conception to minimise the risk of neural tube defects in the fetus. Optimal prepregnancy counselling will also include a review of body weight, smoking, blood pressure control and the use of oral medications such as ACE inhibitors and statins.

### Management of diabetes during pregnancy

As in all forms of diabetes, women with GDM should receive nutritional counselling. Individualisation of medical nutrition therapy depending on maternal weight and height is recommended. For women who are obese (body mass index above 30 kg/m$^2$), a 30–33% calorie restriction (to 25 kcal/kg actual weight per day) has been shown to reduce hyperglycaemia and plasma triglycerides with no increase in ketonuria. Restriction of carbohydrates to 35–40% of calories has been shown to decrease maternal glucose levels and improve maternal and fetal outcomes. Moderate physical exercise has been shown to lower maternal glucose concentrations in women with GDM.

Insulin therapy has most consistently been shown to reduce fetal morbidities when added to nutritional therapy. The selection of pregnancies for insulin therapy is based on measures of maternal glycaemia with or without assessment of fetal growth characteristics.

When maternal glucose levels are used, insulin therapy is recommended when the diet fails to maintain self-monitored whole-blood glucose levels below 5.3 mmol/l (fasting), 7.8 mmol/l (1 hour postprandial) or 6.7 mmol/l (2 hours postprandial). Appropriate values for plasma glucose levels are 5.8 mmol/l, 8.6 mmol/l and 7.2 mmol/l, respectively. The goal of insulin therapy during pregnancy is to achieve glucose profiles similar to those of pregnant women without diabetes.

Insulin lispro, insulin aspart, regular insulin and isophane insulin are well studied in pregnancy and regarded as safe and efficacious. Insulin regimens during pregnancy must be continuously modified as the woman progresses from the first to the third trimester and insulin resistance rises. In a select group of women, use of a subcutaneous continuous insulin infusion using a pump may improve control.

Oral glucose-lowering agents have generally not been recommended during pregnancy. The biguanide metformin functions mainly by decreasing hepatic glucose output. It crosses the placenta and cord levels are even higher than maternal levels. Studies of women with polycystic ovary syndrome who used metformin at 1.5–2.5 g/day throughout pregnancy have illustrated the relative safety of the drug in the second and third trimesters. The use of metformin in women with type 2 diabetes in pregnancy to reduce insulin levels needs further investigation.

Glibenclamide, a sulphonylurea, is minimally transported across the human placenta. Several studies have concluded that it is as safe and efficacious as insulin in type 2 diabetes mellitus. Success rates for achieving glycaemic control with glibenclamide are about 80%. The drug has been shown to be safe in breastfeeding, with no transfer into human milk.

Many women with diabetes take antihypertensives such as ACE inhibitors or statins as part of their treatment. ACE inhibitors are contraindicated in the second and third trimesters of pregnancy as they interfere with normal fetal renal development, causing oligohydramnios and fetal growth restriction. Methyldopa is the drug of choice, although therapeutic doses of atenolol and nifedipine may be considered as safe alternatives in pregnant women. The use of statins is contraindicated during pregnancy.

### Monitoring of pregnant women with diabetes

Maternal monitoring is directed at detecting hyperglycaemia that is severe enough to increase risks to the fetus. Women are advised to self-monitor blood glucose levels every day. For women treated with insulin, success depends on the glycaemic targets that are set and achieved. The frequency and timing of home glucose monitoring should be individualised. Good glycaemic control requires attention to both preprandial and postprandial glucose levels. Urine glucose monitoring is not useful in GDM. Blood pressure and urine protein should be monitored to detect hypertensive disorders.

Increased surveillance of pregnancies at risk is appropriate, particularly when fasting glucose levels exceed 5.8 mmol/l or the pregnancy progresses past term. Assessment for fetal growth by ultrasonography, particularly in the early third trimester, may aid in identifying fetuses that can benefit from maternal insulin therapy.

### Long-term therapeutic considerations in women with gestational diabetes mellitus

Maternal glycaemic status should be checked after at least 6 weeks have passed since delivery. If glucose levels are normal postpartum, reassessment of glycaemia should be undertaken at least every 3 years. Women with impaired fasting glucose or impaired glucose tolerance in the postpartum period should be tested for diabetes annually. These women should receive intensive dietary and lifestyle advice and be counselled on the need for family planning. Oral contraceptives may be used in those with prior histories of GDM. Women should be advised to seek medical attention if they develop symptoms suggestive of diabetes mellitus.

Children of women with GDM should be followed closely for the development of obesity and/or abnormalities of glucose tolerance.

## Sample questions relating to the placenta

### EXTENDED MATCHING QUESTIONS

#### Questions 1–6

■ *Instructions: These questions relate to embryology. For each item below, select the* **single** *best option from the list of options (A–M). Each option may be used once, more than once or not at all.*

OPTIONS

▷ **A** Amnion
▷ **B** Blastocyst
▷ **C** Blastomere
▷ **D** Chorion
▷ **E** Cytotrophoblast
▷ **F** Decidua
▷ **G** Morula
▷ **H** Syncytiotrophoblast
▷ **I** Trophoblast
▷ **J** Zona fasciculate
▷ **K** Zona glomerulosa
▷ **L** Zona pellucida
▷ **M** Zona reticularis

1 ▶ The conceptus up to the 16-cell stage

2 ▶ 16 or more cell stage, with fluid filled cavities

3 ▶ A cell of the blastocyst

4 ▶ Layer surrounding the oocyte

5 ▶ Derived from the outer cell layer of the blastocyst

6 ▶ Pregnancy endometrium

### MULTIPLE CHOICE QUESTIONS

7 ▶ During early development of an embryo from the fertilisation of the oocyte:

    **A** ▷ First cleavage division takes place in the ampulla
    **B** ▷ First cleavage occurs within 12 hours
    **C** ▷ Cell divisions are regular at every 6 hours
    **D** ▷ All blastomeres are totipotent
    **E** ▷ The embryo enters the uterus at the 16-cell stage

8 ▶ During early development of an embryo from the fertilisation of the oocyte:

    **A** ▷ The outer cell mass forms the placenta
    **B** ▷ The inner cell mass develops into the fetus
    **C** ▷ In the preimplantation phase, new trophoblast develops from the outer cell mass
    **D** ▷ The inner and outer cell masses are in direct contact
    **E** ▷ The process is driven by glucose

9 ▶ Regarding decidualisation:

    **A** ▷ The process occurs when the embryo enters the uterine cavity
    **B** ▷ Decidualisation entails local change only
    **C** ▷ There is suppression of the maternal defence system
    **D** ▷ Decidualisation regulates trophoblast invasion
    **E** ▷ The uterine cavity becomes fluid filled

10 ▶ Regarding the process of attachment of the embryo:

    **A** ▷ The zona pellucida is retained
    **B** ▷ The endometrial epithelium is destroyed
    **C** ▷ Attachment is complete by day 12
    **D** ▷ Trophoblast cells destroy endometrial cells with which they come into contact
    **E** ▷ Vascular endothelial growth factor is made by the trophoblast

11 ▶ Regarding the placenta:

    **A** ▷ The cytotrophoblast is the outer cell layer
    **B** ▷ The syncytiotrophoblast has distinct cells
    **C** ▷ The cytotrophoblast has multinucleated cells
    **D** ▷ Lacunae form before implantation is complete
    **E** ▷ The trophoblast penetrates into the myometrium

12 ▶ The placenta:

    **A** ▷ has an anchoring role from day 13
    **B** ▷ reaches its ultimate form by week 12
    **C** ▷ reaches full thickness by week 10
    **D** ▷ weighs less than the fetus from week 12 onwards
    **E** ▷ weighs one-quarter of the fetus at term

13 ▶ Regarding placental development:

    **A** ▷ The extraembryonic mesoderm of the primary stem villi vascularises
    **B** ▷ Villi forming from a primary villus are collectively known as a lobule
    **C** ▷ There are 100 lobules in a placenta
    **D** ▷ Twenty-five lobules make up one cotyledon
    **E** ▷ All lobules are formed by week 10

14 ▶ Regarding immunotolerance of pregnancy:

    **A** ▷ Trophoblastic cells are exposed to maternal allogenic immune responses

    **B** ▷ There is enlargement of the uterine stromal cells

    **C** ▷ There is a uterine-specific population of natural killer cells

    **D** ▷ Tubal ectopic pregnancies show poor trophoblast invasion

    **E** ▷ Deficient decidua produces poor trophoblastic invasion

15 ▶ Regarding immunotolerance of pregnancy:

    **A** ▷ Fetal cells that enter the maternal circulation do not provoke a reaction

    **B** ▷ Trophoblast is always negative for major histocompatibility complex class 1 expression

    **C** ▷ Syncytiotrophoblast expresses major histocompatibility complex class 2

    **D** ▷ Human leucocyte antigen G expression is only expressed by trophoblast invading the decidua

    **E** ▷ CD8+ regulatory T-cells are not present in the pregnant uterus

16 ▶ Regarding perfusion of the intervillous spaces of the placenta with maternal blood:

    **A** ▷ Simple diffusion is more efficient in early pregnancy than in late pregnancy

    **B** ▷ Nonpolar molecules diffuse across the placenta

    **C** ▷ Urea diffuses across the placenta

    **D** ▷ Diffusion of oxygen across the placenta is dependent on the thickness of the terminal villi

    **E** ▷ Only the maternal side changes as pregnancy progresses

17 ▶ Regarding perfusion of the intervillous spaces of the placenta with maternal blood:

    **A** ▷ Oxygen transfer is promoted by a rise in fetal pH

    **B** ▷ Blood flow through the placenta increases transport of oxygen across the placenta

    **C** ▷ Glucose is transported across the placenta by specific carriers

    **D** ▷ Some amino acids are synthesised within the trophoblast

    **E** ▷ All amino acid uptake by the placenta is used for fetal growth

18 ▶ Regarding perfusion of the intervillous spaces of the placenta with maternal blood:

    **A** ▷ Water is exchanged at the placenta only

    **B** ▷ There is a large hydrostatic force pushing water from the mother to the fetus

    **C** ▷ Iron diffuses down its concentration gradient

    **D** ▷ Calcium diffuses down its concentration gradient

    **E** ▷ Sodium diffuses across in a co-transport system only

19 ▶ Regarding amniotic fluid:

    **A** ▷ It has a volume of 50 ml at week 8

    **B** ▷ There is no production after week 34

    **C** ▷ The creatinine concentration of amniotic fluid increases towards term

    **D** ▷ The amnion arises between the ectodermal and endodermal layers

    **E** ▷ The amnion contains lymphatics

20 ▶ Human chorionic gonadotrophin:

    **A** ▷ is secreted by the cytotrophoblast

    **B** ▷ is secreted from day 7 post fertilisation

    **C** ▷ has three amino acid chains

    **D** ▷ rises rapidly until week 12

    **E** ▷ binds to luteinising hormone receptors in the corpus luteum

21 ▶ Regarding molar pregnancies:

    **A** ▷ They contain no fetal tissue

    **B** ▷ A complete mole has 46 chromosomes in each cell

    **C** ▷ A complete mole contains maternally derived chromosomes

    **D** ▷ A partial mole has 23 chromosomes in each cell

    **E** ▷ Moles contain highly invasive placental tissue

## Sample questions relating to the hypothalamus, the pituitary, adrenal and thyroid glands and the pancreas

### EXTENDED MATCHING QUESTIONS

#### Questions 1–9

▪ *This question relates to hormones of the pituitary gland. For each item below, choose the **single** best option from the list of options (A–F). Each option may be used once, more than once or not at all.*

OPTIONS

▷ **A** Adrenocorticotrophin
▷ **B** Follicle-stimulating hormone
▷ **C** Growth hormone
▷ **D** Luteinising hormone
▷ **E** Prolactin
▷ **F** Thyroid-stimulating hormone

1 ▶ Antagonises the actions of insulin

2 ▶ Is a nongonadotrophin glycoprotein

3 ▶ Increases the concentration of free fatty acids in the blood

4 ▶ Has a similar structure to growth hormone

5 ▶ Its release is controlled by dopamine

6 ▶ Has a peak release in the early morning

7 ▶ Its secretion is inhibited by somatostatin

8 ▶ Its secretion is induced by high concentrations of estrogen

9 ▶ Stimulates ovarian follicles

### MULTIPLE CHOICE QUESTIONS

10 ▶ Regarding hypothalamic hormones:

    **A** ▷ They are all peptides
    **B** ▷ Only the release of corticotrophin-releasing hormone follows a circadian rhythm
    **C** ▷ They have a long half-life
    **D** ▷ Thyrotrophin-releasing hormone (TRH) increases prolactin release
    **E** ▷ TRH stimulates the release of thyrotrophin-stimulating hormone

11 ▶ Regarding the adrenal gland:

    **A** ▷ Norepinephrine mainly increases glycogenolysis
    **B** ▷ Cortisol stimulates gluconeogenesis
    **C** ▷ Ninety-five percent of cortisol is bound to albumin
    **D** ▷ The zona reticularis secretes androgenic hormones
    **E** ▷ Epinephrine is released on stimulation by sympathetic postganglionic cholinergic neurons

12 ▶ Regarding aldosterone:

    **A** ▷ Angiotensinogen stimulates aldosterone production
    **B** ▷ Aldosterone decreases the excretion of $K^+$
    **C** ▷ The plasma $K^+$ concentration directly stimulates aldosterone production
    **D** ▷ Aldosterone mainly acts in the proximal convoluted tubule
    **E** ▷ Aldosterone increases the excretion of $H_2O$

# Genetics

# CHAPTER 18

# Single-gene and chromosome abnormalities

*Katrina Tatton-Brown*

## Chromosomes, genes and cell division

### CHROMOSOMES

Each human somatic cell has 23 pairs of chromosomes that are distinguished according to their length and pattern of light and dark bands. Each chromosome has a centromere (a constriction along its length), which divides the chromosome into short and long arms known as the p and q arms, respectively (Figure 18.1). When the short and long arms are of approximately equal length, the chromosome is known as a metacentric chromosome. When the centromere divides the chromosome into two arms where one arm is obviously longer than the other, the chromosome is known as a submetacentric chromosome. When the centromere is situated at the top of the chromosome, the chromosome is known as an acrocentric chromosome.

The first 22 pairs of chromosomes are known as autosomes and have been designated the numbers 1 through to 22 depending upon the decreasing relative length of the chromosome pairs. The composition of the 23rd pair of chromosomes, the sex chromosomes, determines a person's gender with female individuals having two X chromosomes and male individuals having an X and a Y chromosome.

In the creation of germ cells, the number of chromosomes is halved so that each ovum and spermatozoon contains only one chromosome from each pair. Germ cells therefore have 23 chromosomes, known as the haploid number, whereas somatic cells have 46 chromosomes, referred to as the diploid number.

### GENES

Each chromosome is composed of tightly coiled threads of DNA organised around proteins called histones (Figure 18.1). A gene is a specific sequence of DNA that carries the instructions for the construction of a protein (see Chapter 5 for further information on the structure of DNA and protein synthesis). The human genome is estimated to contain approximately 25 000 genes.

### MEIOSIS

When somatic cells divide, they go through a process known as mitosis, whereby the cell duplicates its DNA and cleaves to generate two identical daughter cells also with 23 pairs, or the diploid number, of chromosomes (Figure 18.2). By contrast, when germ cells divide to produce ova or sperm, they undergo meiosis. Meiosis is unique to the germ cells and is essential to reduce the somatic diploid number of 46 chromosomes to the haploid number of 23 chromosomes (Figure 18.3). This reduction ensures that, when fertilisation occurs, the zygote has 46 chromosomes rather than 92, which would be the result of fertilisation involving two diploid germ cells.

Meiosis consists of two consecutive division cycles that are designated meiosis I and meiosis II.

### Meiosis I

Chromosomes duplicate at the beginning of meiosis I. Homologous chromosomes, now consisting of identical

271

FIGURE 18.1 **Structure of a chromosome**

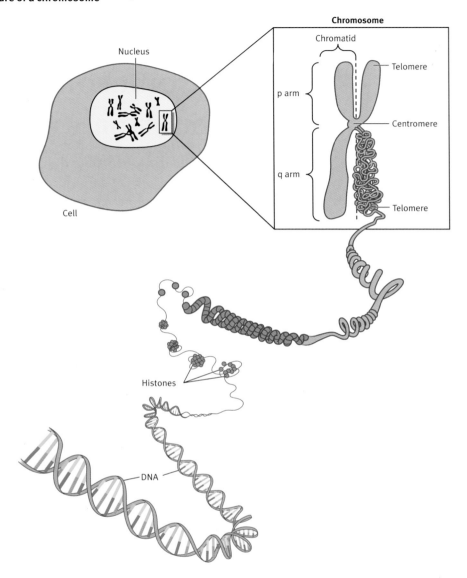

sister chromatids, align and reciprocal exchange of genetic material occurs between homologous but nonidentical chromatids. This process, known as recombination, enables the mixing of paternally and maternally inherited genes, ensuring that children inherit unique gene combinations. Following recombination, the pairs of duplicated chromosomes align at the spindle equator and one duplicated chromosome from each pair, consisting of two sister chromatids, is pulled to either pole of the cell before cyto-

kinesis generates two daughter cells. Therefore, at the end of meiosis I each daughter cell has 23 chromosomes, each consisting of two chromatids (Figure 18.3).

### *Meiosis II*

The phases of meiosis II resemble those of mitosis except that, as each chromosome is already duplicated at the beginning of meiosis II, there is no requirement for addi-

FIGURE 18.2 **Mitosis**

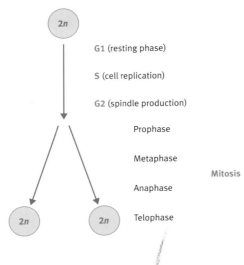

2n = diploid chromosome number

FIGURE 18.3 **Meiosis**

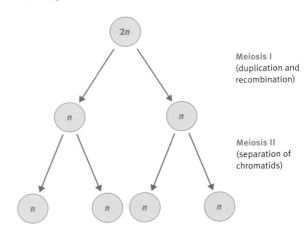

n = haploid chromosome number | 2n = diploid chromosome number

tional replication. Therefore, the single chromosomes align at the spindle equator, the spindle matrix is generated and sister chromatids are pulled to opposite poles of the cell before cytokinesis.

---

**CHROMOSOMES, GENES AND CELL DIVISION**

- There are 46 chromosomes (23 pairs) in each somatic cell; this is the diploid number.
- There are 23 individual chromosomes, one from each chromosome pair, in the ova and sperm; this is the haploid number.
- The chromosomes contain approximately 25 000 genes.
- Genes code for the production of specific proteins.
- Mitosis is the process whereby somatic cells divide. The progenitor cell has 46 chromosomes and each daughter cell has 46 chromosomes.
- Meiosis occurs in the generation of germ cells. It has two distinct phases:
  - During meiosis I, chromosomes duplicate, paternally and maternally inherited chromosomes are recombined and the diploid number is reduced to the haploid number.
  - During meiosis II, splitting of sister chromatids occurs.
  - Therefore, by the end of meiosis, four daughter cells are generated from one dividing germ cell, paternal and maternal genetic material is mixed and each germ cell has only 23 chromosomes.

---

Thus, by the end of meiosis, four daughter cells are generated from each dividing germ cell. Each of these daughter cells should have 23 individual chromosomes, representing one chromosome from each pair of autosomes in addition to an X chromosome in ova and either an X chromosome or a Y chromosome in sperm. As a result of recombination during meiosis I, each germ cell will have a unique combination of both paternally and maternally inherited genes.

Of note, in female meiosis, three of the daughter cells constitute polar bodies and will not survive; only one daughter cell becomes an ovum. By contrast, all four daughter cells produced from male meiosis develop into spermatozoa.

## Chromosome abnormalities

An abnormality of chromosome number is known as aneuploidy. Aneuploidy can result from various mechanisms, including nondisjunction and translocation.

### NONDISJUNCTION

Occasionally, pairs of homologous chromosomes at meiosis I or sister chromatids during mitosis anaphase do not separate and so both chromosomes are passed to one daughter cell and none to the other. One daughter

TABLE 18.1 **Karyotype and clinical features associated with common trisomy conditions**

| Syndrome name | Additional chromosome | Clinical features |
|---|---|---|
| Down syndrome | 21 | Moderate to severe learning difficulties (100%) |
| | | Cardiac problems (40–50%, VSD, ASD, AVSD) |
| | | Hypothyroidism (20–40%) |
| | | Dementia (10–15%) |
| | | Acute lymphoblastic leukaemia |
| Edwards syndrome | 18 | Profound learning difficulties (100%) |
| | | Congenital heart disease (90%, commonly VSD) |
| | | Facial clefts |
| | | Spina bifida |
| | | Clenched hands |
| | | Rocker-bottom feet |
| Patau syndrome | 13 | Profound learning difficulties (100%) |
| | | Congenital heart disease (80%, VSD, ASD) |
| | | Holoprosencephaly (60–70%) |
| | | Microphthalmia/anophthalmia (60–70%) |
| | | Postaxial polydactyly (60–70%) |
| | | Scalp defects |
| | | Cleft lip/palate (60–70%) |
| | | Omphalocele |
| | | Renal anomalies |
| Klinefelter syndrome | X (in an XY individual) | Slightly decreased IQ but within the normal range |
| | | Tall stature |
| | | Infertility |
| | | Transient gynaecomastia |
| Triple X syndrome | X (in an XX individual) | Slightly decreased IQ but within the normal range |
| | | Tall stature |
| | | Normal fertility |
| XYY syndrome | Y (in an XY individual) | Slightly decreased IQ but within the normal range |
| | | Tall stature after puberty |
| | | Behavioural problems |

*(handwritten margin note: duodenal atresia, facial dysmorphism)*

ASD = atrial septal defect  |  AVSD = atrioventricular septal defect  |  VSD = ventricular septal defect

TABLE 18.2 **Maternal age versus risk of chromosome nondisjunction**

| Age (years) | Risk |
|---|---|
| 20 | One in 1500 |
| 30 | One in 900 |
| 34 | One in 500 |
| 36 | One in 300 |
| 38 | One in 200 |
| 40 | One in 100 |
| 42 | One in 60 |
| 45 | One in 30 |

cell therefore has an additional chromosome, a phenomenon known as trisomy, whereas the other is missing one chromosome, known as monosomy.

Common trisomic conditions include Down syndrome (trisomy 21), Edward's syndrome (trisomy 18), Patau syndrome (trisomy 13) and Klinefelter syndrome (47,XXY); Table 18.1 provides an overview of these conditions. Turner syndrome (45,X) is the most common monosomy identified at birth. In addition, mosaic (where only a proportion of cells have the additional chromosome) trisomy 16 and mosaic trisomy 8 are occasionally identified postnatally. Other trisomies and monosomies are rarely seen postnatally as they are not compatible with term development of the fetus.

The risk of chromosome nondisjunction increases with advancing maternal age (Table 18.2).

### Down syndrome

Nondisjunction resulting in three separate copies of chromosome 21 accounts for more than 95% of the total incidence of Down syndrome. Alternative causes include Robertsonian translocations and other chromosome rearrangements.

All individuals with Down syndrome have some degree of learning difficulties, usually moderate. In addition, atrioventricular septal defect is 1000 times more common in children with Down syndrome than in the general population. The facial appearance of children and adults with Down syndrome is characteristic and

consists of upslanting palpebral fissures, epicanthic folds (folds of skin from the upper eyelid continue down to the nasal corner), a flat midface and brachycephaly (short anterior–posterior diameter of the cranium). Other associated features are shown in Table 18.1.

### Edwards syndrome

Edwards syndrome is associated with a poor prenatal and postnatal outcome. The great majority of occurrences are caused by meiotic nondisjunction but, as with Down syndrome, the syndrome can be attributable to unbalanced Robertsonian translocations and other chromosome rearrangements.

Edwards syndrome is usually detected prenatally either through aneuploidy screening methods or through identification of a combination of many associated prenatal anomalies (Table 18.1). Babies with Edwards syndrome who survive to term are likely to die within the first year of life (usually within the first months). Very rarely, children have survived beyond the first year with profound cognitive impairment and associated anomalies described in Table 18.1.

### Patau syndrome

Patau syndrome, caused by an additional copy of chromosome 13, is also associated with a high rate of spontaneous pregnancy loss and, if the baby survives to term, poor postnatal outcome. Most (90%) occurrences of Patau syndrome are caused by nondisjunction of chromosome 13 (the vast majority of which occur during maternal meiosis). The remainder are attributable to unbalanced translocations (primarily Robertsonian translocations).

### Klinefelter syndrome

Individuals with Klinefelter syndrome have an additional sex chromosome, with a karyotype of 47,XXY. Many individuals with Klinefelter syndrome are not diagnosed unless as an incidental finding prenatally during chorionic villus sampling (CVS) or amniocentesis or in adulthood during infertility investigations. As Klinefelter syndrome does not, in general, cause an increase in nuchal translucency (NT) thickness and does not result in features that are evident on the second tri-

FIGURE 18.4 **Reciprocal translocation**

**Parents' chromosomes**

Chromosomes in parent carrying
a balanced translocation

Chromosomes in other parent
(normal arrangement)

**Possible chromosome arrangements in their children[a]**

Normal
chromosome
arrangement

Balanced
translocation

Unbalanced
translocation

Unbalanced
translocation

[a] Other arrangements occur less frequently

mester anomaly scan, the condition is usually not identified prenatally.

### Other sex chromosome abnormalities resulting from nondisjunction

These are illustrated in Table 18.1. The most common examples are a 47,XXX karyotype (triple X syndrome) in female persons and a 47,XYY karyotype in male persons. Triple X syndrome is usually identified incidentally as it causes few problems prenatally or postnatally. There is a suggestion that young boys with 47,XYY are more prone to temper tantrums and defiant behaviour.

### Turner syndrome

In general, girls with Turner syndrome (45,X) have IQ scores 10–15 points lower than their siblings but they attend mainstream school and do not have learning difficulties. Many fetuses with 45,X do not survive to term because of fetal hydrops. Indeed, Turner syndrome should be considered in any fetus with an NT thickness above 4 mm. The attrition rate for conceptions with Turner syndrome is reported to be very high, so if the syndrome is

diagnosed in the first trimester, parents should be advised of a high risk of spontaneous miscarriage.

### TRANSLOCATIONS

#### Reciprocal translocations

Chromosome rearrangements involving the transfer of genetic material between two nonhomologous chromosomes are known as reciprocal translocations (Figure 18.4). The most common reciprocal translocation in humans, t(11;22)(q23;q11), involves chromosomes 11 and 22.

Reciprocal translocations can be either balanced or unbalanced. In general, a balanced exchange of chromosome material does not have phenotypic consequences as the adult or child has a normal amount of genetic material. However, if unbalanced, there will be one chromosome with missing genetic material (a monosomy) and another chromosome with duplicated genetic material (a trisomy), a combination that is usually associated with developmental and other congenital problems.

If a woman with a balanced reciprocal translocation is seen before she conceives, she should be advised that a pregnancy can have four possible outcomes (Figure 18.4):

- A normal pregnancy with a normal karyotype.
- A normal pregnancy with the familial balanced reciprocal translocation.
- A spontaneous miscarriage owing to an unbalanced product of the familial reciprocal translocation.
- A pregnancy that goes to term but the child has a high likelihood of learning difficulties and possibly other congenital anomalies associated with an unbalanced product of the familial reciprocal translocation.

The relative proportion of pregnancies that spontaneously miscarry or go to term with problems depends upon the chromosomes involved and the size of the translocated chromosome segments.

If an unbalanced reciprocal translocation is detected prenatally, it is likely to be associated with fetal anomalies and the parents should be counselled accordingly. If a balanced reciprocal translocation is identified, the parents should be karyotyped to determine whether it is *de novo*. If it is familial and the parent carrying the balanced rearrangement is healthy with no learning or

FIGURE 18.5  **Robertsonian translocation**

other medical difficulties, the baby is unlikely to have problems related to the translocation. However, if the balanced translocation has arisen for the first time in the fetus (it is *de novo*), it may or may not be associated with problems.

### Robertsonian translocations

A Robertsonian translocation is a chromosome rearrangement that involves fusion of the long arms of two acrocentric chromosomes and loss of their short arms (Figure 18.5). The genes contained on the short arms are represented elsewhere and so their loss does not result in any phenotypic effect.

By definition, Robertsonian translocations only involve the five acrocentric chromosomes 13, 14, 15, 21 and 22. The most common Robertsonian translocations are rob(13q;14q), which involves fusion of chromosome 13 to chromosome 14, and rob(14q;21q), which involves fusion of chromosome 14 to chromosome 21. Occasionally, the long arms of two homologous chromosomes may fuse resulting in an isochromosome.

Individuals who are seen before conception to discuss the implications of a balanced Robertsonian translocation for a future pregnancy should be advised of a number of possible outcomes (Figure 18.5):

- A normal pregnancy with a normal karyotype.

- A normal pregnancy associated with a balanced Robertsonian translocation.
- A spontaneous miscarriage attributable to an unbalanced Robertsonian translocation (the fetus will be trisomic or monosomic for one of the component chromosomes).
- A spontaneous miscarriage owing to an imprinting defect.
- A liveborn child with abnormalities; in all instances, these will be attributable to trisomy rather than monosomy, as the latter will always result in spontaneous miscarriage; in the common rob(13q;14q) and rob(14q;21q) translocations, there is a risk of a child with Patau syndrome or Down syndrome, respectively; these risks are higher if the mother carries the balanced translocation (10–15%) than if the father carries it (below 1%).
- A liveborn child with abnormalities associated with an imprinting defect (risk below 0.5%).

Imprinting is the process by which one parental allele is preferentially silenced according to its parental origin. Of the five acrocentric chromosomes, imprinted genes are found only on chromosomes 14 and 15. Imprinting abnormalities associated with Robertsonian translocations are therefore only of concern if one or both of these two chromosomes are involved. Following mitosis, a trisomic conceptus may occur but this may be 'corrected' through trisomy rescue. This reduction of three copies to two copies leaves the cell with an apparently balanced arrangement. However, if both the remaining chromosomes are of the same parental origin (known as uniparental disomy or UPD) and contain imprinted genes, there may be phenotypic consequences.

Babies with maternal UPD14 generally survive to term and are small, have learning difficulties, hypotonia and relative macrocephaly. By contrast, paternal UPD14 tends to result in spontaneous miscarriage, but if babies do survive to term they have severe problems including profound learning difficulties, feeding difficulties and joint contractures.

Paternal UPD15 and maternal UPD15 cause Angelman syndrome and Prader–Willi syndrome, respectively. These are well described syndromes that are both associated with severe learning difficulties. In addition, children with Angelman syndrome have a characteristic facial appearance and an ataxic gait. Children with Prader–Willi syndrome are characteristically poor feeders in the neonatal period but develop an insatiable appetite from childhood onwards. In addition, they may be hypotonic and of short stature.

### CHROMOSOME MICRODELETIONS

Chromosome microdeletions are an important cause of a number of different syndromes illustrated in Table 18.3. Common to all is a 'chromosome phenotype' consisting of learning difficulties, characteristic dysmorphic facial features and congenital anomalies. Microdeletions may be visible with conventional cytogenetic techniques, possibly in association with fluorescence *in situ* hybridisation (FISH), but they are increasingly detected using newer molecular techniques including multiplex ligation-dependent probe amplification (MLPA) and microarray comparative genomic hybridisation (CGH).

## Gene abnormalities

The normal functioning of genes can be disrupted through a number of different mechanisms, including intragenic mutations (missense, frameshift, nonsense and splice site mutations), exon deletions, triplet repeat expansions and whole gene deletions.

### MISSENSE MUTATIONS

Missense mutations are single-base substitutions that have occurred in a coding, critical region of the gene. Without performing functional studies it is often difficult to elucidate the pathogenicity of these single-base substitutions.

### FRAMESHIFT MUTATIONS

Frameshift mutations occur when one or more bases (but not a multiple of three) are inserted or deleted from the usual genetic sequence so disrupting the normal reading frame. Eventually, a variable number of codons along the sequence, a new stop codon will have been generated and the resulting abnormal protein will be prematurely truncated.

### NONSENSE MUTATIONS

A nonsense mutation is a single-base substitution that generates a premature stop codon resulting in a truncated protein. As both frameshift and nonsense mutations result in truncated proteins, they are sometimes referred to together as truncating mutations.

### SPLICE SITE MUTATIONS

Splicing is the process by which introns are removed from the primary transcript and consecutive exons joined together. Splice site mutations affect the nucleotides at the splice site, at the junction between the introns and exons.

### EXON DELETIONS

Exon deletions, alternatively known as partial gene deletions, can occur when one or more exons within a gene are deleted in a process that does not constitute an alternative splicing event.

### TRIPLET REPEAT EXPANSIONS

Triplet repeat conditions result from extensive duplication of a single codon. If such a run of nucleotide triplets increases above a critical threshold, an abnormal phenotype results. Common triplet repeat conditions include fragile X syndrome, Huntington's disease and myotonic dystrophy. Features common to these conditions include variability of phenotype, anticipation (progression in triplet repeat size and phenotype severity as the repeat is passed on to the next generation) and a parent-of-origin effect (the triplet repeat may expand more if passed on by the mother rather than the father or vice versa).

TABLE 18.3 **Common microdeletion syndromes**

| Microdeletion | Syndrome name | Cardinal features |
|---|---|---|
| 1p36 | | Severe learning difficulties<br>Seizures<br>Hypotonia<br>Feeding difficulties<br>Characteristic facial appearance with low-set horizontal eyebrows and deep-set eyes |
| 4p15 | Wolf–Hirschhorn | Severe learning difficulties<br>Low birth weight and postnatal failure to thrive<br>Characteristic facial appearance with 'Greek helmet' profile |
| 5p15 | Cri du chat | Severe learning difficulties<br>Characteristic cat-like cry<br>Characteristic facial appearance with bitemporal narrowing, hypertelorism and downslanted palpebral fissures |
| 7q11 | Williams | Mild to severe learning difficulties<br>Cardiac problems, particularly supravalvular aortic/pulmonary stenosis<br>Renal artery stenosis<br>Characteristic facial appearance with short upturned nose, long philtrum, wide mouth, periorbital fullness<br>'Cocktail party personality' (chatty, interactive behaviour) |
| 8q24 | Langer–Giedion | Contiguous gene deletion syndrome characterised by fine sparse hair, brittle nails, bulbous nose and cone-shaped epiphyses on X-ray (owing to deletion of the *TRPS1* gene) in addition to exostoses and mental restriction (owing to deletion of neighbouring genes including *EXT1*) |
| 17p11 | Smith–Magenis | Severe learning difficulties<br>Severe behavioural problems with self-injuring<br>Sleep problems<br>Characteristic facial appearance with square-shaped face and heavy eyebrows |
| 17p13 | Miller–Dieker | Lissencephaly<br>Characteristic facial appearance with vertical furrowing on the forehead, hypertelorism and short nose with anteverted nares |
| 22q11 | DiGeorge/<br>velocardiofacial/<br>Shprintzen | Mild to moderate learning difficulties<br>Cardiac anomalies, most commonly tetralogy of Fallot, VSD and interrupted aortic arch<br>Short stature<br>Psychiatric disorders<br>Renal anomalies<br>Cleft palate with or without velopharyngeal insufficiency<br>Hypocalcaemia<br>T-cell immune disorder<br>Characteristic facial appearance with tubular nose, narrow palpebral fissures and simple ears |

VSD = ventricular septal defect

**ABNORMALITIES OF CHROMOSOMES AND GENES**

*Common chromosome abnormalities include:*

- nondisjunction (for example Down, Edward's, Patau, Klinefelter and Turner syndromes)
- translocations
  - Robertsonian translocations
  - Reciprocal translocations
- microdeletions (for example DiGeorge, Wolf–Hirschhorn and Williams syndromes).

*Mechanisms that abrogate gene function include:*

- missense mutations
- truncating mutations including frameshift and nonsense mutations
- splice site mutations
- partial gene deletions
- whole gene deletions
- triplet repeat expansions.

FIGURE 18.6 **Autosomal dominant inheritance**

**A** Pattern of inheritance

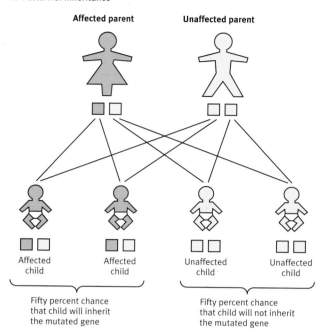

Key

■ Mutated gene     □ Wild type gene

**B** Pedigree

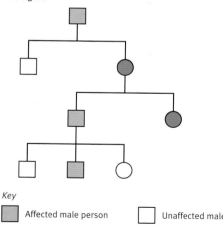

Key

■ Affected male person     □ Unaffected male person

● Affected female person     ○ Unaffected female person

## Principles of inheritance

Genes encode proteins, which are essential to the normal development and functioning of the body. Genes are arranged in pairs, with one gene from each pair being inherited from each parent. Traits determined by a single gene locus generally follow one of four different patterns of inheritance: autosomal dominant, autosomal recessive, X-linked recessive or X-linked dominant inheritance.

### AUTOSOMAL DOMINANT INHERITANCE

Autosomal dominant conditions are caused by disruption of only one gene of a gene pair by any of the previously described mechanisms that abrogate gene function. The children of an individual affected by an autosomal dominant condition have a one in two chance of inheriting the disrupted gene and, therefore, the associated condition (Figure 18.6 A). A few more common autosomal dominant conditions are shown in Table 18.4.

Pedigrees where an autosomal dominant trait has been passed on from generation to generation have several characteristic features (Figure 18.6 B):

- Individuals in each generation are affected.
- Male and female relatives are affected in roughly equal numbers.
- Both men and women can have affected children.

## FIGURE 18.7 Autosomal recessive inheritance

**A** Pattern of inheritance

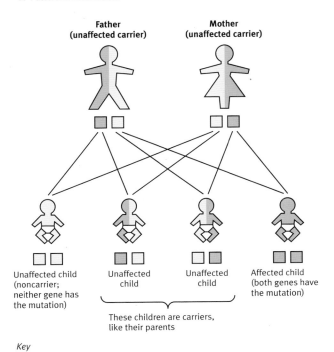

Unaffected child (noncarrier; neither gene has the mutation)

Unaffected child

Unaffected child

Affected child (both genes have the mutation)

These children are carriers, like their parents

*Key*

■ Mutated gene    □ Wild type gene

**B** Pedigree

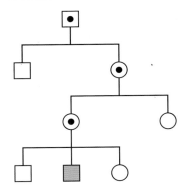

*Key*

■ Affected male person

□ Unaffected male noncarrier

⊡ Unaffected male carrier

⊙ Unaffected female carrier

○ Unaffected female noncarrier

## AUTOSOMAL RECESSIVE INHERITANCE

Autosomal recessive conditions (Table 18.5) are caused by disruption of both genes in a gene pair. Where only one gene is disrupted, the individual is known as a carrier and is healthy.

Individuals with an autosomal recessive condition will only have affected children if they mate with another affected individual or a carrier of the condition. If two carriers have children, the chance of their children being affected by the condition is one in four. There is therefore a three in four chance of having healthy children, of whom two would be anticipated to be carriers and one would be anticipated to have inherited the two normal genes from his or her parents (Figure 18.7 A).

Autosomal recessive conditions should be considered in pedigrees with the following features (Figure 18.7 B):

- Only one generation is affected.
- Parents of affected children are genetically related (consanguineous).

## X-LINKED RECESSIVE INHERITANCE

If a recessive mutation is present within a gene on the X chromosome, male individuals will be affected because they are hemizygous for that gene. However, female individuals who have one mutated copy and one normal copy generally do not manifest features of the disorder. Common X-linked recessive disorders are described in Table 18.6.

Characteristics of X-linked recessive pedigrees include the following:

- Only male individuals are affected, or if female individuals are affected they have a milder phenotype.
- There is no male to male transmission of the condition. If this occurs then the condition cannot be an X-linked recessive condition.
- The condition may seem to skip generations.

## X-LINKED DOMINANT INHERITANCE

An X-linked dominant disorder often manifests so severely in male fetuses that it results in a spontaneous loss of pregnancy or early neonatal death. X-linked dom-

TABLE 18.4 **Common autosomal dominant conditions**

| Condition | Gene | Features |
|---|---|---|
| Tuberous sclerosis | *TSC1/TSC2* | Multisystem disorder characterised by cutaneous (angiofibromata, hypomelanotic macules, shagreen patches), neurological (brain hamartomas causing seizures) and renal (angiomyolipomata) abnormalities; should be strongly suspected prenatally if cardiac rhabdomyosarcomas are identified |
| Marfan syndrome | Fibrillin 1 | Tall stature, arm span to height ratio >1.05, long fingers, dolicocephaly, aortic dilatation and other cardiac anomalies |
| Neurofibromatosis type I | *NF1* | Combination of café-au-lait spots, neurofibromata, axillary and inguinal freckling and optic glioma |
| Breast/ovarian cancer susceptibility | *BRCA1/ BRCA2* | Inherited susceptibility to the development of breast cancer (lifetime risk ~80%) and ovarian cancer (lifetime risk 20–40%) |
| Hereditary nonpolyposis colon cancer | *MLH* | Inherited predisposition to the development of colon and other cancers including endometrial, gastric and ovarian |
| Huntington's disease | Huntingtin | Condition characterised by progressive neurological deterioration with dementia, psychiatric disturbance and movement disorder |
| Autosomal dominant polycystic kidney disease | *PKD1/PKD2* | Systemic disorder with cysts in the kidneys, liver, pancreas and spleen and cardiovascular anomalies including intracranial aneurysms and mitral valve prolapse |
| Achondroplasia | *FGFR3* | Condition characterised by disproportionate short stature with rhizomelic (proximal) shortening and relative macrocephaly |

inant conditions therefore seem to be restricted to female individuals. Examples of X-linked dominant disorders are shown in Table 18.7.

### OTHER FORMS OF INHERITANCE

Occasionally, disorders follow more complex patterns of inheritance including mitochondrial inheritance and imprinting. Disorders resulting from mitochondrial inheritance can only be transmitted through the maternal line. Mitochondrial disorders are caused by a defect in the mitochondrial DNA and include mitochondrial encephalomyopathy with lactic acidosis and stroke-like episodes (MELAS), myoclonic epilepsy with ragged red fibres (MERRF) and Leigh's disease (subacute necrotising encephalomyopathy).

Imprinting is briefly described earlier in this chapter. In summary, it is the process whereby one allele is preferentially silenced according to its parent of origin.

## Prenatal genetics

Screening tests available to pregnant women in the first and second trimesters include a combination of NT ultrasound and/or serum screening. These screening investigations will provide the pregnant woman with a statistical risk of having a baby with trisomy 21, 18 or 13. Such investigations do not provide a definitive diagnosis. If the risk is deemed high, women can proceed to a diagnostic test. In practice, CVS or amniocentesis are the only tests offered at the end of the first and beginning of the second trimester.

### SCREENING TESTS

An overview is provided in Table 18.8.

#### Nuchal translucency ultrasound

The term NT refers to the sonographic appearance of

TABLE 18.5  **Common autosomal recessive conditions**

| Condition | Gene | Features |
|---|---|---|
| Cystic fibrosis | CFTR | Characterised by chronic pulmonary disease and exocrine pancreatic dysfunction |
| Spinal muscular atrophy | SMN | Characterised by symmetrical proximal muscle weakness; life expectancy ranges from infancy to adulthood depending upon the type of spinal muscular atrophy |
| Tay–Sachs disease | HEXA | A GM2 gangliosidosis characterised by a 'cherry-red spot' on the retina and deteriorating motor and cognitive abilities |
| Haemochromatosis | HFE | Excess absorption of iron with deposition in liver, pancreas and skin leading to cirrhosis, diabetes mellitus and bronzed appearance of skin |
| α1-Antitrypsin deficiency | SERPIN A1 | α1-Antitrypsin is a proteinase inhibitor that protects the lungs from elastase; without α1-antitrypsin individuals will develop emphysema at a young age; they may also develop cirrhosis owing to a direct effect of the abnormal α1-antitrypsin on the hepatocytes |
| Congenital adrenal hyperplasia due to 21-hydroxylase deficiency | CYP21A2 | Attributable to abrogation of 21-hydroxylase, required for the synthesis of cortisol; associated with female virilisation and abnormal puberty (precocious in boys) with or without salt wasting |
| Deafness due to mutations in connexin 26 | GJB2 | Most common cause of autosomal recessive nonsyndromic deafness |

TABLE 18.6  **Common X-linked recessive conditions**

| Condition | Gene | Features |
|---|---|---|
| Duchenne muscular dystrophy | Dystrophin | Progressive myopathy affecting proximal muscles; causes early loss of ambulation and death in the third decade owing to respiratory failure |
| Haemophilia A | Factor VIII gene | Attributable to deficiency of factor VIII, an important component of the clotting cascade; affected male individuals have abnormal clotting, with severe haemophilia A leading to spontaneous joint and muscle bleeding |
| Ocular albinism | GPR143 | Hypopigmentation of iris and retina; associated with poor visual acuity, nystagmus, strabismus and abnormal decussation of the optic nerves |
| X-linked adrenoleucodystrophy | ACBD1 | Accumulation of very-long-chain fatty acids in the adrenal glands and brain; results in progressive cognitive deterioration and adrenal failure |
| Fragile X syndrome | FMR1 | Caused by expansion of a CGG repeat; results in learning difficulties and characteristic facial appearance |

CGG = cytosine-guanine-guanine trinucleotide

TABLE 18.7  **X-linked dominant conditions**

| Condition | Gene | Features |
|---|---|---|
| Incontinentia pigmenti | NEMO | Initially presents as blistering lesions following Blaschko lines; these later become hyperpigmented and eventually appear as atrophic streaks |
| Rett syndrome | MECP2 | Associated with cognitive regression and severe learning difficulties; other characteristic features include hand wringing and stereotypical movements |

subcutaneous fluid at the back of the fetal neck between weeks 11 and 14 of gestation (Figure 18.8). An increased NT thickness is associated with chromosomal abnormalities, a wide range of cardiac defects, single-gene defects including Noonan syndrome (syndrome of short stature, cardiac defects, learning difficulties and clotting abnormalities primarily associated with mutations within the *PTPN11* gene) and some skeletal dysplasias.

Chromosome trisomy attributable to nondisjunction occurs more frequently with increasing maternal age (Table 18.2). Many pregnancies are now screened for chromosomal abnormalities by use of an algorithm that combines NT thickness and maternal age. This algorithm will give the pregnant woman the statistical likelihood of her pregnancy being affected with trisomy 21, 18 or 13. It does not provide a statistical risk for abnormalities other than the three trisomies.

## Combined test

The combined test uses information derived from the NT scan and two serum biochemical markers: pregnancy-associated plasma protein A (PAPP-A) and beta human chorionic gonadotrophin (β-hCG). Data from prospec-

tive studies suggest that use of NT measurement in isolation will detect approximately 70–75% of trisomy 21 pregnancies with a false-positive rate of 5%. By contrast, combining NT scanning with β-hCG and PAPP-A testing increases the trisomy 21 detection rate to nearer 90%.

## Other screening tests

Other screening options are shown in Table 18.8 and include the triple test, quadruple test, integrated test (which combines first-trimester and second-trimester risk assessment but with nondisclosure of first-trimester results) and sequential test (which involves disclosure of first-trimester results, which in turn determine whether subsequent serum screening is undertaken).

Some babies with trisomy 21 have recently been shown to have an absent or hypoplastic nasal bone on first-trimester ultrasound. Reverse flow in the ductus venosus has also been associated with trisomy 21 (Table 18.8). However, nasal-bone measurement and ductus-venosus blood-flow assessment should be used with caution because they are technically more difficult to perform than NT ultrasound.

TABLE 18.8 **Aneuploidy risk evaluation**

| Test | Effect in trisomy 21 pregnancy | Trisomy 21 detection rate |
|---|---|---|
| **FIRST TRIMESTER** | | |
| NT scan | ↑NT | 70–75% |
| NT scan + nasal-bone measurement | Absent or hypoplastic nasal bone | 80–85% |
| NT scan + assessment of blood flow in the ductus venosus | Absent or reversed A-wave | 80–85% |
| **COMBINED TEST SECOND TRIMESTER** | ↑NT + ↑β-hCG + ↓PAPP-A | 90% |
| Triple screen | ↓α-FP + ↑β-hCG + ↓uE$_3$ | 70% |
| Quadruple screen | ↓α-FP + ↑β-hCG + ↓uE$_3$ + ↑inh | 81% |
| **FIRST AND SECOND TRIMESTERS** | | |
| Integrated | ↑NT + ↓PAPP-A + quadruple screen | 86% |
| Sequential | ↑NT + ↓PAPP-A + quadruple screen but quadruple screen is only undertaken if NT scan and PAPP-A indicate a high risk | 95% |

↑ = increase  |  ↓ = decrease  |  α-FP = alphafetoprotein  |  β-hCG = beta-human chorionic gonadotrophin  |  inh = inhibin  |  NT = nuchal translucency  |  PAPP-A = pregnancy-associated plasma protein A  |  uE$_3$ = unconjugated estradiol

FIGURE 18.8 **Nuchal translucency scan showing an increase in subcutaneous fluid behind the baby's neck**

FIGURE 18.9 **Ultrasound-guided chorionic villus sampling showing a first-trimester placenta with a chorionic villus sampling needle in place**

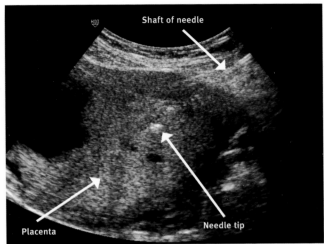

## DIAGNOSTIC TESTS

Diagnostic tests are undertaken if an increased aneuploidy risk is identified through screening, if the maternal age is advanced, if fetal abnormalities are identified on routine screening or if there is a family history of a genetic or chromosomal abnormality. The most commonly used diagnostic tests include measurement of maternal cell-free fetal DNA (cffDNA), CVS and amniocentesis.

### Cell-free fetal DNA in maternal blood

cffDNA in maternal blood is predominantly of placental origin and probably released during apoptosis of placental cells. During the early weeks of pregnancy, cffDNA constitutes 3.4% of the total cell-free DNA in maternal plasma but this figure doubles in later pregnancy. Current clinical applications for cffDNA measurement include gender determination and fetal rhesus D blood typing.

### Chorionic villus sampling

Following reports of possible fetal-limb abnormalities following early CVS, this investigation is currently performed no earlier than week 11 of gestation. CVS involves the aspiration of placental tissue (Figure 18.9). Chorionic

villi consist of two cell layers: the outer rapidly dividing and invading cytotrophoblast and the inner mesenchymal core. As the cytotrophoblast is actively dividing, it can be used in the direct evaluation of metaphases. This 'direct' result is usually available 2–3 days following the procedure. In addition to a direct preparation, a culture from the inner mesenchyme is also established. Cultures usually take 1–3 weeks before cells can be harvested and a result obtained. The mesenchymal core is usually considered to be more representative of the fetal cells than the cytotrophoblast as the latter cell line is established earlier in the process of fetoplacental differentiation. If an abnormal result is obtained from the direct preparation, it is therefore wise to wait for the results of the culture as the abnormality may be confined to the cytotrophoblast layer.

Confined placental mosaicism, where a chromosome abnormality is present in placental but not fetal tissue, is observed in a small (approximately 1.5%) number of CVS samples. Confined placental mosaicism should be considered if the CVS karyotype shows only a proportion of the cells to be affected with an abnormal karyotype or if the identified karyotype is not anticipated to be associated with fetal viability. If an abnormal karyotype is present in the placenta but not in the fetus, this may compromise placental functioning, resulting in restricted fetal growth and structural anomalies known to be associated with impaired blood supply.

### Amniocentesis

Amniocentesis is performed after week 15 of gestation. The amniocytes, cells derived from fetal skin, urinary tract and gastrointestinal tract, are aspirated and cultured. As the aspirate does not contain any rapidly dividing cells, a direct preparation is not available. Cells cultured from amniocytes are usually available to harvest 1–3 weeks after the procedure has been performed.

### Chorionic villus sampling versus amniocentesis

In the past, the miscarriage rate associated with CVS was reportedly higher than that associated with amniocentesis. However, increased use of, and expertise with CVS in recent years mean that the miscarriage rates quoted for amniocentesis and CVS are now more equal (in the order of 1%), although the exact figure depends upon the expertise at the centre where the procedure is undertaken. This equalisation of miscarriage rates has altered prenatal obstetric practice such that, in many centres, CVS is now performed in preference to amniocentesis. This is because CVS can be performed earlier in gestation, whereas amniocentesis cannot be performed until later in pregnancy. An additional advantage that CVS has over amniocentesis is the availability of a rapid result from a direct preparation.

However, cultured amniocytes are fetal cells and as such allow a direct assay of fetal chromosomes/genes. Therefore, if mosaicism is reported following an amniocentesis, this is probably a true reflection of a mosaic state in the fetus. By contrast, CVS involves assaying the placental cells and so there must always be a residual concern that any abnormal result is attributable to confined placental mosaicism, although the risk of this is low.

### Cordocentesis

Fetal blood, taken from the umbilical vein, may be sampled from week 18 of gestation. Before week 18, the vein is considered too small for cordocentesis. In addition to genetic/chromosomal investigations, which can be undertaken in cultured lymphocytes, fetal blood sampling is an important means of assessing anaemia and diagnosing prenatal infection. Disadvantages of cordocentesis include the associated miscarriage rate (1–2%)

and the technical demands of the procedure.

## CYTOGENETIC METHODS IN PRENATAL DIAGNOSIS

An overview of these methods is provided in Table 18.9.

### Conventional cytogenetic analysis

Before the advent of molecular techniques, chromosomes were exclusively analysed microscopically. To do this, cells (from blood, amniotic fluid, placenta, tumour or other tissues) are cultured, arrested midmitosis, lysed and then fixed before a specific banding agent is added. Banding techniques include the commonly used Giemsa banding (or G-banding) technique but alternative banding patterns can be generated using other techniques such as reverse banding (R-banding), quinacrine banding (Q-banding) or centromeric banding (C-banding).

### Fluorescence in situ hybridisation

In general, FISH is performed on interphase chromosomes and consists of a DNA probe labelled with a fluorophore. The probe is designed to anneal to one specific chromosome region and can be visualised using fluorescent microscopy.

FISH is useful in the following situations:

- detection of whole-chromosome aneuploidies (there will be three or one rather than two signals for a given chromosome)
- investigation of chromosome microdeletions not detectable with conventional G-banding methods (a specific FISH probe will be unable to anneal to the deleted region and so only one signal will be visualised)
- cytogenetic evaluation of structurally abnormal chromosomes such as derivative chromosomes associated with unbalanced or balanced Robertsonian or reciprocal translocations
- characterisation of supernumerary marker chromosomes.

Supernumerary marker chromosomes are identified in less than 1% of pregnancies and without FISH it is often very difficult to determine the origin of the chromosome material.

TABLE 18.9 **Comparison of the laboratory methods that may be employed in the analysis of chorionic villus sampling/amniocentesis**

| Test | Uses | Advantages | Disadvantages |
|---|---|---|---|
| FISH | Rapid aneuploidy detection<br><br>Evaluation of unbalanced translocations | A good technique for investigating predictable unbalanced chromosome rearrangement | Expensive<br><br>Labour-intensive |
| QF-PCR | Rapid aneuploidy detection | Rapid results<br><br>Cheap | Will usually only identify abnormal dosage involving chromosomes 13, 18 or 21 |
| MLPA | Rapid aneuploidy detection<br><br>Evaluation of unbalanced translocations | Rapid results | Limited genomic coverage |
| Array-CGH | Rapid aneuploidy detection<br><br>Detection of microdeletions<br><br>Detection of microduplications | Rapid results<br><br>Information about gene dosage throughout the genome | New assay, so unclear whether abnormal results are pathogenic variants or polymorphisms |

Array-CGH = microarray comparative genomic hybridisation  |  FISH = fluorescence *in situ* hybridisation  |  MLPA = multiplex ligation-dependent probe amplification  |  QF-PCR = quantitative fluorescence polymerase chain reaction

### Quantitative fluorescence polymerase chain reaction

As ultrasound and biochemical screening tests for fetal aneuploidy become more widely available, so the demand for a rapid, cost-effective diagnostic method has increased. Quantitative fluorescence polymerase chain reaction (QF-PCR) is now commonly used and involves amplification with fluorescent primers that target highly polymorphic short tandem repeats (STRs, consisting of repetitive sequences of one, two, three or maybe four bases) specific to the chromosomes of interest. In most centres, QF-PCR is restricted to investigating trisomy 13, 18 and 21 and possibly the sex chromosomes (primarily to identify 45,X) as abnormalities of these chromosomes account for 80% of clinically significant aneuploidies diagnosed in the prenatal setting.

The main advantages of QF-PCR are the speed with which results are available (1–2 days) and the relative cost-effectiveness compared with conventional cytogenetic techniques. The main disadvantage is that, in general, only STRs from chromosome 13, 18 and 21 are amplified and so other more complex chromosome rearrangements or abnormal dosage of other chromosomes are not identified.

### Multiplex ligation-dependent probe amplification

MLPA is a relatively new technique designed to detect dosage abnormalities (deletion or duplication) of specific genes, chromosome regions or whole chromosomes. It is different from QF-PCR in that it is the probe and not the DNA that is amplified and quantified.

Each MLPA probe consists of two oligonucleotides (short DNA sequences) that are designed to anneal to specific adjacent target DNA sequences. If both target sequences are present, the two annealed probes will be joined with a ligase and amplified using polymerase chain reaction (PCR). A computer programme calculates the relative quantities of the PCR products, which are compared with those of a control sample, and the result is presented as a ratio. A ratio of 1.0 indicates that both alleles are present; a ratio of 0.5 indicates that one allele is deleted and a ratio of 1.5 suggests that one allele is duplicated.

### Microarray comparative genomic hybridisation

Array-CGH uses DNA from the person being tested and compares it with that of a control person. Test and reference DNA are labelled with different coloured fluorophores, conventionally red and green. A prepared chip is used where each of many hundreds of different wells contains a unique sequence of DNA, either in the form of an oligonucleotide or in the form of a bacterial artificial chromosome (BAC). Target DNA sequences can vary in size from 25–85 base pairs (the oligonucleotides) to 80–200 base pairs (the BAC sequences). The spacing of the DNA sequences along the human genome will also vary from chip to chip such that some chips provide denser genomic coverage than others.

The huge advantage of array-CGH is that it can detect DNA dosage imbalance over the whole genome in a single simultaneous assay. The technique is therefore very good for identifying aneuploidies, microdeletions and microduplications.

## Genetics of gynaecological malignancies

Inherited gynaecological malignancies are rare. However, germline mutations within specific cancer-predisposing genes have been identified in a small minority of families with ovarian cancer or endometrial cancer.

### OVARIAN CANCER

The lifetime risk of developing ovarian cancer in the general population is in the order of one in 70. A small proportion of ovarian cancers are attributable to a familial predisposition, and the breast cancer susceptibility genes BRCA1 and BRCA2 together account for 6–8% of ovarian cancers. To a lesser extent, the mismatch repair genes MSH2, MLH1, MSH6 and PMS2 have been identified in families with ovarian cancer, usually in association with many other cancer types.

### BRCA1 and BRCA2

Alterations within the BRCA1 and BRCA2 genes are associated with an increased susceptibility to developing breast and ovarian cancer. In general, if a woman is found to have a mutation within the BRCA1 gene, she has a 60–90% lifetime risk of developing breast cancer and a 40–60% lifetime risk of developing ovarian cancer. A mutation within BRCA2 is also associated with a high lifetime risk (45–85%) of developing breast cancer but the risk of developing ovarian cancer (10–30%) is lower than that associated with BRCA1. However, the overall contribution of BRCA1 and BRCA2 to the prevalence of female breast cancer is less than 2%.

### Mismatch repair genes

Alterations within the mismatch repair genes MSH2, MLH2, MSH6 and PMS2 are associated with a spectrum of tumour types that most commonly include colorectal, endometrial, gastric and ovarian cancers. Together this tumour predisposition syndrome is known as hereditary nonpolyposis colon cancer (HNPCC). Mutations within one of these mismatch repair genes confer a lifetime risk of developing ovarian cancer in the order of 4%. This is a two- to three-fold increase over the lifetime risk of developing ovarian cancer in the general population.

### Surveillance and management of increased ovarian cancer susceptibility

Where a familial susceptibility to ovarian cancer has been identified, it is important to consider what kind of surveillance can be offered to carrier family members. Ovarian cancer screening is currently controversial and while many centres will offer a combination of serum CA125 measurement and ovarian ultrasonography, there is no consensus of opinion as to how frequently the tests should be undertaken. Some clinicians even argue that no screening would be preferable to that currently on offer, given that both CA125 and ultrasonography screening are associated with high rates of false-positive results (leading to unnecessary anxiety and possibly surgical intervention) and false-negative results (meaning that ovarian cancers are not being detected).

Indeed, given the limitations of current ovarian cancer screening, some women who are found to have a germline mutation in BRCA1 or BRCA2 opt for a bilateral salpingo-oophorectomy (BSO). This has the advantage of nearly eliminating their ovarian cancer risk (there is a small residual risk, equivalent to 1%, of primary peritoneal ovarian cancer) and halving their breast cancer risk but it also has the disadvantage of precipitating an abrupt menopause. Current practice is to advise carriers of *BRCA* mutations who have completed their family to consider BSO as a method of managing their breast and ovarian cancer risk.

## ENDOMETRIAL CANCER

An inherited susceptibility to uterine cancer (lifetime risk approximately 50%) is conferred by the mismatch repair genes associated with HNPCC. Unfortunately, screening (for example by use of Pipelle biopsy) is neither optimal nor universally available and so women are advised to monitor the regularity of periods and act if postmenopausal bleeding occurs. Some women will consider a prophylactic hysterectomy.

In addition, a predisposition to endometrial cancer is associated with Peutz–Jegher syndrome and Cowden disease. Peutz–Jegher syndrome, caused by mutations within the gene encoding serine/threonine protein kinase 11 (*LKB1*), is associated with pigmented macules of the mucous membranes and skin, gastrointestinal polyps and a predisposition to cancers including gastrointestinal cancer (lifetime risk approximately 30%) and endometrial cancer (lifetime risk approximately 40%). Cowden disease is caused by germline mutations within the gene encoding phosphatase and tensin homologue (*PTEN*). It is characterised by multiple hamartomas and an increased risk of breast, thyroid and endometrial cancers. The lifetime risk of endometrial cancer in *PTEN* carriers has not yet been ascertained.

## Sample questions relating to single-gene and chromosome abnormalities

### EXTENDED MATCHING QUESTIONS

#### Questions 1–3

■ *This question relates to autosomal dominant mutations. For each item below, choose the **single** best option from the list of options (A–F). Each option may be used once, more than once or not at all.*

OPTIONS

▷ **A** Marfan syndrome
▷ **B** Neurofibromatosis type 1
▷ **C** Breast/ovarian cancer susceptibility
▷ **D** Hereditary nonpolyposis colon cancer (HNPCC)
▷ **E** Autosomal dominant polycystic kidney disease
▷ **F** Achondroplasia

**1** ▶ Condition characterised by a combination of café-au-lait spots and neurofibromata

**2** ▶ Condition characterised by tall stature and aortic dilatation

**3** ▶ Systemic disorder with cysts in the liver, pancreas and spleen

### MULTIPLE CHOICE QUESTIONS

**4** ▶ Regarding chromosomes:

   **A** ▷ Humans have 23 pairs of autosomal chromosomes
   **B** ▷ The centromere always lies at the centre of each chromosome
   **C** ▷ The p arm is the long arm
   **D** ▷ Submetacentric chromosomes have the centromere at the top of the chromosome
   **E** ▷ The numbering of chromosomes is done according to their length

**5** ▶ Nondisjunction:

   **A** ▷ results in aneuploidy
   **B** ▷ occurs because of chromosome nonseparation in meiosis II
   **C** ▷ occurs because sister chromatids fail to separate during mitotic anaphase
   **D** ▷ causes trisomies
   **E** ▷ causes monosomies

**6** ▶ The following pregnancy outcomes are possible if a parent has a balanced reciprocal translocation:

   **A** ▷ A normal pregnancy with the child having a normal karyotype
   **B** ▷ A normal pregnancy with the child having a balanced translocation
   **C** ▷ A spontaneous miscarriage because the child has a balanced translocation
   **D** ▷ A term pregnancy with the child having an increased chance of developmental delay because of a balanced translocation
   **E** ▷ A term pregnancy with the child having an increased chance of developmental delay because of an unbalanced translocation

**7** ▶ Regarding common trisomic conditions:

   **A** ▷ Ninety-five percent of Down syndrome occurrences are caused by nondisjunction
   **B** ▷ All individuals with Down syndrome have some learning difficulties
   **C** ▷ Patau syndrome is associated with holoprosencephaly
   **D** ▷ Patau syndrome is associated with diaphragmatic hernias
   **E** ▷ Edwards syndrome is associated with blindness

**8** ▶ Regarding common trisomic conditions:

   **A** ▷ Individuals with Down syndrome have a ten-fold increased risk of atrioventricular septal defect
   **B** ▷ People with Down syndrome are scaphocephalic
   **C** ▷ Patau syndrome is associated with polydactyly
   **D** ▷ Patau syndrome is associated with duodenal atresia
   **E** ▷ Edwards syndrome is associated with acute lymphoblastic anaemia

**9 ▶** Regarding Klinefelter syndrome:

**A** ▷ It is usually picked up on ultrasound
**B** ▷ It is associated with short stature
**C** ▷ Those affected are infertile
**D** ▷ Those affected develop gynaecomastia
**E** ▷ Those affected are more likely to be homosexual

**10 ▶** Regarding autosomal recessive diseases:

**A** ▷ Both inherited genes are affected
**B** ▷ If both parents are carriers, then 50% of children will have the condition
**C** ▷ If both parents are carriers, then 75% of children will be normal or carriers
**D** ▷ There is an increased risk of these diseases in consanguineous marriages
**E** ▷ They usually skip a generation

**11 ▶** Regarding screening tests for trisomy 21:

**A** ▷ The triple test has a trisomy 21 detection rate of 60%
**B** ▷ The combined test includes a nuchal translucency scan and measurement of beta-human chorionic gonadotrophin and pregnancy-associated plasma protein A (PaPP-A)
**C** ▷ The combined test has a trisomy 21 detection rate of 80%
**D** ▷ The quadruple test includes a measurement of PaPP-A
**E** ▷ The quadruple test is carried out in the first trimester

**12 ▶** Regarding diagnostic tests:

**A** ▷ Cell-free fetal DNA is measured to determine the rhesus status of the fetus
**B** ▷ Chorionic villus sampling is best carried out after week 13 of gestation
**C** ▷ Cytotrophoblast cells are more representative of fetal cells than the placental mesechyme
**D** ▷ Direct cell preparation is used in amniocentesis
**E** ▷ Cordocentesis is only done after week 22 of gestation

# Immunology

CHAPTER 19    Basic immunology

CHAPTER 19

# Basic immunology

*Sharon Cookson and Ian Sargent*

## Organisation of the immune system

The main function of the immune system is to protect the host from invasion by infectious organisms. Immune responses are comprised of:

- rapid, nonspecific reactions against foreign invaders (innate immunity)

- antigen-specific reactions that 'recognise' the pathogenic organism both during initial infection and upon subsequent contact with the same organism (adaptive immunity).

The innate immune response is mediated principally by macrophages and neutrophils and by soluble circulating molecules such as complement proteins. The adaptive immune response is mediated by T cells and B cells.

The innate and adaptive arms of the immune system must interact to generate an effective immune response. Cytokines are key molecules that control this interaction.

Table 19.1 and Table 19.2 provide an overview of innate compared with adaptive immunity and of the cells of the immune system, respectively.

## Innate immune response

### CELLS OF THE INNATE IMMUNE SYSTEM

#### Phagocytes

Phagocytes are derived from the bone marrow and their primary function is to engulf, ingest and destroy (phagocytose) exogenous or endogenous particles such as infectious agents and cellular debris. Phagocytes are attracted by chemokines and activated by cytokines that have been secreted by antigen-specific T cells. Thus, the innate and adaptive arms of the immune system are intrinsically linked.

**TABLE 19.1 Comparison of innate and adaptive immunity**

| Parameter of comparison | Innate | Adaptive |
|---|---|---|
| Response time | Hours | Days |
| Specificity | Limited | Diverse |
| Memory | None | Efficient |
| Response to repeat infection | Identical to primary response | Much more rapid and vigorous than primary response |
| Cellular components | Phagocytes, natural killer cells | T cells, B cells |
| Humoral components | Complement | Antibody |

TABLE 19.2 **Immune cells in adult blood**

| Type of cell | Proportion of total leucocytes |
|---|---|
| **NEUTROPHILS** | 50–70% |
| **LYMPHOCYTES** | 20–40% |
| T cells | 70–85%[a] |
| B cells | 10–15%[a] |
| Natural killer cells | 10%[a] |
| **MONOCYTES** | 1–6% |
| **EOSINOPHILS** | 1–3% |
| **BASOPHILS** | <1% |
| **DENDRITIC** cells | <1% |

[a] Proportion of total lymphocytes

There are two basic types of phagocyte:

- the monocyte/macrophage lineage
- granulocytes, which may be subdivided into neutrophils, mast cells, basophils and eosinophils.

Each cell type has distinct effector functions. Monocytes are short-lived cells that circulate in the blood for a few hours before migrating into tissues and differentiating into mature macrophages. They express three distinct receptors for the crystallisable fragment (Fc) region of immunoglobulin G (IgG): Fc gamma receptor I (FcγRI; high affinity), FcγRII (medium affinity) and FcγRIII (CD16; low affinity).

Tissue macrophages are long-lived. They bind to microorganisms via their Fc receptors if the pathogen is coated with antibody or via their complement receptors if the bacteria have been opsonised with complement. Following binding, macrophages phagocytose and kill microorganisms. Internalised microorganisms can be processed and presented as peptides to T cells, thus triggering the adaptive arm of the immune response.

Dendritic cells are an additional phagocytic cell type derived from monocytes or from lymphoid lineages. This is the only cell type whose sole function is to capture, process and present antigen to T cells, that is, they are 'professional' antigen-presenting cells (APCs).

Neutrophils are the most abundant type of circulatory phagocyte, comprising the majority of leucocytes in the blood. These cells recognise and kill invading microorganisms (mainly bacteria), either by phagocytosis or by the release of granules and cytotoxic substances, which can occur when neutrophils are activated through their Fc or complement receptors. Neutrophils are short-lived, surviving only a few days; once they have phagocytosed material and destroyed it, they die.

Mast cells are located in the skin, mucosal surfaces and around blood vessels. They are phagocytic and express Fc receptors specific for the antibody immunoglobulin (IgE). Activation results in the release of a wide range of mediators including histamine, heparin, prostaglandin and a variety of cytokines and chemokines, which induce or control inflammation in the surrounding tissues.

Basophils are phenotypically similar to mast cells and also have receptors for IgE. They circulate in the blood and may not be phagocytic.

Eosinophils are a highly specialised group of leucocytes. They principally reside in tissues such as the respiratory and gut subepithelia, where they attach to the surface of parasites such as schistosomes. Following attachment, the eosinophils degranulate and release proteins that damage the parasite membrane. Degranulation releases cytokines, which amplify the immune response.

### Natural killer cells

Natural killer (NK) cells bridge the innate and adaptive arms of the immune system. NK cells are large granular lymphocytes that represent a morphologically distinct population and display cytotoxic activity against a wide range of tumour cells and virally infected cells. They can distinguish these targets from normal cells by means of two different types of receptor on their surface:

- FcγRIII (CD16) receptors, which attach to specific antibodies bound to tumour cells or virally infected cells in a process called antibody-dependent cell-mediated cytotoxicity
- killer cell immunoglobulin-like receptors (KIRs), a heterogeneous group that includes both activating and inhibitory cell surface receptors that engage class I major histocompatibility complex (MHC) molecules on target cells.

Healthy cells expressing self-MHC class I molecules are protected from NK cell lysis but some disease processes (for example many tumours) cause a downregulation of MHC class I. The cytolytic activity of NK cells is regulated by KIRs that detect the absence of MHC class I expression on target cells.

The mechanisms for NK cell killing resemble those for cytotoxic T cells described later in this chapter. Like phagocytes, NK cells can be activated by cytokines, such as interleukin-2 (IL-2) and interferon gamma (IFN-γ), secreted from activated T cells.

## COMPLEMENT SYSTEM

The complement system consists of a series of approximately 20 serum proteins that together constitute almost 10% of the total serum proteins, thereby making it one of the major immune defence systems of the body. The major function of the complement system is to remove or destroy antigen. Activation of complement has three main consequences:

- lysis of microorganisms, enveloped viruses and *Plasma membrane* infected cells by damaging the plasma membrane
- opsonisation, that is, coating of foreign particles with complement protein fragments; phagocytes expressing receptors for these complement components are then able to bind to the target and phagocytose it
- triggering of the complement cascade (forming a bridge between the adaptive and innate immune responses).

Complement components are largely designated by numerals (C1–C9) and activated in a cascade such that a small initial stimulus can rapidly cause a large effect. Many cells express receptors for one or more complement products. When activated, a component is able to cleave the next component in the sequence into two or more fragments:

- the minor fragments (designated the suffix 'a', as in C3a) diffuse from the site of activation and are able to initiate a local inflammatory response by binding to specific receptors
- the major fragment (designated the suffix 'b', as in C3b) binds to the target cell membrane.

## Mechanism of complement activation

Complement may be activated by one of three pathways, depending upon composition of the initial stimulus:

- classic pathway — *adaptive*
- alternative pathway ⎫ *innate*
- lectin pathway. ⎭

Central to all three is cleavage of the most abundant complement protein, C3, followed by activation of the lytic sequence (Figure 19.1).

The classic pathway is initiated by the binding of antibody to antigen, with the antibody being either IgG or immunoglobulin (IgM) bound to the surface of a pathogen. Formation of an antigen–antibody complex causes a conformational change in the Fc portion of the antibody that exposes a binding site for the first complement component, C1q.

The alternative pathway does not require antibody. It is activated by the binding of C3b to hydroxyl and amine groups on the surface of pathogens, including many Gram-positive and Gram-negative bacteria. This path-

FIGURE 19.1  **Pathways of complement activation**

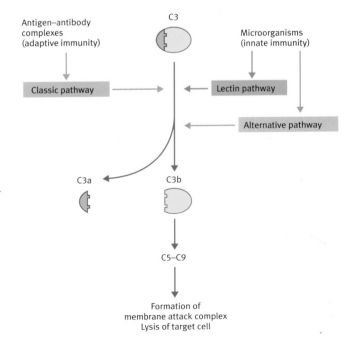

way is relatively inefficient because its activation requires high concentrations of the various components.

The mannose-binding lectin pathway is more efficient than the alternative pathway. It is initiated by the binding of lectin to glycoproteins or carbohydrates on the surface of pathogens, including Gram-positive and Gram-negative bacteria.

All three pathways of activation converge at the final lytic sequence. Here, C5, C6, C7, C8 and C9 sequentially interact to form a membrane attack complex, which binds to the membrane of the target forming a trans-membrane channel through which salts and water can flow, resulting in lysis of the target cell.

The classic pathway links to the adaptive immune system because its activation requires that the host has previously encountered the target and has generated an antibody response to it. The alternative and lectin pathways are considered to be part of the innate immune system because they are activated by microorganisms rather than antibody.

The importance of complement is readily apparent in individuals who lack particular components. For example, classic-pathway deficiencies result in tissue inflammation and individuals with C3 deficiencies are subject to overwhelming bacterial infections.

## LIMITATIONS OF INNATE IMMUNITY

Although innate immunity can provide a line of defence against many common microorganisms, such as bacteria, yeasts and parasites, there are many more-sophisticated pathogens, such as viruses or intracellular microorganisms, that the cells of the innate immune system cannot recognise or effectively destroy. This limitation has been addressed by the evolution of the adaptive immune system as a more versatile and adaptable means of host defence.

# Adaptive immune response

Adaptive immune responses are mediated by lymphocytes that have the capacity to recognise foreign antigens and distinguish them from self-antigens. In many instances this mechanism confers lifelong protective immunity against re-infection with the same pathogen, which can be intracellular or extracellular.

There are two basic lymphocyte categories: bursa-equivalent cells (B cells) and thymus-derived cells (T cells) (Table 19.2).

## B CELLS

B cells are so called because of their similarity to lymphocytes found in the bursa of Fabricius organ in birds. B cells develop in the bone marrow, are found in all lymphoid tissues and represent up to 15% of the circulating lymphoid pool. Antibodies on the surface of B cells serve as antigen receptors and binding initiates a series of events whereby antigen is internalised, degraded, complexed with MHC class II molecules and returned to the cell surface. This peptide–MHC complex can then be presented to antigen-specific T cells, which secrete cytokines and induce clonal B cell proliferation and differentiation into antibody-producing plasma cells.

### Antibodies

Antibodies, also known as immunoglobulins, are a particularly effective means of combating extracellular organisms such as bacteria, and are efficient at neutralising circulating viruses. In mammals, there are five distinct classes of immunoglobulin (Table 19.3): IgG, IgM, IgA, IgE and IgD. All are made up of a unit comprising two identical light chains and two identical heavy chains but they differ in size, charge, carbohydrate content and amino acid sequence (Figure 19.2). It is the type of heavy chain that determines the class and subclass of antibody; for example, IgM has a mu heavy chain, whereas IgA1 and A2 have alpha 1 and alpha 2 heavy chains, respectively.

Different parts of an antibody have distinct functions. The antigen-binding fragment (Fab) region comprises the amino-terminal domains of each heavy and light chain (referred to as the variable region) and forms the antigen-binding site, thereby determining the antibody's antigen specificity. The other part of the antibody, the Fc region, comprises the carboxy-terminal domains of each heavy and light chain (referred to as the constant region). The Fc region determines which effector function will be activated.

All immunoglobulin isotypes, with the exception of IgD, are bifunctional in that they do not only recognise and bind antigen but they also exhibit one or more effector functions.

TABLE 19.3 **Properties and biological activities of immunoglobulin isotypes**

| Property | IgM | IgG | IgA | IgE | IgD |
|---|---|---|---|---|---|
| Heavy chain | Mu | Gamma | Alpha | Epsilon | Delta |
| Normal serum level (mg/ml) | 1.5 | 13.5 | 3.0 | 0.0003 | 0.03 |
| Activates classic complement pathway | + | + | – | – | – |
| Binds to phagocyte Fc receptors | ? | + | – | – | – |
| Present on membrane of mature B cells | + | – | – | – | + |
| Transported in mucosal secretions | – | – | + | – | – |
| Induces mast cell degranulation | – | – | – | + | – |
| Crosses placenta | – | + | – | – | – |

Fc = crystallisable fragment | Ig = immunoglobulin | + = yes | – = no | ? = not known

IgM comprises 5–10% of the serum immunoglobulin pool. It is secreted from plasma cells as a pentamer and is largely confined to the intravascular pool. IgM is the first antibody formed in a primary response to an antigen and is also the first antibody to be synthesised by the newborn baby, but it is unable to cross the placenta. This immunoglobulin is a potent activator of the classic pathway of complement owing to its five complement-binding sites.

IgG comprises 70–80% of the serum immunoglobulin pool. It is the predominant antibody of secondary immune responses and equilibrates between the intravascular and extravascular pools. There are four subclasses with unique effector functions:

- IgG1, IgG3 and IgG4 readily cross the placenta and have an important role in protecting the developing fetus.
- IgG1 and IgG3 are extremely efficient in activating complement via the classic pathway, IgG2 less so.
- IgG1 and IgG3 bind with high affinity to Fc receptors on phagocytic cells and thereby mediate opsonisation.

IgA constitutes 10–20% of the serum immunoglobulin pool. It is the predominant antibody in secretions such as saliva, tears and mucus of the bronchial, digestive and genitourinary tracts. Breast milk is also rich in secretory IgA, which protects the newborn against infection during the first few months of life. IgA participates in secondary immune responses. IgA-containing immune complexes opsonise antigens and induce phagocytosis through Fc receptors. Binding of secretory IgA to microbial antigens prevents their attachment to mucosal cells, thus inhibiting infection and colonisation.

IgE achieves very low serum levels. It binds with high affinity to specific receptors on mast cells and basophils. Cross-linkage of bound IgE by antigen causes degranulation and release of a range of pharmacologically active mediators. IgE can give rise to a variety of allergic manifestations.

IgD comprises less than 0.5% of the serum immunoglobulin pool. It has no known effector functions as a serum protein; instead, it functions as a transmembrane antigen receptor on mature B cells.

### Vaccination

The importance of antibody to host defence comes into play when considering the crucial role it plays during vaccination. During infection, a primary antibody response is launched to eliminate the pathogen. This also leads to the generation of long-lived antigen-specific memory B cells, which are restimulated upon subsequent exposure to the same pathogen, resulting in a faster and much more intense secondary response.

FIGURE 19.2 **Structure of immunoglobulins**

**A** Immunoglobulin M

**B** Immunoglobulin G

**C** Immunoglobulin A

Cα = alpha heavy chain |
Cδ = delta heavy chain |
Cε = epsilon heavy chain |
C$_H$ = heavy chain of the
constant region |
C$_L$ = light chain of the
constant region |
Cμ = mu heavy chain |
Fab = antigen-binding
fragment |
Fc = crystallisable fragment |
V$_L$ = light chain of the
variable region |
V$_H$ = heavy chain of the
variable region

*Reproduced by permission:*
*Immunology.* 6th ed. Roitt IM,
Brostoff J, Male D. St Louis: Mosby;
2002.

**D** Immunoglobulin E

**E** Immunoglobulin D

It is important to realise that antibodies do not recognise the whole microorganism but particular parts of antigens called epitopes. Successful vaccine development therefore relies upon modification of a pathogen so that it retains its antigenicity (that is, it is still able to generate a primary antibody response) but is innocuous. In essence then, a vaccine essentially replaces the initial infection but still leads to the generation of memory B cells. This consequently provides immunity to vaccinated individuals such that when they are exposed to the microorganism in question, they are able to mount a quick and effective secondary response, leading to protection from and elimination of the pathogen.

## T CELLS

T cells are the principal mediators of the adaptive immune response and exhibit a wide variety of effector functions including target-cell lysis and cytokine release, which can cause proliferation, differentiation or activation of many different cells of the immune system. Antigen recognition takes place through the T cell receptor (TCR).

Two types of TCR have been characterised:

- alpha/beta TCRs, which are expressed on more than 95% of circulating T cells
- gamma/delta TCRs, which are rarely expressed on peripheral-blood T cells but are present on populations of T cells in mucosal surfaces (small intestine, pregnant uterus) and liver.

### T cell maturation

Alpha/beta T cells are generated in the bone marrow and recognise nonself antigens that are presented by self-MHC class I or class II molecules on the surface of APCs. This specificity is the result of a rigorous selection process.

Following TCR gene rearrangement in the thymus, immature T cells (thymocytes) that recognise self-MHC molecules expressed on cortical epithelial cells with high affinity are positively selected. Those cells that are not selected undergo death by apoptosis.

As the thymocytes migrate to the deeper cortex, they increase their expression of TCR and the cell surface molecules CD3, CD4 and CD8. Those TCRs that recognise self-antigens with high affinity are deleted by a process called negative selection. T cells at this stage of maturation go on to express TCRs at high density and to lose either CD4 or CD8, becoming single-positive (positive for either CD4 or CD8) mature thymocytes.

The mature cells leave the thymus and travel to the secondary lymphoid tissues and periphery, where they have the potential to function as one of the following, depending on whether they express CD4 or CD8:

- T helper (Th) cells, which are CD4-positive and MHC class II restricted
- cytotoxic T (Tc) cells, which are CD8-positive and MHC class I restricted.

T cells that express a gamma/delta TCR are also generated from bone marrow precursors but differ from T cells that express alpha/beta TCRs in their specificity (they are MHC-unrestricted) and expression of CD4 and CD8 (they are predominantly double-negative).

The mechanism by which T cells become committed to one or the other of these two TCR cell types is largely unknown.

### CD4-positive T cells

CD4 is a transmembrane protein that is expressed on T cells and macrophages. It serves as a cell adhesion molecule, facilitating TCR/CD3-mediated signal transduction upon binding of MHC class II molecules on APCs.

CD4-positive T cells can be categorised as Th1 or Th2 cells according to the pattern of cytokines they secrete (Figure 19.3 A):

- Th1 cells produce IFN-γ and IL-2, which activate macrophages and CD8-positive T cells, promoting cell-mediated immunity.
- Th2 cells secrete IL-4 and IL-5, which stimulate B cells to produce antibody, promoting humoral (that is, antibody-mediated) immunity.

Following stimulation by antigen, naïve CD4-positive T cells produce IL-2 and subsequently polarise towards a Th1 or Th2 phenotype, depending on signals received during and after activation (Figure 19.3A). IFN-γ and IL-12 enhance Th1 development, whereas IL-4 promotes differentiation into Th2 cells. The type of APC and the antigen dose may also have a role. It is likely that the polarisation to a Th1 or Th2 immune response occurs

FIGURE 19.3 **Generation of Th1 and Th2 CD4-positive subsets**

**A** Nonpregnant women

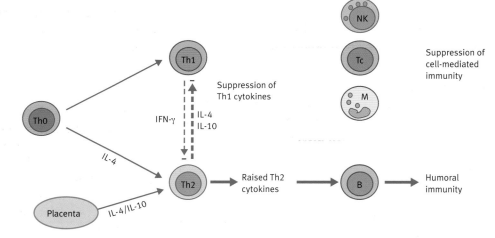

**B** Pregnant women (normal pregnancy)

B = B cell |
GM-CSF = granulocyte–macrophage colony-stimulating factor |
IFN-γ = interferon gamma |
IL = interleukin | M = macrophage |
NK = natural killer cell |
Tc = cytotoxic T cell |
Th = T helper cell |
TNF-α = tumour necrosis factor alpha

through the complex interaction of various factors, rather than on the basis of any single criterion.

Other CD4-positive T cell types are Th3, Th0 and type 1 regulatory T (Tr1) cells:

- Th3 cells produce high amounts of transforming growth factor beta (TGF-β).
- Th0 cells express both Th1 and Th2 cytokines.
- Tr1 cells secrete high levels of IL-10 (and little or no IL-2 and IL-4) leading to immune suppression.

### CD8-positive T cells

CD8 serves as a cell adhesion molecule by binding to MHC class I, thereby stabilising the interaction of a class I restricted T cell with a target cell or APC. CD8 expression predominantly identifies a subset of T cells called Tc cells. These can kill tumour cells or virally infected cells following appropriate priming and activation.

In addition to their cytotoxic activity, CD8-positive T cells can also secrete distinct patterns of cytokines. As with CD4-positive cells, CD8-positive precursors can be driven toward a type 1 cytotoxic (Tc1) phenotype by IL-12 and IFN-γ, whereas IL-4 induces the generation of Tc2 cells. Both of these phenotypes retain cytolytic function.

## CYTOKINES

Cytokines are molecules produced by a variety of cell types, including monocytes, macrophages, lymphocytes, endothelial cells, fibroblasts and tissue epithelia, and provide a link between the innate and adaptive immune responses. Although they are often described as hormone-like, cytokines differ from hormones in that their effects are predominantly exerted at a local level. Cytokines are low-molecular-weight proteins that act at very low concentrations by binding to specific cell surface receptors.

A cytokine may act in one of three ways:

■ in an autocrine fashion by binding to receptors on the membrane of the cell that secreted it
■ in a paracrine fashion by binding to receptors on cells in the immediate vicinity
■ in an endocrine fashion by binding to distant cells.

Cytokines can be subdivided into categories (such as interferons, interleukins, chemokines, growth factors) according to their primary function, although there is considerable overlap between these groups.

### Interferons

This family of molecules was first recognised by their ability to inhibit viral replication. They are produced early in infection and are pivotal in controlling the spread of a virus until adaptive immunity has had a chance to develop.

IFN-α and IFN-β are produced by virally infected leucocytes and fibroblasts, respectively.

IFN-γ is a product of activated Th1 and NK cells. It has the following functions:

■ antiviral effects
■ increasing the expression of both MHC class I and MHC class II molecules
■ activating macrophages and NK cells
■ promoting cytotoxic susceptibility of target cells
■ polarising Th0 cells to the Th1 phenotype.

### Interleukins

Interleukins are a large and diverse group of cytokines with a wide range of functions. They are predominantly secreted by lymphocytes. The most important immunoregulatory interleukins are listed in Table 19.4.

### Proinflammatory cytokines

Two cytokines are principally responsible for the early inflammatory reaction that occurs in response to microbial invasion:

■ IL-1, produced by macrophages and B cells, activates lymphocytes (T cells, B cells and NK cells) and increases the expression of adhesion molecules on endothelial cells.
■ Tumour necrosis factor alpha (TNF-α) exerts similar effects to IL-1 but is primarily produced by macrophages and activated T cells.

Macrophages are stimulated to produce IL-1 and TNF-α by oxidative stress or by endotoxins such as bacterial lipopolysaccharide.

### Chemokines

Chemokines are a group of chemotactic cytokines that are involved in cell migration, activation and chemotaxis. They diffuse from the site of production (for example tissue leucocytes, endothelium) to form a concentration gradient along which circulating leucocytes can migrate towards the stimulus.

Specific chemokine receptors are selectively expressed on particular populations of leucocytes and this is what determines which cells a chemokine will attract. Some receptors (for example chemokine C-C motif receptor 5 or CCR5) are expressed preferentially by Th1 cells, while others (such as CCR3 and CCR4) are characteristic of Th2 cells.

### Growth factors

Growth factors are required for the differentiation of haematopoietic cells. Granulocyte–macrophage colony-stimulating factor (GM-CSF), released by macrophages, T cells

TABLE **19.4** Biological activities of the most important interleukins

| Name | Cells secreting this interleukin | Biological function |
| --- | --- | --- |
| IL-1 | Macrophages and monocytes | Has proinflammatory effects |
| IL-2 | T cells | Acts as a growth factor for T cells |
| | | Stimulates proliferation and differentiation of T cells |
| | | Increases the cytolytic activity of NK cells |
| IL-4 | Th2 cells | Promotes proliferation and differentiation of B cells |
| | | Upregulates B-cell HLA class II expression |
| IL-10 | T cells, B cells, monocytes and mast cells | Has potent anti-inflammatory effects |
| | | Inhibits the synthesis of IL-2 and IFN-$\gamma$ by Th1 cells |
| | | Regulates growth and differentiation of B cells |
| | | Enhances expression of HLA class II |
| IL-12[a] | Macrophages, dendritic cells and B cells | Enhances the cytolytic activity of CD8$^+$ T cells and NK cells |
| | | Directs the immune response towards a Th1-type bias by inducing the secretion of IFN-$\gamma$, IL-2 and TNF-$\alpha$ |

[a] Secretion strongly induced by bacteria, bacterial products and certain parasites. | CD8$^+$ = CD8-positive | HLA = human leucocyte antigen | IFN = interferon | IL = interleukin | NK = natural killer | Th = T helper | TNF-$\alpha$ = tumour necrosis factor alpha

and fibroblasts, induces the development of nonlymphoid cells such as granulocytes and activates macrophages and eosinophils. TGF-$\beta$ modulates the immune response by inhibiting the proliferation of T and B cells and suppressing the activities of macrophages and NK cells.

## MAJOR HISTOCOMPATIBILITY COMPLEX

T cells cannot respond to protein antigens unless they have been processed and presented as short peptides, complexed with MHC molecules, on the surface of an APC. The MHC is conventionally divided into three sub-regions: class I, class II and class III. Class I and class II molecules are closely related in structure and function, whereas class III molecules show little structural similarity. The genes that encode the human MHC, also known as human leucocyte antigen (HLA), have been mapped to chromosome 6p21.3.

### Class I major histocompatibility complex

There are two major groups of class I MHC antigens:

- 'classic' class I molecules (HLA-A, HLA-B and HLA-C)
- 'nonclassic' class I molecules (HLA-E, HLA-F and HLA-G).

The classic molecules are constitutively expressed on most nucleated cells. They are highly polymorphic, with over 500 *HLA-A*, over 900 *HLA-B* and over 300 *HLA-C* alleles being described.

The nonclassic molecules have a limited polymorphism and their tissue expression is also limited. HLA-E and HLA-F are expressed on a variety of adult and fetal tissues, while HLA-G is predominantly restricted to the invasive extravillous cytotrophoblast tissue of the placenta.

Class I molecules present peptides of eight to nine amino acids in length, predominantly derived from within the cell cytoplasm (endogenous antigens, such as viruses), to CD8-positive T cells. The Tc cells are then able to kill the infected cells and eliminate the pathogen.

### Class II major histocompatibility complex

The MHC class II region encodes more than 30 proteins, including HLA-DR, HLA-DQ and HLA-DP. These antigens are highly polymorphic (with over 800 alleles having been described) and are expressed on specialised APCs including monocytes, macrophages, B cells and dendritic cells.

Compared with the peptide-binding groove of class I molecules, the class II peptide-binding groove is more open-ended, allowing longer peptides of 15–24 amino acids to bind. Class II molecules present antigenic peptides derived from outside the cell (exogenous antigens) to CD4-positive T cells.

### Class III major histocompatibility complex

The MHC class III region contains a large number of genes, most of which encode a diverse range of serum and plasma proteins. These include the complement components C2 and C4 and complement factor Bf, some heat shock proteins (HSP70, HSP71 and HSP72) and the proinflammatory cytokine TNF-α.

## Transplantation

Transplantation refers to the act of transferring cells, tissues or organs from one site to another. It is the only treatment for end-stage organ failure but its success largely depends upon the level of disparity between graft donor and recipient. There are four main types of transplant:

- An autograft is tissue transferred from one part of the body to another in the same individual, for example skin grafting in people with burns.
- An isograft is tissue transferred between genetically identical individuals, for example monozygotic twins.
- An allograft is tissue transferred between genetically different members of the same species.
- A xenograft is tissue transferred between different species, for example the graft of a pig heart into a human.

Thus, autografts and isografts are usually accepted by the host but allografts and xenografts are recognised as foreign by the recipient's immune system and, unless treated, will be rejected. This latter phenomenon is principally attributable to recipient T cells recognising allogeneic MHC antigens, a process known as allorecognition.

### ALLORECOGNITION

The immune response against a transplanted organ is much more vigorous than the response seen against a pathogen. Since isolated MHC antigens in themselves are considered to be poor immunogens that do not induce graft rejection, other factors in addition to MHC incompatibility must be responsible for the allograft response.

The presence of MHC-incompatible dendritic cells (passenger dendritic cells) in a recently transplanted graft has been shown to be of crucial importance in this context. These cells can present donor-derived peptides in the binding groove of donor MHC molecules and, being professional APCs, they are able to activate naïve T cells (that is, T cells that have never encountered antigen before).

In addition, the strength of the alloresponse is attributable to the fact that the normal T cell repertoire contains a high proportion of T cells that are capable of recognising the MHC molecules on the graft as foreign and reacting against them.

It is important to note that minor histocompatibility antigens can also be targets of rejection even when the MHC is identical between donor and recipient. The most important example is the histocompatibility antigen H-Y, which is encoded by the Y chromosome and hence expressed only on male cells.

### GRAFT-VERSUS-HOST DISEASE

In certain circumstances, for example during bone marrow transplantation, it is the graft that initiates a rejection response against the recipient. Immune-competent donor T cells that reside in the graft recognise the recipient's MHC and/or minor histocompatibility antigens as being foreign and initiate an immune response against the host. This reaction is known as graft-versus-host disease and can be prevented by careful matching of the donor and recipient, removal of all T cells from the graft and effective immunosuppression.

## TYPES OF REJECTION

### Hyperacute rejection

Hyperacute rejection occurs within minutes to hours of connecting the host's circulation to the transplanted organ. It is defined as a severe immunological response to the graft, mediated by preformed, naturally occurring antibodies that react against antigens expressed on donor cells. For example, it may occur as a result of ABO blood group incompatibility or, because the recipient has been sensitised to the donor MHC (for example by a previous transplant). Antibody binding initiates an immunological cascade, with complement activation, increased vascular leakage, activation of the coagulation process and increased expression of adhesion molecules; the end result is rapid destruction of the graft.

### Acute rejection

Acute rejection is normally seen days to weeks after transplantation. It is caused by donor leucocytes (so-called passenger leucocytes) migrating out of the graft and initiating a primary immune response. Activated recipient T cells then migrate to the organ and initiate tissue damage by the induction of delayed (type IV) hypersensitivity reactions and by the generation of Tc cells.

### Chronic rejection

Chronic rejection occurs months to years after transplantation. It is less understood than hyperacute or acute rejection. Occlusion of blood vessels, macrophage infiltration and smooth muscle proliferation lead to blockage of the blood vessels and ischaemia of the graft.

## METHODS TO PREVENT REJECTION

Two major methods are employed to minimise graft rejection:

- donor and recipient matching
- use of immunosuppressive drugs.

Table 19.5 provides an overview of drugs that are commonly used to prevent graft rejection.

### Human leucocyte antigen matching

Human MHC class I and class II antigens display extensive polymorphism and the chances of matching an unrelated donor and recipient at all of the class I and class II gene loci is extremely remote. However, the strength of graft rejection inversely correlates with the degree of HLA matching: the better the match, the lower the chance of rejection. Moreover, differences at class II loci are more detrimental to graft survival than differences at class I. Thus, a single class II difference has been shown to have the same effect on the graft as that observed when there are three or four class I mismatches. When both class I and class II antigens are mismatched, rejection is greatly accelerated.

## Hypersensitivity

An immune response provides the host with protection from a wide range of pathogens. However, some immune responses can have deleterious effects, resulting in tissue damage. Such an excessive or inappropriate reaction is referred to as hypersensitivity. Hypersensitivity reactions may be distinguished by the type of immune response generated (Figure 19.4). It is important to note that most hypersensitivity reactions involve a range of mechanisms and are not restricted to a single type.

TABLE 19.5 **Immunosuppressive drugs**

| Drug name | Mechanism of action |
|---|---|
| Azathioprine | Inhibition of nucleic acid synthesis in all mitotic cells |
| Corticosteroids (e.g. prednisolone) | Prevention of the generation of cytotoxic effector cells; general anti-inflammatory effects |
| Ciclosporin A and tacrolimus | Blocking of T cell activation |
| Sirolimus | Inhibition of T cell proliferation |
| Anti-CTLA-4 antibodies | Promotion of unresponsiveness in alloreactive T cells |

CTLA-4 = cytotoxic T lymphocyte antigen 4

## IMMEDIATE (TYPE I) HYPERSENSITIVITY

This is mediated by antigens (allergens) that enter the body via inhalation or ingestion (Figure 19.4 A). The allergens bind to and cross-link IgE antibodies that are bound to Fc receptors on the surface of tissue mast cells or blood basophils. This leads to cell activation and the release of histamine (degranulation). The primary effects may be localised ('weal and flare reaction') or systemic depending on the degree of mediator release.

Type I hypersensitivity includes severe anaphylactic reactions to peanuts, bee venom and penicillin as well as the atopic diseases of asthma and hay fever.

## ANTIBODY-MEDIATED (TYPE II) HYPERSENSITIVITY

Type II reactions are mediated by IgG or IgM antibodies that react against antigen bound to specific cells or tissues (Figure 19.4 B). The antibodies interact with the Fc receptors on a range of effector cells including platelets and neutrophils, causing activation of the complement system and damage to target cells.

Examples include transfusion reactions and haemolytic disease of the newborn.

FIGURE 19.4 **Hypersensitivity reactions**

**A** Immediate (type I)

**B** Antibody-mediated (type II)

**C** Immune complex (type III)

**D** Delayed-type (type IV)

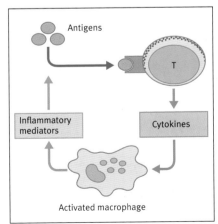

C = complement | Ig = immunoglobulin |
Fc = crystallisable fragment |
K = K cell (responsible for antibody-dependent cell-mediated cytotoxicity) |
T = T cell

*Reproduced by permission: Immunology.* 6th ed. Roitt IM, Brostoff J, Male D. St Louis: Mosby; 2002.

## IMMUNE COMPLEX (TYPE III) HYPERSENSITIVITY

*IgG, IgM*

Type III hypersensitivity is caused by failure of phagocytes to clear immune complexes (Figure 19.4 C). The immune complexes then initiate an inflammatory response via complement activation and histamine and proinflammatory cytokine release. The magnitude of the reaction depends upon both the quantity and the location of the immune complexes. Much of the tissue damage stems from the release of lysosomal enzymes by granulocytes as they attempt to phagocytose complexes that are bound to vessel walls.

This type of hypersensitivity is found in persistent infections (for example leprosy and viral hepatitis), autoimmune disease (for example rheumatoid arthritis and systemic lupus erythematosus) and following inhalation of antigen (for example farmer's lung and pigeon fancier's lung).

## DELAYED-TYPE (TYPE IV) HYPERSENSITIVITY

This is a localised inflammatory reaction caused by the recruitment of antigen-specific T cells to a site of antigen deposition (Figure 19.4 D); it develops over 24–72 hours. There are three variants:

- contact hypersensitivity
- tuberculin-type hypersensitivity
- granulomatous hypersensitivity.

Contact hypersensitivity occurs at the point of contact with an allergen (for example nickel, chromate). It is characterised by an eczema-like reaction within 72 hours.

Tuberculin-type hypersensitivity is induced by soluble antigens from organisms such as *Mycobacterium tuberculosis* and *M. leprae*. It results in a localised inflammatory response in the form of a swelling at the tuberculin injection site.

Granulomatous hypersensitivity develops over 21–28 days. Persistence of antigen leads to chronic stimulation of T cells and the release of cytokines such as TNF-α. This results in the formation of epithelioid cell granulomas. The most important forms of type IV hypersensitivity clinically occur in many chronic diseases including tuberculosis, leprosy and Crohn's disease.

## The fetus as an allograft

Pregnancy presents an immune paradox in that half of the fetus's genetic component is derived from the father and therefore the mother would be expected to mount a graft rejection response directed against paternal antigens expressed on the placenta. The fact that this does not happen in normal pregnancy shows that there must be mechanisms that have evolved to prevent rejection of the placenta and hence the fetus by the maternal immune system.

### THE TWO IMMUNOLOGICAL INTERFACES OF PREGNANCY

It is the placenta, not the fetus, that forms the interface with the mother. There are two main interfaces (see Figure 19.5).

Interface 1 is formed by the extravillous cytotrophoblast, which invades from the tips of the chorionic villi into the decidua in the early stages of pregnancy to anchor the placenta to the uterine wall. It subsequently invades the spiral arteries that supply maternal blood to the intervillous space, displacing the endothelium and destroying the muscle layer, thereby remodelling the arteries to increase blood flow to the developing placenta (see Chapter 14). This therefore forms a tissue–tissue interface, which plays an important role in the first trimester of pregnancy.

Interface 2 is that between the surface of the chorionic villi (the syncytiotrophoblast) and the maternal blood, across which the exchange of gases and nutrients occurs. This is a tissue–blood interface and is more important in the second and third trimester. The second interface is extended throughout the mother's circulation in two ways. Firstly, there is shedding of cellular and microparticulate syncytiotrophoblast debris, DNA and mRNA from the surface of the placenta into the mother's blood throughout pregnancy and, secondly, there are haemorrhages of fetal blood across the placenta. Thus, fetal red blood cells and leucocytes can be found in the maternal circulation as early as in the first trimester, which has immunological implications.

FIGURE 19.5  **The two immune interfaces of pregnancy**

**Interface 1**

Extravillous cytotrophoblast
and decidua

**Interface 2**

Syncytiotrophoblast and
maternal blood

**Extended interface 2**

Syncytiotrophoblast debris and fetal
blood cells in the maternal circulation

DC = dendritic cell  |  E = endothelial cell  |  L = lymphocyte  |  M = macrophage  |  Mo = monocyte  |  NK = circulating natural killer cell  |  S = decidual stromal cell  |
SPA = spiral artery  |  STBM = syncytiotrophoblast microparticle  |  Tx = extravillous cytotrophoblast  |  uNK = uterine (decidual) natural killer cell

*Reproduced with permission from*: Trends Immunol. 27:399–404. Sargent IL, Borzychowski AM, Redman CW. Copyright Elsevier 2006.

### IMMUNE INTERACTIONS AT INTERFACES 1 AND 2

#### Interaction between invasive extravillous cytotrophoblast and maternal immune cells in the decidua (interface 1)

The invasive extravillous cytotrophoblast comes into intimate contact with maternal immune cells in the decidua. Some 40% of maternal cells in the decidua are bone-marrow-derived. They are comprised of T cells (approximately 10%), macrophages (approximately 20%) and dendritic cells (approximately 2%); there are also some reports of T cells that express gamma/delta TCRs. There are virtually no B cells. However, by far the largest immune cell population (up to 70%) are a specialised form of NK cell.

Decidual NK cells stain brightly positive for a marker called CD56 (an adhesion molecule) but are negative for CD16, an Fc receptor found on all other NK cells. The phenotype of these decidual NK cells differs from that of most other NK cells in that, instead of being cytotoxic (for the surveillance of tumours and virally infected cells), activated decidual NK cells produce cytokines, chemokines and angiogenic factors that facilitate trophoblast invasion. The close interaction between the invasive extravillous trophoblast and decidual NK cells suggests that these cells may have a key role in maternal–fetal immune interactions.

#### Interaction between the syncytiotrophoblast and maternal immune cells in the blood (interface 2)

The syncytiotrophoblast is the epithelium that covers the surface of the human placenta. However, it functions as endothelium as it lines the placental side of the intervillous space through which the maternal blood flows. It is therefore in contact with the full range of maternal blood cells including T cells, B cells, NK cells, monocytes and polymorphonuclear leucocytes.

### EXPRESSION OF MAJOR HISTOCOMPATIBILITY COMPLEX ANTIGENS BY THE TROPHOBLAST AT INTERFACES 1 AND 2

Central to the nature of the maternal–fetal immune response is the expression of MHC antigens (the key molecules that stimulate graft rejection) by the trophoblast (see Table 19.6).

Extravillous cytotrophoblast cells are MHC class I positive but they have a pattern of expression that is unique to this cell type. Unlike any other cell in the body, they do not express the highly polymorphic classic class I antigens HLA-A or HLA-B, which are the principal stimulators of graft rejection. However, they do express the classic class I antigen HLA-C. In addition, they express the nonpolymorphic, nonclassic class I MHC antigens HLA-E and HLA-G.

In contrast to the extravillous cytotrophoblast, the syncytiotrophoblast is completely negative for class I MHC expression, making it almost unique in the human body, with the exception of red blood cells. The syncytiotrophoblast is therefore unlikely to stimulate the maternal immune system.

Neither the invasive extravillous cytotrophoblast nor the syncytiotrophoblast expresses class II MHC antigens.

Immune interactions in the decidua seem to be predominantly between trophoblast and NK cells rather than T cells, as occurs in graft rejection. The functions of trophoblast HLA-G, HLA-E and HLA-C are as follows.

#### Human leucocyte antigen G

HLA-G has four different membrane-bound forms (HLA-G1, HLA-G2, HLA-G3 and HLA-G4) and three

TABLE 19.6 **Major histocompatibility complex antigens expressed by the trophoblast**

| Tissue | HLA-A[a] | HLA-B[a] | HLA-C[a] | HLA-E[b] | HLA-G[b] |
|---|---|---|---|---|---|
| Adult and fetal tissues | + | + | + | + | – |
| Extravillous cytotrophoblast (interface 1) | – | – | + | + | + |
| Syncytiotrophoblast (interface 2) | – | – | – | – | – |

[a] Polymorphic | [b] monomorphic | HLA = human leucocyte antigen | + = antigen is expressed | – = antigen is not expressed

soluble forms (HLA-G5, HLA-G6 and HLA-G7), which do not contain transmembrane or cytoplasmic domains that would anchor them to the cell surface. Thus, HLA-G can mediate its effects both locally (mainly via the membrane-bound form HLA-G1) and systemically (mainly via the soluble form HLA-G5).

HLA-G is almost always expressed on the extravillous cytotrophoblast, which suggests that it is fundamental to reproduction. In stark contrast to the highly polymorphic HLA-A and HLA-B molecules, HLA-G displays very little polymorphism (only four alleles have been identified that encode slightly modified proteins). Such limited polymorphism ensures that paternal HLA-G molecules are almost identical to the maternal ones and therefore unlikely to induce an alloreactive maternal T cell response during pregnancy.

HLA-G isoforms have a peptide-binding groove and should therefore be able to present peptides in a similar way to polymorphic classic class I molecules; this has indeed been demonstrated for both HLA-G1 and soluble HLA-G5. However, the low polymorphism in HLA-G limits the diversity of peptides it can bind. The binding of peptides might therefore be necessary to ensure the stability of the HLA-G molecule rather than for it to be involved in antigen presentation.

HLA-G has been shown to interact with both CD4-positive and CD8-positive T cells. Rather than activating the T cells, however, HLA-G induces apoptosis of CD8-positive T cells via a pathway that involves Fas and Fas ligand and suppresses the proliferation of CD4-positive T cells and Tc cells.

HLA-G interacts with NK cells via their KIRs. To date, three KIRs have been identified that interact with HLA-G: KIR2DL4 and the immunoglobulin-like transcripts ILT-2 and ILT-4. These receptors are also expressed on monocytes, macrophages and dendritic cells.

The result of the interaction between HLA-G and the cells of the innate immune system is not the production of an immune response that attacks the placenta but one that facilitates implantation, trophoblast invasion and placentation. On interacting with HLA-G-expressing trophoblast, the decidual NK cells produce a range of immunoregulatory molecules (see Figure 19.6) including:

- cytokines (IFN-γ, IL-10, TGF-β1, metalloproteinase inhibitor 1)
- chemokines (IL-8, IFN-γ-inducible protein 10)
- angiogenic factors (vascular endothelial growth factor, placenta growth factor).

These promote and regulate trophoblast invasion.

### Human leucocyte antigen E

HLA-E is also expressed on the invasive cells of the extravillous cytotrophoblast as well as on most other cells in the body. Like HLA-G, it is virtually monomorphic and only presents a small repertoire of peptides. The primary peptides that HLA-E binds are derived from the leader sequence of other HLA class I molecules, such as HLA-A, HLA-B, HLA-C and HLA-G.

FIGURE 19.6 **Interactions between decidual natural killer cells and extravillous cytotrophoblast at interface 1**

HLA = human leucocyte antigen | KIR = killer cell immunoglobulin-like receptor | NKG2A = natural killer cell receptor group 2A | NK = natural killer

### Human leucocyte antigen C

The expression of HLA-C on the extravillous trophoblast is counterintuitive as it is polymorphic and might therefore be expected to stimulate T-cell-mediated graft rejection. Indeed, differences in HLA-C alone between graft and donor are sufficient to trigger a graft rejection response. However, as for HLA-G, the primary interaction of HLA-C seems to be not with T cells but with NK cells (Figure 19.6). This interaction is also believed to stimulate the production of beneficial cytokines, chemokines and angiogenic factors.

## MATERNAL IMMUNOREGULATION IN PREGNANCY

The extravillous cytotrophoblast and syncytiotrophoblast do not seem to stimulate classic acquired (T cell and B cell) immune responses because of their pattern of MHC expression. However, fetal leucocytes that enter the maternal circulation express HLA-A, HLA-B and HLA-C antigens and therefore have the potential to stimulate both antibody-mediated and cell-mediated immunity.

### Antibody production

The mother is able to make antibodies to paternal HLA-A, HLA-B and HLA-C antigens. This occurs in around 15% of first pregnancies and 60% of subsequent pregnancies by the same father. However, these antibodies do not seem to harm the pregnancy in any way. Harm is a real possibility as one of the major functions of the placenta is to transport maternal antibodies to the fetal circulation (Figure 19.7 A). In this process, maternal IgG antibodies in the mother's blood bind to Fc receptors on the surface of the syncytiotrophoblast and are actively transported into the chorionic villus, where they enter the fetal circulation. The maternal antibodies provide immediate protection for the fetus against infections to which the mother has been exposed. Only IgG antibodies are transported in this way; IgM, IgE, IgA or IgD are not.

The potentially harmful antibodies against paternal HLA molecules are filtered out by the placenta before they reach the fetal blood (Figure 19.7 B). The antibodies are transported across the syncytiotrophoblast but they then bind to paternal HLA antigens expressed on the macrophages and endothelium of the chorionic villus. Here, the

FIGURE 19.7 **Transport of antibodies across the placenta**

A Passive transfer of immunity

B Placental barrier to antifetal (paternal) antibodies

DAF = decay-accelerating factor | HLA = human leucocyte antigen | IgG = immunoglobulin G

immune complexes formed are cleared by the macrophages, and complement regulatory factors (for example decay-accelerating factor) inhibit complement activation. Thus, none of the harmful antibodies enter the fetal circulation.

One situation where this mechanism breaks down is in haemolytic disease of the newborn or rhesus disease (see Figure 19.8). This occurs when a mother makes IgG antibodies to antigens present on the surface of her infant's red blood cells. These antibodies are transferred across the placenta into the fetal circulation and cause the destruction of fetal erythrocytes. The most commonly involved antigen in such a condition is rhesus D (RhD).

During her first pregnancy with an RhD-positive baby, an RhD-negative mother is not exposed to significant numbers of fetal RhD-positive erythrocytes. However, at delivery, separation of the placenta allows fetal blood to enter the mother's circulation (Figure 19.8 A). These fetal red blood cells are then recognised by the maternal immune system, leading to the production of RhD-specific memory B cells postpartum (Figure 19.8 B).

The first incompatible child is therefore usually unaffected, but activation of such cells during a subsequent pregnancy with an RhD-positive fetus results in the formation of IgG anti-RhD antibodies, which cross the placenta and damage fetal red blood cells (Figure 19.8 C). The consequences of this process to the fetus are wide-

**FIGURE 19.8  Haemolytic disease of the newborn (rhesus isoimmunisation)**

**A** First birth  **B** Postpartum    **C** Subsequent pregnancy

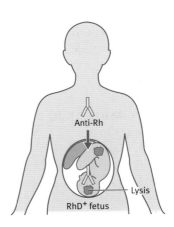

B = B cell  |  RhD⁺ = rhesus D positive  |  RhD⁻ = rhesus D negative

*Reproduced by permission: Immunology. 6th ed. Roitt IM, Brostoff J, Male D. St Louis: Mosby; 2002.*

ranging and sometimes fatal. Symptoms include mild to severe anaemia, impaired platelet function and dysfunction of the liver and spleen.

The incidence of haemolytic disease of the newborn due to RhD incompatibility has fallen dramatically following the introduction of RhD prophylaxis, where anti-RhD antibodies are administered to RhD-negative mothers immediately following the delivery of RhD-positive babies. These antibodies bind to any fetal erythrocytes that may have entered the mother's circulation and destroy them before they can cause sensitisation.

### Cell-mediated immunity

In contrast to antibody-mediated immunity, maternal cell-mediated immune responses to paternal antigens during pregnancy are depressed. This is thought to be the result of changes in the Th1/Th2 balance in pregnancy.

As described previously, following stimulation by antigen, naïve CD4-positive T cells polarise to a Th1 or Th2 phenotype depending on the signals they receive during activation. In nonpregnant individuals, responses may go in either direction, allowing them to mount both cell-mediated (Th1) and antibody-mediated (Th2) responses (Figure 19.3 A). However, in pregnancy this equilibrium is altered because the placenta produces Th2-promoting

cytokines, such as IL-4 and IL-10, as well as progesterone, which inhibits Th1 responses (Figure 19.3 B). Thus, the bias in normal pregnancy is towards Th2 immunity, with suppression of cell-mediated immunity (in particular suppression of IFN-γ production). This leaves the pregnant woman with her antibody-mediated immunity intact and thus she is still able to fight infection.

Clinical evidence for a shift towards Th2 and away from Th1 responses in normal pregnancy includes:

- temporary remission of rheumatoid arthritis (Th1-mediated) during pregnancy
- exacerbation of diseases caused by intracellular pathogens (for example herpes and malaria) during pregnancy
- worsening of systemic lupus erythematosus (Th2-mediated) during pregnancy.

### Maternal inflammatory response to pregnancy

While being a useful working model, the Th1/Th2 model is too simplistic to fully explain the immune changes in pregnancy. It has recently been found that during pregnancy there is activation of the mother's innate immune system (monocytes, granulocytes and NK cells) with increased production of Th1 cytokines, IL-12, IL-18 and

TNF-α. However, as mentioned previously, IFN-γ production is not stimulated and there is reduced T cell activity. This must be the pivotal point. It is thought that this inflammatory response is triggered by the release of factors, possibly apoptotic microparticulate debris, from the surface of the placenta into the maternal circulation. This material does not express MHC antigens and cannot stimulate T cells.

## IMMUNE MECHANISMS IN DISORDERS OF PREGNANCY

If immune mechanisms are important for facilitating trophoblast invasion, then defects in these mechanisms

FIGURE 19.9 **Interaction between trophoblast and decidual natural killer cells**

A Normal pregnancy

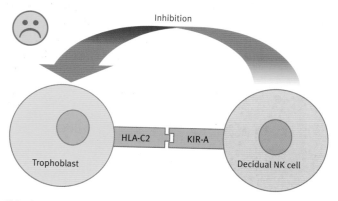

B Pre-eclampsia

HLA = human leucocyte antigen | KIR = killer cell immunoglobulin-like receptor | NK = natural killer

would be expected to lead to disorders such as recurrent implantation failure, miscarriage and pre-eclampsia.

### Major histocompatibility complex expression at the maternal–fetal interface

HLA-G is expressed as early as at the two-cell embryo stage in humans. Embryos that produce soluble HLA-G are more likely to implant than those that do not, as shown by studies that measured soluble HLA-G secreted into the culture supernatant by embryos obtained through *in vitro* fertilisation. In addition, HLA-G expression has been reported to be reduced on the invasive extravillous cytotrophoblast in women with recurrent spontaneous abortions and in pre-eclampsia.

HLA-C may also have an important role in miscarriage and pre-eclampsia. HLA-C is polymorphic and individuals express one of two major subtypes: HLA-C1, which mediates the activation of NK cells, or HLA-C2, which mediates their inhibition. Similarly, individuals have KIR receptors belonging to one of two different subtypes: KIR-A receptors, which inhibit NK cells, or KIR-B receptors, which activate NK cells. Thus, a pregnancy where the trophoblast expresses an HLA-C1 subtype and the maternal decidual NK cells express KIR-B receptors will result in activation of the decidual NK cells to produce the cytokines, chemokines and angiogenic factors required for trophoblast invasion (Figure 19.9A). However, a combination of the HLA-C2 and KIR-A subtypes would lead to inhibition of the decidual NK cells and poor trophoblast invasion (Figure 19.9B). The latter two subtypes have been found to be more common in pre-eclampsia and recurrent miscarriage.

Whether there is altered trophoblast HLA-E expression in these conditions is not known.

### Balance between type 1 and type 2 T helper cells and inflammatory responses

If a shift to Th2-type immune responses is important for the success of normal pregnancy, then it might be expected that this shift does not occur to the same extent in recurrent miscarriage and pre-eclampsia. This is indeed the case, with IFN-γ production being significantly increased compared with normal pregnancy. The maternal systemic inflammatory response is also significantly increased in pre-eclampsia, as defined by a range of markers (including IFN-γ, C-reactive protein). This exaggerated inflammatory response leads to endothelial dysfunction in the mother, which is the cause of the maternal syndrome (including hypertension, proteinuria, oedema and disseminated intravascular coagulopathy). This inflammatory response seems to be centred on NK cells rather than T cells.

### Antiphospholipid antibodies

The presence of lupus anticoagulant and anticardiolipin antibodies in maternal blood is closely related to the risk of miscarriage. Lupus anticoagulant antibodies inhibit coagulation by inhibiting the conversion of prothrombin to thrombin. They are present in 2–5% of the normal obstetric population but have an 85–95% risk of fetal mortality. Anticardiolipin antibodies develop against certain phospholipid components (β2-glycoprotein) of cell membranes and are found in 15% of women with a miscarriage. During differentiation into syncytiotrophoblast, trophoblasts express cell membrane phospholipids that can bind anti-β2-glycoprotein antibodies. These interfere with trophoblast cell maturation, resulting in defective placentation. Low-dose heparin and aspirin, alone or in combination, may improve pregnancy outcome. These antibodies can also be transferred to the fetus, where they may cause transient autoimmune thyroiditis, myasthenia gravis and autoimmune thrombocytopenia.

### IMMUNOTHERAPY

The possibility that immune mechanisms may be involved in implantation failure, recurrent miscarriage and pre-eclampsia has lead to the use of immunotherapy as a possible way of preventing these disorders. Three main approaches have been used.

### Paternal and third-party leucocyte immunisation

This treatment is based on the premise that in women with implantation failure or recurrent miscarriage, exposure of the maternal immune system to paternal antigens during implantation and early pregnancy fails to trigger the necessary facilitating immune response. By analogy with the finding that pretransplant blood transfusions significantly increase renal allograft survival, it has been argued that injection of a preparation of paternal or third-party leucocytes into the mother on one or more occasions before conception will stimulate the appropriate immune response and lead to successful pregnancy. This is a controversial area. There is little scientific basis for this treatment and meta-analysis of the published studies has shown little benefit.

### Intravenous immunoglobulin therapy

Given the controversies surrounding leucocyte immunotherapy, treatment with intravenous immunoglobulin (IVIg) has been used as a safer alternative. IVIg is produced from pooled human plasma obtained from multiple donors and is used as an immunomodulator in many diseases including autoimmune conditions, transplantation and cancer. It is proposed that it contains antibodies that are beneficial to pregnancy survival by downregulating B-cell and NK-cell function. However, data regarding its ability to prevent miscarriage are conflicting and a number of adverse effects have been reported. This area requires further study.

### Treatment with antibodies against tumour necrosis factor alpha

Anti-TNF-α antibodies are used to treat inflammatory conditions such as rheumatoid arthritis and ankylosing spondylitis. It has therefore been proposed that the risk of implantation failure and miscarriage might be modulated by anti-TNF-α antibodies, provided these events are indeed attributable to an excessive Th1 response.

While good success rates for this treatment are claimed, there is no strong scientific support and anti-TNF agents have been reported to be associated with the development of granulomatous disease, lymphoma, systemic lupus erythematosus and congestive cardiac failure.

A Cochrane review has concluded that immunotherapy provides no significant beneficial effect over placebo in improving the livebirth rate.

## FURTHER READING

KINDT T J, GOLDSBY R A, OSBORNE B A. *Kuby Immunology*. 6th ed. New York: WH Freeman; 2007.

HIBY S E, WALKER J J, O'SHAUGHNESSY K M, REDMAN C W, CARRINGTON M, TROWSDALE J *et al.* Combinations of maternal K I R and fetal HLA-C genes influence the risk of preeclampsia and reproductive success. *J Exp Med* 2004;200:957–65.

MOFFETT A, LOKE C. Immunology of placentation in eutherian mammals. *Nat Rev Immunol* 2006;5:584–94.

HVIID T. HLA-G in human reproduction: aspects of genetics, function and pregnancy complications. *Hum Reprod Update* 2006;12:209–32.

# Sample questions relating to basic immunology

## EXTENDED MATCHING QUESTIONS

### Questions 1–3

■ *This question relates to immune cells. For each item below, select the **single** best option from the list of options (A–M). Each option may be used once, more than once or not at all.*

OPTIONS

▷ **A**  Monocytes
▷ **B**  Macrophages
▷ **C**  Dendritic cells
▷ **D**  Neutrophils
▷ **E**  Mast cells
▷ **F**  Basophils
▷ **G**  Eosinophils
▷ **H**  Natural killer cells
▷ **I**  CD4-positive T helper cells type 1
▷ **J**  CD4-positive T helper cells type 2
▷ **K**  CD8-positive cytotoxic T cells
▷ **L**  Gamma/delta T cells
▷ **M**  B cells

**1** ▶  Most abundant in the decidua

**2** ▶  Most effective at antigen presentation

**3** ▶  Express killer cell immunoglobulin-like receptors

### Questions 4–6

■ *This question relates to humoral immunity. For each item below, select the **single** best option from the list of options (A–M). Each option may be used once, more than once or not at all.*

OPTIONS

▷ **A**  Immunoglobulin G
▷ **B**  Immunoglobulin M
▷ **C**  Immunoglobulin A
▷ **D**  Immunoglobulin E
▷ **E**  Immunoglobulin D
▷ **F**  Complement protein C1q
▷ **G**  Complement protein C3
▷ **H**  Complement protein C5
▷ **I**  Complement protein C6
▷ **J**  Complement protein C7
▷ **K**  Complement protein C8
▷ **L**  Complement protein C9
▷ **M**  Decay-accelerating factor

**4** ▶  Found in high levels in breast milk

**5** ▶  Most abundant complement component

**6** ▶  Primarily important in allergic reactions

### Questions 7–9

■ *This question relates to cytokines. For each item below, select the **single** best option from the list of options (A–N). Each option may be used once, more than once or not at all.*

OPTIONS

▷ **A**  Interleukin-1
▷ **B**  Interleukin-2
▷ **C**  Interleukin-4
▷ **D**  Interleukin-10
▷ **E**  Interleukin-12
▷ **F**  Tumour necrosis factor alpha
▷ **G**  Interferon alpha
▷ **H**  Interferon beta
▷ **I**  Interferon gamma
▷ **J**  Granulocyte–macrophage colony-stimulating factor
▷ **K**  Transforming growth factor beta
▷ **L**  Chemokine C-C motif receptor 3 (CCR3)
▷ **M**  Chemokine C-C motif receptor 4 (CCR4)
▷ **N**  Chemokine C-C motif receptor 5 (CCR5)

**7** ▶  Primarily produced by type 1 regulatory T cells

**8** ▶  Upregulates class I major histocompatibility complex expression

**9** ▶  Stimulates the development of nonlymphoid cells

### Questions 10–21

■ *This question relates to phagocytes. For each item below, select the **single** best option from the list of options (A–G). Each option may be used once, more than once or not at all.*

OPTIONS

▷ **A**  Basophils
▷ **B**  Dendritic cells
▷ **C**  Eosinophils
▷ **D**  Mast cells
▷ **E**  Monocytes
▷ **F**  Neutrophils
▷ **G**  Tissue macrophages

10 ▶ Attach to parasites

11 ▶ Circulate in the blood for a few hours only

12 ▶ Die after phagocytosing

13 ▶ Differentiate into mature macrophages

14 ▶ Express antibody specifically for immunoglobulin E

15 ▶ Have both Fc and complement receptors

16 ▶ The sole function is to capture, process and present antigen to T cells

17 ▶ Have three receptors for immunoglobulin G

18 ▶ Are long-lived

19 ▶ Are located in the skin and mucosal surfaces

20 ▶ Most abundant circulating phagocyte

21 ▶ Release heparin

## Questions 22–33

■ *This question relates to immunoglobulins. For each item below, select the* **single** *best option from the list of options (A–E). Each option may be used once, more than once or not at all.*

OPTIONS

▷ **A** Immunoglobulin A
▷ **B** Immunoglobulin D
▷ **C** Immunoglobulin E
▷ **D** Immunoglobulin G
▷ **E** Immunoglobulin M

22 ▶ Binds to phagocytes

23 ▶ Can cause hypersensitivity reactions

24 ▶ Crosses the placenta

25 ▶ Has five complement-binding sites

26 ▶ Has the highest concentration in serum

27 ▶ Has the lowest concentration in serum

28 ▶ Induces mast cell degradation

29 ▶ Present in equal concentrations in the intra- and extravascular pools

30 ▶ Secreted into breast milk

31 ▶ First antigen formed in a primary response

32 ▶ Most effective at activating the classic complement pathway

33 ▶ Transported in mucosal secretions

## MULTIPLE CHOICE QUESTIONS

34 ▶ When comparing the innate and adaptive immune responses:

   **A** ▷ The innate response has some memory
   **B** ▷ Natural killer cells belong to the adaptive immune response
   **C** ▷ The innate response to repeat infection is identical to the primary innate response
   **D** ▷ The adaptive response requires several days to become effective
   **E** ▷ Complement is the humoral component of the innate response

35 ▶ Phagocytes:

   **A** ▷ are derived from the spleen
   **B** ▷ are divided into two categories
   **C** ▷ act on endogenous and exogenous particles
   **D** ▷ are released upon activation by cytokines
   **E** ▷ work independently of the adaptive immune response

36 ▶ Natural killer cells:

   **A** ▷ are phagocytes of the macrophage lineage
   **B** ▷ play a role in both the adaptive and the innate immune responses
   **C** ▷ are cytotoxic against tumour cells and virally infected cells
   **D** ▷ attack cells that express an excess of major histocompatibility complex class I molecules
   **E** ▷ are activated by cytokines

**37 ▶ The complement system:**

A ▷ is made up of 20 proteins
B ▷ constitutes 1% of the serum proteins
C ▷ causes damage to bacterial cell walls
D ▷ is activated by the adaptive immune response
E ▷ contains major fragments designated the suffix 'a'

**38 ▶ Regarding the complement system:**

A ▷ All pathways require the cleavage of complement protein C3
B ▷ The classic pathway is activated by antibodies to immunoglobulin G only
C ▷ In the classic pathway, an antigen–antibody complex causes increased release of complement component C1q
D ▷ The classic pathway requires previous encounter with the antigen
E ▷ Deficiencies in the classic pathway result in overwhelming bacterial infections

**39 ▶ Regarding the complement system:**

A ▷ The alternative pathway is activated by complement binding to antigens
B ▷ The alternative pathway requires antibody for activation
C ▷ The mannose-binding lectin pathway is part of the adaptive immune response
D ▷ In the final lytic sequence, all three pathways converge
E ▷ The final lytic sequence creates a channel in the membrane of the target cell through which salts and water can flow

**40 ▶ Antibodies:**

A ▷ are effective against bacteria
B ▷ are not effective against viruses
C ▷ are divided into six classes
D ▷ have two light chains
E ▷ have one heavy chain

**41 ▶ Regarding antibodies:**

A ▷ The type of heavy chain determines the class of antibody
B ▷ The carboxy terminus is the antigen-binding site
C ▷ All immunoglobulins are bifunctional
D ▷ Immunoglobulin G has four heavy chain subtypes
E ▷ Immunoglobulin E has two different heavy chain subtypes

**42 ▶ Immunoglobulin M:**

A ▷ comprises 30% of the serum immunoglobulin pool
B ▷ is the first antibody formed in a primary response
C ▷ exists in mucosal membranes
D ▷ activates the alternative complement pathway
E ▷ crosses the placenta

**43 ▶ Regarding immunoglobulin G (IgG):**

A ▷ It is the most common serum immunoglobulin
B ▷ It has six subclasses
C ▷ IgG2 crosses the placenta
D ▷ IgG4 activates complement via the classic pathway
E ▷ IgG1 mediates opsonisation

**44 ▶ Immunoglobulin A:**

A ▷ is characteristic of a primary immune response
B ▷ induces phagocytosis
C ▷ is secreted into the saliva
D ▷ crosses the placenta
E ▷ is secreted into breast milk

**45 ▶ Regarding T cells:**

A ▷ They mediate the adaptive immune response
B ▷ They mediate antigen recognition
C ▷ They have three classes of receptors
D ▷ Ninety-five percent of T cells express the alpha/beta T cell receptor
E ▷ Beta/gamma T cell receptors are present on the pregnant uterus

**46 ▶ Regarding T cells:**

A ▷ They recognise antigens presented by major histocompatibility complex (MHC) class II molecules
B ▷ Thymocytes are selected if they recognise nonself-MHC molecules in the thymus
C ▷ Negative selection is used against all nonselected thymocytes
D ▷ CD4-positive cells remain in the thymus
E ▷ Gamma/delta T cells express CD8

**47** ▶ Regarding single-positive (CD4- or CD8-positive) T cells:

A ▷ CD4 is a transmembrane protein
B ▷ They recognise major histocompatibility complex class I molecules
C ▷ CD4 type 2 T helper cells release interferon
D ▷ CD8 cells kill tumour cells
E ▷ CD8 cells kill virally infected cells

**48** ▶ Regarding interferons (IFNs):

A ▷ They are proteins
B ▷ They inhibit bacteria
C ▷ They are produced early in infection
D ▷ IFN-$\alpha$ is produced by fibroblasts
E ▷ IFN-$\beta$ is produced by natural killer cells

**49** ▶ Regarding interleukins (ILs):

A ▷ They are secreted by leucocytes
B ▷ IL-2 stimulates proliferation and differentiation of T cells
C ▷ IL-4 is produced by type 1 T helper cells
D ▷ IL-10 is secreted by mast cells
E ▷ IL-12 enhances the cytolytic activity of CD4-positive T cells

**50** ▶ Regarding cytokines:

A ▷ Interleukin-1 activates complement
B ▷ Activated T cells produce tumour necrosis factor alpha (TNF-$\alpha$)
C ▷ TNF-$\alpha$ production is stimulated by endotoxins
D ▷ CD8-positive cells are categorised into type 1 and type 2 T helper cells
E ▷ Type 2 T helper cells promote the antibody response to bacterial infection

**51** ▶ Regarding cytokines:

A ▷ Granulocyte–macrophage colony-stimulating factor induces the development of nonlymphoid cells
B ▷ Transforming growth factor beta activates the proliferation of T cells
C ▷ Chemokines are involved in cell migration
D ▷ Chemokines attract complement
E ▷ Chemokines are equally distributed in a given tissue

**52** ▶ Class II major histocompatibility complex molecules:

A ▷ have limited polymorphism
B ▷ present longer peptides than class I molecules do
C ▷ are expressed on B cells
D ▷ present antigen to CD8-positive cells
E ▷ present peptides that are mostly exogenous antigens

**53** ▶ Regarding maternal and fetal immune interactions:

A ▷ There is an interface between the extravillous cytotrophoblast and the myometrium
B ▷ There are specialised natural killer cells in the maternal decidua
C ▷ Decidual natural killer cells are cytotoxic
D ▷ T cells make up the majority of decidual cells
E ▷ Passive maternal immunity is important to the fetus in the third trimester

**54** ▶ Regarding the interface between chorionic villi and maternal blood:

A ▷ It is important in the third trimester
B ▷ It allows passage of nonblood fetal cells into the maternal system
C ▷ It is the site of maternal–fetal haemorrhage
D ▷ Fetal leucocytes are found in the maternal system from the second trimester on
E ▷ It leaves the placenta in contact with all maternal blood cells

**55** ▶ Regarding the expression of major histocompatibility complex (MHC) antigens by trophoblasts:

A ▷ Class I MHC expression is found on the syncytiotrophoblast
B ▷ Class I MHC expression is found on the invasive extravillous cytotrophoblast
C ▷ Class II MHC expression is found on the syncytiotrophoblast
D ▷ Class II MHC expression is found on the invasive extravillous cytotrophoblast
E ▷ Extravillous cytotrophoblasts are unique in not expressing class I human leucocyte antigen A

**56** ▶ Regarding trophoblast human leucocyte antigen G (HLA-G):

- **A** ▷ It has a similar structure to other major histocompatibility complex class II molecules
- **B** ▷ There are four types
- **C** ▷ It displays extensive polymorphism
- **D** ▷ Paternal and maternal HLA-G molecules are very similar
- **E** ▷ It induces the proliferation of CD4-positive T cells

**57** ▶ Regarding trophoblast human leucocyte antigens (HLAs):

- **A** ▷ HLA-G molecules present peptides in a similar way to classic major histocompatibility complex class II molecules
- **B** ▷ HLA-G induces CD8-positive T cells
- **C** ▷ HLA-E is expressed on the invasive extravillous cytotrophoblast
- **D** ▷ HLA-C is polymorphic
- **E** ▷ HLA-C is expressed on the extravillous trophoblast

**58** ▶ Regarding abnormal maternal immune responses to a pregnancy:

- **A** ▷ Human leucocyte antigen G is poorly expressed on the invasive extravillous cytotrophoblast in women with recurrent miscarriages
- **B** ▷ In pre-eclampsia, there is a greater shift to the production of CD4-positive type 2 T helper cells than normal
- **C** ▷ The maternal systemic inflammatory processes are decreased in pre-eclamptic pregnancies
- **D** ▷ The presence of maternal lupus anticoagulant antibodies is associated with an 85–95% risk of fetal mortality
- **E** ▷ Maternal anticardiolipin antibodies cause poor placentation

# Microbiology

# CHAPTER 20

# Microbiology

*Susan Hopkins and Daniel Brudney*

## Classification and identification of microorganisms

A systematic approach is required to classify the different forms of microorganisms that can cause disease. A variety of methods can be used but a clinically useful classification is as follows:

- viruses (covered in Chapter 21)
- bacteria
  - Gram-positive bacteria
  - Gram-negative bacteria
  - spirochaetes
  - mycobacteria
  - 'unusual' bacteria
- fungi
- protozoa.

## General bacteriology

### TAXONOMIC CLASSIFICATION OF BACTERIA

#### Subdivision by Gram staining

The majority of clinically important pathogenic bacteria can be visualised under a light microscope with the aid of the Gram stain (named after the Danish bacteriologist Hans Christian Gram). The Gram stain is the most widely used stain in medical microbiology and remains the bedrock of laboratory diagnosis. It allows rapid division of bacteria into two categories, namely Gram-positive and Gram-negative, according to the degree of staining.

The process of Gram staining is illustrated in Figure 20.1. First, the clinical specimen is placed on a slide and

FIGURE 20.1 **Gram stain procedure**

**A** Specimen preparation    **B** Staining with crystal violet    **C** Fixation with Gram's iodine solution    **D** Decolourisation    **E** Staining with safranin

dried (Figure 20.1 A). Crystal violet, which stains bacterial cell walls, is added to the slide (Figure 20.1 B), followed by the addition of Gram's iodine solution as a fixative (Figure 20.1 C). The iodine forms a complex with the crystal violet, binding it more tightly to the cell wall. A decolouriser (a mixture of acetone and ethanol) is then added (Figure 20.1 D). This washes the crystal violet–iodine complex out of Gram-negative cell walls. Gram-positive cell walls have a thicker peptidoglycan layer and lack an outer lipopolysaccharide layer. These properties allow Gram-positive bacteria to retain the crystal violet–iodine dye and to resist washing with the decolouriser. Gram-positive bacteria therefore appear purple. Now, a counter stain such as safranin is added (Figure 20.1 E). The decolourised Gram-negative bacteria take up this stain, making them appear pink. Figure 20.1 E shows a mixture of Gram-positive (purple) and Gram-negative (pink) bacilli, which can be viewed under the light microscope.

## Subdivision by morphological and biochemical characteristics

Gram-positive and Gram-negative bacteria can be further subdivided according to their morphological and biochemical characteristics. The principal subdivisions include:

- morphology (shape) on microscopy
  - cocci (spherical)
  - bacilli (rod-shaped)
- $O_2$ requirements
  - aerobes (grow in the presence of $O_2$)
    - obligate aerobes (require $O_2$ to grow)
    - facultative anaerobes (can grow in the presence or absence of $O_2$)
  - anaerobes (require the exclusion of $O_2$ to grow).

By combining the appearance on microscopy after Gram staining with the growth characteristics (aerobic/anaerobic), a rapid initial putative identification may be made as shown in Table 20.1.

TABLE 20.1 **Identification of bacteria on the basis of their morphology, Gram stain and $O_2$ requirements**

| $O_2$ requirements | Gram-positive bacteria | | Gram-negative bacteria | |
| --- | --- | --- | --- | --- |
| | **COCCI** | **BACILLI (RODS)** | **COCCI** | **BACILLI (RODS)** |
| Obligate aerobes (require the presence of $O_2$ to grow) | *Micrococcus* spp. | *Nocardia* spp.<br><br>(*Mycobacterium tuberculosis*) [a] | *Neisseria meningitidis*<br><br>*Neisseria gonorrhoeae* | *Pseudomonas aeruginosa*<br><br>*Bordetella pertussis* |
| Facultative anaerobes (can tolerate aerobic and anaerobic conditions) | *Staphylococcus* spp. (e.g. *S. aureus*)<br><br>*Streptococcus* spp.<br><br>*Enterococcus* spp. | *Corynebacterium* spp. (e.g. *C. diphtheriae*)<br><br>*Listeria monocytogenes*<br><br>*Bacillus* spp. | There are no common pathogens within the group of facultative anaerobic Gram-negative cocci | *Escherichia coli*<br><br>*Klebsiella* spp.<br><br>*Enterobacter* spp.<br><br>*Citrobacter* spp.<br><br>*Haemophilus influenzae* (coccobacillus) |
| Obligate anaerobes (require the exclusion of $O_2$ to grow) | *Peptostreptococcus* spp. | *Clostridium* spp. (e.g. *C. tetani*, *C. difficile*)<br><br>*Actinomyces israelii*<br><br>*Lactobacillus* spp.<br><br>*Propionibacterium* spp. | *Veillonella parvula* | *Bacteroides* spp.<br><br>*Fusobacterium* spp. |

[a] Weakly Gram-positive, stains better with Ziehl–Neelsen stain | spp. = two or more species

Biochemical properties and growth characteristics can also help to further subdivide related bacteria. For example, Gram-negative bacteria can be broadly divided upon their ability to ferment glucose:

- Enterobacteriaceae are glucose fermenters
- pseudomonads and related organisms are glucose nonfermenters.

Gram-negative organisms will grow well on the majority of laboratory media but they are best identified on MacConkey agar. MacConkey agar contains bile salts and is selective for enteric bacteria. It is also an indicator medium, allowing differentiation between:

- lactose fermenters (for example *Escherichia coli*, *Klebsiella* species), which produce a pink colour
- lactose nonfermenters (for example *Pseudomonas aeruginosa*, *Serratia* species), which produce a pale yellow colour.

## TOXIN-MEDIATED EFFECTS OF BACTERIA

The pathogenic potential of several bacteria is enhanced by the production of either exotoxins or endotoxins. Exo-

TABLE 20.2 **Important exotoxins**

| Organism | Exotoxin | Action | Clinical significance |
|---|---|---|---|
| *Staphylococcus aureus* | Toxic shock syndrome toxin 1 | Polyclonal T-cell activation<br>Cytokine release<br>Fever and shock | Toxic shock syndrome |
| | Enterotoxins A–E | Vomiting | Food poisoning |
| | Epidermolytic toxin | Intraepidermal blisters and desquamation | Scalded skin syndrome |
| | Panton–Valentine leucocidin | Lysis of leucocytes | Invasive, pyogenic and necrotising infections |
| *Streptococcus pyogenes* | Streptococcal pyrogenic exotoxins A and B | Endothelial damage<br>Fever | Tissue oedema |
| | Streptolysin O | Lysis of erythrocytes and leucocytes | Poststreptococcal rheumatic fever |
| *Clostridium* spp. | *C. tetani* toxin | Sustained neuronal discharge | Motor spasms |
| | *C. botulinum* toxin | Neuromuscular blockade | Botulism (food poisoning, wound botulism) |
| | *C. difficile* toxins A and B, binary toxin | Cytotoxicity | Pseudomembranous colitis (association with the use of broad-spectrum antibiotics) |
| *Corynebacterium diphtheriae* | Diphtheria toxin | Inhibition of protein synthesis | Diphtheria |
| *Vibrio cholerae* | Cholera enterotoxin | Activation of adenylate cyclase and gastrointestinal water loss | Cholera (torrential diarrhoea) |
| *Shigella dysenteriae* | Shiga toxin | Inhibition of protein synthesis and cell death | Bacterial dysentery |
| Verocytotoxigenic *Escherichia coli* | Verocytotoxin | Inhibition of protein synthesis and cell death | Bacterial dysentery<br>Haemorrhagic colitis |

spp. = two or more species

**TABLE 20.3** Comparison of exotoxins and endotoxins

| Parameter of comparison | Exotoxins | Endotoxins |
| --- | --- | --- |
| Producing organisms | Mostly Gram-positive organisms (and a few Gram-negative organisms) | Only Gram-negative organisms |
| Chemical composition | Proteins | Lipopolysaccharide |
| Source | Manufactured in bacterial cytoplasm | Bacterial outer-membrane component |
| Release | Secreted from cell | Released from membrane as vesicles (blebs) during bacterial cell death |
| Biochemical properties | Heat-labile<br><br>Denatured by formaldehyde | Heat-stable<br><br>Not denatured by formaldehyde |
| Antigenicity | Neutralised by specific antibodies; therefore immunity can be developed | Poorly antigenic; only partially neutralised by specific antibodies |

toxins are proteins secreted by bacteria. Some important exotoxins are listed in Table 20.2. The properties of exotoxins and endotoxins are compared in Table 20.3.

## Important pathogenic bacteria and associated disease states

This section considers bacterial pathogens of the female urogenital tract and a variety of other bacterial infections that are of relevance to obstetrics or gynaecology.

### STREPTOCOCCACEAE

These are Gram-positive cocci that are facultative anaerobes. They typically grow in chains or pairs. Biochemically, streptococci can be distinguished from other Gram-positive cocci by a negative catalase test (failure to hydrolyse hydrogen peroxide to $O_2$ and $H_2O$).

There are numerous genera within the Streptococcaceae. Most pathogens fall into one of two main genera:

- *Streptococcus*
- *Enterococcus*.

### Classification of Streptococcaceae

The classification of streptococci is complicated by the presence of three overlapping methods of subdividing the group, namely on pattern of haemolysis, on serologic (Lancefield) group and on biochemical reactions (Table 20.4).

Haemolysis is visualised by culture of streptococci on blood agar:

- Clear zones of haemolysis surrounding the colonies indicate complete haemolysis (beta-haemolysis).
- Green zones around the colonies indicate partial haemolysis (alpha-haemolysis).
- Lack of zones around the colonies (also referred to as gamma-haemolysis) indicates the presence of a nonhaemolytic strain.

Lancefield serotyping (developed by Rebecca Lancefield) is based on the fact that different streptococci have different cell wall antigens (polysaccharides). This allows rapid differentiation of streptococci by agglutination. The method is very useful for subdividing beta-haemolytic streptococci. Although some alpha-haemolytic streptococci also possess Lancefield group antigens, this method is not recommended for these organisms.

Finally, streptococci can be subdivided on the basis of biochemical properties. For example, enterococci hydrolyse bile salts (as detected by use of the aesculin test), whereas most streptococci do not.

**TABLE 20.4  Classification and diseases of Streptococcaceae**

| Species | Distinguishing microbial tests | Normal habitat | Disease |
|---|---|---|---|
| **ALPHA-HAEMOLYSIS STRAINS** | | | |
| Viridans-type streptococci,[a] e.g. *Streptococcus mitis, S. mutans, S. anginosus, S. bovis* | Optochin-resistant, not bile soluble | Normal flora of oropharynx, gastrointestinal tract and genitourinary tract | *S. mitis*: endocarditis<br><br>*S. mutans*: dental caries, endocarditis<br><br>*S. anginosus* (also known as *S. milleri*): deep-tissue abscesses<br><br>*S. bovis*: association with colonic carcinoma |
| *Enterococcus* spp.,[a] e.g. *E. faecalis, E. faecium* | Aesculin-positive | Part of bowel flora | Urinary tract infection, biliary/abdominal sepsis, endocarditis (rare) |
| *S. pneumoniae* | 'Draughtsman' appearance of colonies, lancet-shaped diplococci on Gram stain, optochin-sensitive, bile-soluble | Commensal of the oropharynx | Pneumonia, meningitis, otitis media, sinusitis |
| **BETA-HAEMOLYSIS STRAINS** | | | |
| *S. pyogenes* | Lancefield group A | Asymptomatic carriage in the oropharynx | Pharyngitis/tonsillitis ('strep throat'), cellulitis/erysipelas, necrotising fasciitis, toxic shock syndrome, poststreptococcal phenomena (rheumatic fever, glomerulonephritis, scarlet fever) |
| *S. agalactiae* | Lancefield group B | Normal flora of lower gastrointestinal tract and female genital tract; 30% of pregnant women are carriers | Early-onset neonatal infection (bacteraemia, meningitis, pneumonia), late-onset neonatal infection (meningitis), maternal infection (urinary tract infection, chorioamnionitis, septic miscarriage) |
| *S. equisimilis* *S. dysgalactiae* | Lancefield groups C and G | May be mucosal commensals | As for group A streptococci but usually less virulent |
| **GAMMA-HAEMOLYSIS STRAINS** | | | |
| Viridans-type streptococci[a] | Optochin-resistant, not bile-soluble | Normal flora of oropharynx, gastrointestinal tract and genitourinary tract | *S. mitis*: endocarditis<br><br>*S. mutans*: dental caries, endocarditis<br><br>*S. anginosus* (also known as *S. milleri*): deep-tissue abscesses<br><br>*S. bovis*: association with colonic carcinoma |
| *Enterococcus* spp.[a] | Aesculin-positive | Part of bowel flora | Urinary tract infection, biliary/abdominal sepsis, endocarditis (rare) |

[a] Strains from these species may in fact be alpha- or gamma-haemolytic; any one strain will show only one type of haemolysis but there may be variation among different strains of the same species | spp. = two or more species

### Streptococcus pyogenes (Lancefield group A)

This *Streptococcus* species possesses a variety of virulence factors, including exotoxins (see Table 20.2), that make it a significant pathogen. Some of the infections and clinical syndromes associated with *S. pyogenes* are described in Table 20.4.

#### Skin and soft-tissue infections
*S. pyogenes* is highly infectious and virulent and can be spread by contact with an infected person or with fomites. People with a microbiological diagnosis of *S. pyogenes* skin or throat infection who are admitted to hospital should be isolated until they have received 48 hours of appropriate antibiotic treatment.

#### Necrotising fasciitis
This is an important invasive streptococcal infection. It is characterised by necrosis spreading through the fascia and fat, with rapid progression to systemic toxicity, shock and death unless aggressively managed. Bacteria gain entry to the subcutaneous layer, often through minor and sometimes unnoticed trauma, but this may also occur as a postsurgical complication. Characteristically, the site of infection is erythematous or purple with marked pain, often progressing to bullae formation and skin necrosis. Affected people may show features of an associated toxic shock syndrome.

Two types of necrotising fasciitis have been identified; they are defined by the organisms involved:

- Necrotising fasciitis type 1 is polymicrobial; typical organisms include anaerobes, Gram-negative bacteria (Enterobacteriaceae), streptococci and staphylococci.
- Necrotising fasciitis type 2 is caused by group A streptococci (with or without a concomitant staphylococci infection).

Treatment should be prompt and aggressive and requires a multidisciplinary approach between physicians, surgeons and microbiologists that involves:

- resuscitation
- immediate surgical debridement (pus and necrotic tissue should be sent for microscopy and culture)
- broad-spectrum intravenous antibiotics (including

streptococcal cover):
  - ○ intravenous benzylpenicillin 1.2 g every 4 hours
  - ○ intravenous clindamycin 600 mg four times/day
  - ○ intravenous ciprofloxacin 400 mg twice/day.

Repeated surgical exploration and debridement may be required. Treatments such as hyperbaric $O_2$ therapy and intravenous immunoglobulin may have a role, although convincing evidence of their effectiveness is currently lacking.

People with necrotising fasciitis should be isolated until cultures are negative for *S. pyogenes*.

#### Toxic shock syndrome
Persons with invasive streptococcal disease, including necrotising fasciitis, may also develop toxic shock syndrome. This is mediated by toxins produced by *S. pyogenes*, particularly streptococcal pyogenic exotoxins A and C. Affected people are unwell with evidence of a marked systemic inflammatory response and shock, often with few superficial signs of infection. Rapid identification and antibiotic treatment are required to avoid progression to organ failure and death.

### Streptococcus agalactiae (Lancefield group B)

*S. agalactiae* (commonly referred to as group B streptococcus or GBS) is part of the normal flora of the lower gastrointestinal tract, the throat and, most importantly, the female genital tract. Carriage of GBS occurs in up to 30% of women during pregnancy but may be intermittent.

#### Group B streptococcal disease and pregnancy
About 60% of babies born to mothers colonised with GBS will themselves become colonised during passage through the vagina. Several factors increase the probability of the baby acquiring GBS:

- premature birth (before week 37 of gestation)
- prolonged rupture of membranes (lasting for more than 18 hours)
- intrapartum fever (over 38 degrees C)
- previous infant with GBS disease
- heavy maternal carriage of GBS.

GBS infection in babies can be divided into early-onset and late-onset disease. Early-onset neonatal disease occurs in infants of women colonised with GBS, with the infection being transmitted either during delivery or by retrograde spread of GBS from the vagina into the amniotic fluid. The disease may develop within a few hours to a few days postpartum and may present as bacteraemia, meningitis or pneumonia. The incidence of early-onset neonatal GBS disease in the UK is estimated to be 0.5 in 1000 births.

Prompt treatment of the infant is required, including administration of antibiotics active against GBS, such as intravenous benzylpenicillin. However, there remains a significant morbidity amongst survivors, with neurological sequelae such as blindness and mental restriction having been reported in those with meningitis.

In disease occurring in older infants (late-onset neonatal disease), GBS is usually not acquired at delivery but through another source (for example contact with other children, relatives or hospital staff who are carriers of GBS). The most common presentation is meningitis with bacteraemia.

In pregnant women, ascending infection with GBS can result in urinary tract infection. Infection of the amniotic fluid may result in chorioamnionitis and miscarriage. Invasive GBS infection may also cause postpartum sepsis with bacteraemia.

### Group B streptococcal disease in other groups of people

In healthy men and nonpregnant women, GBS rarely causes infection. However, it may cause invasive disease in elderly people with other underlying conditions or a degree of immunosuppression. Presentations include septicaemia, pneumonia, cellulitis, osteomyelitis and septic arthritis.

### Maternal screening for group B streptococci and peripartum prophylaxis

Current UK guidelines on the peripartum prophylaxis of GBS disease, published by the Royal College of Obstetricians and Gynaecologists,[1] differ from those in the USA in that they do not advocate the routine antenatal screening of all pregnant women for carriage of GBS. This is because the current evidence base is insufficient to determine with certainty its clinical efficacy and its cost-effectiveness in the UK population. Therefore, a risk-based approach is used to determine which women should receive prophylactic antibiotics peripartum.

Women with one or more of the following risk factors should receive antibiotics:

- GBS disease in a previous baby or pregnancy
- GBS found incidentally in the vagina or urine at any time during pregnancy
- prolonged rupture of membranes at term (more than 18 hours)
- preterm rupture of membranes in labour (before week 37 of gestation)
- preterm rupture of membranes with known GBS (whether in labour or not)
- intrapartum temperature (more than 38 degrees C).

The following antibiotic regimens are used for prophylaxis during labour:

- intravenous benzylpenicillin 3 g at onset of labour or in the presence of any of the previously mentioned risk factors, followed by intravenous benzylpenicillin 1.5 g every 4 hours until delivery
- intravenous clindamycin 900 mg every 8 hours until delivery (in people with penicillin allergy).

## STAPHYLOCOCCACEAE

These are facultatively anaerobic Gram-positive cocci that typically appear as clusters, like bunches of grapes, when viewed using the Gram stain technique. In Table 20.5, the features of staphylococci are compared with those of streptococci.

The genus *Staphylococcus* contains a number of species that are classified mainly upon their ability to clot plasma, which signifies the presence of the extracellular enzyme coagulase:

- *S. aureus* is coagulase-positive
- coagulase-negative staphylococci include *S. epidermidis*, *S. haemolyticus*, *S. capitis* and *S. saprophyticus*.

### Staphylococcus aureus

The following features aid the differentiation of *S. aureus* from the other (coagulase-negative) staphylococci in the laboratory:

TABLE 20.5 **Comparison of staphylococci and streptococci**

| Parameter of comparison | Staphylococcaceae | | Streptococcaceae | | |
|---|---|---|---|---|---|
| Gram stain and morphology | Gram-positive cocci in clusters | | Gram-positive cocci in pairs or chains | | |
| Catalase test [a] | Positive | | Negative | | |
| Colonisation site | Skin and mucous membranes | | Oropharynx, oral mucosa, gastrointestinal tract, genitourinary tract | | |
| | COAGULASE-POSITIVE STAPHYLOCOCCI (S. AUREUS) | COAGULASE-NEGATIVE STAPHYLOCOCCI | STREPTOCOCCI [b] | PNEUMOCOCCI [c] | ENTEROCOCCI |
| Infections | Skin and soft-tissue infections, bacteraemia, endocarditis, osteomyelitis and septic arthritis | Device-associated infections | Skin and soft-tissue infections, bacteraemia, endocarditis, osteomyelitis and septic arthritis, pharyngitis ('strep throat') | Pneumonia, meningitis, sinusitis | Urinary tract infections, abdominal/biliary sepsis |
| First-line antibiotics | Flucloxacillin (meticillin-sensitive strains); vancomycin (meticillin-resistant strains) | Flucloxacillin (meticillin-sensitive strains); vancomycin (meticillin-resistant strains) | Penicillin | Penicillin | Amoxicillin, teicoplanin |

[a] Hydrolysis of hydrogen peroxide | [b] excepting pneumococci | [c] *Streptococcus pneumoniae*

- positive coagulase test
- positive DNase test, indicating the production of a nuclease enzyme that can break down DNA
- presence of surface protein A (detected by agglutination).

*S. aureus* may form part of the normal flora of the nose, skin and perineum. It may be spread from person to person by direct contact (for example on unwashed hands) or via fomites. *S. aureus* may, however, also cause disease. Its virulence may be enhanced by the production of exotoxin (see Table 20.2).

### Meticillin-resistant staphylococcus aureus

*S. aureus* can gain resistance to all beta-lactam antibiotics by mutations in the cellular proteins targeted by these drugs (the penicillin-binding proteins). If this occurs, the strain is referred to as meticillin-resistant

*S. aureus* (MRSA); meticillin is a beta-lactam antibiotic used previously in laboratory testing but not in clinical practice. MRSA is a major problem in hospitals, where the pressure of antibiotic therapy helps select out meticillin-resistant strains. Like all strains of *S. aureus*, MRSA may be spread from person to person by direct contact or by fomites. People may be asymptomatic carriers of MRSA or develop the same range of infections caused by meticillin-sensitive *S. aureus*.

MRSA infections will not respond clinically to any of the beta-lactam antibiotics (flucloxacillin, other penicillins, cephalosporins, carbapenems). The bacteria may, however, still be sensitive to other antibiotics, such as glycopeptides (vancomycin, teicoplanin), tetracyclines, rifampicin and fusidic acid. However, the pharmacokinetic and pharmacodynamic properties of these antibiotics render them suboptimal when compared with flucloxacillin.

Measures for the prevention of MRSA carriage are therefore important to reduce the number of MRSA infections. Several measures can be adopted:

- prevention of spread between people
  - spacing hospital beds adequately
  - handwashing/use of alcohol hand gels between patients
  - cleaning of equipment (e.g. stethoscopes) between patients
- identification of patients colonised with MRSA
  - screening of patients for MRSA carriage
- decolonisation of patients with known carriage of MRSA (especially before elective surgical procedures)
  - body washes containing chlorhexidine gluconate
  - shampoo containing chlorhexidine gluconate
  - mouthwash containing chlorhexidine gluconate
  - nasal mupirocin.

Although MRSA infection remains more common in hospitals, an increasing proportion of infections is found in the community, sometimes in people with little history of contact with healthcare facilities. This trend emphasises the need to screen asymptomatic patients for MRSA.

UK guidelines recommend a risk factor approach to MRSA screening that favours the screening of patients at high risk for MRSA carriage (for example frequent hospital attenders, people from nursing or residential homes, intravenous drug users) with swabs of the nose and perineum.[2] However, national policy from the Department of Health states that all patients admitted for elective surgery (including day surgery) and those admitted through emergency departments should be screened for MRSA carriage with at least a nasal swab.[3]

## Coagulase-negative staphylococci

This large group of related staphylococci is part of the normal flora of human skin and mucosal surfaces. In general, these species are of low pathogenicity and are largely opportunistic pathogens. They are frequent contaminants of microbiological specimens and are only associated with disease in a few specific circumstances (in particular infection associated with devices such as central venous catheters or prosthetic heart valves).

## LISTERIA

The genus *Listeria* comprises six species, of which *L. monocytogenes* is the most significant pathogen of humans and the cause of listeriosis. *L. monocytogenes* bacteria are short, nonsporing, Gram-positive rods that are facultative anaerobes. They produce beta-haemolysis on blood agar. Certain groups of people are at increased risk of listeriosis, namely newborn babies, the elderly, people with an underlying immunosuppressive condition and pregnant women.

### Pathogenesis and transmission of Listeria monocytogenes

*L. monocytogenes* is a common environmental organism found in soil, water and the faeces of many animals. Because it can tolerate wide pH and temperature ranges, it is capable of multiplying in foods that have been refrigerated for a prolonged period. Food-borne outbreaks have been associated with contaminated milk and soft cheese, undercooked meat and unwashed, uncooked vegetables.

*L. monocytogenes* is an intracellular pathogen. This allows it to 'hide' within phagocytic cells and evade the host's immune responses.

### Clinical presentations of Listeria infection

#### Infection during pregnancy

During pregnancy, infection with *L. monocytogenes* is frequently asymptomatic in the mother or may produce a mild febrile illness with associated conjunctivitis, headache and sore throat. The incubation time varies from 3 to 30 days and is occasionally even longer. Colonisation of the mother's bowel and genital tract with *L. monocytogenes* may occur.

Maternal listeriosis during gestation may result in fetal infection. Infection can occur at any point during pregnancy. In early gestation, infection may result in spontaneous miscarriage. In later gestation, fetal infection may cause premature labour and stillbirth. The infant may go on to develop neonatal listeriosis. However, about 5% of maternal infections occur without fetal infection.

Diagnosis of maternal disease may be made by cultures of blood, high vaginal swabs, midstream urine and stool samples. Amniotic fluid may be discoloured or contain meconium and may also be culture-positive for *L. monocytogenes*.

### Neonatal infection

Early neonatal listeriosis occurs soon (within less than 2 days) postpartum and represents infection contracted *in utero*. The infant is usually septicaemic with evidence of disseminated disease and multisystem involvement. The mortality is high (up to 60%).

Late neonatal listeriosis occurs more than 5 days postpartum and is probably the result of infection during delivery from the maternal genital tract or of hospital cross-infection (for example via healthcare workers). It typically presents as meningitis. Examination of the cerebrospinal fluid may show a predominance of lymphocytes or monocytes. Gram staining of the cerebrospinal fluid may show the organisms. The mortality rate is approximately 10%.

### Listeriosis in nonpregnant people

In adults and children older than 1 month, listeriosis is rare and is usually associated with an underlying immunosuppressive condition or old age. A number of presentations are recognised, including meningitis and bacteraemia.

People with meningitis may actually have little evidence of meningism and may present with focal brainstem signs. Progression of infection is more rapid in people with an underlying immunosuppressive condition. As with newborn babies, the cerebrospinal fluid may show a mostly lymphocytic picture.

Primary bacteraemia presents most often in people with underlying haematological malignancy or immunosuppression secondary to organ transplant. Bacteraemia may occur secondary to *L. monocytogenes* endocarditis.

### Treatment of listeriosis

The antibiotic of choice in the treatment of listeriosis is intravenous amoxicillin at high doses. Long courses of up to 3 weeks are required. Gentamicin is also active against *L. monocytogenes* but does not cross the blood–brain barrier well enough to treat meningitis. *L. monocytogenes* is intrinsically resistant to cephalosporins.

## ENTEROBACTERIACEAE

The Enterobacteriaceae are Gram-negative rods that ferment glucose. The clinically relevant Enterobacteriaceae belong to one of two groups:

- Commensal bacteria form part of the normal bowel flora and some may form part of the flora of the vaginal tract.
- Overt pathogens produce virulence factors making them capable of severe invasive infection. The discovery of these in clinical specimens should always be considered significant. *Salmonella typhi* and *S. paratyphi* are the causative organisms of typhoid fever. Other members of this group (for example *Shigella*, other *Salmonella* species) cause gastroenteritis.

Clinically important Enterobacteriaceae are listed in Table 20.6.

### Infections associated with commensal Enterobacteriaceae

### Urinary tract infections

*Escherichia coli* is the most common cause of acute, uncomplicated urinary tract infection in the community. Women are more susceptible to urinary tract infections than men owing to the short length of the urethra. Organisms may be transferred from the perianal region to the vulval region and then spread in a retrograde manner back up the urethra into the normally sterile urinary tract.

In hospitals, a number of other Enterobacteriaceae in addition to *E. coli* may cause urinary tract infection,

TABLE 20.6 **Clinically important Enterobacteriaceae**

| Gastrointestinal commensals | Overt pathogens |
| --- | --- |
| *Escherichia coli* | *Salmonella typhi* |
| *Klebsiella oxytoca* | *Salmonella paratyphi* |
| *Klebsiella pneumoniae* | *Salmonella enteritidis* |
| *Proteus mirabilis* | *Shigella* spp. |
| *Enterobacter* spp. | *Campylobacter* spp. |
| *Citrobacter* spp. | |

spp. = two or more species

especially in people who are catheterised or have undergone instrumentation of the urinary tract.

Diagnosis is best made on a clean-catch, midstream urine to culture the organisms. A urine dipstick is a useful screening test, with the presence of leucocytes and nitrites being specific for urinary tract infection. Simple urinary tract infections may be treated with an appropriate oral antibiotic (such as trimethoprim or nitrofurantoin). Urinary tract infections associated with catheterisation require removal of the infected catheter.

During pregnancy, women may be at increased risk of urinary tract infection. In addition, urinary infection may be asymptomatic (asymptomatic bacteriuria). Asymptomatic bacteriuria is estimated to occur in 2–5% of pregnant women. This is important as untreated urinary tract infection may progress to pyelonephritis (infection of the kidneys) and increases the risk of preterm birth. Therefore, current guidelines recommend the screening of asymptomatic women in early pregnancy with midstream urine and the treatment of women with infection.

### Biliary tract infections
The bowel Enterobacteriaceae may also cause infection of the biliary tree, such as cholangitis or cholecystitis. This is by retrograde spread from the gut, usually in the presence of a structurally abnormal biliary tract (for example obstruction by a tumour) or a nidus for infection (for example biliary calculi).

### Neonatal sepsis and meningitis
*E. coli* is also an important cause of neonatal sepsis. Like GBS, neonatal infection with *E. coli* is acquired during passage through the maternal genital tract. Bacteraemia may present quite nonspecifically in newborn babies, with fever, drowsiness and poor muscle tone ('floppy' infant). Likewise, meningitis may present without classic signs of meningism.

Prompt antibiotic treatment of suspected neonatal sepsis should be initiated, with antibiotics to cover GBS and Enterobacteriaceae, for example intravenous benzylpenicillin and gentamicin. Cultures of blood, urine and, if indicated, cerebrospinal fluid should be taken before antibiotic therapy to guide future management.

### Wound infections
The Enterobacteriaceae may be responsible for wound infections in people who have undergone abdominopelvic surgery, especially procedures involving the gastrointestinal or genitourinary tracts. People with impaired immunity, including those with diabetes, are particularly at risk.

### Septicaemia
Finally, the Enterobacteriaceae are an important cause of bacteraemia and sepsis syndrome, the most common causative agent being *E. coli*. Gram-negative organisms may produce endotoxins, which are responsible for many of the pathological effects of Gram-negative sepsis.

Blood cultures are important to identify the causative organism and guide antimicrobial therapy. Imaging and culture of other sites may identify the source of sepsis. Management involves initial resuscitation and supportive measures. Empirical antibiotics should be started while awaiting the results of cultures. Empirical broad-spectrum antibiotics should include Gram-negative cover, such as co-amoxiclav or a third-generation cephalosporin such as ceftriaxone.

New resistance patterns are emerging in Gram-negative organisms, such as extended-spectrum beta-lactamase production. Therefore, consideration should be given to the use of aminoglycosides (for example gentamicin or amikacin) or carbapenems (for example ertapenem or meropenem) in people with prior exposure to co-amoxiclav or cephalosporins.

## PSEUDOMONADS AND OTHER NONFERMENTERS

This group comprises a mixture of glucose-nonfermenting, lactose-nonfermenting Gram-negative rods. Some of the clinically important members of this group are shown in Table 20.7.

The members of this group are mostly environmental organisms, being widely found in the soil, water and hospital environment. However, they are largely of low pathogenicity and, with a few exceptions, normally only cause infections in the hospital setting. Infections usually occur in people who have an underlying immunosuppressive condition (for example diabetes, leukaemia), an indwelling device (for example a catheter, an intravenous line) or an underlying chronic disease (for example bronchiectasis) and in those who are severely unwell (for example people in intensive care). Members of this group of bacteria do not usually cause infection in otherwise healthy persons.

## NEISSERIA

This genus comprises two significant pathogens, namely *Neisseria meningitidis* (also called meningococcus) and *Neisseria gonorrhoeae* (also called gonococcus). Bacteria of the *Neisseria* genus are aerobic Gram-negative diplococci (cocci found in pairs). They are often seen within neutrophils on the Gram stain but extracellular organisms may also be seen. They do not grow on plain agar and may need richer media, such as chocolate agar (containing heated horse blood). All *Neisseria* species give positive catalase and oxidase tests. The various species can be differentiated on the basis of the different sugars they ferment.

### Neisseria meningitidis (meningococcus)

Meningococci are part of the normal flora of the nasopharynx in about 10% of the population. They can be divided into 13 serogroups. The most common serogroups associated with disease are serogroups A, B, C and W135. The most common disease-associated serogroup in the UK is serogroup B. Many factors determine whether carriers will go on to develop disease, including bacterial factors (virulence of the strain), host factors (differing immunity) and environmental factors (overcrowding).

Clinical presentations include bacteraemia and meningitis.

### Bacteraemia

After a usually quite short incubation period (2–5 days), affected people develop fever. They may develop a petechial or purpuric rash (nonblanching), which often spreads rapidly and indicates underlying disseminated intravascular coagulation. People with bacteraemia rapidly progress to septic shock, which is driven by the production of bacterial endotoxin. Mortality is high and rapid diagnosis and appropriate management are paramount.

### Meningitis

Affected persons may present with signs and symptoms of meningitis without septicaemia, although one may rapidly progress to the other. People with meningitis are febrile,

TABLE 20.7 **Principal pseudomonads and nonfermenters**

| Organism | Associated infections |
| --- | --- |
| *Pseudomonas aeruginosa* | Hospital-acquired pneumonia |
| | Ventilator-associated pneumonia |
| | Pneumonia in people with chronic respiratory disease (e.g. bronchiectasis) |
| | Cellulitis (in people with burns, ulcers or underlying immunosuppressive condition) |
| | Catheter-/device-associated urinary tract infection |
| | Otitis externa |
| *Stenotrophomonas maltophilia* | Rare cause of hospital-associated infections, especially associated with indwelling devices |
| *Burkholderia cepacia* | Lower respiratory tract infection (in cystic fibrosis) |
| *Burkholderia mallei* and *B. pseudomallei* | Glanders |
| | Melioidosis |
| *Acinetobacter baumannii* | Ventilator-associated pneumonia |
| | Wound infections (in people with underlying immunosuppressive condition) |
| | Device-associated urinary tract infections |

with a subacute onset of headache, photophobia, nausea, vomiting and neck stiffness. Inflammatory markers in the blood are raised. Lumbar puncture helps to confirm the diagnosis. The cerebrospinal fluid will show a raised protein count, a low glucose level and a raised white blood cell count, with neutrophils being the predominant cell type. The Gram-negative diplococci may be visible within the neutrophils on the Gram stain. *N. meningitidis* may be cultured from the cerebrospinal fluid.

### Management of meningococcal infections

Early diagnosis and rapid administration of appropriate antibiotics are key to ensure the best possible outcome. In the community, general practitioners should administer intramuscular benzylpenicillin upon suspicion of meningococcal infection. In the hospital setting, high-dose intravenous benzylpenicillin may be used. However, in practice, intravenous ceftriaxone is more commonly given as empirical treatment as this has better activity against other organisms that may cause a similar presentation.

People with meningococcal septicaemia deteriorate rapidly and often require management in the intensive care unit. Contacts of an affected person (including healthcare workers) should be traced and offered prophylaxis with ciprofloxacin or rifampicin.

### Neisseria gonorrhoeae (gonococcus)

*N. gonorrhoeae* is the causative organism of gonorrhoea. Gonorrhoea is the second most common sexually transmitted bacterial infection in the UK and is rising in incidence in younger age groups. Unlike meningococcus, gonococcus does not form part of the normal flora in humans and is always considered a pathogen when found in clinical samples. Accurate laboratory diagnosis is required to differentiate it from other *Neisseria* species as a diagnosis of gonorrhoea has important public health implications in terms of informing and screening potential contacts.

### Sample collection and incubation

*N. gonorrhoeae* rapidly undergoes autolysis if incubated in unfavourable conditions. Therefore, clinical samples should be inoculated directly onto appropriate incubation media at the bedside. Where this is not possible, use of special transport media is required while the specimen is taken to the laboratory.

The organism should be incubated on selective media, such as Thayer–Martin agar, to prevent overgrowth of vaginal or rectal flora from clinical samples. It is a fastidious organism that requires a humid atmosphere and supplementation with $CO_2$.

The clinical aspects of this infection are covered in Chapter 22.

## CHLAMYDIA, MYCOPLASMA AND UREAPLASMA

Bacteria of these genera lack a standard bacterial cell wall and therefore are not stainable by the Gram method. They are mainly intracellular pathogens and contain both DNA and RNA. Diagnosis is predominantly by serology, cell culture or nucleic acid amplification techniques. However, *Mycoplasma hominis* can grow on blood agar plates and in blood culture media.

Table 20.8 provides an overview of infections caused by these three genera. Infection with *C. trachomatis* is discussed in detail in Chapter 22.

### SPIROCHAETACEAE

These are long and slender bacteria that are between 0.1 and 0.6 micrometres in diameter and 5–250 micrometres long. They are not usually visible by Gram stain microscopy because of their size but may be visualised on dark-ground or phase-contrast microscopy as spiral or spring-like organisms. This key feature is attributable to axial filaments that run lengthwise and allow the bacteria to rotate around their longitudinal axis. Table 20.9 outlines key species and their disease states.

### Syphilis

Syphilis is caused by *Treponema pallidum* subspecies *pallidum*. These are spirochaetes that do not stain by Gram staining and are difficult to culture in the laboratory. They must therefore be identified by use of special staining techniques and by serology to detect host antibodies against the organism. Several other treponemal species cause nonvenereal infections in humans, including *T. pallidum* subspecies *pertenue* and *T. pallidum* subspecies *endemicum*, the causative agents of yaws and bejel, respectively.

TABLE 20.8 **Overview of** *Chlamydia*, *Mycoplasma* **and** *Ureaplasma*

| Genus | Species | Route of transmission | Manifestations |
|---|---|---|---|
| Chlamydia | C. trachomatis A–C | Hand to eye, fomites | Ocular trachoma (blindness) |
| | C. trachomatis D–K | Sexual | Urethritis, cervicitis, pelvic inflammatory disease, epididymo-orchitis |
| | C. trachomatis L1–L3 | Sexual | Lymphogranuloma venereum |
| | C. pneumoniae | Aerosol | Pneumonia |
| | C. psittaci | Birds, cats | Pneumonia, miscarriage, endocarditis |
| Mycoplasma | M. pneumoniae | Aerosol | Pneumonia, Raynaud's disease, monoarticular or migratory arthritis, aseptic meningitis |
| | M. hominis[a] | Human reservoir/endogenous from urogenital tract | Vaginitis, urethritis, pelvic inflammatory disease, arthritis, postpartum fever |
| | M. genitalium[a] | Human reservoir/endogenous from urogenital tract | Urethritis |
| Ureaplasma | U. urealyticum[a] | Human reservoir/endogenous from urogenital tract | Urethritis, prematurity |

[a] Variably implicated in genitourinary disease, miscarriage, chorioamnionitis and low birth weight

### Epidemiology of syphilis

Syphilis is now relatively uncommon in developed countries, owing to the advent of effective antimicrobial therapy. However, it remains a very important disease worldwide with high prevalences in some countries and increased prevalences in particular social groups including homosexual men and prostitutes. The long latent course and social stigma associated with infection mean that many of those infected are not tested and diagnosed, leading to underestimation of the true incidence.

The clinical aspects of this infection are covered in Chapter 22.

### MYCOBACTERIACEAE

Mycobacteria are obligately aerobic, nonmotile, nonsporing, rod-shaped bacteria between 2–4 micrometres in length. Their cell wall is made up of 60% lipids and also contains peptidoglycan. With the exception of tuberculosis, disease by mycobacteria occurs predominantly in people with underlying immunosuppression, as outlined in Table 20.10. The reservoir of tuberculosis is humans and spread is from person to person through droplet inhalation. Other mycobacteria are ubiquitous in nature, particularly in soil and water.

### Tuberculosis

*Mycobacterium tuberculosis* complex is composed of five distinct species: *M. tuberculosis*, *M. bovis*, *M. ulcerans*, *M. microti*, *M. africanum*. However, any disease caused by these organisms is referred to as tuberculosis.

### Epidemiology

The prevalence of tuberculosis continues to rise in the UK and recent reports state that approximately 15 out of 100 000 people are infected in England, Wales and Northern Ireland. Nearly half the burden of disease occurs in London with rates approaching 50/100 000 population. The rates peak in the 25–29-year-old age group and are approximately three times higher in those not born in the UK. Approximately 60% of people reported to be infected have pulmonary disease.

Only 60% of infections reported in 2005 were con-

**TABLE 20.9 Overview of spirochaetal organisms**

| Genus | Route of transmission | Species | Disease | Manifestations |
|---|---|---|---|---|
| *Treponema* | Person to person | *T. pallidum* ssp. *pertenue* | Yaws | Papillomatous skin lesions, periostitis, gummata |
| | | *T. carateum* | Pinta | Papulosquamous skin lesions, achromic skin lesions |
| | | *T. pallidum* ssp. *endemicum* | Bejel, nonvenereal or endemic syphilis | Oral mucosal lesions, mucus patches, condylomata lata, gummata |
| | | *T. pallidum* ssp. *pallidum* | Syphilis | Primary, secondary, cardiovascular, neurological and gummatous syphilis |
| *Leptospira* | Soil and water, excreted in urine from animal reservoirs | *L. interrogans* | Weil's disease | Jaundice, hepatosplenomegaly, renal failure, fever, meningitis |
| *Borrelia* | Tick, louse | *B. burgdorferi* | Lyme disease (ixodid ticks) | Erythema migrans, meningitis, arthritis, pancarditis, splenomegaly, lymphadenopathy, myelitis |
| | | *B. hermsii* *B. recurrentis* | Relapsing fever (tick/louse) | Fever, headache, myalgia, constitutional symptoms |

ssp. = subspecies

firmed by culture. Of those that were culture-positive, 8.7% were resistant to at least one first-line drug; however, less than 1% were multidrug-resistant (defined as resistance to isoniazid and rifampicin).

### Diagnosis

Laboratories identify the organism by use of fluorochrome (for example auramine) stains and confirm the result by use of the traditional Ziehl–Neelsen stain (staining mycobacteria pink with carbol fuchsin). A positive smear is indicative of $10^5$ organisms/ml.

Culture is performed either in liquid culture media, where the organisms are detected on the basis of the metabolism of substances, or in solid media such as Löwenstein–Jensen slopes, where the organisms appear as small buff-coloured colonies.

Nucleic-acid amplification techniques allow identification of *M. tuberculosis* DNA directly from clinical or cultured specimens. These techniques can also be used to assess the relatedness of organisms through DNA fingerprinting and to identify common mutations related to drug resistance.

Histology findings include caseating granulomas with multinucleate giant cells. Staining of formalin-fixed tissues may also demonstrate the organisms.

### Clinical features

The clinical features are predominantly related to the organ involved. Pulmonary disease presents with cough, haemoptysis and evidence of consolidation, nodules or fibrosis on chest radiograph. Genitourinary disease may be the result of dissemination from a primary haematogenous focus in the endosalpinx and may result in a granulomatous mass (mimicking cancer), chronic pelvic inflammatory disease or primary infertility related to pyosalpinx. Chronic peritonitis may also develop. Miliary disease is the traditional term (pathological 'millet seeds') for disseminated haematogenous disease. Lymphadenopathy, hepatosplenomegaly, skeletal disease and meningitis are other manifestations of disease. Systemic features such as fever, weight loss and night sweats may occur with any presentation.

TABLE 20.10 **Overview of mycobacteria**

| Species | Risk factors for infection | Manifestations | Treatment |
|---|---|---|---|
| *Mycobacterium tuberculosis* complex (*M. tuberculosis, M. bovis, M. ulcerans, M. microti, M. africanum*) | Immunosuppressive condition, HIV, arrival in the UK from countries of high prevalence (sub-Saharan Africa, Asia) | Pulmonary disease, lymphadenopathy, osteomyelitis, meningitis, cerebral tuberculomas | Rifampicin, isoniazid, pyrazinamide and ethambutol for 2 months, followed by rifampicin and isoniazid for a further 4 months |
| *M. avium* complex (*M. avium* and *M. intracellulare*) | COPD, emphysema, smoking, alcoholism, previous granulomatous disease, HIV infection, immunosuppressive condition, children | Pulmonary disease, disseminated disease,[a] lymphadenitis[a] | Clarithromycin, ethambutol, rifamycins (rifampicin/rifabutin) for 12 months or until culture-negative |
| *M. kansasii, M. chelonae, M. fortuitum* | Immunosuppressive condition, HIV infection, presence of central venous catheter, nosocomial outbreak related to contaminated fluids | Pulmonary, bacteraemic, disseminated, cutaneous, bone and joint disease | Treatment for at least 12–18 months according to antimicrbial sensitivities likely to include macrolide and/or quinine |
| *M. abscessus* | Immunosuppressive condition, HIV infection, presence of central venous catheter, nosocomial outbreak related to contaminated fluids | Pulmonary, disseminated or localised cutaneous disease | Amikacin, cefoxitin, clarithromycin |
| *M. marinum* | Swimming pool and fish tank environments | Cutaneous disease | As for *M. avium* complex; treatment for 3 months |
| *M. leprae* | Endemic in Asia, Africa, Latin America | Skin, upper respiratory system, eyes, testis, peripheral nerves (destructive lesions) | Dapsone, clofazimine and rifampicin for 6 months to 2 years |

[a] In people with impaired immunity or HIV infection and in children | COPD = chronic obstructive pulmonary disease

## Treatment

Studies demonstrate that 6 months of treatment with rifampicin, isoniazid and pyrazinamide is effective. However, with rising resistance, particularly to isozianid, standard treatment in the UK is now recommended to consist of four drugs (rifampicin, isoniazid, pyrazinamide and ethambutol hydrochloride) for 2 months, de-escalating to rifampicin plus isozianid for a further 4 months if the strain is known to be sensitive to these drugs, de-escalating to rifampicin, isoniazid and ethambutol hydrochloride for a further 7 months if drug sensitivities are unknown, or de-escalating to rifampicin plus ethambutol for a further 10 months if the strain is resistant to isoniazid.

Adverse effects include:

- orange colouring of body secretions (urine, tears, sweat) and hepatotoxicity for rifampicin
- hepatotoxicity and peripheral neuropathy (reduced in high-risk groups by the addition of pyridoxine hydrochloride) for isoniazid
- hepatotoxicity, arthralgia and raised levels of uric acid/gout for pyrazinamide
- optic neuritis (colour vision) and renal impairment for ethambutol hydrochloride.

## Infection control

People with pulmonary tuberculosis and positive smears are moderately infectious. Pragmatic contact tracing should be performed among close contacts, including hospital contacts who spent approximately 8 hours in the same environment. Contact tracing involves tuberculin skin testing and/or interferon gamma testing in certain groups, obtaining a clinical history for tuberculosis symptoms and performing a chest radiograph. People with suspected open (pulmonary) tuberculosis who are admitted to hospital in a neutral or negative pressure side room, usually for the first 2 weeks of treatment.

# Actinomycosis

Actinomycosis is an indolent, slowly progressive infection caused by anaerobic or microaerophilic bacteria. It is most commonly caused by the Gram-positive rod *Actinomyces israelii*. Other *Actinomyces*, *Arcanobacterium*, *Actinobaculum* and *Propionibacterium* species are also implicated. Evidence suggests that many infections are polymicrobial in nature.

## EPIDEMIOLOGY

Infection may occur at any age and most series have reported more infections in men than in women. The incidence has diminished in the last 50 years owing to better antimicrobial therapy and better dental hygiene.

## RISK FACTORS

Disease requires disruption of the mucosal barrier. Oral and cervicofacial disease is associated with dental procedures, oral surgery and head and neck radiotherapy. Abdominal disease is often preceded by diverticulitis or appendicitis. There is a strong association between pelvic actinomycosis and intrauterine contraceptive devices. Immunosuppression due to steroid use, haematological cancers, transplants or HIV infection is also associated with disease.

## CLINICAL DISEASE

The clinical presentation is subacute with fever, weight loss and night sweats.

### Orocervicofacial disease

Orocervicofacial disease presents as a soft-tissue swelling or mass lesion, often in association with recent surgery or manipulation. Extension to any contiguous structure may occur including to carotid vessels, cranium, cervical spine or trachea. Lymphatic spread and associated lymphadenitis are uncommon.

### Perimandibular disease

Perimandibular disease is the most common presentation. It is often associated with dental infection. The fascial planes in the perimandibular area are contiguous allowing unrestricted bacterial growth, although osteomyelitis is rare.

### Thoracic disease

Thoracic disease accounts for about 15% of the total incidence of actinomycosis, with aspiration from the oropharynx being the most common source. Haemoptysis and a productive cough as well as the generic symptoms may occur. There are no specific radiographic changes, although mass lesions, hilar adenopathy, pneumonia, pleural effusions or thickenings or cavitatory disease (multiple small rather than large) may occur. Extension to a soft-tissue chest wall mass or a sinus is classic evidence of actinomycosis. Mediastinal or bony extensions are rare.

### Abdominal disease

Abdominal disease presents either as an abscess or as a firm tumour-like lesion. Enterocutaenous or intra-abdominal sinuses may occur and adenopathy is rare. Perforated appendicitis is the most common predisposing event (65% of abdominal infections). It rarely presents as a complication of Crohn's disease or ulcerative colitis. All intra-abdominal organs may be affected.

### Pelvic disease

Pelvic disease is most commonly caused by ascending uterine infection associated with intrauterine devices (30% in a recent series). On average, an intrauterine device has been in place for 8 years in pelvic disease. A pelvic mass or a 'frozen pelvis' mimicking malignancy or endometriosis is most commonly present. Disease frequently results in hydroureter or hydronephrosis.

### Other manifestations

Central nervous system, musculoskeletal and disseminated disease are rare but have all been reported.

### DIAGNOSIS

The presence of sulphur grains on histopathology specimens is diagnostic. Gram staining shows nonsporing, branching, filamentous Gram-positive rods. Culture of an organism associated with actinomycosis from a sterile site is also diagnostic, although these organisms are slow-growing and usually take 5–7 days to grow in anaerobic conditions. Molecular techniques, especially 16S ribosomal polymerase chain reaction, are particularly useful for the identification of these and other difficult-to-grow organisms.

### TREATMENT

Ideally, treatment is with penicillin (intravenously then orally) for a prolonged period (6–12 months). Erythromycin, doxycycline and clindamycin are reasonable in penicillin-allergic people. Percutaneous drainage and appropriate surgical debulking are useful adjuncts to antibiotic treatment.

## Mycosis

Table 20.11 provides an overview of diseases caused by yeast-like fungi. Box 20.1 lists important mycology terms for clinicians.

### CANDIDA

There are more than 150 species of *Candida* but less than a dozen are considered to be frequent human pathogens. *C. albicans* is the most frequent organism isolated in human disease.

### Clinical manifestations

#### Mucous membrane infection
*Candida* species can affect all mucous membranes and most commonly affect the oral or vaginal mucosa. They can also affect the oesophagus and the gastrointestinal tract.

Risk factors for oral candidiasis include treatment with inhaled steroids, cancer and severe HIV-related immunosuppression (AIDS). Those for vaginal candidiasis include diabetes mellitus, antibiotic therapy, pregnancy and, according to some studies, the oral contraceptive pill. Estimates are that the majority of women will have at least one episode of vaginal thrush during their lifetime, often in association with recognised risk factors.

#### Cutaneous syndromes
Cutaneous syndromes most commonly occur in warm moist areas such as intertriginous zones, with examples including balanitis, perianal rash and nappy rash. However, *Candida* species can also affect nails (causing paronychia) and hair follicles (causing folliculitis).

#### Invasive disease
Deep-organ involvement, such as hepatosplenic candidiasis, endocarditis, pneumonia, intracerebral disease and involvement of the bone and joints, is extremely rare in immunocompetent individuals. However, these syndromes may occur in immunocompetent persons in intensive care, particularly postoperatively after extensive intra-abdominal surgery.

### Treatment of Candida infections

Mucous-membrane and limited cutaneous disease can be treated by use of oral nystatin, topical clotrimazole or miconazole. Deep or recurrent disease requires oral azole therapy (for example fluconazole, itraconazole). Invasive disease or nonresponsive disease usually requires intravenous amphotericin.

TABLE 20.11 **Yeast-like fungi: diseases and diagnostic methods**

| Organism name | Geographical site | Diseases | Diagnostic methods |
|---|---|---|---|
| *Candida albicans* and other *Candida* species | Worldwide | Oral thrush, vaginitis, cutaneous candidiasis, invasive and disseminated disease (including eye, heart, bone, joint, hepatosplenic disease) | Gram stain, calcifluor white stain, germ-tube formation, chromogenic agar, PCR |
| *Histoplasma capsulatum* | Endemic in Ohio and Mississippi valleys (but has been found worldwide) | Acute pulmonary disease (similar to influenza), cavitatory pulmonary disease, disseminated disease (in people with impaired immunity) | Histoplasma antigen, histoplasma antibody, PCR |
| *Penicillium marneffei* | Southeast Asia (particularly in people infected with HIV) | Skin, lung, disseminated | Gram stain, galactomannan antigen |
| *Cryptococcus neoformans* | Worldwide (in people with impaired immunity) | Meningitis, cryptococcoma, pulmonary, skin (umbilicated lesions) | India ink stain, cryptococcal antigen |
| *Blastomyces dermatitidis* | Endemic in southeastern and central US states | Pneumonia, reactivation pneumonia, chronic skin nodules, osteomyelitis, arthritis, CNS disease | KOH wet mount preparation, Gömöri methenamine–silver stain, serology, PCR |
| *Coccidioides* | Southern US states, Central and South America | Pneumonia, chronic skin nodules, osteomyelitis, arthritis, CNS disease | KOH wet mount preparation, PAS stain, serology, skin testing |
| *Paracoccidioides* | Central and South America | Most infections subclinical; skin, lymphadenitis, mucosal, adrenal lesions | KOH wet mount preparation, Gömöri methenamine–silver stain, serology |
| *Pneumocystis jirovecii* (previously *P. carinii*) | Worldwide (particularly in people with impaired immunity, especially those infected with HIV) | Predominantly pulmonary disease, rarely disseminated | Grocott methenamine–silver stain in tissue, Giemsa stain, immunofluorescence, PCR |
| *Aspergillus* spp. | Worldwide (in people with impaired immunity) | ABPA, infection associated with foreign body/surgery (e.g. catheter-associated, burns-related, prosthetic-valve endocarditis), infection associated with impaired immunity (invasive pulmonary aspergillosis, rhinosinusitis, disseminated and cerebral aspergillosis) | Gram stain, calcifluor white stain, galactomannan antigen, *Aspergillus* antibody, PCR |
| Agents of mucormycosis (many species, most frequently *Rhizopus* spp. and *Rhizomucor* spp.) | Worldwide, but predominantly related to severely impaired immunity | Rhinocerebral, pulmonary, gastrointestinal, CNS, cutaneous | KOH preparation, Grocott methenamine–silver stain or PAS stain in tissue |

ABPA = allergic bronchopulmonary aspergillosis | CNS = central nervous system | KOH = potassium hydroxide | PAS = periodic acid–Schiff stain | PCR = polymerase chain reaction | spp. = two or more species

**IMPORTANT MYCOLOGY TERMS FOR CLINICIANS**

**Anamorph:** a fungus forming only asexual spores

**Asexual spores:** spores formed by mitosis

**Blastospore:** an asexual spore formed by budding (e.g. *Cryptococcus neoformans*, *Candida* species)

**Conidium (plural: conidia):** an asexual spore usually produced at the tip or side of a hypha

**Dimorphic:** capable of producing both hyphae and yeast (e.g. the agents of coccidioidomycosis, blastomycosis, histoplasmosis, sporotrichosis and chromoblastomycosis)

**Germ tube:** a hypha emerging from a yeast-like structure, characteristic of *Candida albicans* cells placed on specialised culture medium

**Hypha (plural: hyphae):** the tubular element that forms the body of a fungus

**Mould:** filamentous fungus (a colony on agar generally appears fuzzy rather than smooth)

**Mucormycosis:** infection by moulds of the order Mucorales

**Pseudohyphae:** a string of budding cells (e.g. those formed by most *Candida* species)

**Yeast:** technically, a fungus of the family Saccharomycetaceae, including *Saccharomyces cerevisiae* (baker's yeast); the terms yeast-form and yeast-like are generally used to denote fungi that reproduce by budding

**Zygomycosis:** a broad term that includes infection caused by fungi belonging to the taxonomic groups Mucorales, Phycomycetes, *Basidiobolus* and Entomophthorales

Nearly all *C. albicans* strains are sensitive to azole therapy. However, azole therapy may fail where resistance has developed or where other *Candida* species (for example *C. glabrata*) are present that are commonly resistant to azoles. If a person is nonresponsive to standard therapy, consideration should be given to culturing the pathogen, identifying which species is present, performing sensitivity testing and consulting a fungal expert.

## Protozoal disease

### TRICHOMONIASIS

Infection with *Trichomonas vaginalis* is covered in Chapter 22.

### MALARIA

There are four species of *Plasmodium*, the protozoan that causes malaria: *P. falciparum*, *P. vivax*, *P. ovale* and *P. malariae*. The majority of deaths are caused by *P. falciparum*. Mixed infection can occur. Two RCOG guidelines (Green-top 54A and 54B) [4,5] on the prevention and treatment of malaria in pregnancy were published in 2010.

#### Life cycle of Plasmodium species

The parasite enters the host's bloodstream as a *Plasmodium* sporozoite after a bite from an infected *Anopheles* mosquito. The *Plasmodium* sporozoites then migrate to the liver, where they multiply in the hepatocytes and mature to schizonts, each containing hundreds of merozoites. They are then released as merozoites into the blood. Within red blood cells, the merozoites first become ring trophozoites and then mature to red blood cell schizonts. The red blood cell schizonts then burst and release further merozoites to infect further red blood cells. Some of these merozoites may develop into male and female gametocytes and circulate in the blood until taken up as a blood meal by the biting mosquito. The male and female gametocytes then complete their lifecycle in the midgut of the *Anopheles* mosquito, where they develop into sporozoites.

#### Epidemiology

Approximately 40% (2.5 billion) of the world's population is at risk of malaria. More than 500 million become ill and one million die from the disease each year. One in five childhood deaths in Africa is related to malaria. Malaria occurs in over 100 countries and large areas of Central and South America, Africa, the Middle East, the Indian subcontinent and Southeast Asia are considered to be endemic malaria zones.

HIV infection has no effect on the frequency or severity of malaria.

Several genetic traits alter the risk of malaria, as outlined in Table 20.12.

## Malaria and pregnancy

Malaria occurs more frequently in pregnant women than in age-matched nonpregnant women. Pregnant women are more likely to have recurrent malaria, develop severe complications and die from the disease.

Malaria makes a large but unquantifiable contribution to the incidence of low birth weight in the developing world and is a major cause of morbidity and mortality in infants and children. Malaria occurs more frequently in women who have had one or two pregnancies than in those who have had more than two pregnancies. Younger maternal age and the second trimester of pregnancy carry the highest risks of acquisition. The prevention of malaria in pregnancy reduces the incidence of severe maternal anaemia by 38%, that of low birth weight by 43% and that of perinatal mortality by 27%.[6] Placental malaria occurs when erythrocytes infected with *P. falciparum* accumulate in the intravillous spaces; the number of parasites in peripheral blood can be minimal making diagnosis difficult.

It is important to obtain a travel history in all pregnant women with unexplained fever and anaemia. Fever may also be absent or low-grade and is unlikely to follow the typical quartian or tertian cycle. Splenomegaly tends to regress in the second half of pregnancy.

## Treatment of malaria

Classification of malaria according to disease severity is used to guide treatment decisions, with severe malaria defined by the World Health Organization as parasitaemia of more than 2% or evidence of complications. The following complications are commonly seen in severe malaria:

- severe anaemia (haemoglobin concentration below 7 g/dl)
- acute pulmonary oedema
- hypoglycaemia (aggravated by parenteral quinine)
- cerebral malaria presenting as impaired consciousness and seizures that may be misdiagnosed as eclampsia
- disseminated intravascular coagulation

**TABLE 20.12  Genetic traits that alter the risk of malaria**

| Genetic trait | Effect on malaria risk |
|---|---|
| Sickle-cell trait | In children under 5 years significantly reduced risk of *Plasmodium falciparum* infection, reduced parasite densities and reduced number of hospital admissions |
| Alpha thalassaemia | Increased susceptibility to *P. vivax* and significantly reduced *P. falciparum* multiplication |
| Beta thalassaemia | Reduced parasite multiplication within red blood cells |
| Absence of Duffy factor | No invasion of *P. vivax* |
| Ovalocytes | Diminished invasion, poor intraerythrocytic growth and diminished cytoadherence |

- acute renal failure (blackwater fever due to intravascular haemolysis).

### Drug treatment during pregnancy

Drugs should be used at adequate doses and according to the clinical condition and local resistance patterns. Consult the RCOG Green-top guideline for details on dosing recommendations for malaria treatment in pregnancy:[4,5]

- Artemisinins seem to be safe in the second and third trimesters. Intravenous artesunate is the treatment of choice in severe malaria. However, if it is unavailable, immediate treatment with intravenous quinine should be initiated before consulting an expert.
- Quinine can be used in all trimesters of pregnancy. Resistance is rare but can occur in Southeast Asia and parts of Africa. Oral quinine is the treatment of choice in uncomplicated malaria. Adverse effects are more frequent with parenteral administration and include hypoglycaemia and cardiac arrhythmias (during infusion the person should therefore be placed on a cardiac monitor).
- Clindamycin should be used as an adjunct treatment in *P. falciparum* malaria.
- Chloroquine can be used safely at any time during pregnancy but resistance is common. It should not

be used to treat *P. falciparum* malaria but can be used in pregnancy to treat non-falciparum malaria (i.e. *P. vivax*, *P. ovale* and *P. malariae*).

- Primaquine, tetracycline, doxycycline and halofantrine are contraindicated during pregnancy.

Recurrence of malaria is common in pregnancy and resistance frequently reduces the usefulness of antimalarials. Primaquine (for eradication of *P. vivax* or *P. ovale* hypnozoites) is contraindicated in pregnancy, so a woman who becomes pregnant following treatment should take weekly chloroquine prophylaxis until after delivery.

### Travel to malaria zones during pregnancy

Pregnant women should be strongly discouraged from travelling to malaria zones because of the high risk of infection and complications. If travel is unavoidable, pregnant women should be advised to take clothing precautions, to use the insect repellent *N,N*-diethyl-*m*-toluamide (DEET) at a concentration of up to 50% and to use impregnated nets to avoid mosquito bites.

### Chemoprophylaxis during pregnancy

Chloroquine and proguanil hydrochloride are safe in all trimesters of pregnancy but give poor protection in many geographical areas because of the presence of drug-resistant *P. falciparum* strains. Proguanil hydrochloride in pregnancy should be supplemented with 5 mg/day of folic acid.

Mefloquine is the recommended drug of choice for prophylaxis in the second and third trimester for chloroquine-resistant areas. Only one study has suggested an increased risk of stillbirth but this was at five times the recommended dose; other published studies have not found this event.

Doxycycline is contraindicated in pregnancy.

Evidence on the safety of atovaquone and proguanil hydrochloride in pregnancy is lacking.

Women of childbearing age should be advised to allow time following the completion of certain antimalarials before seeking to conceive:

- mefloquine: 3 months
- doxycycline: 1 week
- atovaquone and proguanil hydrochloride: 2 weeks.

## Postsurgical infections

Surgery places individuals at risk of infection from several possible sources as summarised in Table 20.13. This section will now focus on surgical site infections. Pneumonia and urinary tract infections are discussed elsewhere in this chapter.

### SURGICAL SITE INFECTIONS

Surveys have revealed that surgical site infections contribute up to 9% of all hospital-acquired infections, making them important causes of morbidity and mortality among hospitalised individuals.

The risk of surgical site infection varies according to a number of factors:

- patient factors
  - older age
  - impaired immunity
  - diabetes mellitus
  - smoking
  - poor nutritional state
- operative factors
  - preoperative skin preparation (including shaving and antisepsis)
  - length of operation
  - design of the theatre (including ventilation)
  - type of surgery (clean, clean–contaminated, contaminated, dirty)
  - adequate sterilisation of instruments
  - surgical technique
  - presence of foreign material at operative site.

The common causative organisms include *Staphylococcus aureus* and *Streptococcus pyogenes* (group A streptococcus), which enter the wound from the surrounding skin or from the environment. In abdominal and pelvic surgery, the integrity of the bowel may be compromised and the wound may become contaminated with perineal and bowel flora, including Enterobateriaceae.

### DIAGNOSIS AND TREATMENT OF SURGICAL SITE INFECTIONS

Surgical site infections may present with erythema, pain and purulent discharge from the operative site. In wounds closed by primary intention, there may be dehiscence of the wound. Affected people may display signs of a systemic inflammatory response, such as fever, tachycardia and, in severe infections, hypotension. In severe infections or in infections that fail to respond rapidly to appropriate antibiotics, the possibility of an abscess, either superficially under the wound or deeper within the abdominopelvic cavity, should be considered. Imaging may be required to diagnose an abscess.

Wound swabs for culture and sensitivities should be taken prior to commencement of antibiotics. Empirical antibiotics should be targeted against the likely organisms. Therefore, an antistaphylococcal antibiotic such as flucloxacillin is an appropriate first-line agent. If the individual is colonised at other sites with MRSA, an antibiotic with activity against MRSA should be used, such as teicoplanin or doxycycline. Both of these agents are also appropriate in individuals with a history of penicillin allergy. In abdominopelvic surgery, the possible presence of a broader range of pathogens means that an antibiotic with activity against a broader spectrum of Gram-negative organisms should be used, such as co-amoxiclav. Oral antibiotics may be appropriate in the outpatient setting for mild infections if the individual has no systemic compromise. In severe infections associated with a systemic inflammatory response, prompt intravenous antibiotics should be given.

Consideration should be given to adjunctive therapies. For example, in necrotic, poorly healing wounds, local debridement will remove infected tissue while leaving well vascularised tissue, aiding antibiotic delivery and the treatment of the infection. If an abscess is present, drainage should be performed, either in theatre or percutaneously via a radiologically inserted drain.

## PRINCIPLES OF ANTIMICROBIAL PROPHYLAXIS AND PERIOPERATIVE CARE

A number of strategies are available to reduce rates of surgical site infections. UK-wide campaigns, such as the NHS programme, 'Saving Lives' [www.clean-safe-care. nhs.uk/index.php?pid=2], have brought these together into care bundles. The principal interventions are best considered during three stages of an individual's hospital admission, namely preoperatively, perioperatively and postoperatively, as summarised in Table 20.14.

Prophylactic antimicrobials have been shown to reduce the postoperative incidence of surgical site infec-

TABLE 20.13  **Summary of the aetiology and pathogenesis of common postsurgical infections**

| Focus of infection | Pathogenesis | Common causative organisms | Preventative strategies |
|---|---|---|---|
| Surgical site infections | Organisms enter the wound from the skin and environment, or from bowel and perineal flora in the case of abdominopelvic surgery | *Staphylococcus aureus*,[a] *Streptococcus pyogenes*,[a] Enterobacteriaceae (e.g. *Escherichia coli*)[b] | Appropriate perioperative care  Prophylactic antibiotics  Surgical technique |
| Hospital-acquired pneumonia | Prolonged periods of bed rest perioperatively prevent full tidal breathing; this may be exacerbated by pain following abdominopelvic surgery | Enterobacteriaceae (e.g. *E. coli*, *Klebsiella pneumoniae*), *Pseudomonas aeruginosa*, *S. aureus* | Early mobilisation after surgery  Physiotherapy  Adequate analgesia  Avoidance of sedative agents that may suppress ventilation |
| Catheter-associated urinary tract infections | Prolonged catheterisation postoperatively in bed-bound individuals, leads to colonisation of the catheter and ascending infection | Enterobacteriaceae (e.g. *E. coli*, *Proteus* spp.), *P. aeruginosa* | Early removal of catheter after surgery and use of alternative devices (e.g. convenes, incontinence pads, bedside commodes)  Prophylactic antibiotics for catheter insertion in high-risk patients |

[a] Any surgical site  |  [b] abdominopelvic surgery  |  spp. = two or more species

TABLE 20.14 **Interventions to reduce the risk of surgical site infections**

| Stage | Intervention | Rationale |
|---|---|---|
| Preoperative | MRSA screening and decolonisation | Requires specific antimicrobial prophylaxis; decolonisation may reduce incidence of postoperative infection |
| | Hair removal, using a clipper with a disposable head (not shaving) | Reduces skin trauma and microabrasions, reducing bacterial colonisation and infection |
| Perioperative | Antimicrobial prophylaxis | Reduces the postoperative incidence of surgical site infections, deep abscesses, pelvic infection and bacteraemias |
| | Glucose control (less than 11 mmol/l) | Reduces wound infections in individuals with diabetes |
| | Maintenance of normothermia (temperature above 36° C) | Reduces infection rates |
| Postoperative | Good wound care and dressing | Physical barrier to gross contamination; allows early detection and treatment of infection |

MRSA = meticillin-resistant *Staphylococcus aureus*

tions, deep abscesses, pelvic infection and bacteraemias. The antibiotic(s) given should have an adequate spectrum of activity to cover the pathogens expected at the surgical site. For example, in abdominopelvic surgery, co-amoxiclav would kill Gram-positive, Gram-negative and anaerobic organisms, all of which may be found colonising this anatomic site.

A number of other factors may also influence the choice of antibiotic therapy, including:

- presence of drug allergies (for example a history of beta-lactam allergy)
- local resistance patterns
- previous colonisation with resistant organisms (for example MRSA, when an antibiotic such as teicoplanin with activity against MRSA should be included in the regimen).

An initial dose of antibiotic should be given intravenously, ideally no more than 30 minutes prior to the skin incision. The aim is to achieve optimal tissue concentrations of the antibiotic to maximise efficacy. If an antibiotic is administered more than 3 hours before surgery, tissue levels may have declined, significantly reducing its effectiveness. A single dose of antibiotic should therefore be administered at the induction of anaesthesia.

For most surgical procedures, additional doses of antibiotics or prolonged postoperative courses do not offer any increased benefit over a single-dose regimen. Furthermore, prolonged administration of prophylactic antibiotics significantly increases the risks of *Clostridium difficile* colonisation and infection and the subsequent carriage of multidrug-resistant organisms. Therefore, single-dose antimicrobial practice is advocated.

Although strong evidence is lacking, longer antibiotic treatment may be appropriate in the following situations:

- prolonged surgery – consider additional doses to cover the duration of surgery
- major intraoperative blood loss (more than 1500 ml) – consider additional doses of antibiotic after fluid replacement
- implant surgery – consider completing up to 24 hours of surgical prophylaxis.

## PRINCIPLES OF WOUND CARE

Postoperative wound care aims to reduce the likelihood of surgical site infection and to detect an infection early, allowing prompt treatment. Dressings offer a physical barrier, protecting the wound from gross environmental contamination until granulation has begun. If the wound is discharging, then the dressing should be regularly inspected and changed. A wet, dirty dressing may encourage infection. If nonabsorbable sutures are used, timely removal is essential. A suture represents foreign

TABLE 20.15  **Infection control in practice**

| Route of transmission | Example organisms | Infection control precautions |
|---|---|---|
| Droplet (e.g. coughing) | *Mycobacterium tuberculosis*, influenza virus | Isolation in negative-pressure room (sucks air into room, preventing 'escape' of pathogens) |
| | | Face mask when seeing patient |
| Aerosol (e.g. from nebulisers, ventilators, air conditioners) | Gram-negative bacilli (hospital-acquired pneumonia), *Legionella pneumophilia* | Equipment design and maintenance (closed systems) |
| | | Sterilisation/disposal of equipment between uses |
| | | Sterilisation and surveillance of ventilation systems |
| Contact (e.g. person to person on hands) | MRSA, group A streptococci, *Clostridium difficile*, multidrug-resistant *Acinetobacter*, *Pseudomonas aeruginosa*, norovirus | Isolation in side room or cohort bay |
| | | Sleeves rolled up and watches off wrists (arms 'bare to the elbows') |
| | | Barrier nursing (apron and gloves when entering patient room; disposal after use) |
| | | Alcohol gel after seeing patient (wash with soap and water if diarrhoeal illness) |
| | | Disinfection of equipment after use on patient |
| | | Disinfection and decontamination of room once patient discharged |
| Inoculation (e.g. sharps injury) | HIV, hepatitis B virus | Universal precautions, disposal of equipment in sharps bins |
| | | Clearly defined procedures and responsibilities in case of a needlestick incident |

MRSA = meticillin-resistant *Staphylococcus aureus*

material in the wound and a possible nidus of infection. Delayed removal may precipitate infection.

Regular inspection of the wound should be performed, particularly in the early postoperative period, to look for any possible signs of infection. Various tools have been developed to aid nursing care of the postsurgical wound and to trigger prompt antibiotic therapy when appropriate.

## Infection control

Table 20.15 provides examples of infections that require special precautions, listing their means of transmission and appropriate isolation procedures.

### REFERENCES

1. Royal College of Obstetricians and Gynaecologists. *Prevention of Early Onset Neonatal Group B Streptococcal Disease*. Green-top Guideline No. 36. London: RCOG; 2003 [www.rcog.org.uk/womens-health/clinical-guidance/prevention-early-onset-neonatal-group-b-streptococcal-disease-green].

2. COIA J E, DUCKWORTH G J, EDWARDS D I, FARRINGTON M, FRY C, HUMPHREYS H, *et al*. Guidelines for the control and prevention of methicillin-resistant *Staphylococcus aureus* (MRSA) in healthcare facilities. *J Hosp Infect* 2006;66 Suppl 1:1–44.

3.  Department of Health. MRSA screening – operational guidance. London: Department of Health; 2008 [http://www.dh.gov.uk/en/Publicationsandstatistics/Lettersandcirculars/Dearcolleagueletters/DH_086687]

4.  Royal College of Obstetricians and Gynaecologists. *The Prevention of Malaria in Pregnancy.* Green-top Guideline No. 54A. London: RCOG; 2010 [www.rcog.org.uk/prevention-malaria-pregnancy-green-top-54A].

5.  Royal College of Obstetricians and Gynaecologists. *The Diagnosis and Treatment of Malaria in Pregnancy.* London: RCOG; 2010 [www.rcog.org.uk/diagnosis-and-treatment-malaria-pregnancy-green-top-54B].

6.  Guyatt H L, Snow R W. Impact of malaria during pregnancy on low birth weight in sub-Saharan Africa. *Clin Microbiol Rev* 2004;17:760–9.

# Viral infections in pregnancy

*Philip Rice*

## Introduction

Viral infections in pregnancy present significant problems in respect of diagnosis, management and prevention despite all the advances in diagnostic techniques, anti-viral agents and vaccination to try and mitigate their impact. This chapter provides a broad overview of the current state of knowledge in all of these areas.

## Varicella zoster virus

Varicella or chickenpox is the name given to the primary infection with varicella zoster virus (VZV). One attack confers lifelong immunity; reinfection is extremely rare. Zoster or shingles is the clinical manifestation of virus reactivation.

General characteristics of the virus include:

- herpesvirus; single strain
- enveloped, double-stranded DNA
- spread by droplet transmission and person-to-person contact
- incubation period 10–21 days (median 14 days)
- preventable by vaccination (live attenuated)
- treatable with antivirals (aciclovir, valaciclovir).

### CLINICAL FEATURES

Chickenpox is an easy clinical diagnosis. It presents with a widespread rash restricted principally to the centre of the body and upper parts of the limbs, with a centripetal distribution. The rash consists of crops of lesions at all stages of development (macule, papule, vesicle, pustule and scab) present at the same time.

Zoster is restricted to one side of the body and very often to one or occasionally two dermatomes. When an affected person presents, the lesions are generally all at the same stage of development and are often associated with pain or altered sensation of the affected area. Occasionally, a rash does not appear; this is referred to as zoster sine herpete.

### EPIDEMIOLOGY

The epidemiology of primary VZV infection varies in different parts of the world. In temperate climates, it is a disease mainly of childhood such that over 95% of adults are immune. However, with the increased use of nursery-based child care, infections are increasingly being seen at a younger age. In tropical countries, primary VZV infection is far less common in childhood and, as a result, adult susceptibility can be 30–50%; for example, in Sri Lanka, the Caribbean and the Philippines.

### VARICELLA IN PREGNANCY

The risk that varicella poses to the developing fetus was examined in a large UK–German study that involved over 1700 women with varicella or zoster in pregnancy.[1] In this study, the risk of giving birth to a baby affected by *in utero* infection was highly dependent on the trimester and gestational age at which the woman developed the rash (Table 21.1). All babies with congenital varicella syndrome were born to mothers who developed varicella during the first 20 weeks of gestation; the period with

TABLE 21.1   **Risk of congenital varicella syndrome by trimester of pregnancy**[1]

| Gestational age at which maternal varicella developed | Number of infected infants/number of varicella pregnancies (%) | Number of symptomatic infants/number of varicella pregnancies (%; 95% confidence interval) |
|---|---|---|
| Weeks 0–12 | 15/339 (4.4) | 2/472 (0.4; 0.05–1.5) |
| Weeks 13–20 | 28/334 (8.4) | 7/351 (2.0; 0.8–4.1) |
| After 20 weeks | 55/277 (19.9) | 0/468 (0) |

the highest risk was the first half of the second trimester. Although the serological assays used were imperfect, the study provides the best estimates of infection risk available to date. Case reports of congenital varicella syndrome in pregnancies where the mother acquired varicella infection after week 20 of gestation are rare.

Confirmation of the diagnosis of varicella embryopathy requires the following:

- confirmed diagnosis of maternal varicella
- presence of features consistent with varicella embryopathy
- immunological evidence of *in utero* infection.

### Diagnosis of maternal varicella during pregnancy

When a pregnant woman presents with a rash that is clinically suspected to be a manifestation of chickenpox, VZV-specific immunoglobulin G (IgG) will normally be undetectable because the woman usually presents within 3 days of symptom onset, whereas the antibody becomes detectable on day 4. Thus, the diagnosis of chickenpox can be confirmed by use of both acute and convalescent serum samples or by taking a current blood sample and collecting some vesicle fluid and cell scrapings for the detection of VZV antigens by immunofluorescence or polymerase chain reaction (PCR). The detection of the virus in the absence of antibody confirms a primary infection.

It is always good practice to confirm what may seem to be a very easy clinical diagnosis as it is more difficult to confirm varicella syndrome later in pregnancy.

FIGURE 21.1 **Pathologenesis of varicella embryopathy**

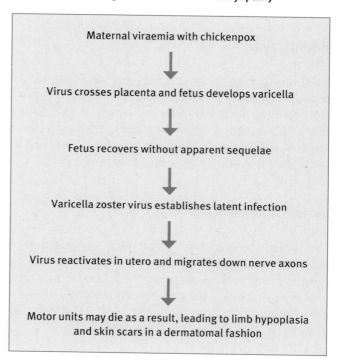

### Clinical features of varicella embryopathy

These include skin scarring and/or changes in skin pigmentation, limb hypoplasia, rudimentary digits, muscle atrophy, chorioretinitis, cortical atrophy and multiple areas of echogenicity of the liver. The development of the cutaneous, limb and neurological features is thought to be related to a reactivation of VZV *in utero* (Figure 21.1). The extent of fetal symptoms depends upon the degree of virus reactivation such that if a fetal VZV viraemia develops, the clinical outcome is disseminated zoster with the attendant risks of central nervous system disease.

## Immunological evidence of in utero infection

*In utero* infection can be demonstrated in one of two ways:

- persistence of VZV-specific IgG at 1 year of age
- detection of VZV-specific immunoglobulin M (IgM) in the newborn baby or infant.

As VZV IgM assays generally lack sensitivity, the former criterion is used in clinical practice. Alternatively, if the child presents with clinical zoster reactivation before the age of 1 year, this implies that *in utero* infection must have occurred.

### USE OF VARICELLA ZOSTER IMMUNE GLOBULIN

To minimise the risks of varicella in pregnancy, any pregnant woman in contact with chickenpox or zoster who does not have a history of previous infection should have blood taken and tested for VZV-specific IgG within 48 hours. If the sample is shown to be antibody-negative and the last contact with varicella or zoster was within the previous 10 days, varicella zoster immune globulin (VZIG) should be administered. Although this may not prevent maternal infection, especially if given late (more than 96 hours after contact), it should at least ameliorate the woman's illness. This is very important as pregnant women are at increased risk of developing life-threatening varicella pneumonia, in particular if infected during the third trimester.

It is important to remember, however, that antibody testing is not necessary to confirm previous infection/immunity if a woman has a reliable history of chickenpox or indeed zoster. In fact, in such women antibody testing may be misleading as the tests for VZV-specific IgG lack the required sensitivity to detect every individual who has been infected with VZV. Sole reliance on antibody testing could also lead to overuse of VZIG.

VZIG may also be effective in preventing fetal infection, even if given as late as 10 days after virus exposure and even if the mother goes on to develop chickenpox. Only when the maternal rash develops, signalling the onset of viraemia, is the placenta infected with VZV. The presence of intravascular virus-specific IgG at this time should therefore mitigate the risk of fetal exposure. This is indeed borne out by the study mentioned previously,[1] which demonstrated that varicella embryopathy did not occur among any of the 97 fetuses whose mothers developed varicella after postexposure prophylaxis with VZIG. Regardless of the caveats on the sensitivity of VZV-specific IgM assays, this study also found that the prevalence of VZV IgM among these fetuses was significantly lower than that among asymptomatic infants whose mothers did not receive prophylactic VZIG. Finally, none of the infants born to the 366 mothers who developed zoster during pregnancy had varicella embryopathy. This is as expected because zoster is rarely accompanied by viraemia and even if viraemia were to occur, it would be counteracted by maternal VZV IgG.

### Use of varicella zoster immune globulin at term

If maternal varicella develops at the end of pregnancy, the fetus can potentially be exposed to VZV without the benefit of passive protection through maternal antibody. Thus, if maternal infection occurs within 7 days of delivery, the baby is recommended to receive VZIG. Reports of infant mortality in the order of 30% are exaggerated but the risk of mortality is significant and probably lies at around 1–2%.

### PRENATAL DIAGNOSIS AND OTHER PROPHYLACTIC MEASURES

Several problems regarding the management of pregnancy-related chickenpox remain unresolved. As the congenital defects may be severe and potentially disabling owing to the possibility of viral reactivation with variable timing and extent, it is important that the value of prenatal diagnosis is explored more extensively.

Prenatal diagnosis is difficult because the virus is restricted largely to nervous tissue; it is not always shed in urine and does not always reactivate to produce skin lesions. This makes PCR detection of viral DNA in amniotic fluid less sensitive than it is for other herpesviruses such as cytomegalovirus (CMV). Given a transmission rate of VZV of 20–50%, depending on the trimester during which maternal infection takes place, the sensitivity of amniotic fluid diagnosis by PCR is relatively low.

Some have proposed antenatal screening for VZV IgG to vaccinate susceptible women postpartum. However, because of the low risk of adverse outcomes, this may not be necessary if varicella vaccine is added to the childhood immunisation schedule.

# Cytomegalovirus

CMV is the most common congenital infection and is said to complicate approximately 0.5% of all pregnancies. Both primary and recurrent infection (by reactivation of the woman's endogenous strain or reinfection with a different one) may lead to congenital infection.

General characteristics of the pathogen include:

- herpesvirus; multiple strains
- enveloped, double-stranded DNA
- spread by person-to-person contact through contact with infected body fluids
- incubation period approximately 3–4 weeks
- not preventable by vaccination
- treatable with antivirals (ganciclovir, valganciclovir, foscarnet sodium).

## EPIDEMIOLOGY

Sources of virus and routes of transmission of CMV infection are summarised in Table 21.2.

The women at highest risk of primary infection are those who are already mothers and have their first child attending a daycare nursery. By the same token, daycare nursery workers who do not adopt good infection control measures are at substantial risk, as are teenagers.

The reasons for these groups being at high risk are principally related to how the virus is acquired and where it is shed. The most effective mode of transmission is via breastfeeding. Asymptomatic infection of the infant then takes place, followed shortly afterwards by urinary excretion of the virus. Indeed, approximately 30–40% of infants below the age of 5 years excrete the virus in urine at some time; this explains why the annual seroconversion rate can be as high as 10–20% in daycare nursery workers. Teenagers are at increased risk because they are more likely to be unexposed and nonimmune at their young age; they can then become infected as a result of sexual exposure.

Migrant African and Asian women are mainly at risk of reinfection as prevalence of past infection at childbearing age is more than 95% among these ethnic groups compared with a prevalence of approximately 40–50% in Caucasian women.

## CYTOMEGALOVIRUS IMMUNITY

It is important to remember that there is no such thing as CMV immunity; in fact, the level of protection that a previous infection affords against infection with a different strain of CMV is only about 60–70%. There is an increased risk of placental transmission if conception occurs within 6 months of a primary infection.

## CLINICAL FEATURES OF MATERNAL INFECTION

A primary or recurrent CMV infection is often asymptomatic. If symptoms do occur, they usually comprise vague lethargy and malaise associated with a moderate fever of approximately 1–3 weeks' duration. Often, investigation of symptomatic individuals reveals a biochemical hepatitis with an alanine aminotransferase level of up to 5–8 times the normal value as well as lymphocytosis or lymphopenia. The monospot test for glandular fever is very often negative.

## CLINICAL FEATURES OF FETAL INFECTION

The clinical features of congenital CMV infection are rarely apparent at birth and reveal themselves later in infancy as a failure to thrive or a failure to reach developmental milestones at the appropriate times. Only 5–10% of babies infected *in utero* are symptomatic at birth. These babies are often small for their gestational age and can have microcephaly, hepatitis, splenomegaly and thrombocytopenia (Table 21.3). A chronic respiratory illness may also be a presenting feature. The prognosis for babies who are symptomatic at birth is poor; 10% die, 60% have hearing loss, 35% have or develop cerebral palsy and 15% have retinitis.

TABLE 21.2 **Sources of cytomegalovirus infection and routes of transmission**

| Source of virus | Route of transmission |
| --- | --- |
| Breast milk | Breastfeeding |
| Urine | Nappies, socially |
| Saliva | Socially |
| Genital secretions | Sexual activity, birth |
| Blood, organs | Iatrogenic |

**TABLE 21.3 Clinical findings in babies with congenital cytomegalovirus infection who are symptomatic at birth**

| Clinical feature | Symptom prevalence (%) |
|---|---|
| Petechiae | 76 |
| Jaundice | 67 |
| Hepatosplenomegaly | 60 |
| Sensorineural hearing loss | 56 |
| Microcephaly | 53 |
| Small for gestational age | 50 |
| Hypotonia | 27 |
| Retinitis | 10–15 |

The majority (90–95%) of infected newborn babies are asymptomatic at birth and in this group the prognosis is much better. Overall, 7–15% of newborn babies develop hearing loss, 2–10% experience restricted mental development, 1–2% develop retinitis and less than 1% show signs of cerebral palsy in later life. Therefore, given a risk of placental transmission of 30–60% depending on the gestational age at which maternal infection occurs, the overall risk with a primary infection of having a baby that is to a greater or lesser degree clinically affected is approximately 20–30%. Recurrent CMV infection is thought to pose a lower risk of transmission.

## CYTOMEGALOVIRUS TESTING

The diagnosis of congenital CMV infection is very straightforward if the syndrome is suspected within the first 3 weeks of life but this is an unusual event in ordinary clinical practice. In such instances, a urine or blood specimen may be tested for the virus (by use of cell culture/PCR or PCR). As the minimum incubation period of CMV is 3 weeks, a positive result indicates that *in utero* infection has occurred.

However, congenital CMV infection is rarely suspected clinically at birth, so the best way to confirm or refute a congenital infection is now by testing neonatal blood, taken within 7 days of birth, for CMV DNA by PCR. Because of the sensitivity of PCR, this test has excellent negative and positive predictive values. Infected babies, although often shedding large quantities of virus

in urine, should be treated in exactly the same manner as other babies on the ward or neonatal unit. Adherence to normal handwashing recommendations is extremely effective in preventing transmission to healthcare workers. Indeed, healthcare workers are at no greater risk of acquiring CMV than the general public if they adhere to good infection control practices.

If infection is suspected in a pregnant woman because of a compatible clinical illness and/or ultrasound features in the fetus, close liaison between the obstetrician and microbiologist is essential as the diagnosis of CMV infection is often difficult and time is critical as gestation advances. One of the difficulties is the unreliability of the available tests for CMV IgM. These tests lack both sensitivity and specificity, so that a low IgM titre may actually be significant and high IgM titre may be seen to persist for many months and even more than 1 year. If ultrasound scan findings are suggestive of congenital CMV, the demonstration of CMV IgG seroconversion, while definitive, is an unusual event even with recourse to a booking blood sample as both IgG and IgM antibodies are commonly present at booking. Thus, it is essential that maternal serum samples be tested by a CMV IgG avidity assay. This is a much more specific and sensitive test for primary infection. In addition, it can distinguish primary from nonprimary infections and this very often helps to resolve diagnostic uncertainty related to low-level IgM reactivity, which often proves to be of no significance.

### Cytomegalovirus immunoglobulin G avidity assay

The CMV IgG avidity assay measures the strength (avidity) with which virus-specific IgG binds to the antigen. The maturation of antibody avidity is always a time-dependent process and the development of high-avidity CMV IgG takes on average 3–4 months. An exception are people with an immunocompromising condition, in whom the maturation of the IgG response is significantly prolonged. The CMV IgG avidity assay is an enzyme immunoassay (EIA) in which two different plates with attached virus antigen are incubated with virus-specific IgG from the person under investigation. A denaturing agent, most often 6–8 mol/l urea, is then added to one set. This agent breaks the weak bonds between the antigen and immature or low-avidity antibody but not between the antigen and high-avidity antibody. Finally, an avidity index is obtained by comparing the CMV-specific IgG signals of both plates. A low avidity index indicates a current primary infection, whereas a high avidity index indicates a past infection or, at worst, a recurrent infection.

### PRENATAL DIAGNOSIS OF CONGENITAL CYTOMEGALOVIRUS INFECTION

Prenatal diagnosis of CMV is now relatively straightforward provided that there is good communication between obstetrician and microbiologist and sufficient time has elapsed for transplacental transmission, fetal infection and replication of the virus to take place so that that the virus is detectable in the amniotic fluid. If more than 6 weeks have elapsed after maternal diagnosis, it may be possible to attempt an amniocentesis early at weeks 16–18 of gestation, even though urinary excretion of CMV is not guaranteed. This would allow an earlier termination of the pregnancy if the result were positive.

However, at this stage, PCR quantification of CMV DNA in amniotic fluid at week 16 of gestation is only approximately 50% sensitive. Even if the test is delayed until at least week 21 of gestation to allow sufficient urine excretion of CMV to occur, the results produce occasional false negatives, which may necessitate a repeat sample. If one sees compatible fetal ultrasound findings (for example echogenic bowel, smallness for gestational age, microcephaly) in a pregnant woman with a confirmed CMV infection, it is important to remember that the two are almost always linked.

### TREATMENT OF CYTOMEGALOVIRUS

There are currently no antiviral treatments licensed to treat either mothers with an active CMV infection or babies *in utero* with confirmed infection. However, intravenous ganciclovir is being used to treat symptomatic newborns and infants in an effort to stop virus replication in the inner ear, which is the underlying mechanism of continued sensorineural hearing loss.

## Parvovirus B19

Parvovirus B19 infection (so called because the virus was discovered by accident in well B19 in an EIA plate during investigations into hepatitis B virus) is an infection of childhood that occurs in winter–spring epidemics with a periodicity of 3–4 years. It typically attacks children aged 5–15 years and is commonly seen in outbreaks among children of primary school age. This infection has several synonyms, namely fifth disease, slapped-cheek syndrome and erythema infectiosum. It is unique among viral exanthems in that once a child presents with the hallmark symptoms of rash and joint pains, they are no longer infectious. This is because the symptoms result from antigen–antibody complexes deposited in the skin and synovial tissues. People who have been in close contact with a symptomatic child are potentially infectious before they themselves present with symptoms and may transmit the virus to others. Against this background, one would probably conclude that this is a very infectious virus but in fact only 60–70% of adults are immune.

General characteristics of the pathogen include:

- parvovirus
- single-stranded DNA
- spread by droplet transmission and person-to-person contact
- time from exposure to becoming infectious 7 days
- time from exposure to becoming symptomatic 18–21 days
- not preventable by vaccination
- not treatable with antivirals
- *in utero* treatment with blood transfusion
- an animal counterpart exists in dogs; does not cross species barrier.

### CLINICAL FEATURES

The clinical features are usually a mild febrile illness followed by a rash. The rash may affect the face, giving the appearance of slapped cheeks, or appear on other parts of the body in a lacy reticular pattern. Very often it is itchy and exacerbated by hot showers. Another cardinal feature is arthralgia, which typically affects the small joints (fingers and wrists) as well as ankles, elbows and knees. The arthralgia occurs in 80% of women but in only 10% of children. It resolves within a few weeks but can occasionally persist for many months.

## EPIDEMIOLOGY

When parvovirus B19 infection occurs in outbreaks, for example in schools or healthcare settings, the attack rates are often high (approximately 25–50%). However, because of the nature of the illness, by the time an outbreak is recognised, the vast majority (over 75%) of people have either already had the illness or have at least already been infected. Another reason for the high attack rates in outbreaks is that 20–30% of infected people develop no symptoms; this is true for adults and even more so for children. Infection control precautions are therefore actually of little use, although handwashing may reduce the risk to an individual who has escaped infection during a localised outbreak. In schools, it would also seem that susceptible staff are as much at risk as are the children. Thus, a pregnant woman in an outbreak area may be advised to wash her hands, but the decision of whether to send her off work until the outbreak is over is difficult because most of the transmission has already taken place by the time the outbreak has been noticed. Furthermore, in large community-wide epidemics, the attack rate in the susceptible general population can be 10%.

In household infection, an attack rate of 45% has been described. Thus, the infectivity of parvovirus B19 is lower than that of varicella, where the household attack rate is 90%.

## PARVOVIRUS B19 INFECTION IN PREGNANCY

The risk that acute parvovirus B19 poses during pregnancy is one of fetal loss or the development of fetal anaemia and hydrops. The general understanding is that parvovirus infects red blood cell precursors via attachment to a blood group antigen called P globoside, which is common throughout the world. Once infected, the production of red blood cells is shut down and the fetus develops anaemia with an appropriate cardiac compensation. However, as the P globoside is also expressed by cardiac myocytes, cardiac contractility may also be compromised. If infection occurs in the first trimester, there is an excess risk of fetal loss of approximately 10–12%; later, in the first 8 weeks of the second trimester, the risk

of miscarriage progressively reduces to be replaced by a 3% risk of fetal hydrops.

If a woman experiences acute parvovirus B19 infection after week 20 of gestation, there is a very low risk to her fetus, although it may become infected *in utero*. The lower risk of fetal affection is undoubtedly attributable to the development of a fetal immune response as well as transfer of maternal IgG to neutralise virus infectivity.

## PARVOVIRUS TESTING AND TREATMENT

Laboratory confirmation of acute parvovirus B19 infection is made by detection of virus-specific IgM and IgG. Diagnosis of fetal infection is achieved by two approaches: maternal serology when the fetus has miscarried or hydrops is diagnosed, virus detection in amniotic fluid and/or fetal blood. It is very important to remember that parvovirus B19 IgM persists for only 2–3 months, so by the time a woman presents with a hydropic fetus, the virus-specific IgM antibodies have disappeared and very often the maternal serology is useful only to exclude parvovirus as a causative agent on the basis of a negative result for virus-specific IgG. If IgM is undetectable but parvovirus IgG is present at the time fetal hydrops is diagnosed, it may be possible to demonstrate seroconversion by comparison with the booking blood. Moreover, if fetal blood is being sampled for the purpose of confirming or refuting anaemia, this may also be tested for parvovirus DNA by PCR. If infection is confirmed, the viral load is very often high (more than 109 virus particles/ml of either amniotic fluid or blood).

Treatment involves an intrauterine blood transfusion, which is often successful at the first attempt, although approximately 20% of fetuses with hydrops will recover spontaneously. Babies who are born to mothers with parvovirus B19 infection in pregnancy suffer no harm in the long term.

## Herpes simplex virus

Herpes simplex is a viral disease caused by one of two types of herpes simplex virus. The type 1 virus (HSV-1) usually causes oral herpes with cold sores or blisters, whereas the type 2 virus (HSV-2) is linked with genital herpes. Herpes viruses cycle between remission and active disease lasting 2–21 days. With time, the infection becomes latent and the virus resides in the sensory nerves for life.

General characteristics of the pathogen include:

- herpesvirus; two types
- enveloped, double-stranded DNA
- spread by person-to-person contact through contact with infected body fluids
- incubation period approximately 1–3 weeks
- not preventable by vaccination
- treatable with antivirals (aciclovir, valaciclovir, penciclovir, famciclovir, ganciclovir, foscarnet sodium).

## EPIDEMIOLOGY OF GENITAL HERPES

Both HSV-1 and HSV-2 are spread through intimate contact. While HSV-2 continues to be the type most commonly encountered in the genital tract, HSV-1 now accounts for approximately 30% of new genital infections in people presenting to genitourinary medicine clinics. This is attributable to the increased susceptibility in childhood and genital exposure in teenage and later years to virus shed orally. The prevalence of HSV-2 infection differs depending on the country of origin and the ethnic group. For example, in the USA and UK, the prevalence rates of HSV-2 antibody in the general population are 21% and 5%, respectively. Asymptomatic genital or oral infection is the norm as less than 10% of seropositive individuals report symptoms at the time of primary infection. In addition, the majority of infections are acquired in the asymptomatic phase of a reactivation, just before lesions appear.

An HSV infection should be regarded as a latent viral infection primarily of nervous tissue that, upon reactivation, results in the virus passing down the axon to the sensory nerve endings in the skin, where a lytic infection occurs and the virus is shed to the exterior and potentially to another susceptible host.

## GENITAL HERPES IN PREGNANCY

HSV infection during pregnancy very rarely causes disseminated intrauterine infection leading to fetal death. The risk depends on the type and the timing of the infection.

Three types of HSV infection may be seen:

- primary infection, where genital tract infection takes place in an individual who has not previously been infected with either type of HSV
- initial infection, where infection of the genital tract with one HSV type takes place in the presence of antibody to the opposing HSV type; for example, a woman may have antibody to HSV-1 and experience cold sores on her lips but is now having an initial infection with HSV-2 and is antibody-negative to that virus type
- recurrent infection, where virus of one type is present at the same time as its antibody.

In the largest study to date examining the risk of HSV infection in pregnancy, it was demonstrated that infection occurs throughout pregnancy, divided equally between all three trimesters; the incidence of HSV infection in pregnancy was 1.3%, with one-third of infections attributable to HSV-1. The incidence varied when stratified by antibody status at booking. Among women who were seronegative for both HSV-1 and HSV-2, the incidence was 3.7%, compared with 1.3% among those with pre-existing antibody against HSV-1 and 0% in women with pre-existing antibody to HSV-2.[2] This indicates an important phenomenon, namely virus interference. It is likely that women with HSV-2 antibodies have had a previous genital infection and as such their sacral plexus is already latently infected. Such a state renders it almost impossible for another virus, in this case HSV-1, to set up a second latent infection in the same tissue.

In addition, the study found no illness among the newborn babies of women who had seroconverted by the onset of labour,[2] indicating that passive antibody transfer is protective. There were no differences in the rates of fetal death, stillbirth, neonatal death, spontaneous miscarriage or early delivery between women who completely seroconverted during the pregnancy and those who remained uninfected.[2] (It should be noted that this study used a Western blot to detect antibody. This technique is much less sensitive than an EIA, so it is not possible to extrapolate these findings to settings where EIAs are used to confirm or refute suspected acute infections.)

The situation is very different among women who are actively seroconverting during the last 6 weeks of pregnancy, because maternal infection at such a late stage in pregnancy presents a much higher risk to the newborn baby. The transmission rate is approximately 40% with a primary or initial infection with genital herpes at the time of delivery but is less than 1% with recurrent attacks of infection.

The incubation period is 1–3 weeks (median 12 days) and there is a nonmaternal source identified in one-third of cases. Importantly, in this group the incubation period may be prolonged to up to 28 days. Most mothers have no lesions at delivery as the majority of primary or initial infections are symptomless or missed.

## NEONATAL HERPES

Neonatal disease is classified broadly into three distinct disease syndromes depending on the extent of the disease and spread of the virus, namely:

- skin/eye/mouth lesions
- neurological disease
- disseminated infection, sometimes presenting as hepatitis and/or multiorgan failure.

The mortality is extremely high if newborn babies are not treated because the diagnosis is not considered but even in those who are treated promptly the morbidity is still significant. The highest-risk pregnancies are those where the woman is antibody-negative for both HSV types at booking; in such circumstances, the incidence of neonatal herpes is 54/100 000 live births, compared with 12/100 000 live births among women who are antibody-positive for both types – a more than four-fold difference.

## PREVENTION OF NEONATAL HERPES

Clearly, it is essential that the management of women in labour with suspected active HSV infection is in favour of reducing the risk to the newborn but it is now generally accepted that women who present with confirmed reactivation of genital HSV during labour or within the last 6 weeks of pregnancy do not need to have a caesarean section unless there are other considerations. However, if the episode cannot be confirmed to be a reactivation, a caesarean section should be performed because of the poor neonatal outcomes if virus transmission occurs. There is a slight caveat to this in that reactivated HSV-1 seems to transmit more efficiently than reactivated HSV-2 for reasons that are currently unknown.

If the episode is one of reactivation, a vaginal delivery is advised, with swabs and other body samples (blood, urine, faeces, throat, conjunctiva and surface skin) collected from the baby at birth and submitted for PCR/virus culture. The newborn is watched for any signs of infection and if these develop and/or the laboratory reports detection of HSV, then intravenous aciclovir is commenced immediately.

The management of a primary or initial infection is very different. If delivered by caesarean section, the newborn baby is swabbed and watched for clinical and/or laboratory evidence of infection. If the membranes have been ruptured for more than 4 hours or a vaginal delivery is unavoidable and primary/initial genital HSV infection is suspected, swabs are taken and postexposure intravenous aciclovir is started as soon as possible after birth.

Appropriate management of serodiscordant couples remains contentious. Prophylactic administration of aciclovir to the uninfected partner reduces the risk of acquisition by approximately 75%, but if the woman is pregnant and her partner suffers from genital HSV, the usual advice is to use condoms or preferably abstain from sexual intercourse for the last 6 weeks of the pregnancy.

## Rubella virus

Rubella virus, as described by McAlister Gregg in 1941, was the first virus to be discovered as cause of a congenital infection syndrome. In Australia in the early 1940s, there had been an extensive outbreak of rubella and many babies he was seeing in his ophthalmology clinics had unilateral and bilateral cataracts in association with other, mainly cardiac, defects. Many of the mothers gave a history of rash/rubella in early pregnancy and so the study of congenital virus infections was born.

General characteristics of the pathogen include:

- togavirus; single strain
- enveloped, single-stranded RNA
- inactivated by detergents
- spread by droplet transmission and close person-to-person contact
- incubation period 13–20 days
- preventable by vaccination (live attenuated)
- not treatable with antiviral agents.

TABLE 21.4 **Prevalence of rubella virus infection by country of birth**

| Country of birth | Prevalence of infection (%)[a] |
|---|---|
| African country | 10 |
| India or Pakistan | 10 |
| Sri Lanka | 17 |
| UK | 1.20 |

[a] Among women who booked at St George's Hospital London in 1999

## RUBELLA VACCINATION

Because of the severity of congenital rubella syndrome, it was one of the defining moments of disease prevention by vaccination when, in the 1970s, rubella vaccine was introduced into childhood vaccination programmes. In countries with well-developed vaccine programmes, rubella vaccine has been hugely successful at reducing the incidence of congenital rubella syndrome such that now it has been all but eliminated from these countries. However, from a global perspective, congenital rubella syndrome is an enormous problem. Approximately 250 000 affected babies are born annually in association with large epidemics. This is because 10–15% of adults are susceptible and remain at risk of becoming infected in pregnancy. This is borne out by studies of the prevalence of rubella antibody in pregnant women when they have their booking bloods taken. Stratified by country of birth, it is clear that countries without rubella vaccine in their childhood immunisation schedules have a much higher rate of adult infections (Table 21.4).

In the mid 1990s, outbreaks of rubella were reported in UK universities and army camps with some spill-over into pregnant women. It is essential that countries with rubella vaccine in their childhood vaccination schedule maintain a high (more than 90%) uptake, as recommended by the World Health Organization. Otherwise, there is a risk of creating a cohort of young girls who, when they reach childbearing age, have a much greater chance of being susceptible and also of being exposed to the virus. Exactly this scenario occurred in Greece and the UK now runs a nationwide measles, mumps and rubella (MMR) vaccine catch-up campaign to counteract the effects of the decade-long suboptimal uptake second-ary to unsubstantiated fears over MMR vaccine being linked to autism.

## RUBELLA IN PREGNANCY

A clinical illness of rubella should be considered and appropriate investigations performed in any pregnant woman who presents with a viral-type exanthem.

It is also very important to remember that a pregnant woman who reports contact with an individual possibly infected with rubella should have blood taken to check for rubella IgG, even if a previous positive IgG result is available. The rationale for this is that errors may be made in result transcription or sample identification when screening large numbers of serum samples, for example in an antenatal setting, and the result issued previously may have been false-positive. Only in cases where the woman has had two previous positive tests or a documented seroconversion to rubella vaccine is it not necessary to screen for antibody.

## CLINICAL FEATURES OF MATERNAL INFECTION

The typical clinical picture of rubella infection is that of a viral upper respiratory tract infection with coryzal symptoms associated with fever and malaise. This is followed by lymphadenopathy (occipital/cervical/postauricular) and a maculopapular rash over the entire body. Akin to parvovirus B19 infection, joint pains are a prominent feature in up to 70% of infections. These may persist for days to a month or more and are attributable to the deposition of antigen–antibody complexes in the synovial membranes. However, in up to 25% of infections, the disease may be so mild or asymptomatic that it may go unnoticed by the woman and her doctor or midwife.

## RUBELLA TESTING IN PREGNANCY

The laboratory diagnosis of maternal rubella is based on the serological response. Normally, because the rash is so abrupt in onset, the pregnant woman presents to her doctor or midwife within 1 or 2 days of its appearance. At this stage, if the rubella IgG result is negative, acute rubella is almost certainly the diagnosis as there has been insufficient time for this antibody to develop. The test for rubella-specific IgM is often also negative at this time. Convalescent serology from approximately 5 days after rash onset is therefore necessary. If there are ultrasound findings compatible with a possible diagnosis of congenital rubella syndrome in the fetus, a rubella IgG avidity assay may also be employed if there are no earlier samples from the woman.

## CLINICAL FEATURES OF FETAL INFECTION

Congenital rubella syndrome results from infection during the first trimester. Some 20% of affected fetuses miscarry. Of the remaining fetuses, 80% will have hearing loss, 60% will develop a neurological deficit, 60% have heart defects (for example patent ductus arteriosus, pulmonary-valve stenosis, ventricular septal defect), 40% have purpura and 30% have or develop cataracts and/or glaucoma. In later life, bony abnormalities become apparent, as does diabetes mellitus.

## PRENATAL DIAGNOSIS

Prenatal diagnosis is really only useful if infection occurs between weeks 12 and 20 of gestation, because maternal infection before week 12 almost always results in a badly affected fetus with multiple abnormalities as detailed previously. By contrast, infection after week 20 of gestation only very rarely leads to a clinically affected fetus. It is between these two times that rubella transmission *in utero* carries an approximately 15–20% risk of retinopathy (not necessarily sight-threatening) and sensorineural hearing loss. However, as neither of these is detectable ultrasonographically, PCR on amniotic fluid may be attempted. This has a sensitivity and specificity of over 90%. Testing of chorionic villus samples may give false-positive results because of the persistence of maternal rubella virus RNA. If rubella virus RNA is detected in amniotic fluid, it proves fetal infection but it does not prove clinical affection.

Before the advent of rubella virus PCR, the diagnosis of fetal infection was only possible by measuring the fetal IgM response at week 23 of gestation. Although the fetal IgM response is very reliable, it does not indicate whether the fetus has a hearing or vision deficit and use of this test instead of rubella virus PCR would delay the diagnosis and therefore a potential termination of pregnancy.

## REFERENCES

1. ENDERS G, MILLER E, CRADOCK-WATSON J, BOLLEY I, RIDEHALGH M. Consequences of varicella and herpes zoster in pregnancy: prospective study of 1739 cases. *Lancet* 1994;343:1548–51.

2. BROWN ZA, SELKE S, ZEH J, KOPELMAN J, MASLOW A, ASHLEY RL, *et al.* The acquisition of herpes simplex virus during pregnancy. *N Engl J Med* 1997;337:509–15.

CHAPTER 22

# Infections in obstetrics and gynaecology

*Phillip E Hay*

## Spectrum of genitourinary infections in women

Genitourinary infections are among the most common medical presentations in women. The most common symptomatic infections are bacterial vaginosis, vulvovaginal candidiasis (thrush) and urinary tract infections. Sexually transmitted infections such as chlamydia and gonorrhoea may be symptomatic or asymptomatic but, if causing pelvic inflammatory disease (PID), are a threat to a woman's future fertility. Viral infections can persist for long periods of time, with human papillomavirus (HPV) causing cervical, vulval and anal cancers and herpes simplex virus (HSV) persisting for life. Worldwide, HIV infection is predominantly sexually acquired and in some parts of the world as many as a third of pregnant women are now infected. Clinicians need to be aware of the way that HIV alters the manifestations of, and host susceptibility to, other infections.

Infections can adversely affect the mother during pregnancy, lead to congenital abnormality in the fetus, prematurity or neonatal infection and cause morbidity in the mother in the postnatal period. As in nonpregnant women, many infections can be silent or present with few symptoms.

The spectrum of infections that are important in pregnancy can be summarised by the acronym STORCH[5]:

- S – syphilis
- T – toxoplasmosis
- O – other
  - bacterial vaginosis
  - *Trichomonas vaginalis*
  - group B streptococcus
  - *Escherichia coli*
  - *Ureaplasma urealyticum*
  - *Haemophilus influenzae*
  - varicella zoster virus
  - *Listeria monocytogenes*
- R – rubella
- C – cytomegalovirus
- H[5] – HSV, HIV, hepatitis B virus, HPV and human parvovirus.

## Lower genital tract infections

The changes in physiology that occur during a woman's lifetime affect the susceptibility to, and site of, infection. At birth, the newborn girl is exposed to high levels of estrogen and progesterone from the mother and the vagina of the newborn is lined with stratified squamous epithelium. It is possible for *T. vaginalis* to be transmitted at birth but the infection usually clears spontaneously. In children, the vagina is lined with a simple cuboidal epithelium. The pH is neutral and the vagina is colonised by organisms similar to skin commensals. Under the influence of estrogen at puberty, stratified squamous epithelium develops and lactobacilli become the predominant organisms. This is accompanied by a drop in pH to a

**TABLE 22.1 Differential diagnosis of the principal causes of abnormal vaginal discharge**

| Symptoms and signs | Candidiasis | Bacterial vaginosis | Trichomoniasis | Cervicitis |
|---|---|---|---|---|
| Itching or soreness | ++ | – | +++ | – |
| Smell | May be 'yeasty' | Offensive, fishy | May be offensive | – |
| Colour | White | White or yellow | Yellow or green | Clear or coloured |
| Consistency | Curdy | Thin, homogeneous | Thin, homogenous | Mucoid |
| pH | <4.5 | 4.5–7.0 | 4.5–7.0 | <4.5 |
| Method of confirmation | Microscopy and culture | Microscopy | Microscopy and culture | Microscopy, tests for *Clamdia trachomatis* and *Neisseria gonorrhoeae* |

++ = moderate to severe | +++ = severe | – = none

level of approximately 3.5–4.5. Following the menopause, atrophic changes occur with a return to bacterial flora similar to that of the skin. The pH again rises to 7.0.

## PHYSIOLOGICAL DISCHARGE

Normal vaginal discharge is white, becoming yellowish on contact with air owing to oxidation. It consists of desquamated epithelial cells from the vagina and cervix, mucus originating mainly from the cervical glands, bacteria and fluid formed as a transudate from the vaginal wall. More than 95% of the bacteria present are lactobacilli. The acidic pH is maintained through the production of lactic acid by the vaginal epithelium metabolising glycogen and by the lactobacilli. Physiological discharge increases in midcycle owing to increased mucus production from the cervix. It also increases in pregnancy and sometimes when women start a combined oral contraceptive pill. Sometimes, a cervical ectropion is associated with excess mucus production causing persistent discharge. This can be treated with cervical cautery.

An overview of the differential diagnosis of abnormal vaginal discharge is provided in Table 22.1.

## VAGINAL CANDIDIASIS

Over 75% of women have at least one episode of vaginal candidiasis in their lifetime. At any time, 25% of women are colonised with *Candida* species in the vagina and a minority get symptoms. The organism is carried in the gut, under the nails, in the vagina and on the skin. *C. albicans* is found in more than 80% of affected women. *C. glabrata*, *C. krusei* and *C. tropicalis* account for most of the remaining 20%. Sexual acquisition is rarely important, although the physical trauma of intercourse may be sufficient to trigger an episode in a predisposed person. Vaginal candidiasisis is estrogen-dependent and therefore rarely seen in prepubertal girls or postmenopausal women.

Factors predisposing to vaginal candidiasis include the following:

- immunosuppression
  - HIV infection
  - immunosuppressive therapy, e.g. steroids
- diabetes mellitus
- vaginal douching, bubble bath, shower gel, tight clothing, tights
- increased estrogen levels
  - pregnancy
  - high-dose combined oral contraceptive pill
- underlying dermatosis, e.g. eczema
- broad-spectrum antibiotic therapy.

It should be noted that the role of tight clothing is anecdotal, described before the era of evidence-based medicine.

### Clinical features

Vaginal candidiasis is characterised by the following symptoms:

- itching, soreness and redness of the vagina and vulva
- curdy white discharge, which may smell yeasty but not unpleasant
- may be accompanied by fissures and excoriations.

Not all vaginal *Candida* infections present in the same way; in some women there may be itching and redness with a thin watery discharge. The pH of vaginal fluid is usually normal (between 3.5 and 4.5). The diagnosis can be confirmed by microscopy and culture of the vaginal fluid. Asymptomatic women from whom a *Candida* species is grown on culture do not require treatment.

Recurrent *Candida* infection or *Candida* infection not responding to treatment is relatively uncommon. If the clinical picture suggests the presence of treatment-resistant *Candida* infection, the correct diagnosis is often HSV infection, vulvodynia or a dermatological condition such as eczema or lichen sclerosis.

### Treatment

As a general rule, it is better to use a topical treatment than a systemic therapy. This minimises the risk of systemic adverse effects. Vaginal creams and pessaries can be prescribed at a variety of doses and for variable durations. However, some women have a preference for oral therapy, particularly if required at the time of menstruation. Treatment options include the following:

- clotrimazole pessary 500 mg given as a single dose
- oral fluconazole 150 mg tablet given as a single dose (only active against *C. albicans* strains).

Longer courses of treatment are needed when there are predisposing factors that cannot be eliminated, such as steroid therapy.

In pregnancy, treatment with a topical agent such as clotrimazole 100 mg/day for 7 days gives superior cure rates. Oral azoles are not recommended in pregnancy.

### Complications and pregnancy

Genuine recurrent infection with a *Candida* species can be suppressed with weekly fluconazole 150 mg for a 6-month period. If resistance to treatment is shown clinically and *in vitro*, new antifungal agents such as voriconazole can be administered. Alternatively, boric acid applied intravaginally can be used.

Complications are uncommon. In some women, a severe episode of vaginal candidiasis can trigger long-term vulvodynia. Candidiasis has not generally been associated with complications in pregnancy, although in one study treatment of asymptomatic vaginal candidiasis was associated with fewer preterm births.

### BACTERIAL VAGINOSIS

Bacterial vaginosis is the most common cause of abnormal vaginal discharge in women of childbearing age. Its reported prevalence has varied widely from as low as 5% in a selected group of asymptomatic college students to 50% of women in a large study in Uganda. Studies in antenatal clinics and gynaecology clinics show a prevalence of approximately 12% in the UK.

Bacterial vaginosis is more common in black women and those who have an intrauterine contraceptive device (IUCD). In addition, it is probably more common in women with sexually transmitted infections, although bacterial vaginosis has also been reported in virgin women and may be particularly common in lesbian women. The condition often arises spontaneously around the time of menstruation and may resolve spontaneously in midcycle.

Previously, a variety of names had been used for this condition, including nonspecific vaginitis, *Gardnerella* vaginitis and anaerobic vaginosis. When bacterial vaginosis develops, the predominantly anaerobic organisms that may be present at low concentration in the vagina increase in concentration up to a thousand-fold. This is accompanied by a rise in vaginal pH to between 4.5 and 7.0 and ultimately the lactobacilli may disappear.

The organisms classically associated with bacterial vaginosis are:

- *Gardnerella vaginalis*
- *Bacteroides* (*Prevotella*) species
- *Mobiluncus* species
- *Mycoplasma hominis*.

Novel organisms such as *Atopobium vaginae* have been identified by use of molecular techniques and a biofilm consisting predominantly of *Gardnerella* species and *A. vaginae* has been described.

### Clinical features

The typical symptom of bacterial vaginosis is an offensive fishy-smelling discharge that is characteristically thin, homogenous and adherent to the walls of the vagina. It may be white or yellow. The smell is particularly noticeable around the time of menstruation or following intercourse. However, semen itself can give off a weak fishy smell.

In clinical practice, the diagnosis is commonly made using the composite (Amsel) criteria:

- vaginal pH above 4.5
- release of a fishy smell on addition of alkali (10% potassium hydroxide)
- characteristic discharge on examination
- presence of 'clue cells' on microscopy.

Clue cells are vaginal epithelial cells so heavily coated with bacteria that the border is obscured.

Bacterial vaginosis can also be diagnosed from a Gram-stained vaginal smear. Large numbers of Gram-positive and Gram-negative cocci are seen, with reduced or absent large Gram-positive bacilli (lactobacilli). Culture of a high vaginal swab yields mixed anaerobes and a high concentration of *G. vaginalis*. However, *G. vaginalis* can be grown from up to 50% of women with normal vaginal flora. Its presence is not, therefore, diagnostic of bacterial vaginosis.

### Treatment

Bacterial vaginosis will resolve on treatment with antibiotics with good antianaerobic activity such as the following:

- metronidazole 400 mg twice/day for 5 days or metronidazole 2 g as a single dose
- metronidazole vaginal gel (0.75%) 5 g/night for 5 nights
- clindamycin cream (2%) 5 g/night for 3–7 nights.

Initial cure rates are greater than 80% but up to 30% of women relapse within 1 month of treatment.

### Complications

It is now established that women with bacterial vaginosis are at increased risk of second-trimester miscarriage and preterm delivery during pregnancy. This may result in perinatal mortality or cerebral palsy. Studies in which bacterial vaginosis in pregnant women has been treated with metronidazole or clindamycin have produced conflicting results, so current guidelines do not recommend routine screening and treatment in pregnancy.

Treatment of bacterial vaginosis with metronidazole before termination of pregnancy has been shown to reduce the number of subsequent incidents of endometritis and PID.

In some women, the vaginal flora is in a dynamic state, with bacterial vaginosis developing and remitting spontaneously. Women with symptoms of recurrent bacterial vaginosis can become frustrated as the condition responds rapidly to treatment with antibiotics but may also relapse rapidly. Our inability to alter this process reflects our current lack of knowledge of the factors that trigger bacterial vaginosis. Regular treatment with 0.75% metronidazole gel twice week reduces the rate of recurrence.

### TRICHOMONIASIS

*Trichomonas vaginalis* is a sexually transmitted infection that can be carried asymptomatically for several months before causing symptoms. It is diagnosed in approximately 1% of women attending genitourinary medicine clinics but is highly prevalent in many tropical countries, with a 25% prevalence rate reported in rural Uganda. In men, trichomoniasis is often carried asymptomatically but may present as nongonococcal urethritis.

### Clinical features

Trichomoniasis is characterised by the following symptoms:

- vulvovaginitis, which can be severe, with inflammation sometimes extending out onto the vulva and adjacent skin
- purulent green or yellow discharge, sometimes with an offensive smell
- punctate haemorrhages can occur on the cervix, giving the appearance of a 'strawberry cervix'.

Many affected women also develop bacterial vaginosis.

The diagnosis is confirmed by culture, preferably in a specific medium such as Feinberg–Whittington medium.

Nucleic acid amplification tests (NAATs) promise a greater diagnostic sensitivity once they become available. Microscopy of vaginal secretions mixed with saline has a 60% sensitivity for detecting the organism. Numerous polymorphonuclear cells are seen and the motile organism is identified from its shape and the presence of four moving flagellae.

## Treatment

Treatment of trichomoniasis involves the following antibiotics:

- metronidazole either 2 g as a single dose or 400 mg twice/day for 5 days
- tinidazole 2 g as a single dose, which is more expensive but occasionally works when metronidazole has failed.

The woman should be advised to send her sexual partner(s) for treatment before resuming intercourse together.

## Complications

T. vaginalis has occasionally been identified in the upper genital tract of women with PID but the organism is probably not an important cause of upper genital tract pathology. It can also be isolated from the bladder.

Occasionally, persistent trichomoniasis is seen. This may be attributable to poor compliance with medication, poor absorption, reinfection or, rarely, a treatment-resistant organism. The usual approach is to use higher doses of metronidazole, initially 400 mg three times/day orally, increasing to 1 g twice/day given per rectum or intravenously. Only a limited number of alternatives are available, including arsphenamine pessaries and clotrimazole, which has an inhibitory effect on T. vaginalis.

## Pregnancy

Pregnant women symptomatic for trichomoniasis should be treated with a 5-day course of metronidazole. Although T. vaginalis infection is a risk factor for preterm birth, treatment of asymptomatic infection has not been shown to improve outcome.

## OTHER CONDITIONS AFFECTING THE LOWER GENITAL TRACT

Occasionally, one encounters a true bacterial vaginitis that is caused by a Streptococcus strain or another organism not classically associated with this condition. It responds to appropriate antibiotic therapy such as co-amoxiclav 375 mg three times/day for 7 days.

The retention of tampons or foreign bodies in the vagina is rarely associated with toxic shock syndrome. An overgrowth of toxin-producing staphylococci causes systemic shock with fever, diarrhoea, vomiting and an erythematous rash. There is a 10% mortality rate. More frequently, a foreign body or retained tampon merely causes an offensive discharge.

### Bartholin abscess

The Bartholin glands are situated on either side of the vagina and open into the vestibule. Cysts can develop if the opening becomes blocked. These present as painless swellings. If they become infected, a Bartholin abscess develops. Examination reveals a hot, tender abscess adjacent to the lower part of the vagina. Surgical treatment is required. This is usually done by marsupialisation. Culture may yield a variety of organisms including Neisseria gonorrhoeae, streptococci, staphylococci, mixed anaerobic organisms and E. coli.

### Infestations

Pubic lice and scabies are transmitted by close bodily contact. Pubic lice (Phthirus pubis) attach their eggs to the base of the pubic hair. Their claws only attach to thick body hair, so that they can also colonise the axillae and eyelashes. Infected individuals may report small itchy papules or notice debris from the lice in their underwear. Lice are treated by application of topical agents such as malathion, carbaryl or permethrin. Treatment should be repeated after 7 days and be supplied for partners to use simultaneously.

Scabies (Sarcoptes scabiei) causes an intensely itchy papular rash. It may be confined to the genital area initially if acquired during intercourse. It responds to applications of malathion or permethrin. Symptoms may take up to 6 weeks to resolve completely.

## Upper genital tract infections

Ascending infection of the female upper genital tract is broadly termed pelvic inflammatory disease (PID) and includes endometritis, parametritis, salpingitis and oophoritis. These infections usually spread from the vagina or cervix through the uterine cavity. Lymphatic spread may also occur, either parametrially or along the surface of the uterus. Although rare, salpingitis has occurred in women who have been sterilised. Infection can also spread from the bowel or be blood-borne.

PID is an important condition because it results in tubal damage producing ectopic pregnancy and tubal factor infertility. As many as 20% of affected women may be left with chronic pelvic pain. PID is common. Approximately 12.5% of a cohort of women born in the 1950s in Sweden had at least one episode of PID before the age of 25 years. The symptoms and signs may be mild and subtle, with many women being unaware of the significance of mild pelvic pain for their future fertility. On the other hand, many women are now aware of these complications and seek reassurance about their future fertility when they receive a diagnosis of PID. The best information available is from a study in Lund, Sweden, that was started in the 1960s. In that study, 8% of women had tubal factor infertility following a single episode of PID, rising to approximately 50% after three episodes.

Many different organisms have been cultured from women with PID but the condition is often triggered by either *Chlamydia trachomatis* or *Neisseria gonorrhoeae*. *Mycoplasma genitalium* has also been implicated in PID (in men it causes nongonococcal urethritis) and, like *C. trachomatis* and *N. gonorrhoeae*, it is probably sexually transmitted. Tests for detecting *M. genitalium* are not available routinely but NAATs are being developed. The organism is difficult to culture and requires a specialised medium for growth. Endogenous anaerobes such as *Bacteroides* species or *Mycoplasma hominis* often come in as secondary invaders and are responsible for subsequent tubal abscess formation.

## INFECTIONS ASSOCIATED WITH CHLAMYDIA TRACHOMATIS AND NEISSERIA GONORRHOEAE

### Chlamydia

Infection with *C. trachomatis* is the most common sexually transmitted bacterial infection in industrialised countries. As many as 10% of women of childbearing age are infected in inner cities in the UK. The prevalence is highest among women under 25 years.

The infection is asymptomatic in approximately 50% of men and 80% of women. In men, *C. trachomatis* is the most important cause of nongonococcal urethritis. In women, it causes cervicitis and PID as well as other complications that will be discussed later on. The organism can infect the rectum but severe proctitis is only caused by lymphogranuloma venereum (LGV) strains. In addition, genital strains can colonise the throat and can also cause conjunctivitis.

There is now a national chlamydia screening programme in the UK targeting women below the age of 25 years with the aim of reducing the incidence of PID and tubal factor infertility.

### Bacteriology

*C. trachomatis* is an obligate intracellular pathogen. The species has been subdivided into several serovars:

- serovars A–C cause trachoma, infecting the conjunctiva
- serovars D–K cause genital infections
- serovars L1–L3 cause LGV.

*C. trachomatis* has a complex life cycle. The infectious form is known as an elementary body. This gains entry to host cells by binding to specific cell surface receptors. Once inside the cell, the elementary bodies differentiate into so-called reticulate bodies. These are the metabolically active form of the organism and can be detected within inclusion bodies. Heavily infected cells die. Damage to the epithelial surface is mainly caused by the inflammatory response to infection and can manifest as cervicitis and PID.

### Diagnosis

Chlamydial infection is now diagnosed by NAAT. Self-collected vaginal swabs provide sensitivity equivalent to clinician-collected endocervical swabs, allowing the use of self-collected swabs for screening. In women, first-pass urine testing has a lower sensitivity than vaginal swab testing but in some settings urine samples are obtained more easily. Serological tests are insensitive and non-specific but high levels of antibody are found in 60% of women with tubal factor infertility.

## Treatment

The following treatments are effective for an uncomplicated chlamydial infection:

- azithromycin 1 g as a single dose
- doxycycline 100 mg twice/day for 7 days
- ofloxacin 400 mg once/day for 7 days
- erythromycin 500 mg twice/day for 14 days (used in pregnancy).

The partner(s) should also receive treatment for *C. trachomatis* and be screened fully for sexually transmitted infections before sexual intercourse is resumed.

### Gonorrhoea

In developed countries, the incidence of gonorrhoea has declined in the last two decades; the prevalence in women of childbearing age is now less than 1%. The spectrum of disease in women is similar to that associated with *Chlamydia* infection. However, chronic asymptomatic infection is common, with 50% of affected women having no symptoms or signs of infection. By contrast, approximately 90% of affected men are symptomatic. The most common presentation in men is severe urethritis with green urethral discharge and dysuria. Women and homosexual men may also present with proctitis, characterised by purulent discharge, bleeding and rectal pain.

   *N. gonorrhoeae* may also be carried in the throat or cause an exudative tonsillitis. In addition, it can cause conjunctivitis in adults.

## Bacteriology

*N. gonorrhoeae* colonises columnar or cuboidal epithelia. In chronic infection, there is a complex interaction with the host immune system. In the presence of an effective antibody response, the expression of antigenic cell surface proteins changes over time, preventing the development of protective immunity.

## Diagnosis

Reliable serological tests for *N. gonorrhoeae* have not been developed. In genitourinary medicine clinics, a presumptive diagnosis is made on observation of typical Gram-negative intracellular diplococci on smears of urethral, cervical or rectal swabs. *N. gonorrhoeae* is a fastidious organism that requires a $CO_2$ concentration of 7%, specific media such as blood agar and antibiotics to inhibit the growth of other organisms. It may fail to grow on culture, especially if transport to the laboratory is delayed. NAATs are available but may have poor specificity. Obtaining a culture remains essential to allow testing for antibiotic sensitivity.

## Treatment

The following treatments are effective in sensitive strains of *N. gonorrhoeae*:

- amoxicillin 3 g with probenecid 2 g as a single dose
- ciprofloxacin 500 mg as a single dose
- spectinomycin 2 g as a single dose (intramuscularly)
- cefixime 400 mg as a single dose
- ceftriaxone 250 mg as a single dose (intramuscularly).

The choice of treatment is dictated by local sensitivity patterns, history of recent travel and cost. Strains resistant to antibiotics emerge rapidly where antibiotic use is not controlled adequately. Chromosomal mutations conferring reduced sensitivity to penicillin emerge slowly in an incremental way, with high-level resistance to penicillin being mediated by a plasmid. The first such plasmid described enables production of the enzyme penicillinase (penicillinase-producing *N. gonorrhoeae* or PPNG strains). Strains with chromosomal mutations conferring resistance to quinolone antibiotics are also seen worldwide.

   Following treatment, two sets of culture should be performed as tests of cure because of the possibility of antibiotic resistance and occasional treatment failures. Tests of cure should include rectal swabs because infection can spread to the rectum regardless of whether anal intercourse has occurred.

   It is important to treat partners for gonorrhoea before sexual intercourse is resumed. In addition, more than 50% of women infected with *N. gonorrhoeae* have a concomitant chlamydial infection. Chlamydial treatment should therefore also be prescribed as a matter of routine for all women with gonorrhoea and their partners.

### Cervicitis

Mucopurulent cervicitis is a clinical diagnosis made on detection of purulent mucus at the cervical os, which is often accompanied by contact bleeding. It can be confused with a benign ectropion but the latter does not usually bleed heavily unless swabbed very vigorously. Women with cervicitis may present with postcoital bleeding or complaining of a purulent vaginal discharge. Many, however, are asymptomatic. The condition is often caused by a sexually transmitted agent, with the male partner having nongonococcal urethritis. Tests for *C. trachomatis* and *N. gonorrhoeae* should be performed. If ulceration is present, an HSV test should be obtained.

The treatment is the same as for chlamydial infection, unless a specific organism is detected.

Chronic cervicitis produces scarring. In addition, nabothian follicles (mucus-containing cysts of up to 1 cm in diameter) are often present following chronic cervicitis.

### Pelvic inflammatory disease

As infection ascends into the uterus, endometritis develops. Plasma cells are seen on endometrial biopsy and, in women with chronic chlamydial infection, germinal centres may develop.

The first stage of salpingitis involves mucosal inflammation with swelling, redness and deciliation. Polymorphonuclear cells invade the submucosa, followed by mononuclear cells and plasma cells. Inflammatory exudate fills the lumen of the tube and adhesions develop between mucosal folds. Inflammation extends to the serosal surface and pus exudes from the fimbriae to the ovaries and their adnexae. At laparoscopy, the tubes in mild salpingitis are swollen and red. In more severe forms of salpingitis, they are fixed to adjacent structures by fibrin exudate and adhesions. With pelvic peritonitis, all the organs are congested with multiple adhesions producing an inflammatory mass. The omentum usually confines the infection to the pelvis. The infection causes considerable tissue destruction. Tubal or tubo-ovarian abscesses may develop.

Subsequent scarring may lead to the fimbriae being drawn into the ends of the fallopian tubes, with the result that they adhere to and seal the ends of the tubes. The uterus and tubes may be pulled back into the pelvis by adhesions, becoming fixed and retroverted. Accumulation of fluid within the tube causes a hydrosalpinx; the affected tube expands and swells. If infected, a pyosalpinx results. Pelvic adhesions organise, matting together the pelvic organs. Some recovery of the ciliated epithelium within the tubes usually occurs.

#### Clinical features

As infection extends into the uterus, the fallopian tubes and the ovaries, it causes pelvic pain and deep dyspareunia. Endometritis may cause intermenstrual bleeding and it is common for women with PID to have an associated urinary tract infection.

The diagnosis of PID is made on the basis of the following findings:

- a history of pelvic pain and deep dyspareunia
- cervical motion tenderness (often called cervical excitation) on examination, with or without uterine and adnexal tenderness
- a lower genital tract infection such as bacterial vaginosis, trichomoniasis or cervicitis
- pyrexia, a raised neutrophil count and a raised erythrocyte sedimentation rate (in more severe forms of PID)
- an adnexal mass (present in 20% women, usually those who are most unwell systemically).

At best, the clinical diagnosis is 70–80% accurate. Laparoscopy is regarded as the gold-standard for diagnosis. In early salpingitis, however, the inflammation may not be visible from the serosal surface of the tubes. The important differential diagnoses are shown in Table 22.2. The most important diagnosis to exclude acutely is ectopic pregnancy.

When PID is suspected, endocervical swabs should be taken for detection of *C. trachomatis* and *N. gonorrhoeae*. A high vaginal swab should be taken for detection of *T. vaginalis* and bacterial vaginosis. Laparoscopy should be performed if the clinical diagnosis is uncertain, if drainage of an abscess might be required or if there is no improvement after 24–48 hours of intravenous antibiotic treatment in a systemically unwell woman.

#### Treatment

Ambulant women with mild symptoms can be treated as outpatients. The antibiotic regimen should cover both

TABLE 22.2 **Findings at laparoscopy in women with suspected pelvic inflammatory disease**

| Diagnosis at laparoscopy | Proportion of women (%) |
| --- | --- |
| Salpingitis/pelvic inflammatory disease | 65 |
| Normal findings | 22 |
| Appendicitis | 3 |
| Endometriosis | 2 |
| Bleeding corpus luteum | 2 |
| Ectopic pregnancy | 2 |
| Miscellaneous | 4 |

*C. trachomatis* and *N. gonorrhoeae* as well as anaerobic organisms.

Current guidelines recommend the following two oral regimens:

- a single dose of intramuscular ceftriaxone 250 mg, doxycycline 100 mg twice/day for 14 days and metronidazole 400 mg twice/day for 14 days
- ofloxacin 400 mg twice/day for 14 days and metronidazole 400 mg twice/day for 14 days.

However, with increasing quinolone resistance of *N. gonorrhoeae*, it is advisable to include ceftriaxone in any treatment regimen.

Women who are systemically unwell or in whom a tubal abscess is suspected should be admitted for intravenous antibiotic treatment and may require laparoscopy to definitely establish the diagnosis. One recommended regimen comprises intravenous cefoxitin and doxycycline followed by oral doxycycline and metronidazole for 14 days. Another uses intravenous clindamycin and gentamicin followed by 14 days of oral doxycycline and metronidazole or 14 days of oral clindamycin. It is essential that sexual partners are screened for *C. trachomatis* and *N. gonorrhoeae* and prescribed appropriate antibiotic treatment before intercourse is resumed.

### Other complications of chlamydia and gonorrhoea

Intra-abdominal spread of *C. trachomatis* or *N. gonorrhoeae* can cause periappendicitis (which mimics appendi-

citis) or perihepatitis; the latter is termed Fitz-Hugh–Curtis syndrome. Women and, rarely, men with this syndrome present with pyrexia and right hypochondrial pain and tenderness. They are frequently misdiagnosed as having cholecystitis. Careful examination usually elicits signs of salpingitis. At laparoscopy, fine 'violin string' adhesions are seen between the liver capsule and the visceral peritoneum. Treatment is a 3-week course of antibiotics for chlamydia and gonorrhoea depending on the identified cause.

Disseminated infection with *C. trachomatis* may cause Reiter syndrome (sexually acquired reactive arthritis) in about 1% of infected individuals. There is usually an asymmetrical oligoarthritis affecting large joints of the lower limb. In Reiter syndrome, the arthritis is accompanied by uveitis and a rash that, if florid, may be similar to psoriasis. It is associated with the presence of human leucocyte antigen haplotype B27 and there is overlap with other seronegative spondarthritides.

Disseminated infection with *N. gonorrhoeae* presents as a septic oligoarthritis that usually affects the small joints of the hand or wrist, often accompanied by a scanty papular rash. It is rare but occurs more often in women than men because of the larger proportion of asymptomatic and untreated infections in women.

### Pregnancy and vertical transmission of chlamydia and gonorrhoea

Genital infection with *C. trachomatis* or *N. gonorrhoeae* during pregnancy can cause chorioamnionitis and women with such infections probably have a two- to three-fold increased risk of preterm birth. Although data on the safety of azithromycin in pregnancy are limited, this drug is now commonly used for the treatment of chlamydia because it is better tolerated than erythromycin. Cephalosporins should be used for gonorrhoea. Quinolones, doxycycline and tetracyclines are contraindicated in pregnancy. Because of altered drug pharmacokinetics in pregnancy, a test of cure should be performed 6 weeks after treatment. If performed earlier, DNA from dead organisms may be detected leading to unnecessary concern about treatment failure.

Newborn babies usually acquire infection as they pass through an infected birth canal. Both *C. trachomatis* and *N. gonorrhoeae* cause ophthalmia neonatorum. Affected infants develop keratoconjunctivitis, which can progress to corneal scarring and blindness if not treated promptly. The diagnosis of ophthalmia neonatorum is confirmed by taking conjunctival swabs for the detection of *C. trachomatis* by direct fluorescent antibody assay or DNA amplification assay and for the detection of *N. gonorrhoeae* by culture. The mother and her sexual partner(s) should also be screened and receive appropriate treatment. *C. trachomatis* may cause pneumonitis in the first few months of life. Babies with ophthalmia neonatorum should therefore receive systemic therapy with erythromycin.

## OTHER CAUSES OF ENDOMETRITIS

### *Tuberculosis*

*Mycobacterium tuberculosis* can spread through the genital tract via the blood or lymphatics. Nearly always, another organ is also affected by tuberculosis, usually the lung. Granulomata develop in the fallopian tubes and subsequently in the other genital organs. Infection may remain subclinical, presenting ultimately with amenorrhoea, infertility or chronic low-grade pelvic pain. The endometrium is involved in up to 80% of affected women and the ovaries in 20–30%. Abnormal uterine bleeding is a presenting symptom in 10–40% of affected women. The examination is often normal but an adnexal mass or fixing of the pelvic organs may be detected. The diagnosis can be confirmed by obtaining endometrial tissue from biopsy or from dilatation and curettage. The detection rate is greatest towards the end of the menstrual cycle. Even so, endometrial biopsy does not have a 100% sensitivity.

As the presentation may be subtle, a high index of suspicion is essential. A Mantoux test or Heaf test should be reactive in women with active tuberculosis unless they have an immunosuppressing condition. A chest X-ray should be performed to look for evidence of pulmonary tuberculosis. Bilateral tubal calcification may be seen on abdominal X-ray after chronic infection. Treatment should be supervised by a physician with expertise in tuberculosis.

### *Actinomycosis*

This infection is almost exclusively seen in women with an IUCD. It can be detected on cervical cytology and careful monitoring is required if there are no clinical features to suggest PID. If there is any history of pelvic pain, the IUCD should be removed and antibiotic treatment with penicillin initiated. If undetected, actinomycosis can progress to widespread pelvic involvement with an inflammatory mass and fixing of the pelvic organs. For further information on the clinical features, diagnosis and treatment of actinomycosis see chapter 20.

## Genital ulcer disease

The diagnosis of genital ulcers can be a considerable challenge for the clinician. The following list provodes an overview of potential infectious and noninfectious causes of genital ulcer disease:

- Infectious causes
  - Herpes simplex virus
  - Primary syphilis
  - Lymphogranuloma venereum
  - Chancroid
  - Donovanosis
  - HIV
- Noninfectious causes
  - Aphthous ulcers
  - Trauma
  - Skin disease, e.g. lichen sclerosus et atrophicus
  - Behçet syndrome
  - Other multisystem disorders, e.g. sarcoidosis
  - Dermatitis artefacta.

In the UK, HSV infection (discussed in Chapter 21) is by far the most common cause. It is essential, however, to take an adequate sexual and travel history as there are many other sexually transmitted causes of genital ulcers that are common in tropical countries.

Among the noninfectious causes, malignancy, particularly squamous cell carcinoma, may arise on a background of lichen sclerosus et atrophicus or vulval intraepithelial neoplasia. In addition, multisystem disorders such as Behçet syndrome, systemic lupus erythematosus and sarcoidosis may be associated with genital ulceration. It is therefore advisable to arrange for a biopsy if there is any doubt about the diagnosis.

Simple aphthous ulcers can occur on the genital mucosa in the same way as in the mouth. HIV infection may present with genital ulceration, particularly in the form of persistent atypical herpetic ulcers. The presentation of other infections is modified by immunosuppression.

## SYPHILIS

At present, the incidence of syphilis is rising in European countries including the UK. The disease is most common in the tropics and in homosexual men. The correct microbiological diagnosis can be difficult and referral to an appropriate specialist may be required.

Syphilis is a systemic sexually transmitted infection caused by *Treponema pallidum*. *In vitro*, *T. pallidum* subspecies *pallidum*, the causative organism of venereal syphilis, cannot be distinguished from *T. pallidum* subspecies *pertenue*, which causes yaws, *T. pallidum* subspecies *endemicum*, which causes endemic syphilis (also called bejel), and *T. pallidum* subspecies *carateum*, which causes pinta. These three tropical treponematoses are not sexually transmitted but are spread by skin-to-skin contact or fomites, often affecting children and household contacts. A description of them is beyond the scope of this chapter. Clinicians in the UK must be aware that they occur in sub-Saharan Africa, in the Caribbean and most of the humid tropics (yaws), in desert regions (endemic syphilis) and in isolated parts of Central and South America (pinta). Following such an infection, the serological tests for syphilis may remain positive for life, causing diagnostic confusion. The tropical treponematoses have become less common following mass treatment campaigns in the 1950s and 1960s but they still occur.

### Clinical features

The first manifestation of venereal syphilis is the chancre, a painless ulcer that arises at the entry site of *T. pallidum*. Some people have multiple chancres. In addition, the regional lymph nodes become enlarged. The time between infection and appearance of the chancre is usually 3–6 weeks and it heals without treatment after a few weeks. Many women do not notice chancres because these often develop on the cervix.

Secondary syphilis can arise as the primary chancre is healing or up to 6 months thereafter. It is a systemic disease that most often manifests as a nonitchy maculopapular rash. The rash is symmetrical and often involves the palms of the hands and soles of the feet. Intertriginous areas, particularly the perianal area, may show more florid, wart-like lesions called condylomata lata. On mucosal surfaces, mucous patches and lines of ulcers (snail track ulcers) may develop. There may also be generalised lymphadenopathy. Other manifestations include alopecia, arthritis and meningitis. A sensorineural deafness can occur early in the infection owing to destruction of the hair cells in the inner ear.

Resolution of secondary syphilis is followed by a period of latency. The infection can only be detected on serological testing as there are no outward manifestations. There is a potential for lesions of secondary syphilis to recur for up to 2 years and during such a relapse the infection can be transmitted to a sexual partner. This period is therefore called early latent syphilis.

Primary and secondary syphilis are not generally life-threatening. The importance of timely diagnosis rests on the risks of late tertiary syphilis (neurosyphilis or cardiovascular syphilis) and transmission from a mother to a fetus.

Approximately 10% of men and 5% of women develop neurosyphilis if not treated in the early stages. Neurosyphilis can manifest within 5 years of infection in the form of meningovascular syphilis, the presenting symptom often being a stroke. Meningovascular syphilis may subsequently progress to tabes dorsalis or general paresis of the insane. Approximately 20% of people with syphilis will develop cardiovascular syphilis, presenting with thoracic aortic aneurysm or aortic regurgitation often many years after the primary infection.

Vertical transmission may severely affect the newborn baby and even cause fetal death. Surviving babies at risk should be fully evaluated (this should include a lumbar puncture) and receive intravenous penicillin. Less severe congenital infection may present during late childhood with symptoms including eighth-nerve deafness, interstitial keratitis and abnormal teeth. The risk of congenital infection is greatest (as high as 70%) in mothers with primary and secondary syphilis during the pregnancy but vertical transmission can even occur in pregnancies where the primary infection of the mother dates back 5–10 years. The effects of late congenital syphilis are not prevented unless the mother is treated before week 20 of gestation.

TABLE 22.3 **Syphilis serology: interpretation of results**

| EIA | TPPA | RPR | IgM | Interpretation |
|---|---|---|---|---|
| Positive | Positive | Titre >1:8 | Positive | Early syphilis |
| Positive | Negative | Negative | N/A | Biological false-positive reaction |
| Positive | Positive | Titre <1:8 | Negative | Late or treated treponemal infection [a] |

[a] IgM assays have a poor sensitivity and specificity, so the diagnosis could also be one of incubating early syphilis. | EIA = enzyme immunoassay | IgM = immunoglobulin M | RPR = rapid plasma reagin | TPPA = *Treponema pallidum* particle agglutination

## Diagnosis

The diagnosis of primary syphilis is traditionally made by visualising the spirochaetes with dark-field microscopy. Polymerase chain reaction (PCR) tests are becoming available. Serological tests for syphilis (Table 22.3) should be requested but these can be negative in early primary syphilis, so repeat serological testing should be performed if clinical suspicion is high. Most laboratories routinely perform an enzyme immunoassay, which detects both immunoglobulin G (IgG) and immunoglobulin M (IgM) antibodies against *T. pallidum*. If this screening test is positive, specific treponemal tests such as the *T. pallidum* haemagglutination (TPHA) test or the *T. pallidum* particle agglutination (TPPA) assay are performed. A test for nonspecific treponemal antibodies, such as the venereal disease research laboratory (VDRL) test or the rapid plasma reagin (RPR) test, is used in addition. These tests are diluted serially to report a titre such as one in 64. Chancres on the cervix may be misdiagnosed as cervical carcinomas. If there is any doubt, biopsies must be taken.

In secondary syphilis, the VDRL test is usually positive at a titre of one to 32 or greater. Dark-field microscopy of material from mucosal patches or condylomata lata can also be performed.

Owing to the possibility of false-positive test results or labelling errors, it is traditional to start treatment only after a second confirmatory test. However, in pregnancy it is better not to risk a treatment delay while waiting for a repeat test if the serological tests are unequivocally positive. Following treatment of primary or secondary syphilis, the VDRL titre should fall two-fold every 3 months, becoming negative within 2 years.

## Treatment

The antibiotic of choice for the treatment of syphilis is penicillin. In early syphilis (primary, secondary and early latent syphilis), the following formulations can be used:

- benzathine benzylpenicillin 2.4 megaunits as a single dose (intramuscularly)
- procaine benzylpenicillin 1.2 megaunits/day to 600 000 units/day for 10 days (intramuscularly).

Alternatives to penicillin are:

- azithromycin 2 g single dose or 500 mg/day for 10 days
- ceftriaxone 500 mg/day for 10 days (intramuscularly)
- doxycycline 100 mg two times/day for 14 days
- erythromycin 500 mg four times/day for 14 days.

However, erythromycin is rarely used because macrolide resistance has been documented in several outbreaks.

If the infection has been present for more than 2 years, the treatment duration is extended to 21 days for penicillin regimens (benzathine benzypenicillin given as 3 injections at 7-day intervals) and 28 days for oral regimens. Only intravenous penicillin or high doses of procaine benzylpenicillin (2.4 megaunits/day) combined with probenecid (500 mg four times/day) produce acceptable levels of penicillin in the central nervous system to treat neurosyphilis.

In the first 24 hours after treatment, fever, malaise and exacerbation of symptoms (including rash) may occur. This is the Jarisch–Herxheimer reaction, which has been attributed to the release of proinflammatory cytokines following death of the infectious organisms. Paracetamol is usually sufficient to reduce the symptoms.

Partner notification is essential to prevent the spread of syphilis. In addition, the sexual history should be reviewed. In some cases, partners from a few years previ-

TABLE 22.4 **Treatment for bacterial genital ulcers**

| Antibacterial agent | Primary syphilis | Lymphogranuloma venereum | Chancroid | Donovanosis |
|---|---|---|---|---|
| Azithromycin | Active but resistance occurs | Active but resistance is common | 1 g single dose | Not recommended |
| Ceftriaxone | Active but not fully evaluated | Not recommended | 250 mg single dose | Not recommended |
| Ciprofloxacin | Not active | Not reliable | 500 mg twice/day for 3 days | 750 mg twice/day for ≥21 days |
| Co-trimoxazole | Not active | Not recommended | May be used but resistance is common in some areas | 960 mg twice/day for ≥21 days |
| Doxycycline | 100 mg twice/day for 14 days | 100 mg twice/day for 21 days | Not recommended | 100 mg twice/day for ≥21 days |
| Erythromycin | 500 mg four times/day for 14 days [a] | 500 mg four times/day for 21 days | 500 mg four times/day for 7 days | 500 mg four times/day for 21 days minimum |
| Penicillin | Procaine benzylpenicillin 600 000 units/day for 10 days or single dose benzathine benzylpenicillin 2.4 mega units | Not recommended | Not recommended | Not recommended |

[a] Rarely used – macrolide resistance has been documented in several outbreaks

ously should be contacted if possible. Children may also need to be tested for syphilis, as well as siblings of individuals with suspected congenital infection. This may be arranged most easily with the help of a genitourinary medicine clinic.

### Treatment in pregnancy

In pregnancy, the absorption of erythromycin is unreliable. In penicillin-allergic pregnant women, intravenous treatment with erythromycin or desensitisation to penicillin should be considered.

Treatment after week 20 of gestation will not necessarily prevent occurrence of the late sequelae of congenital syphilis, as inflammation in the teeth, inner ear and cornea can already occur *in utero*. Therefore, treatment of pregnant women should be initiated after one positive test without delay. In a mother with a high load of organisms, a Jarisch–Herxheimer reaction can precipitate pre-

term labour. These women should be advised to attend a labour ward if contractions start. When preterm birth occurs, the fetus is usually severely affected by congenital syphilis.

### TROPICAL GENITAL ULCER DISEASE

Sexually transmitted infections causing genital ulcer disease present considerable diagnostic difficulty. Sometimes, more than one infecting agent may be present. Most of the aetiological agents cannot be cultured in standard microbiological media. Histological examination of tissue is sometimes the only means of confirming the diagnosis. In many resource-poor tropical countries, a syndromic approach is taken to the treatment of genital ulcers. Recommended treatments are shown in Table 22.4.

### Lymphogranuloma venereum

Lymphogranuloma venereum (LGV) is caused by serovars L1–L3 of C. trachomatis. It is found in the Far East, sub-Saharan Africa and South America. In the early stages of infection, a small superficial ulcer may appear that slowly increases in size but often remains undetected. More obvious is the enlargement of lymph nodes, forming buboes. In the groin region, such buboes may become compressed by the inguinal ligament, leading to a characteristic finding called the groove sign. The buboes can also become matted together and discharge pus. Women may develop a severe proctocolitis that can progress to fistulae and strictures. Rectal infection presenting as proctocolitis has also become common in homosexual men in Europe and the USA.

The diagnosis of LGV can be confirmed serologically by a complement fixation test.

### Chancroid

Chancroid is an infection caused by Haemophilus ducreyi. The geographical distribution is similar to that of LGV. The illness starts with small shallow ulcers that are usually multiple and painful. The edges are irregular and there is localised lymphadenopathy. The sores may persist for several months and the glands can suppurate through the skin.

It may be difficult to obtain a positive culture. The organism requires a specialised culture medium, which should ideally be inoculated directly from the person under investigation. NAATs are not commercially available but are offered by many reference laboratories. They are more sensitive than culture. Identification of the Ducreyi bacillus in biopsy tissue confirms the diagnosis if it cannot be done microbiologically.

### Granuloma inguinale

Granuloma inguinale (donovanosis) is an infection caused by Klebsiella granulomatis (previously known as Calymmatobacterium granulomatis). It is endemic in India, Papua New Guinea and southern Africa. The disease course is usually slowly progressive, starting with the formation of discrete papules on the skin or vulva. The papules can enlarge to form 'beefy red' painful ulcers, which slowly spread around the genitalia and perineum. As they heal, fibrosis can ensue and cause genital lymphoedema and elephantiasis. The diagnosis is best confirmed by biopsy or tissue crush preparation. Donovan bodies are visible as intracellular 'safety pin' bacteria with bipolar distribution of chromatin.

## Other viral infections

### HUMAN PAPILLOMAVIRUS INFECTION

More than 100 different types of HPV have been described, with around 20–30 infecting the anogenital tract. These strains are mainly sexually transmitted through skin-to-skin contact and penetrative intercourse is not necessary for infection to occur. Infection with genital HPV is the most common sexually transmitted infection in Europe and developing countries, with a lifetime risk of 80% such that almost everyone is at risk of a genital HPV infection at some point in their lives. It is therefore not possible to define high-risk groups for HPV infection. Infection is often asymptomatic (80%) and transient, in the majority (80%) being cleared spontaneously after 9–18 months by the immune system.

Genital HPV types can be divided into high-risk and low-risk types according to oncogenic potential. Low-risk types cause genital warts and low-grade lesions. HPV-6 and HPV-11 are the most common low-risk types found in over 90% of genital warts. High-risk HPV types cause anogenital neoplasia. HPV-16 and HPV-18 are the most common high-risk types and are found in over 70% of cervical cancers. Other high-risk types also found in genital cancers include HPV-45, HPV-31, HPV-33, HPV-35, HPV-52 and HPV-58. Only persistent infections with high-risk types may become malignant.

In one study, genital warts developed in nearly two-thirds of people within 3 months of starting a relationship with a partner who had visible genital warts. There is less information on the role of asymptomatic shedding of HPV in those with subclinical lesions. The virus can infect the skin of the vulva and perineum, the vagina, cervix and rectum. Orogenital contact possibly leads to warts developing in the mouth or lips. Warts are frequently multiple and slowly increase in size. They can spread directly to the perianal skin without anal intercourse being practised.

The same strains can affect the larynx of a newborn baby (rarely) but do not usually spread to normal skin.

The majority (99.7%) of squamous cell carcinomas of the cervix contain DNA sequences from oncogenic HPV strains. It is thought that the viral proteins E6 and E7 bind to the tumour suppressor proteins p53 and pRB. This leads to dysregulation of the cell cycle and cell proliferation.

Most women infected with HPV-16 or HPV-18 do not develop cancer. It is estimated that 5% of high-risk infections result in cervical cancer in unscreened populations and 1–2% in screened women. The real burden of HPV-related neoplasia is borne by developing countries without cervical screening programmes. Worldwide, there are over 500 000 new cases of cervical cancer annually, 80% of which occur in the developing world.

Other risk factors for anogenital neoplasia exist, such as smoking, but by far the greatest risk is posed by high-risk HPV infection. Vaccines against HPV are now licensed, with a bivalent vaccine targeting HPV-16 and HPV-18 (this vaccine also provides a degree of protection against several other oncogenic strains) and a quadrivalent vaccine targeting HPV-6 and HPV-11 in addition to HPV-16 and HPV-18. In clinical trials, these vaccines were highly effective in preventing high-grade cervical intraepithelial neoplasia associated with the target viruses.

### Treatment of genital warts

The following approaches are available for the treatment of genital warts:

- physical methods such as weekly cryotherapy
- podophyllotoxin applied twice/day for 3 days, repeated after 4 days as needed for up to four courses
- imiquimod applied three times/week for up to 16 weeks
- surgical treatment employing lasers, electrocautery or scissor excision; this is used for intractable cases.

People with impaired immunity such as those with HIV infection or underlying malignancies are particularly difficult to treat.

Women with warts on the cervix should be referred for colposcopic assessment. Recent sexual partners should be examined for evidence of genital warts and also other infections. Traditionally, people with warts have been advised to use barrier methods of contraception during treatment and for the subsequent 3 months. We do not know enough about the risks of transmission from asymptomatic carriers of HPV to allow evidence-based recommendations to be made. The role of condoms can be discussed in the general context of protecting against both acquisition and transmission of sexually transmitted infections with new partners.

Immune-based therapies with interferon or topical application of imiquimod, a cream that stimulates local cytokine release, may be helpful for people with genital warts. Nucleotide analogues, a new class of antiviral drugs, are active against HPV and may become useful for its treatment.

### MOLLUSCUM CONTAGIOSUM

Molluscum contagiosum virus is a poxvirus that produces painless lesions of up to 5 mm in diameter. The lesions have a pearly appearance and a dimple in the centre. They can be mistaken for genital warts and affected people should be warned not to pick at them because the fluid from the vesicles is infectious. Molluscum contagiosum is common in childhood and clears after a few months. Adults may acquire the virus during sexual intercourse. The infection resolves with cryotherapy or following curettage and application of phenol. In individuals with suppressed immunity, widespread large confluent lesions may develop. In HIV-infected individuals, these resolve with immune restitution following initiation of antiretroviral treatment.

### AIDS

AIDS is caused by infection with HIV, a retrovirus. It is a particularly devastating disease because of the stigma of sexual transmission and the risk of vertical transmission to children. Even if a child is not infected, the death of one or both parents threatens his/her development and survival in many parts of the world. The prevalence is greatest in sub-Saharan Africa, where in several cities as many as a third of pregnant women are infected. A resurgence in tuberculosis has occurred hand in hand with the AIDS epidemic.

HIV-related immunodeficiency can manifest itself in any organ system; in people with HIV infection, a high index of suspicion is therefore required because the infection can alter many other disease processes.

### Natural history of HIV infection

In 20% of those infected with HIV, an acute seroconversion illness develops within a few weeks of infection. The clinical features include fever, generalised lymphadenopathy, a macular erythematous rash, pharyngitis and conjunctivitis. A steady decline in immune function over the first few years may manifest itself in the form of opportunistic infections that are not life-threatening, including recurrent oral and vaginal candidiasis, single-dermatome herpes zoster (shingles), frequent and prolonged episodes of oral or genital herpes and persistent warts. Furry white patches on the sides of the tongue, termed oral hairy leucoplakia, may come and go. This is pathognomonic of immunodeficiency. Persistent generalised lymphadenopathy may be present. Skin problems include seborrhoeic dermatitis, folliculitis, dry skin, tinea pedis and a high frequency of allergic reactions.

Without antiretroviral treatment, the median time to the development of AIDS is 10 years. Essentially, AIDS is defined by the onset of life-threatening opportunistic infections or malignancies associated with immunodeficiency. The most common presentations are listed in Table 22.5.

### Virology

HIV is a retrovirus that contains two single strands of RNA. The world pandemic is predominantly caused by HIV-1. HIV-2 infection originating in West Africa tends to progress to AIDS more slowly and is less infectious. To gain entry into a human cell, the viral outer membrane protein gp120 binds to the CD4 receptors that are present on T helper lymphocytes, macrophages, dendritic cells and microglia. Coreceptors, such as the chemokine C-C motif receptor 5 (CCR5), are also used to enhance viral entry. The enzyme reverse transcriptase carried within the virus particle enables the production of proviral DNA in infected cells. Once proviral DNA has been integrated into the host genome, viral peptides are transcribed. Specific viral protease enzymes cleave these before the daughter virus particles are assembled.

TABLE 22.5 **Common AIDS-presenting illnesses**

| Affected body system | Presenting illness |
|---|---|
| Pulmonary | *Pneumocystis* pneumonia |
| | Tuberculosis (pulmonary or extrapulmonary) |
| Neurological | Cerebral toxoplasmosis |
| | Cryptococcal meningitis |
| | AIDS dementia |
| Gastrointestinal | Diarrhoea and wasting syndrome[a] |
| | Oesophageal candidiasis |
| Ophthalmic | Cytomegalovirus retinitis |
| Malignancy | Kaposi sarcoma |
| | Non-Hodgkin lymphoma |
| Systemic | *Mycobacterium avium* complex infection |

[a] May be attributable to infection with *Cryptosporidium*, *Microsporidium* or *Isospora* species

### Diagnosis

HIV infection is diagnosed by detection of antibodies to gp120. During seroconversion, p24 antigen is detectable in the serum before antibodies are produced. Rapid tests using a fingerprick of blood or a buccal sample are increasingly being used for diagnosis, particularly in outreach settings.

The disease is monitored by measuring the level of CD4 lymphocytes in peripheral blood. A normal lymphocyte count lies above 500 cells/mm$^3$. There is a 10% risk of AIDS developing within 1 year when the CD4 lymphocyte count drops to 200 cells/mm$^3$. This is the level at which primary prophylaxis against *Pneumocystis jirovecii* pneumonia is recommended. Using PCR technology, it is also possible to measure the concentration of viral RNA in the plasma. A high level of more than 100 000 particles/ml predicts rapid disease progression.

Where there is access to effective antiretroviral therapy, treatment is now highly successful with a near-normal life expectancy predicted. Widespread testing with minimal pretest discussion is now advocated because failure to test and diagnose early increases the risk of late presentation with potentially irreversible complications.

### Treatment

Two treatment strategies are used:

- antiretroviral therapy
- prophylaxis against opportunistic infections in individuals with suppressed immunity.

Antiretroviral drugs targeting reverse transcriptase or viral proteases were the first classes to be developed and are most widely used in initial treatment. Newer drugs, including fusion inhibitors, entry inhibitors and integrase inhibitors, target other stages of the viral lifecycle. The aim of therapy is to reduce the level of virus in the plasma to zero with a combination of antiretroviral agents. First-line regimens usually comprise two nucleoside or nucleotide reverse transcriptase inhibitors (NRTIs) combined with a nonnucleoside reverse transcriptase inhibitor (NNRTI). Protease inhibitors are used instead of the NNRTI if there is resistance or another reason not to use an NNRTI.

If treatment is successful, the immune system partially recovers with a rise in the CD4 count and the risk of opportunistic infection is decreased. If total suppression of viral replication is not achieved, resistant strains of virus will inevitably arise within the treated person over the course of a few months. This is because reverse transcription is inherently inaccurate, leading to a high rate of mutation. With each cycle of replication of the virus, which takes 48 hours, single point mutations arise that will confer reduced sensitivity to antiviral agents.

Unfortunately, HIV infects long-lived memory cells from which the virus can rapidly reseed the body on cessation of therapy. Eradication, and thus cure, is unlikely even after several years of treatment.

If immunodeficiency has already occurred, treatment and prevention of opportunistic infections are needed. This may include co-trimoxazole to prevent *Pneumocysis* pneumonia and, in individuals with severely suppressed immunity and CD4 counts below 50 cells/mm$^3$, azithromycin and valganciclovir to prevent disseminated *Mycobacterium avium* complex infection and cytomegalovirus infection, respectively. Regular administration of antifungal agents may be necessary to control oral and vaginal candidiasis.

The prognosis has improved dramatically for those with access to treatment. AIDS is now regarded as a treatable chronic disease with a near normal life expectancy. Increased morbidity and mortality from cancers other than the traditional AIDS-related ones and cardiovascular disease are starting to be recognised.

Of note, antiretroviral drugs, particularly some of the protease inhibitors, have many potential interactions with other drugs through effects on the cytochrome P450 enzymes. This includes an increase in the rate of breakdown of the synthetic estrogens present in oral contraceptive pills.

### Transmission

In most developing countries, HIV is principally spread through vaginal intercourse, with approximately equal numbers of men and women being infected. In developed countries, the majority of infections have been acquired through homosexual sex or intravenous drug use, although the incidence of heterosexual transmission is increasing. Genital infections, including genital ulcer disease, chlamydia and gonorrhoea, are risk factors for HIV transmission and acquisition. Bacterial vaginosis may also be a risk factor and is very common in some African countries, with a prevalence of 50% or greater. Good control of sexually transmitted infections should reduce the incidence of HIV infection.

### HIV infection in pregnancy

Vertical transmission occurs in 25–40% of affected pregnancies if no interventions are used to reduce the risk. It is thought that a minority of fetuses are infected during gestation. These babies can present with AIDS in the neonatal period. The majority are infected during parturition. Transmission through breastfeeding occurs in up to 15% of pregnancies. Transmission by this route may occur even after several months of breastfeeding. The risk of vertical transmission is increased if there is a high HIV viral load or a preterm delivery. The role of genital infections in vertical transmission is still being assessed. Many children infected with HIV will survive into adolescence.

Combined interventions that have been shown to reduce the risk of vertical transmission of HIV include:

- avoidance of breastfeeding (or continuation of maternal antiretroviral therapy if breastfeeding)
- elective caesarean section
- prescription of antiviral medication during the latter half of the pregnancy and to the newborn for 4 weeks.

If pregnant women with a viral load of less than 50 copies/ml start combination antiretroviral therapy at week 20 of gestation, the risk of transmission is below 1% even with a vaginal delivery, so this option is increasingly being taken up. Currently, efavirenz is avoided in women who plan a pregnancy because its use is associated with teratogenicity in rhesus macaque monkeys. The dose of some protease inhibitors may need to be modified owing to altered pharmacokinetics in the second and third trimesters of pregnancy.

In many developing countries, the risk of infant death from gastroenteritis in formula-fed infants is greater than the risk of HIV acquisition from breastfeeding. Transmission is more likely if breastfeeding is mixed with bottle-feeding or if juice is added as this can induce damage to the gut, increasing the likelihood of virus penetrating the mucosa. Studies report low rates of transmission from breastfeeding mothers who continue to take antiretroviral therapy during lactation.

### Impact of HIV infection on gynaecological health

HPV infection flourishes in individuals with suppressed immunity. Genital warts often persist despite aggressive surgical treatment. Chronic HPV infection can result in the development of cervical carcinoma, anal and vulval intraepithelial neoplasia and Bowen's disease. Because of these risks, most physicians perform cervical cytology annually in women with HIV infection. Persistent atypical warty lesions of the skin or vulva should be biopsied.

Other infections can also be more persistent in HIV-infected individuals. There is limited evidence that PID requires longer courses of antibiotics in women with HIV. Careful follow-up is certainly indicated. Postpartum endometritis is common in this group of women and HSV infection has been implicated occasionally. Eruptions of secondary genital herpes may become widespread, severe and persist for weeks if not diagnosed and treated. Genital herpes often presents as deep, painful ulceration.

Although all HIV-infected women are urged to use condoms to prevent transmission of the infection to others, they should also be advised to use a more reliable form of contraception if they do not wish to become pregnant. Only depot medroxyprogesterone acetate and IUCDs are known to work reliably in women receiving antiretroviral drugs.

Preconceptional advice is important for women with HIV. Antiretroviral medication may need modifying. If the partner is HIV-negative, the couple should use artificial insemination. Infertility treatment is available at a limited number of centres.

## Urinary tract infection

Most women experience urinary tract infections at some point in their lives. They are considerably more common in young women than young men. This is generally attributed to the urethra being so much shorter in women, allowing organisms easier access to the bladder. Older men develop more infections as a consequence of prostatic enlargement. Urinary tract infections occurring in childhood require investigation to exclude congenital abnormality. If not detected, chronic pyelonephritis causes renal failure in adulthood.

The majority of infections in sexually active women are benign. It is thought that the vagina and, particularly, the periurethral area become colonised by pathogens, most often *E. coli*. During intercourse, the organisms can be pushed into the urethra, which is also traumatised, and from there ascend into the bladder. A short course of antibiotics will eliminate the infection from the bladder but does not usually stop periurethral colonisation. Broad-spectrum antibiotics such as amoxicillin, which are active against lactobacilli, disturb normal vaginal flora further and it is therefore preferable to use trimethoprim, nitrofurantoin or quinolones, which have less effect on lactobacilli.

Women with a urinary tract infection (cystitis) present with dysuria, suprapubic pain and urinary frequency. The differential diagnosis involves the distinction between internal dysuria, arising from the bladder or urethra, and external dysuria, in which urine causes stinging on contact with the vagina and vulva. The latter is usually attributable to vaginitis or HSV infection. Cystitis may be accompanied by an offensive smell from the urine, nocturia and, in severe cases, haematuria. Unilateral or bilateral loin pain and tenderness indicate pyelonephritis. Systemic features include fever, rigors, vomiting and malaise. Gram-negative septicaemia may ensue. Hospital admission is required in severe or systemic infection for close monitoring and treatment with intravenous antibiotics.

### DIAGNOSIS AND TREATMENT

Urine should be tested initially with a dipstick that incorporates tests for leucocyte esterase and nitrite. If both of these are positive, a presumptive diagnosis of urinary tract infection can be made in symptomatic women and treatment can be initiated while the culture is being performed. A pure growth of at least $10^8$ organisms/l is interpreted as confirming an infection. Polymorphs are usually present.

Subsequent treatment will of course depend on antibiotic sensitivities reported. The majority of urinary tract infections are caused by *E. coli*. Other common pathogens include *Proteus mirabilis, Staphylococcus saprophyticus* and *Klebsiella* species. All these organisms have the potential to develop resistance to antibiotics. The choice of treatment therefore depends on local sensitivity patterns, which usually reflect local antibiotic prescribing, and resistance patterns of previous isolates from the person to be treated. Optimal antibiotic treatment for uncomplicated infections is a 3-day course of antibiotics.

Investigation is indicated if infections are persistently recurring or if complications such as pyelonephritis occur. A plain abdominal X-ray, requested as a kidney, ureter and bladder (KUB) X-ray, and ultrasound examination of the renal tract are usually sufficient for screening.

Women who experience frequent urinary tract infections in relation to sexual intercourse can be prescribed treatment for 3–6 months with low-dose antibiotics. Those that are used most commonly are trimethoprim 100 mg at night, ciprofloxacin 125 mg at night or nitrofurantoin 100 mg at night. These can be taken every night or only following sexual intercourse. Such long-term treatment should enable periurethral colonisation to disappear. Postmenopausal women benefit from treatment with topical estrogen to reverse atrophic change.

Self-help measures include attention to hygiene and wiping front to back after defaecation. Regular drinking of cranberry juice, which inhibits adherence of coliform bacteria to epithelial cells, might also be of benefit.

## Puerperal sepsis/postpartum endometritis

In the 19th century, sepsis accounted for 50% of maternal deaths. Improvements in hygiene, aseptic techniques and our understanding of socioeconomic status and appropriate use of antibiotics mean that it is now uncommon in industrialised countries. However, it remains a major cause of maternal morbidity and mortality in developing countries, accounting for 10% of maternal deaths.

After delivery, the uterus and genital tract contain blood and products of conception – an environment highly conducive for the growth of microorganisms. The risk of infection is increased in the following scenarios:

- preterm birth associated with chorioamnionitis
- emergency caesarean section
- prolonged rupture of membranes.

A single dose of prophylactic antibiotics should be given before a caesarean section to reduce the risk of postpartum infection.

Infection is usually polymicrobial, influenced by bacteria colonising the vagina (*E. coli*, beta-haemolytic group B and group G streptococci, *Staphylococcus aureus* and *Citrobacter* and *Fusobacterium* species). Fortunately, the classic puerperal fever associated with group A streptococcus is now a rare event. The organism is often identified in severe infections. Invasive group A streptococcus infection associated with necrotising fasciitis and fulminant streptococcal toxic shock syndrome carries the highest risk of maternal mortality.

Postpartum endometritis may present with fever, purulent discharge and uterine tenderness, usually within a few days of delivery. Septicaemia and septic shock can occur if the early signs of infection are neglected.

### TREATMENT

A structured approach to management, as in the Surviving Sepsis Campaign, is associated with improved outcomes. This includes the use of broad-spectrum antibiotics, intravenous fluids and low-dose steroids. Before starting antibiotic treatment, cultures should be obtained from the vagina, urine and blood. Occasionally, uterine evacuation may be required. The choice of antibiotic depends on local guidelines and liaison with microbiologists. Initial therapy is often with clindamycin and an aminoglycoside, or with metronidazole and an aminoglycoside with or without ampicillin.

## FURTHER READING

HOLMES K K, SPARLING P F, STAMM W E, PIOT P, WASSERHEIT J N, COREY L et al. Sexually Transmitted Diseases. 4th ed. New York: McGraw Hill; 2007.
The most comprehensive reference source on sexually transmitted infections

British Association for Sexual Health and HIV (BASHH) [www.bashh.org.uk].
Includes link to Clinical Effectiveness Group for latest guidelines

British HIV Association (BHIVA) [www.bhiva.org].
Includes links to latest guidelines including management of HIV in pregnancy

Royal College of Obstetricians and Gynaecologists (RCOG) [www.rcog.org.uk].

Centers for Disease Control and Prevention (CDC); Treatment Guidelines for Sexually Transmitted Diseases [www.cdc.gov/std/treatment].

# Sample questions relating to microorganisms and infection control

## MULTIPLE CHOICE QUESTIONS

**1 ▶** Streptococcaceae:

A ▷ are Gram-positive
B ▷ are obligate anaerobes
C ▷ grow individually
D ▷ are positive for the catalase test
E ▷ fall into two main groups

**2 ▶** Necrotising fasciitis:

A ▷ is caused by streptococcal infection
B ▷ involves the fat and fascia
C ▷ can rapidly lead to death
D ▷ is not associated with pain
E ▷ requires immediate surgical debridement

**3 ▶** Regarding *Streptococcus agalactiae* (group B streptococcus or GBS):

A ▷ It is not normally found in the female genital tract
B ▷ Ninety percent of babies born to GBS-positive mothers are infected
C ▷ Premature delivery increases the risk of GBS infection
D ▷ Prolonged rupture of membranes increases the risk of GBS infection
E ▷ Intrapartum maternal fever does not alter the risk of GBS infection

**4 ▶** *Streptococcus agalactiae* (group B streptococcus):

A ▷ should be screened for in all pregnant women
B ▷ can cause miscarriage in pregnancy
C ▷ can cause postpartum sepsis
D ▷ causes infection in otherwise healthy men
E ▷ is more common in the young than the old

**5 ▶** Staphylococci:

A ▷ are Gram-negative
B ▷ are facultative aerobes
C ▷ form clusters
D ▷ are commensals of the gastrointestinal tract
E ▷ are treated with flucloxacillin

**6 ▶** Regarding meticillin-resistant *Staphylococcus aureus*:

A ▷ It is resistant to all beta-lactam antibiotics only
B ▷ It is spread by direct contact
C ▷ Infected people are usually asymptomatic
D ▷ The infection is cleared by nasal mupirocin
E ▷ It is more common in the community than in hospitals

**7 ▶** Meticillin-resistant *Staphylococcus aureus* responds to the following antibiotics:

A ▷ Cephalosporins
B ▷ Flucloxacillin
C ▷ Rifampicin
D ▷ Tetracyclines
E ▷ Vancomycin

**8 ▶** *Listeria monocytogenes*:

A ▷ is Gram-negative
B ▷ is spore-forming
C ▷ is a coccus
D ▷ is an aerobe organism
E ▷ is alpha-haemolytic

**9 ▶** *Listeria monocytogenes*:

A ▷ is found in soil
B ▷ can tolerate a wide range of temperatures
C ▷ is an extracellular pathogen
D ▷ causes encephalitis
E ▷ is best treated with oral amoxicillin

**10 ▶** Regarding the consequences of *Listeria monocytogenes* infection during pregnancy:

A ▷ Ninety-five percent of maternal infection results in fetal infection
B ▷ Infected pregnant women usually remain asymptomatic
C ▷ The infection is known to cause preterm labour
D ▷ The mortality rate of early neonatal listeriosis is higher than 50%
E ▷ Late neonatal listeriosis often presents with septicaemia

**11 ▶** Enterobacteriaceae:

A ▷ are Gram-positive
B ▷ are bacilli
C ▷ ferment glucose
D ▷ are aerobe organisms
E ▷ are all overt pathogens

**12 ▶** Regarding urinary tract infections (UTIs) caused by Enterobacteriaceae:

**A** ▷ *Escherichia coli* is the most common cause of community-acquired UTI

**B** ▷ A dipstick positive for leucocytes and nitrite is diagnostic of a UTI

**C** ▷ Cefalexin is the treatment of choice for community-acquired UTI

**D** ▷ Pregnancy increases the risk of asymptomatic UTI

**E** ▷ A UTI increases the risk of preterm labour

**13 ▶** Regarding enterobacterial infections:

**A** ▷ Enterobacteriaceae only cause cholecystitis if biliary calculi are present

**B** ▷ Enterobacteriaceae are common causes of wound infection in thoracic surgery

**C** ▷ *Escherichia coli* is the most common cause of bacteraemia

**D** ▷ Treatment of bacteraemia should include a cephalosporin

**E** ▷ *E. coli* is the most common cause of neonatal sepsis

**14 ▶** Regarding Gram-negative glucose-nonfermenting bacilli:

**A** ▷ They are rare in the hospital environment

**B** ▷ They are highly pathogenic

**C** ▷ *Pseudomonas aeruginosa* causes ventilator-associated pneumonia

**D** ▷ *P. aeruginosa* causes wound infections in people with impaired immunity

**E** ▷ *Burkholderia cepacia* causes lower respiratory tract infection in people with cystic fibrosis

**15 ▶** The neisseriae:

**A** ▷ are Gram-negative

**B** ▷ are bacilli

**C** ▷ form clusters

**D** ▷ are obligate aerobes

**E** ▷ are negative for the catalase test

**16 ▶** Regarding *Neisseria meningitidis* (meningococcus):

**A** ▷ It is not part of the normal flora in humans

**B** ▷ Infected people develop a slow-spreading petechial rash

**C** ▷ People with meningitis typically have co-existing septicaemia

**D** ▷ The cerebrospinal fluid glucose concentration of infected persons is increased

**E** ▷ Treatment is with penicillin

**17 ▶** *Neisseria gonorrhoeae* (gonococcus):

**A** ▷ is the most common cause of sexually transmitted bacterial infection in the UK

**B** ▷ is not part of the normal human flora

**C** ▷ does not always cause symptoms in men

**D** ▷ causes nondischarging urethritis in men

**E** ▷ causes proctitis after receptive anal intercourse

**18 ▶** Regarding the Spirochaetaceae:

**A** ▷ They are visible on Gram staining

**B** ▷ They have axial filaments that allow them to rotate lengthwise

**C** ▷ They are notoriously difficult to culture

**D** ▷ *Leptospira interrogans* is found in animal urine

**E** ▷ *Borrelia burgdorferi* causes Weil disease

**19 ▶** *Mycobacteria*:

**A** ▷ are obligate aerobes

**B** ▷ are motile

**C** ▷ are nonsporing organisms

**D** ▷ are rod-shaped

**E** ▷ have cell walls that have a lipid content of 90%

**20 ▶** Regarding tuberculosis:

**A** ▷ The incidence is rising in the UK

**B** ▷ It is ten times more likely to occur in people born outside the UK

**C** ▷ It is pulmonary in 90% of cases

**D** ▷ The diagnosis requires a Ziehl–Neelsen stain

**E** ▷ Histologically, it is characterised by caseating granulomas

**21 ▶** Regarding the treatment of tuberculosis:

**A** ▷ Four drugs are now the standard treatment

**B** ▷ It continues unaltered for 6 months

**C** ▷ Rifampicin can cause peripheral neuropathy

**D** ▷ Ethambutol can cause optic neuritis

**E** ▷ People with open pulmonary tuberculosis should be admitted as inpatients

**22 ▶** Regarding actinomycosis:

**A** ▷ It is caused by Gram-positive organisms

**B** ▷ It is most commonly caused by the genus Actinobaculum

**C** ▷ It is more common in women than in men

**D** ▷ Pelvic infection is almost always associated with an intrauterine contraceptive device

**E** ▷ First-line treatment is with long-term cephalosporins

**23** ▷ Regarding the genus *Candida*:

    **A** ▷ It includes more than 100 species

    **B** ▷ It can infect all mucous membranes

    **C** ▷ Infections are less likely to occur in people using inhaled steroids

    **D** ▷ Infections rarely involve an internal organ

    **E** ▷ All infections respond to azole therapy

**24** ▶ Regarding malaria:

    **A** ▷ *Plasmodium falciparum* causes the majority of malaria deaths

    **B** ▷ The disease is carried by *Anopheles* mosquitoes only

    **C** ▷ The sporozoite multiplies in the bloodstream

    **D** ▷ The life cycle is completed in hepatocytes

    **E** ▷ One million people a year die from the disease

**25** ▶ The following reduce the risk of contracting malaria:

    **A** ▷ Absence of Duffy factor

    **B** ▷ Alpha thalassaemia

    **C** ▷ Beta thalassaemia

    **D** ▷ HIV

    **E** ▷ Sickle-cell trait

**26** ▶ Regarding malaria and pregnancy:

    **A** ▷ Pregnant women are more likely than nonpregnant women to contract malaria

    **B** ▷ Malaria is less likely to recur in pregnant women than in nonpregnant women

    **C** ▷ The disease causes a low birth weight

    **D** ▷ The disease causes severe maternal anaemia

    **E** ▷ The disease causes preterm labour

**27** ▶ Regarding infection control:

    **A** ▷ If a microorganism is transmitted by droplets, then a negative-pressure room is required

    **B** ▷ If a microorganism is transmitted by droplets, aprons and gloves should be worn when seeing the infected person

    **C** ▷ Alcohol gel should be used after every contact with an infected person

    **D** ▷ The 'bare below the elbows' policy has not been proven to prevent cross-infection

    **E** ▷ Stethoscopes need not be cleaned between use

# Sample questions relating to viral infections in pregnancy in obstetrics and gynaecology

## EXTENDED MATCHING QUESTIONS

### Questions 1–10

■ *This question relates to viral infections in pregnancy. For each item below, choose the* **single** *best option from the list of options (A–E). Each option may be used once, more than once or not at all.*

**OPTIONS**

▷ **A** Varicella zoster virus

▷ **B** Cytomegalovirus

▷ **C** Parvovirus B19

▷ **D** Herpes simplex virus

▷ **E** Rubella virus

**1** ▶ Causes fetal cataracts

**2** ▶ Causes fetal heart defects

**3** ▶ Causes fetal hydrops

**4** ▶ Causes microcephaly

**5** ▶ Has a poor prognosis in symptomatic newborns

**6** ▶ Has a vaccine that can be used in pregnancy for up to 10 days after infection

**7** ▶ Associated with fetal chorioretinitis

**8** ▶ The most common congenital infection

**9** ▶ Treated by an *in utero* blood transfusion

**10** ▶ Requires a caesarean section if the infection is primary

## MULTIPLE CHOICE QUESTIONS

**11** ▶ Regarding varicella zoster virus:

**A** ▷ The primary infection is also known as chickenpox
**B** ▷ It presents with a rash covering the entire body
**C** ▷ Lifelong immunity occurs after a second infection
**D** ▷ Re-infection is common
**E** ▷ Virus reactivation is known as shingles

**12** ▶ Regarding varicella zoster virus:

**A** ▷ It is a single-strain herpes virus
**B** ▷ It contains single-stranded DNA
**C** ▷ It is spread by person-to-person contact
**D** ▷ The incubation period lasts 1 week
**E** ▷ Infections are preventable by a killed vaccine

**13** ▶ Regarding varicella zoster and pregnancy:

**A** ▷ Infection of the fetus is most likely in the first trimester
**B** ▷ Infection of the fetus is most likely in the second trimester
**C** ▷ Detection of the virus in maternal blood confirms the diagnosis
**D** ▷ If a child presents before the age of 1 year with clinical zoster reactivation, then in utero infection must have occurred
**E** ▷ Varicella zoster immunoglobulin can be given during pregnancy

**14** ▶ The following are features of fetal varicella infection:

**A** ▷ Skin scarring
**B** ▷ Limb hyperplasia
**C** ▷ Chorioretinitis
**D** ▷ Cortical atrophy
**E** ▷ Liver fibrosis

**15** ▶ Regarding cytomegalovirus:

**A** ▷ It is the second most common congenital infection
**B** ▷ Only recurrent infection causes congenital abnormalities
**C** ▷ First-time mothers are at the highest risk
**D** ▷ Breastfeeding is the most effective mode of transmission
**E** ▷ Re-infection is most common in Caucasian women

**16** ▶ Cytomegalovirus:

**A** ▷ is a herpes virus
**B** ▷ contains double-stranded DNA
**C** ▷ has an incubation period of 14 days
**D** ▷ has a live attenuated vaccine
**E** ▷ is treatable with antivirals

**17** ▶ Regarding cytomegalovirus:

**A** ▷ Previous infection affords complete immunity against a different strain
**B** ▷ There is an increased risk of placental transmission if conception occurs within 6 months of a primary infection
**C** ▷ It is usually asymptomatic
**D** ▷ Fever can last for 3 weeks
**E** ▷ The monospot test is positive

**18** ▶ Regarding fetal cytomegalovirus infection:

**A** ▷ The infection is usually symptomatic at birth
**B** ▷ Microcephaly is a common finding
**C** ▷ Sixty percent of those presenting at birth have hearing loss
**D** ▷ Cerebral palsy is rare in symptomatic babies
**E** ▷ Up to 10% of asymptomatic babies are restricted in their mental development

**19** ▶ Regarding parvovirus B19:

**A** ▷ It occurs in summer epidemics.
**B** ▷ Infected individuals who have developed the typical parvovirus rash are not infectious
**C** ▷ It deposits antigen–antibody complexes into the synovial joints
**D** ▷ It causes a slapped-cheek-like rash
**E** ▷ It causes arthralgia, usually of the neck

**20** ▶ Parvovirus B19:

**A** ▷ contains double-stranded DNA
**B** ▷ is spread by droplets
**C** ▷ has an incubation period of 21 days
**D** ▷ has no vaccine
**E** ▷ is treated *in utero* by a fetal blood transfusion

**21** ▶ Parvovirus B19 infection in pregnancy:

**A** ▷ causes fetal anaemia
**B** ▷ causes fetal hydrops
**C** ▷ causes fetal immune suppression
**D** ▷ causes fetal loss
**E** ▷ causes mental restriction in the newborn baby

**22 ▶** Herpes simplex virus:

    **A** ▷ contains double-stranded DNA
    **B** ▷ is spread via infected body fluids only
    **C** ▷ has an incubation period of up to 2 weeks
    **D** ▷ does not have a vaccine
    **E** ▷ is treatable with antivirals

**23 ▶** The rubella virus:

    **A** ▷ contains double-stranded DNA
    **B** ▷ is spread by person-to-person contact
    **C** ▷ has an incubation period of 13–20 days
    **D** ▷ has a killed vaccine
    **E** ▷ is treated with antivirals

**24 ▶** Regarding rubella and pregnancy:

    **A** ▷ Infection should be considered in all women with a viral-type exanthema
    **B** ▷ All women with symptoms should have an immunoglobulin G (IgG) test even if they have previously had a positive IgG test
    **C** ▷ The first symptom is a maculopapular rash
    **D** ▷ Maternal lymphadenopathy is usually present
    **E** ▷ On presentation, most infected women have a positive IgG result

**25 ▶** Regarding first-trimester rubella infections:

    **A** ▷ Fetal hearing loss is common
    **B** ▷ Sixty percent of infected fetuses develop a heart defect
    **C** ▷ Half of infected fetuses develop cataracts
    **D** ▷ Fetal neurological defects are rare
    **E** ▷ Prenatal diagnosis is most important during this trimester

## Sample questions relating to infections in obstetrics and gynaecology

### EXTENDED MATCHING QUESTIONS

### Questions 1–11

■ *This question relates to infectious diseases. For each item below, select the* **single** *best option from the list of options (A–Q). Each option may be used once, more than once or not at all.*

OPTIONS

▷ **A** Actinomycosis
▷ **B** Bacterial vaginosis
▷ **C** *Candida albicans*
▷ **D** Chancroid
▷ **E** *Chlamydia trachomatis*
▷ **F** *Escherichia coli*
▷ **G** Gonorrhoea
▷ **H** Granuloma inguinale
▷ **I** *Haemophilus influenzae*
▷ **J** Herpes simplex virus
▷ **K** HIV
▷ **L** Human papillomavirus
▷ **M** Lymphogranuloma venereum
▷ **N** Molluscum contagiosum
▷ **O** Syphilis
▷ **P** Trichomoniasis
▷ **Q** Tuberculosis

**1 ▶** Forms a chancre

**2 ▶** An infection related to intrauterine contraceptive devices

**3 ▶** Diagnosed by appearance of the Ducreyi bacillus

**4 ▶** The most common sexually transmitted bacterial infection in developed countries

**5 ▶** The most common cause of genital warts

**6 ▶** The most common cause of urinary tract infections

**7 ▶** The most common cause of vaginal discharge

**8 ▶** Usually also present in the lungs when detected in the genital tract

**9 ▶** Has a yeasty smell

**10** ▶ Presents with a green discharge

**11** ▶ Requires the mother to have a caesarean section if primary infection is active at term

## MULTIPLE CHOICE QUESTIONS

**12** ▶ Physiological vaginal discharge:

A ▷ becomes yellow on contact with air
B ▷ contains 99% lactobacilli
C ▷ contains epithelial cells from the vaginal walls
D ▷ always has an acidic pH
E ▷ decreases in amount midcycle

**13** ▶ Vaginal candidiasis:

A ▷ is caused by *Candida albicans* in 95% of presenting women
B ▷ is estrogen-dependent
C ▷ is common in prepubertal girls
D ▷ is more common in women who wear tights
E ▷ is common in patients who use steroids

**14** ▶ Regarding vaginal candidiasis:

A ▷ The vulva is red
B ▷ Discharge is usually offensive
C ▷ Recurrent infections not responding to treatment are common
D ▷ In pregnancy, topical treatment for 7 days is best used
E ▷ If untreated in pregnancy, it is proven to cause preterm delivery

**15** ▶ Regarding bacterial vaginosis:

A ▷ It is caused by aerobic organisms
B ▷ *Gardnerella vaginalis* is a common cause
C ▷ The discharge is offensive
D ▷ Clue cells are seen on microscopy
E ▷ There is an increased risk of second-trimester miscarriage in pregnant women

**16** ▶ Trichomoniasis:

A ▷ causes a green/yellow discharge
B ▷ does not affect the cervix
C ▷ co-exists with bacterial vaginosis
D ▷ is diagnosed microscopically
E ▷ is treated with topical clindamycin

**17** ▶ Regarding infections of the cervix:

A ▷ Human papillomavirus is a sexually transmitted infection
B ▷ Herpes simplex virus 2 leads to wart formation on the cervix
C ▷ *Neisseria gonorrhoeae* affects the squamous epithelium of the cervix
D ▷ *Chlamydia trachomatis* causes follicular cervicitis
E ▷ *Trichomonas vaginalis* causes a strawberry cervix

**18** ▶ Regarding infection of the fallopian tubes:

A ▷ The most common route of infection is via the local lymphatics
B ▷ Tuberculosis invades by the blood-borne route
C ▷ During acute salpingitis, pus forms within the lumen
D ▷ Hydrosalpinx is a long-term consequence of infection
E ▷ Mild inflammation tends to lead to a tubo-ovarian abscess

**19** ▶ *Chlamydia trachomatis*:

A ▷ is the most common cause of sexually transmitted bacterial infection in the UK
B ▷ is more likely to be asymptomatic in men than in women
C ▷ is restricted to the genital tract
D ▷ is the most important cause of nongonococcal urethritis in men
E ▷ causes cervicitis in women

**20** ▶ Regarding *Chlamydia trachomatis*:

A ▷ It is an obligate intracellular pathogen
B ▷ It directly damages epithelial cells by releasing toxic particles
C ▷ Self-collected swabs are as sensitive for the diagnosis as endocervical swabs
D ▷ The infection is treated with metronidazole
E ▷ It is a known cause of preterm labour in pregnant women

**21 ▶** Regarding gonorrhoea:

**A** ▷ The incidence is increasing in the developed world
**B** ▷ It is symptomatic in 90% of men
**C** ▷ It is not known to cause chronic infection in women
**D** ▷ It causes a yellow urethral discharge in men
**E** ▷ It is a known cause of proctitis

**22 ▶** Regarding *Neisseria gonorrhoeae*:

**A** ▷ It is a Gram-positive diplococcus
**B** ▷ It is diagnosed microscopically
**C** ▷ Treatment is standardised to a single dose of cefixime
**D** ▷ Fifty percent of women with *Neisseria gonorrhoeae* also have a *Chlamydia* infection
**E** ▷ Post-treatment swabs should be carried out

**23 ▶** Cervicitis:

**A** ▷ is a clinical diagnosis
**B** ▷ causes purulent discharge seen at the cervical os
**C** ▷ only bleeds if swabbed vigorously
**D** ▷ is rarely caused by a sexually transmitted infection
**E** ▷ causes nabothian follicles if it becomes chronic

**24 ▶** Regarding pelvic inflammatory disease:

**A** ▷ Plasma cells are seen on endometrial biopsy
**B** ▷ It is associated with intermenstrual bleeding
**C** ▷ In salpingitis, plasma cells are the first leucocytes to enter
**D** ▷ Pus leaking from the tubes causes them to adhere to the ovaries
**E** ▷ The omentum is usually unable to confine the infection to the pelvis

**25 ▶** Regarding pelvic inflammatory disease in pregnancy:

**A** ▷ *Chlamydia* infection increases the risk of preterm birth five-fold
**B** ▷ Gonorrhoea can cause chorioamnionitis
**C** ▷ *Chlamydia trachomatis* causes ophthalmia neonatorum
**D** ▷ *Neisseria gonorrhoeae* causes pneumonitis in the first few months of life
**E** ▷ Azithromycin is used to treat gonorrhoea in pregnancy

**26 ▶** Regarding nonherpes genital ulcers:

**A** ▷ Lymphogranuloma venereum is caused by specific serovars of *Chlamydia trachomatis*
**B** ▷ Lymphogranuloma venereum causes severe proctocolitis
**C** ▷ Chancroid is an infection caused by Klebsiella granulomatis
**D** ▷ Chancroid causes inflamed lymph nodes to weep through the skin
**E** ▷ Granuloma inguinale causes elephantiasis

**27 ▶** Regarding syphilis:

**A** ▷ The incidence is decreasing in the UK
**B** ▷ It is most common in women with multiple partners
**C** ▷ It is caused by *Treponema pallidum*
**D** ▷ It produces chancres
**E** ▷ In women it most often causes lesions of the cervix

**28 ▶** Regarding syphilis:

**A** ▷ Chancres require treatment to resolve
**B** ▷ Condylomata lata are perianal lesions of primary syphilis
**C** ▷ Secondary syphilis presents with a systemic rash
**D** ▷ It causes alopecia
**E** ▷ It causes sensorineural deafness

**29 ▶** Syphilis:

**A** ▷ affects the central nervous system (neurosyphilis) twice as often in men as in women
**B** ▷ causes strokes
**C** ▷ causes myocardial infarction
**D** ▷ causes miscarriage in pregnant women
**E** ▷ causes fetal deafness if transmitted during pregnancy

**30 ▶** Regarding syphilis:

**A** ▷ It is caused by *Treponema pallidum* subspecies *pallidum*
**B** ▷ It is usually contracted through sexual contact
**C** ▷ The first-line antibiotic is doxycycline
**D** ▷ It produces a chancre
**E** ▷ Lesions only arise at the site of entry of *Treponema pallidum*

**31 ▶ Regarding syphilis:**

**A** ▷ Primary syphilis has an incubation period of 28 days

**B** ▷ Primary syphilis produces a painful ulcer

**C** ▷ Secondary syphilis presents as a systemic disease

**D** ▷ People with secondary syphilis have a localised rash on their genitals

**E** ▷ The latent phase can last years

**32 ▶ Regarding syphilis:**

**A** ▷ Secondary syphilis presents up to 6 months after healing of the primary chancre

**B** ▷ The infected person is asymptomatic during the latent phase

**C** ▷ Latent syphilis eventually progresses to tertiary syphilis

**D** ▷ Tertiary syphilis is associated with a dissecting aorta

**E** ▷ Tertiary syphilis is associated with tabes dorsalis

**33 ▶ Regarding the human papillomavirus:**

**A** ▷ There are more than 100 types

**B** ▷ Penetrative intercourse is required for infection

**C** ▷ In developed countries the lifetime risk of infection is 70–80%

**D** ▷ Infected women usually have genital warts

**E** ▷ The immune system is inefficient at clearing the virus completely

**34 ▶ The following types of human papillomavirus (HPV) have a low oncogenic potential:**

**A** ▷ HPV-6

**B** ▷ HPV-11

**C** ▷ HPV-16

**D** ▷ HPV-18

**E** ▷ HPV-31

**35 ▶ Regarding human papillomavirus (HPV) and cervical cancer:**

**A** ▷ The majority (99.7%) of squamous cell carcinomas of the cervix contain HPV DNA

**B** ▷ In unscreened populations, 25% of women with HPV of high oncogenic potential develop cervical cancer

**C** ▷ In screened populations, 1% of women with HPV of high oncogenic potential develop cervical cancer

**D** ▷ Smoking is a greater risk factor for cervical cancer than HPV

**E** ▷ All women with cervical warts should be sent for colposcopy

**36 ▶ Molluscum contagiosum:**

**A** ▷ is a poxvirus

**B** ▷ causes red lesions

**C** ▷ does not occur in children

**D** ▷ requires cryotherapy for treatment

**E** ▷ is no longer infectious once the lesions have burst

**37 ▶ Regarding HIV infection:**

**A** ▷ HIV is a retrovirus

**B** ▷ Acute seroconversion in the first few weeks of HIV infection is rare

**C** ▷ There are often several opportunistic infections as the immune system weakens

**D** ▷ AIDS is defined by the onset of life-threatening opportunistic infections or of malignancies associated with immunodeficiency

**E** ▷ Without antiretroviral treatment the median time to the development of AIDS is 5 years

**38 ▶ The following are common AIDS-presenting illnesses:**

**A** ▷ *Pneumocystis* pneumonia

**B** ▷ Cerebral toxoplasmosis

**C** ▷ Cytomegalovirus retinitis

**D** ▷ Kaposi sarcoma

**E** ▷ *Mycobacterium avium* complex infection

**39** ▶ Regarding the treatment of HIV infection:

- **A** ▷ First-line drug treatment involves the use of a nucleoside or nucleotide reverse transcriptase inhibitor and a nonnucleoside reverse transcriptase inhibitor (NNRTI)
- **B** ▷ Protease inhibitors are used if there is resistance to NNRTIs
- **C** ▷ A rise in the CD8 count is a sign that treatment is successful
- **D** ▷ Clotrimazole is used to prevent *Pneumocystis* pneumonia
- **E** ▷ Antifungals are of limited use in people with severe immunodeficiency

**40** ▶ Regarding HIV:

- **A** ▷ The diagnosis is based on finding HIV RNA in the plasma
- **B** ▷ Homosexual intercourse is the most common form of transmission in developed countries
- **C** ▷ In developing countries more men are infected than women
- **D** ▷ Genital infections are more common in HIV-positive people
- **E** ▷ Bacterial vaginosis is a risk factor for transmission

**41** ▶ Regarding vertical HIV transmission:

- **A** ▷ Without intervention this occurs in 50% of pregnancies
- **B** ▷ Infection *in utero* is impossible
- **C** ▷ Babies can present with AIDS in the neonatal period
- **D** ▷ All mothers with HIV or AIDS should have a caesarean section
- **E** ▷ Breastfeeding is permissible in mothers with HIV or AIDS

**42** ▶ Regarding urinary tract infection (UTI):

- **A** ▷ In young girls UTIs need investigation to exclude congenital abnormalities
- **B** ▷ *Escherichia coli* is the most common pathogen in UTIs
- **C** ▷ Sexual intercourse does not increase the risk of a UTI
- **D** ▷ Antibiotics for UTIs stop periurethral infection
- **E** ▷ Amoxicillin has no affect on the lactobacilli in the vagina

**43** ▶ Regarding urinary tract infection:

- **A** ▷ External dysuria is a symptom
- **B** ▷ Haematuria is a sign of severe disease
- **C** ▷ Symptomatic women should be treated without delay
- **D** ▷ Treatment should be commenced based on a dipstick test that is positive for nitrites only
- **E** ▷ A pure growth of at least $10^8$ organisms/l is interpreted as confirming an infection

# Pathology

10

# CHAPTER 23

# Cellular response to disease

*Raji Ganesan*

The ways in which the body responds to disease are universal irrespective of the organ in which these responses take place. These responses form the core general principles of pathology.

## Inflammation and healing of tissues

Cells show a number of reactions to injury, including hypertrophy, hyperplasia and atrophy (Table 23.1). These changes are collectively termed adaptation.

When the capacity of the cell to adapt is exceeded, the cell undergoes a series of changes referred to as cell injury. The degree of the injury dictates whether the cell will recover or progress to cell death.

The causes of cell injury (see Table 23.2) can be interrelated; for example, damage by infectious agents may occur secondary to wound contamination. Whatever the cause of cell injury, the main biochemical changes that occur are the release of $O_2$-derived free radicals, increases in cytoplasmic $Ca^{2+}$ levels, depletion of ATP and defects in cell membrane permeability.

## PATTERNS OF CELL DEATH

Apoptosis, or programmed cell death, is a regulated event that results in cell death during embryogenesis and during physiological events such as ovarian follicular atresia during menopause. A cell undergoing apoptosis shows condensation of chromatin, followed by fragmentation of the nucleus. No proinflammatory mediators are released during apoptosis.

Necrosis is the death of cells in living tissue. It is characterised by cell swelling, death of cell organelles and release of inflammatory mediators. The cytoplasm appears more eosinophilic and the nucleus may show karyolysis (dissolution), pyknosis (shrinkage) and karyorrhexis (fragmentation). Table 23.3 provides an overview of different types of necrosis.

TABLE 23.1 **Cellular adaptations to injury**

| Type of adaptation | Definition | Physiological example | Pathological example |
|---|---|---|---|
| Hypertrophy | Increase in cell size without cell replication | Muscle hypertrophy in athletes | Cardiac muscle hypertrophy in hypertension |
| Hyperplasia | Increase in cell numbers by cell division | Uterine muscle in pregnancy | Bone hyperplasia in Paget's disease of bone |
| Atrophy | Decrease in the size of cells or organs | Involution of the thymus with age | Muscle atrophy in paralysis secondary to loss of innervation |

TABLE 23.2 **Causes of cell injury**

| Cause of cell injury | Example |
|---|---|
| Hypoxia | Inhalation of carbon monoxide |
| Physical injury | Burns |
| Chemical injury | Ingestion of corrosive agents |
| Infectious agent | Viruses |
| Immunological reaction | Graft-versus-host disease |
| Genetic derangement | Cystic fibrosis |
| Nutritional imbalance | Scurvy |

TABLE 23.3 **Types of necrosis**

| Type of necrosis | Example |
|---|---|
| Coagulative necrosis | Myocardial infarction |
| Colliquative necrosis | Cerebral infarction |
| Caseous necrosis | Tuberculous lymphadenitis |
| Gangrene | Clostridial infection |
| Fat necrosis | Acute pancreatitis |

TABLE 23.4 **Main chemical mediators of inflammation**

| Chemical mediator | Source |
|---|---|
| Histamine | Mast cells, platelets |
| Serotonin | Platelets, mast cells |
| Prostaglandins | Leucocytes, platelets, endothelium |
| Cytokines, nitric oxide | Macrophages, endothelium |
| Kinins | Plasma |

## INFLAMMATION

Inflammation is the response of vascularised tissue to injury. It is a complex series of events that includes vascular, chemical and systemic responses, all aimed at restoring the tissue to normality.

The earliest response is vascular constriction, followed by dilatation with slowing of blood flow. In sequence, the red blood cells aggregate, the white blood cells adhere to endothelial cells (margination) and there is an increase in the gaps between endothelial cells. White blood cells emigrate (transmigration) actively through the vessel wall by a process termed diapedesis, where the neutrophils exit the vessels followed by mononuclear cells.

The chemical substances released in this process are referred to as chemical mediators of inflammation and may originate either from plasma or from cells (Table 23.4). Their production is triggered by microbial products or by products of the complement, kinin and coagulation systems.

Chemical mediators generally set off a chain of events. The mediators themselves tend to be short-lived and removed by phagocytes. This system of balances and checks generally ensures that the inflammatory mediators do not cause excess damage.

Acute inflammation may resolve completely, may heal by fibrosis, result in the formation of an abscess or progress to chronic inflammation (Figure 23.1). Chronic inflammation, although difficult to define precisely, is considered to be inflammation of prolonged duration. It can be a continuation of acute inflammation or start *de novo*.

Chronic inflammation is characterised by concurrent tissue destruction and inflammation. The tissue changes include mononuclear cell infiltration, small-vessel proliferation and fibrosis. Granulomatous inflammation is a specific type of chronic inflammation characterised by the presence of granulomas in the diseased tissue. Granulomas are collections of macrophages referred to as epithelioid cells. When the granulomas show loss of

FIGURE 23.1 **Outcomes of acute inflammation**

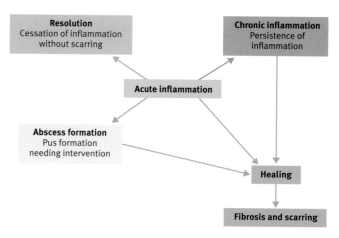

cellular detail with cheese-like material centrally, they are called caseating granulomas; tuberculosis is the classic example. Giant cells (multinucleate cells) are seen and, if the nuclei in these cells are arranged peripherally in a horseshoe shape, the cells are termed Langhans-type giant cells.

Sarcoidosis is the prototypical example of a noncaseating granuloma. Sarcoid granulomas can occur anywhere in the body, with lymph nodes, lung and skin being more common sites. Sarcoidosis can be confirmed by the Kveim test, where a sterile homogenate of sarcoid tissue is injected into the skin of the person undergoing investigation; the subsequent formation of granulomas is indicative of sarcoidosis. In nearly one-third of people with sarcoidosis, the serum level of angiotensin-converting enzyme is raised.

## WOUND HEALING

Replacement of dead tissue by living cells or fibrous tissue is known as wound healing. Labile cells, such as surface epithelial cells, have a great capacity for renewal. Stable cells are generally slow at regeneration but can renew almost completely, with examples including liver and renal tubular cells. Permanent cells, including the cells that constitute the central nervous system, lack regenerative capacity.

Wound healing begins with the formation of granulation tissue followed by growth of new blood vessels and migration of myofibroblasts into the injured tissue. Collagen then accumulates to form a scar. Sometimes, fibroblast proliferation is excessive and results in the formation of a hypertrophic scar or a keloid.

### Wound healing in the skin

Clean surgical incisions with approximated wound margins heal by a process called healing by first intention (also termed primary healing). When there is larger tissue loss, the healing process is referred to as healing by secondary intention (secondary healing). The latter differs from the former mainly by the phenomenon of wound contraction.

### Wound healing in bone

Fractures initially result in the formation of haematomas. The haematomas then become organised into alternating layers of fibrin and blood cells, followed by the removal of dead bone, callus formation and replacement by trabecular bone. Then, depending on the physical forces, the bone undergoes remodelling. Early or excessive movement, infection and pre-existing bone disease affect the healing of fractures.

### Wound healing in the liver

Liver cells can regenerate completely but the liver architecture cannot be satisfactorily replaced.

### Wound healing in muscle

Cardiac and smooth muscle cells are permanent cells; when damaged they are replaced by scarring. Skeletal muscle also has limited capacity for regeneration.

## Disturbances of blood flow

### OEDEMA

The term oedema refers to an abnormal accumulation of fluid in tissues. This may occur as a result of alteration of haemodynamic forces, as in oedema secondary to cardiac failure. Oedema is one of the cardinal features of inflammation, where it results from increased vascular permeability.

### THROMBOSIS

Thrombosis is the pathological process by which a blood clot forms within the uninterrupted vascular system by a complex process involving the endothelium lining the vessels, the platelets and the coagulation or clotting cascade. The thrombus formed can undergo dissolution by fibrinolytic activity and then organisation and recanalisation of vessels occurs with re-establishment of the blood flow. Thrombi can also extend and block the vessel further. They can detach from the site of original formation and embolise to distant sites.

## EMBOLUS

An embolus is a detached fragment of material (solid, liquid or gas) that is seen in a blood vessel distant from its site of origin or entry. Examples include:

- pulmonary embolus (usually the result of deep venous thrombosis of the limbs)
- amniotic fluid embolus (results from entry of amniotic fluid into maternal vessels following a tear in placental membranes)
- air embolus (occurs in deep-sea divers as a result of sudden decompression)
- fat embolus (results from entry of fatty marrow into the circulation following fracture of a long bone).

## INFARCTION

This term describes the necrosis that follows ischaemia secondary to occlusion of the arterial blood supply or ischaemia secondary to occlusion of venous drainage.

## SHOCK

Shock is a condition of circulatory failure that leads to hypoperfusion of vital organs. This can result in irreversible neuronal injury, acute renal tubular necrosis, cerebral damage and eventual death. Shock can have various causes, including:

- myocardial infarction (cardiogenic shock)
- traumatic haemorrhage (hypovolaemic shock)
- Gram-negative septicaemia (toxic shock).

### FURTHER READING

UNDERWOOD J C E, editor. *General and Systemic Pathology.* 5th ed. Edinburgh: Churchill Livingstone; 2009.

KUMAR V, ABBAS A K, FAUSTO N, MITCHELL R. *Robbins Basic Pathology.* 8th ed. Philadelphia: Saunders/Elsevier; 2007.

KURMAN R J. *Blaustein's Pathology of the Female Genital Tract.* 5th ed. New York: Springer-Verlag; 2002.

# Benign gynaecological pathology

*Raji Ganesan*

## Non-neoplastic disease of the female genital tract

Non-neoplastic disease of the female genital tract can be an underlying cause of significant morbidity. The most common conditions include infections, endometriosis and some conditions peculiar to pregnancy.

## Pathology of sexually transmitted infections and tubal damage

A number of organisms can be transmitted through sexual contact. For some of these organisms (for example *Chlamydia trachomatis*), sexual contact is the usual route of transmission, whereas others (for example *Entamoeba histolytica*) are typically spread by different routes but can also be transmitted by sexual contact. Table 24.1 provides an overview of sexually transmitted infections (STIs) and the diseases they can cause.

STIs can be the cause of damage after the initial inflammation subsides; they can also increase the risk for others STIs and the causative organism may cross the maternal–fetal barrier and affect the unborn fetus.

Some STIs, such as gonorrhoea, may result in pelvic inflammatory disease (see also chapter 22). The infection usually begins in the Bartholin gland or other glands in the perineum and then the organism spreads upwards to involve the fallopian tubes with persistent inflammation (pyosalpinx) or chronic damage (hydrosalpinx). The alterations in the fallopian tube can result in infertility and ectopic pregnancy.

Tuberculous salpingitis is common in areas of the world where tuberculosis is prevalent and it is an important cause of infertility in these populations.

TABLE 24.1 **Sexually transmitted infections**

| Organism | Disease caused | Other effects |
|---|---|---|
| *Trichomonas vaginalis* | Vaginitis | None |
| *Treponema pallidum* | Syphilis | Congenital syphilis in fetus |
| *Neisseria gonorrhoeae* | Gonorrhoeal cervicitis | Endometritis, bartholinitis, salpingitis with sequelae such as infertility, ectopic pregnancy |
| *Chlamydia trachomatis* | Urethral syndrome | Bartholinitis, salpingitis with sequelae such as infertility |
| Human papillomavirus (HPV) | Genital wart or condyloma (low-risk types of HPV) | Cervical intraepithelial neoplasia and cervical carcinoma (high-risk types of HPV) |
| HIV | AIDS | Increased susceptibility to other infections and unusual malignancies |

## Pathology of endometriosis

Endometriosis is defined as the presence of endometrial glands and/or stroma outside of the endometrial cavity. The most common sites (in descending order of occurrence) are the ovaries, the rectovaginal septum, the pelvic peritoneum, laparotomy scars and, rarely, the umbilicus or appendix. The presence of endometrial glands and/or stroma in the uterine wall is termed adenomyosis.

Several theories have been put forward to explain the presence of endometrial tissue outside the uterus:

- The retrograde menstruation theory postulates that, during menstruation, endometrial tissue passes through the fallopian tube and implants in the peritoneal cavity.
- The metaplastic theory implies that the lining of the peritoneal cavity can change to endometrial tissue.
- The vascular dissemination theory suggests that endometrial tissue is disseminated by blood and lymphatic vessels. This could explain endometriosis in distant sites such as the lung and nasal cavity.

Endometriosis and adenomyosis can be the underlying cause of pelvic pain, menstrual irregularities and infertility. Endometriotic cysts of the ovaries can be filled with altered blood (fancifully likened to liquid chocolate) and are then called chocolate cysts of the ovary. Malignancies, notably clear cell carcinoma and endometrioid carcinoma, can arise in longstanding endometriosis.

## Pathology of pregnancy

### DISORDERS OF EARLY PREGNANCY

#### Spontaneous miscarriage

Nearly 10–15% of all recognised pregnancies end in spontaneous loss. The causes include defective implantation, genetic or acquired abnormality of the fetus and maternal viral infections such as toxoplasmosis.

#### Ectopic pregnancy

The term 'ectopic pregnancy' is applied to implantation of the fetus in any location other than the uterine cavity. The most common site is the fallopian tube and this is usually secondary to tubal damage. An ectopic pregnancy can end in tubal rupture or extrusion of the contents through the fimbrial end of the tube (tubal miscarriage).

#### Tumours of the villous trophoblast

Hydatidiform mole is a disorder of pregnancy that occurs in about one in 1000 pregnancies in the West; the frequency is significantly higher in the Far East. There are two kinds of mole (Table 24.2):

- complete mole
- partial mole.

TABLE 24.2 **Molar pregnancy**

| Feature | Complete mole | Partial mole |
|---|---|---|
| Karyotype | 46,XX or 46,XY | Triploid  69 |
| DNA | Paternal DNA only | Maternal and paternal DNA |
| Villous morphology | Scalloped outline of villi | Fjord-like outline of villi |
| | Villous oedema | Vessels present contain nucleated red blood cells |
| | Lack of vessels | Less prominent trophoblast |
| | Circumferential trophoblastic hyperplasia | Presence of P57 (a maternally expressed gene product) |
| Serum hCG | Markedly elevated | Slightly elevated |
| Risk of choriocarcinoma | About 2% | Rare |

hCG = human chorionic gonadotrophin

Invasive mole or chorioadenoma destruens is a rare condition in which the chorionic villi invade the myometrium. Although these chorionic villi can be transported to distant sites, they are not capable of growing there.

Choriocarcinoma is a very rare malignancy with a marked propensity to vascular dissemination. The favoured sites of metastasis are the lungs, vagina and brain. The malignancy is very sensitive to chemotherapy.

### Tumours of the extravillous or placental-site trophoblast

Placental-site nodule is a benign condition in which hyalinised nodules of the intermediate-type or placental-site trophoblast continue to remain in the endometrial lining. This can result in persistent bleeding.

Placental-site trophoblastic tumour is a rare malignant tumour of the placental-site or intermediate trophoblast. About 10% of these tumours result in metastases and death. In contrast to diseases of the villous trophoblast, where the serum level of human chorionic gonadotrophin is raised, the marker for tumours of the extravillous or placental-site trophoblast is human placental lactogen.

## DISORDERS OF LATE PREGNANCY

### Toxaemia of pregnancy

Pre-eclampsia of pregnancy is a symptom complex characterised by hypertension, proteinuria and oedema. The exact mechanism of disease is still uncertain. The toxic effects of free oxygen radicals and lipid peroxides on endothelial cells are important factors. The initial pathology seems to be an abnormality of placentation that results in placental ischaemia. This then stimulates the release of vasoconstrictor agents and the inhibition of vasodilator agents. There is reduced uteroplacental perfusion, systemic hypertension and disseminated intravascular coagulation.

The severity of the disease does not correlate with the magnitude of pathological changes. The liver shows subcapsular and intraparenchymal haemorrhages. Haemorrhages can also be seen in the brain, the heart and, typically, the anterior pituitary. Placental infarcts and retroplacental haematomas are seen more often than in normal full-term placentas.

On microscopy, the characteristic feature is fibrinoid necrosis of the uterine spiral arteries with intramural infiltrates of foam cells. This is termed acute atherosis. In the liver, fibrin thrombi are seen in portal capillaries, resulting in peripheral haemorrhagic necrosis. In the kidney, diffuse glomerular lesions are noted with deposition of fibrin in the glomeruli.

### Abnormalities of placentation

Placenta accreta is a disorder of implantation in which the chorionic villi are seen at the interface with the myometrium without any interposed decidua. This may be a primary disorder or occur secondary to implantation on an area of endometrial scarring. Postpartum bleeding may result if this abnormal placenta fails to separate from the uterus. Very rarely, when the chorionic villi penetrate through the full thickness of the uterine wall (placenta percreta), hysterectomy may be the only method to control the bleeding.

When the interface of the fetal surface of the placenta (chorionic plate) is smaller than the maternal surface (basal plate), there is a discordance of placentation referred to as extrachorial placentation. The extrachorial placenta can be classified as circummarginate or circumvallate depending on whether the margin is flat or raised.

The umbilical cord is generally inserted centrally or eccentrically in the placenta. A placenta where the umbilical cord is inserted at the edge is referred to as battledore placenta. Insertion beyond the edge into the membranes is referred to as velamentous insertion of the cord. If there are nodules on the fetal surface of the placenta, particularly around the site of cord insertion, this is called amnion nodosum; it is associated with oligohydramnios.

### Inflammation of the placenta

If the placenta has become infected with a pathogen transmitted through the maternal bloodstream, as may be the case if the mother has listeriosis, a cytomegalovirus infection or toxoplasmosis, the chorionic villi may become inflamed. This condition is known as villitis. By contrast, ascending infections more commonly result in inflammation of the extraplacental membranes, a condition called chorioamnionitis.

## FURTHER READING

UNDERWOOD JCE, editor. *General and Systemic Pathology.* 5th ed. Edinburgh: Churchill Livingstone; 2009.

KUMAR V, ABBAS AK, FAUSTO N, MITCHELL R. *Robbins Basic Pathology.* 8th ed. Philadelphia: Saunders/Elsevier; 2007.

KURMAN RJ. *Blaustein's Pathology of the Female Genital Tract.* 5th ed. New York: Springer-Verlag; 2002.

CHAPTER 25

# Gynaecological neoplasia

*Raji Ganesan*

## General aspects of neoplasia

A neoplasm has been best defined by the eminent British oncologist Sir Rupert Willis as 'an abnormal mass of tissue, the growth of which exceeds and is uncoordinated with that of the normal tissues and persists in the same excessive manner after cessation of the stimuli which evoked the change' (Willis, 1952). Tumours can be benign or malignant and their nomenclature can reflect their origin (Table 25.1).

Characteristics of benign tumours include:

- slow, expansive growth
- presence of a limiting capsule
- microscopic features similar to those of the tissue from which it arises
- inability to spread beyond the tissue of origin
- clinical symptoms related to the size and position of the tumour
- ability to function like tissue of the site of origin.

Characteristics of malignant tumours include:

- rapid growth
- invasion of surrounding tissue
- ability to metastasise
- anaplasia (cell dedifferentiation) characterised by variation in the size of cells and nuclei
- extent of similarity to the parent tissue depends on the degree of differentiation
- abnormal mitotic activity with aberrant mitotic forms.

### SPREAD OF MALIGNANT TUMOURS

Malignant tumours can spread by direct invasion and infiltration of surrounding tissues, by lymphatic and vascular spread and by spread across serous cavities. Typically, carcinomas spread to lymph nodes, osteosarcomas and renal cell carcinomas spread through blood vessels and lobular carcinomas of the breast spread to serous cavities.

TABLE 25.1 **Nomenclature of neoplasms**

| Tissue of origin | Benign | Malignant |
|---|---|---|
| Bone | Osteoma | Osteosarcoma |
| Blood vessels | Haemangioma | Angiosarcoma |
| Smooth muscle | Leiomyoma | Leiomyosarcoma |
| Squamous cells | Papilloma | Squamous cell carcinoma |
| Glands or ducts | Adenoma | Adenocarcinoma |
| Placental tissue | Hydatidiform mole | Choriocarcinoma |
| Germ cells | Mature teratoma | Malignant teratoma |

**TABLE 25.2 Physical and chemical agents and associated cancers**

| Carcinogen | Associated neoplasm |
|---|---|
| Wood dust | Adenocarcinoma of the nose and nasal sinuses |
| Aflatoxin B$_1$ | Hepatocellular carcinoma |
| Asbestos | Mesothelioma |
| Aniline dyes | Bladder cancer |
| Anabolic steroids | Hepatocellular carcinoma |

**TABLE 25.3 Tumour markers used in clinical practice**

| Tumour marker | Neoplasm |
|---|---|
| hCG | Trophoblastic tumours, e.g. choriocarcinoma |
| | Nonseminomatous germ cell tumours |
| AFP | Hepatocellular carcinoma |
| | Yolk sac tumour |
| PSA | Prostatic carcinoma |
| CA125 | Ovarian carcinoma |
| | Primary peritoneal carcinoma |
| CA19-9 | Colonic and pancreatic cancer |

AFP = alphafetoprotein  |  CA = cancer antigen  |  hCG = human chorionic gonadotrophin  |  PSA = prostate-specific antigen

Some malignant tumours, such as basal cell carcinomas and gliomas, have limited or no capacity to metastasise, whereas intravenous leiomyomas are benign tumours that can spread through vascular channels.

## Aetiology of tumours

### GENETIC CAUSES

Cancers that run in families are referred to as familial cancers. In some cases, inheritance of a single genetic mutation increases the risk of developing specific types of cancer. Such single-gene disorders are referred to as inherited cancer syndromes and include familial retino-blastomas, familial adenomatous polyps of the colon, multiple endocrine neoplasia syndrome and von Hippel–Lindau syndrome. However, the role of the inherited risk cannot always be clearly defined in an individual person, as is often the case in people presenting with breast, ovarian or colon cancer.

In a small group of autosomal recessive disorders, predisposition to certain malignancies is conferred by chromosomal or DNA instability. These disorders include xeroderma pigmentosum, ataxia telangiectasia and Bloom syndrome.

### OTHER CAUSES

Cancer-causing genes are commonly referred to as oncogenes. Normal genes may become oncogenic as a result of modification by viruses or other influences (see Chapter 5 for further information).

Oncogenic viruses include human papillomavirus (HPV), which is associated with cervical cancer, Epstein–Barr virus, which is associated with nasopharyngeal carcinoma and lymphomas, and hepatitis B virus, which may cause hepatocellular carcinoma.

Physical and chemical agents that may cause cancer are listed in Table 25.2.

## Signs of cancer

### TUMOUR MARKERS

Tumour markers are biochemical indicators of the presence of a tumour (Table 25.3) and usually comprise a substance that can be detected in blood, plasma or another body fluid. These substances cannot be the primary modalities for the diagnosis of cancer. However, they can be used to screen for cancers, to locate the primary tumour in case of disseminated disease, to evaluate the response to therapy and to serve as an early indicator of relapse.

### PARANEOPLASTIC SYNDROMES

Paraneoplastic syndromes are symptom complexes that occur in people with cancer. They may represent the earliest manifestation of an occult neoplasm or mimic

TABLE 25.4 **Characteristics of vulval intraepithelial neoplasia (VIN)**

| Type of VIN | Classic VIN | Differentiated VIN |
|---|---|---|
| Age group affected | Younger women | Older women |
| Associated condition | Infection with high-risk types of HPV | Lichen sclerosus |
| Tumour grading | Three grades (VIN 1–3) | No further grading |

HPV = human papillomavirus

metastatic disease. Hypercalcaemia is probably the most common paraneoplastic syndrome.

Some paraneoplastic syndromes are characteristic of certain tumours. For example, Cushing syndrome is associated with small-cell carcinoma of the lung, polycythaemia is associated with renal cell carcinoma and carcinoid syndrome is associated with bronchial adenoma.

## Neoplasms affecting women

Cervical carcinoma is a disease that is common in less developed countries. It is caused by HPV, especially by high-risk and intermediate-risk strains. The most common high-risk types are HPV-16 and HPV-18.

Endometrial carcinoma is emerging as a disease of more affluent populations. The most common type is associated with obesity, diabetes and hypertension. This type of endometrial carcinoma is often preceded by a condition termed endometrial hyperplasia.

Tumours of the ovary are among the more common cancers in women. Most ovarian cancers cannot be detected early and no definite preneoplastic state is identified. Risk factors for ovarian cancer include nulliparity and a family history of ovarian or breast cancer. For example, mutations in the *BRCA* gene are known to increase the risk of ovarian cancer and women from families with such a mutation are monitored with imaging and measurement of serum CA125 levels. These mutations also confer an increased risk of cancers of the fallopian tube and the peritoneum.

## PREMALIGNANT CONDITIONS IN THE FEMALE GENITAL TRACT

### Vulva

The most common cancer of the vulva is squamous cell carcinoma. The preinvasive condition is termed vulval intraepithelial neoplasia (VIN). Two distinct types of VIN are recognised (Table 25.4):

- classic VIN (sometimes referred to as usual-type VIN)
- differentiated VIN.

Paget's disease of the vulva is a rare condition that occurs almost exclusively in postmenopausal women. It is histologically characterised by the presence of mucin-containing malignant cells within the epithelium of the vulva. In most women with Paget's disease, there is no association with invasion, although rarely the disease may have spread from an underlying adnexal malignancy.

### Vagina

Vaginal intraepithelial neoplasia is much less common than cervical intraepithelial neoplasia (CIN) or VIN. It is associated with high-risk HPV infection and may coexist with VIN (of the classic type) or CIN, reflecting the multicentric nature of HPV-associated disease.

### Cervix

Cervical squamous cell carcinoma is associated with a number of risk factors including age at first intercourse, number of sexual partners and frequency of intercourse. All of these are interrelated with the major independent risk factor, which is infection with HPV. The other major independent risk factor is cigarette smoking.

There are more than 100 subtypes of HPV. Some of these show a predilection for infecting the lower female genital tract, notably HPV-6, HPV-11, HPV-16 and HPV-18. HPV-6 and HPV-11 are implicated in benign condylomas and are rarely associated with malignancy. HPV-16 and, to a lesser extent, HPV-18 are found in CIN and cervical carcinomas.

The area of the cervix where cancers arise is the transformation zone. In pubertal girls, this is a labile zone and the delicate columnar epithelium undergoes squamous metaplasia when exposed to the acidic environment of the vagina. The term metaplasia refers to the replacement of one adult cell type with another as an adaptive response to cell injury. For example, the normal lining of the bronchus is replaced by squamous epithelium secondary to irritation by cigarette smoke. In the metaplastic epithelium, dysplasia can develop. This is a disturbance of cell development that can progress to invasive carcinoma.

CIN can be recognised in cervical smears and this forms the basis of any cervical screening programme. The aim of such programmes is the reduction of the incidence of cervical carcinoma by detection and treatment of the preneoplastic disease.

The precursor lesion of cervical adenocarcinoma is cervical glandular intraepithelial neoplasia (CGIN). Both cervical adenocarcinoma and CGIN are HPV-related lesions.

### Endometrium

The most common type of endometrial carcinoma is associated with endometrial hyperplasia. This change in the endometrium is associated with unopposed estrogenic stimulation. The source may be endogenous, such as polycystic ovary syndrome or an estrogen-secreting granulosa cell tumour, or exogenous. Obesity is an important cause of a hyperestrogenic state, as there is increased peripheral conversion of androstenedione to estrone by the enzyme aromatase in the fat cells.

Endometrial hyperplasia can be classified as:

- simple (diffuse abnormality showing dilated glands)
- complex (focal abnormality associated with crowding and architectural abnormality of glands)
- atypical (superadded abnormality of cells

characterised by cytological atypia; this is associated with the greatest risk of carcinoma).

## COMMON MALIGNANCIES OF THE FEMALE GENITAL TRACT

### Vulva

Squamous cell carcinoma is the most common epithelial malignancy of the vulva. Its appearance is similar to the appearance of squamous carcinomas anywhere in the body and the tumours are graded by use of a three-tier system on the basis of resemblance to normal squamous cells. The prognosis is determined by the size of the tumour, the depth of invasion, the degree of differentiation and the presence and extent of nodal metastases. The inguinal lymph nodes are commonly affected. Carcinomas invading to a depth of less than 1 mm are sometimes referred to as being superficially invasive and have virtually no risk of metastasis.

### Vagina

Squamous cell carcinoma is the most common malignancy of the vagina. Clear-cell adenocarcinomas occur in young women who have been exposed prenatally (during the first 18 weeks of gestation) to diethylstilbestrol.

Sarcoma botryoides is an embryonal rhabdomyosarcoma of the vagina that occurs in children before the age of 5 years. The name of this malignancy is derived from the fact that, macroscopically, the polypoid mass that fills the vagina of the affected child resembles a bunch of grapes (botryoides means grape-like in Greek).

### Cervix

Histologically, the most common type of cervical cancer is squamous cell carcinoma. Cervical squamous cell carcinomas that are less than 3 mm in depth have a good prognosis.

Other types of cancer that are encountered in the cervix are adenocarcinomas, adenosquamous carcinomas and neuroendocrine carcinomas. Neuroendocrine carcinomas have an unusually poor prognosis owing to early spread. Cervical carcinomas extend by direct spread to contiguous structures such as the bladder and ureter. Local and distant lymph nodes can also be involved.

## Uterus

Endometrial carcinomas can be divided into two types:

- Type 1 (endometrioid carcinoma) occurs in younger women and arises from endometrial hyperplasia.
- Type 2 (serous carcinoma) occurs in older women and is not associated with hyperplasia.

Spread of endometrial carcinoma generally occurs by direct myometrial invasion. Spread to lymph nodes and distant metastasis happen late in the disease. Even with relatively superficial myometrial invasion, serous carcinomas can spread to the peritoneal cavity.

Malignant tumours of the endometrial stroma are called endometrial stromal sarcoma. These tumours are hormone-sensitive and initial recurrences occur locally. After a few local recurrences, endometrial stromal sarcomas tend to spread to extrapelvic sites.

Leiomyosarcoma is an uncommon malignant neoplasm of the smooth muscle of the uterine wall. These tumours recur after removal and most of them eventually metastasise through the bloodstream to distant organs.

## Ovary

A plethora of tumour types is seen in the ovary. These include epithelial tumours, sex cord–stromal tumours, germ cell tumours, miscellaneous tumours and metastatic tumours.

Primary ovarian carcinoma is the most common ovarian malignancy and can be of many different epithelial types. Serous carcinoma accounts for approximately 40% of all ovarian cancers. They are often bilateral. Spread is commonly to the omentum and the peritoneal cavity. The ovarian-cancer-related protein CA125 is used as a marker of serous carcinoma, particularly to aid the early detection of relapse. Other types of primary ovarian carcinoma are mucinous carcinoma, endometrioid carcinoma and clear-cell carcinoma. The last two types have an aetiological association with endometriosis.

The most common malignant sex cord–stromal tumour is the adult type of granulosa cell tumour. Adult-type granulosa cell tumours are usually unilateral and can be haemorrhagic. They are characterised by their propensity for late recurrence.

Germ cell tumours constitute 15–20% of all ovarian tumours. Except for mature cystic teratomas, these tumours are principally seen in children and young adults.

The ovary is a common site for the occurrence of metastatic tumours. Some of these tumours can closely mimic primary cancers of the ovary and their diagnosis poses problems for the pathologist. The most common tumours presenting as metastatic carcinoma are from the uterus, fallopian tube, colon, stomach, biliary tract and pancreas. The classic example of gastrointestinal cancers metastatic to the ovaries is termed Krukenberg tumour; it is characterised by bilateral ovarian enlargement with diffuse infiltration of malignant cells that contain intracellular mucin.

## Fallopian tube

Primary carcinomas of the fallopian tube are often recognised only when they have spread beyond the tubes. They are associated with *BRCA* mutations.

**FURTHER READING**

UNDERWOOD J C E, editor. *General and Systemic Pathology.* 5th ed. Edinburgh: Churchill Livingstone; 2009.

KUMAR V, ABBAS A K, FAUSTO N, MITCHELL R. *Robbins Basic Pathology.* 8th ed. Philadelphia: Saunders/Elsevier; 2007.

KURMAN RJ. *Blaustein's Pathology of the Female Genital Tract.* 5th ed. New York: Springer-Verlag; 2002.

WILLIS RA. *The Spread of Tumors in the Human Body.* 3rd ed. London: Butterworths; 1973.

## Sample questions relating to pathology

### EXTENDED MATCHING QUESTIONS

#### Questions 1–3

■ *For each item below, select the* **single** *correct chemical mediator that it produces from the list of options (A–E). Each option may be used once, more than once or not at all.*

OPTIONS

▷ **A** Histamine
▷ **B** Lysosomal enzymes
▷ **C** Platelet-activating factor
▷ **D** Cytokines
▷ **E** Kinins

1 ▶ Macrophages

2 ▶ Mast cells

3 ▶ Plasma

#### Questions 5–7

■ *This question relates to gestational trophoblastic disease. For each item below, select the* **single** *best option from the list of options (A–E). Each option may be used once, more than once or not at all.*

OPTIONS

▷ **A** Complete hydatidiform mole
▷ **B** Partial hydatidiform mole
▷ **C** Invasive hydatidiform mole
▷ **D** Choriocarcinoma
▷ **E** Placental-site trophoblastic tumour

4 ▶ Has a triploid genotype

5 ▶ Widely disseminated

6 ▶ Molar villi penetrate deep into the myometrium

7 ▶ Both sex chromosomes are paternally derived

#### Questions 8–13

■ *For each type of cancer below, select the* **single** *most commonly used tumour marker from the list of options of options (A–H). Each option may be used once, more than once or not at all.*

OPTIONS

▷ **A** Human chorionic gonadotrophin
▷ **B** Calcitonin
▷ **C** Catecholamines
▷ **D** Alphafetoprotein
▷ **E** Chorioembryonic antigen
▷ **F** Prostate-specific antigen
▷ **G** CA125
▷ **H** CA19-9

8 ▶ Choriocarcinoma

9 ▶ Pancreatic cancer

10 ▶ Primary peritoneal cancer

11 ▶ Prostatic cancer

12 ▶ Ovarian cancer

13 ▶ Hepatocellular carcinoma

### MULTIPLE CHOICE QUESTIONS

14 ▶ Regarding wound healing:

    **A** ▷ Granulation tissue is a mixture of myofibroblasts and capillaries only
    **B** ▷ Healing by first intention occurs only if there is close approximation of the tissue edges
    **C** ▷ A keloid scar is caused by excessive epithelial regeneration.
    **D** ▷ Granulation is the main process of organisation in the healing of bone
    **E** ▷ The hepatic architecture is easily rebuilt after being damaged

**15** ▶ Regarding inflammation:

    **A** ▷ The aim of it is to repair tissues
    **B** ▷ Vascular dilatation is the first response
    **C** ▷ White blood cells diffuse through the cell walls
    **D** ▷ Neutrophils cannot cross the vessel walls
    **E** ▷ Mononuclear cells are the first cells to cross the vessel walls

**16** ▶ Regarding inflammation:

    **A** ▷ Acute inflammation may result in the formation of an abscess
    **B** ▷ Acute inflammation becomes chronic inflammation after 1 week
    **C** ▷ Chronic inflammation can occur as a result of acute inflammation
    **D** ▷ Chronic inflammation involves mast cell infiltration.
    **E** ▷ Granulomas are collections of epithelioid cells

**17** ▶ Regarding malignant spread:

    **A** ▷ Carcinomas spread to lymph nodes
    **B** ▷ Osteosarcomas spread through the blood
    **C** ▷ Renal cancer spreads through lymph nodes
    **D** ▷ Lobular breast cancer spreads to serous cavities
    **E** ▷ Basal cell carcinomas spread through the blood

**18** ▶ Regarding gynaecological neoplasias:

    **A** ▷ Malignant tumours of the vulva are associated with herpes simplex virus
    **B** ▷ Lymph node spread is not a prognostic factor in malignant tumours of the vulva
    **C** ▷ The number of partners a woman has had does not alter her risk of cervical intraepithelial neoplasia
    **D** ▷ Krukenberg tumours arise from the breast
    **E** ▷ Choricarcinomas are trophoblastic

**19** ▶ Regarding gynaecological neoplasias:

    **A** ▷ The most important human papillomavirus types in the aetiology of cervical intraepithelial neoplasia (CIN) are types 14 and 16
    **B** ▷ Smoking is not an independent risk factor for CIN
    **C** ▷ Leiomyosarcomas arise from the stromal cells of the uterus
    **D** ▷ Metastatic ovarian cancer is histologically similar to primary tissue
    **E** ▷ Krukenberg tumours are cystic

# Pharmacology

# CHAPTER 26

# Pharmacokinetics, pharmacodynamics and teratogenesis

*Kevin Hayes*

## Pharmacokinetics

Pharmacokinetics describes what the body does to the drug and encompasses drug absorption, drug distribution (bioavailability and volume of distribution) and drug elimination (clearance is largely renal and hepatic).

### DRUG ABSORPTION

The absorption of a drug depends on its solubility. Lipid-soluble drugs cross membranes and are easily absorbed. Water-soluble drugs do not cross membranes and need to be moved across membranes by carriers (for example, ion channels). Most drugs are given orally unless oral intake is not possible (for example, with an unconscious person) or if oral intake does not allow the drug to be absorbed or causes the drug to be altered or digested (for example, insulin).

### DRUG DISTRIBUTION

Bioavailability is the amount of drug that reaches the systemic circulation unchanged. Intravenous drugs therefore have 100% bioavailability.

Volume of distribution is the theoretical volume of water in which the amount of drug would need to be uniformly distributed to produce the observed blood concentration. Fat-soluble drugs may have an enormous volume of distribution and they may have prolonged duration of action, as they can have a reservoir in fat tissue.

### DRUG ELIMINATION

Both the liver and the kidneys are involved in drug elimination. Drug concentrations are usually increased when impaired hepatic and/or renal function reduces elimination, which increases the risk of adverse effects and toxicity. Most drugs will, therefore, need dose adjustments, level monitoring or avoidance in these circumstances.

Hepatic metabolism generally makes drugs more water soluble to aid elimination. There are two phases of drug elimination in the liver:

- **Phase I:** Metabolism by reduction, oxidation and hydrolysis is principally due to the cytochrome P450 enzyme complex. After metabolism, drugs can become inactive (the vast majority), active (for example, enalapril and diazepam) or toxic (for example, paracetamol).
- **Phase II:** Drugs can be solubilised by conjugation with glucuronate (for example, paracetamol, morphine), acetate (for example, hydralazine, procainamide, isoniazid) or sulphate (for example, oral contraceptives). Once soluble, they are excreted into urine, or bile if the molecular weight is greater than 300 Da.

Renal elimination depends upon glomerular filtration rate and renal function. The determining factors are:

- **Molecular size:** Filtration in the kidney acts on molecules less than 20 000 Da. Very large drugs (for example, heparin) are not renally excreted.

- **Protein binding:** Filtration of highly protein-bound drugs is reduced (for example, warfarin).
- **Active excretion:** Active transport takes place in the proximal convoluted tubule, using anion transporters for acidic drugs (for example, penicillins, cephalosporins, salicylates, furosemide) and cation transporters for basic drugs (for example, morphine, pethidine, amiloride, quinine).
- **Diffusion:** Passive diffusion takes place in the descending limb of the loop of Henle owing to drug concentration gradients.

### PREGNANCY AND PHARMACOKINETICS

Owing to the large physiological changes associated with pregnancy, it is mainly drug handling that is affected rather than intrinsic drug actions. Relevant factors in pregnancy include:

- increased circulating volume (40–50%)
- increased renal blood flow and consequent glomerular filtration rate
- increased third space (amniotic fluid and peripheral oedema)
- relatively increased fat content
- reduced albumin and other binding proteins.

Thus, pregnancy results in increased clearance of most drugs, which reduces serum concentrations and sometimes efficacy (for example, anticonvulsants, lithium, thyroxine). The effect is less marked for protein-bound drugs as the free concentration is less affected because of reduction in albumin levels (for example, warfarin) and for fat-soluble drugs because of the increased fat reservoir (for example, chloroquine).

## Pharmacodynamics

Pharmacodynamics describes what the drug does to the body (drug effect). There are generally four major drug targets: receptors, enzymes, membrane ion channels and metabolic processes.

Ionotropic receptors directly open or close an ion pore in a membrane and metabotropic receptors are indirectly linked to ion channels in plasma membranes via signal transduction by secondary messengers, usually G-coupled

**TABLE 26.1 Examples of drugs with agonistic and antagonistic actions on receptors**

| Drug | Receptor |
|------|----------|
| **AGONISTS** | |
| Salbutamol | $\beta 1$ and $\beta 2$ |
| Methyldopa | $\alpha 2$ |
| Phenylephrine | $\alpha 1$ |
| Pilocarpine | Muscarinic |
| Diazepam | $\gamma$-Aminobutyric acid |
| Morphine | $\mu$-Opioid |
| Cabergoline | Dopamine |
| **ANTAGONISTS** | |
| Atenolol | $\beta 1$ adrenergic |
| Labetalol | $\alpha 1$, $\beta$ adrenergic |
| Doxazosin | $\alpha 1$ adrenergic |
| Tolterodine | Muscarinic |
| Ranitidine | Histamine 2 |
| Cyproterone acetate | Testosterone |
| Metoclopramide | Dopamine |

**FIGURE 26.1 Illustration of muscarinic receptor mode of action**

The signalling molecule acts via a G-protein-coupled receptor to influence intracellular events. An antagonist will block the receptor and hence the signalling molecule's action. | GDP = Guanosine diphosphate | GTP = Guanosine-5'-triphosphate

TABLE 26.2  **Examples of drugs that act by inhibiting enzymes**

| Drug | Enzyme inhibited |
|------|------------------|
| Diclofenac | Cyclooxygenase |
| Ramipril | Angiotensin-converting enzyme |
| Neostigmine | Anti-cholinesterase |
| Zidovudine | Reverse transcriptase |
| Aciclovir | Herpes simplex virus-specific thymidine kinase |
| Warfarin | Vitamin-K-epoxide reductase |
| Methotrexate | Dihydrofolate reductase |

TABLE 26.3  **Examples of drugs acting on membrane ion channels and their effect**

| Drug | Effect |
|------|--------|
| Nifedipine | Calcium blocking |
| Diltiazem | Calcium blocking |
| Verapamil | Calcium blocking |
| Lidocaine | Sodium blocking |
| Amiloride | Sodium blocking |

FIGURE 26.2  **Enzyme block due to warfarin**

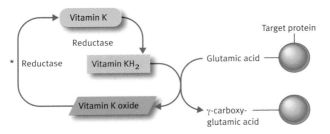

* = step blocked by warfarin

Drugs that interact with enzymes are shown in Table 26.2 and the mechanism of action for warfarin is illustrated in Figure 26.2.

Membrane ion channels are opened or closed by ligands directly binding to them (Figure 26.3). Drugs that perform a ligand-blocking function are shown in Table 26.3.

Metabolic processes such as protein, ribosome and DNA synthesis can be targeted with antibiotics. Table 26.4 shows the targets of metabolism of some antibiotics and, for some of these, their mode of action is illustrated in Figure 26.4.

### DRUG INTERACTIONS

A drug interaction occurs when one drug has an effect on the pharmacokinetics and/or dynamics of another drug used at the same time. An interaction can occur

proteins (Figure 26.1). Drugs can act on receptors agonistically or antagonistically or may occasionally have a mixed effect on receptors. Table 26.1 gives some examples of drugs and their target receptors.

FIGURE 26.3  **Ligand action on membrane ion channels**

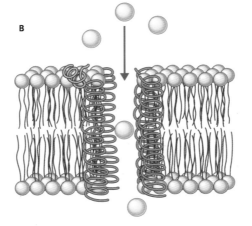

Ligands, which may be drugs, can bind directly to ion channels and **A** close or block them or **B** open them

TABLE 26.4 **Examples of antibiotics that affect metabolic processes**

| Antibiotic | Process affected | Mechanism of action |
|---|---|---|
| Carboplatin | DNA replication | Alkylates DNA |
| Chloramphenicol | Protein synthesis | Inhibits peptidyl transferase |
| Doxycycline | Protein synthesis | Interferes with tRNA binding |
| Erythromycin | Protein synthesis | Interferes with tRNA translocation |
| Gentamicin | Protein synthesis | Interferes with tRNA recognition and/or translocation |
| Paclitaxel | Cell division | Prevents microtubule disassembly |
| Streptomycin | Protein synthesis | Interferes with tRNA recognition |
| Tetracycline | Protein synthesis | Interferes with tRNA binding |
| Vincristine | Cell division | Inhibits microtubule assembly |

FIGURE 26.4 **Mechanism of inhibition of protein synthesis by some antibiotics**

as a result of enzyme induction or inhibition or an individual effect. These effects may be potentiated in the very young and very old and where there is altered renal and hepatic function.

One example of an enzyme inducer is phenytoin, which is a potent inducer of the cytochrome p450 enzyme complex and leads to reduced levels and indeed reduced efficacy of many drugs metabolised in the liver (for example, oral contraceptives, warfarin). Rifampicin, griseofulvin and spironolactone are other examples.

As an example of an enzyme inhibitor, sulphonamides inhibit hepatic metabolism and, therefore, increase drug levels in the plasma levels, which increases the risk of toxicity.

An example of a drug leading to an individual effect is ampicillin. Ampicillin alters the bacterial gut flora and thus leads to a reduced enterohepatic recirculation of estrogens, thus impairing the efficacy of the oral contraceptive pill.

### DRUG MONITORING

All drugs have a dose at which they will be ineffective and a dose at which they may be toxic. Between these levels is known as the therapeutic window of effect (Figure 26.5). Most commonly used drugs do not need monitoring of concentrations; drugs that need monitoring have a narrow therapeutic window (that is, there is little difference between being ineffective and being toxic) or have serious adverse effects or toxicity (for example, gentamicin, lithium, phenytoin).

## Drugs in relation to pregnancy and lactation

There are some general principles to consider when deciding to prescribe for women who are pregnant or breastfeeding:

FIGURE 26.5  **Therapeutic window of effect**

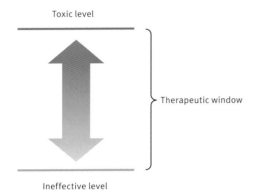

Toxic level

Therapeutic window

Ineffective level

- A woman of reproductive age might be pregnant.
- Always question the need for drug therapy.
- Avoid drugs in the first trimester if possible.
- Ensure that the benefits to the mother outweigh the risks to the fetus (although fetal therapy is a notable exception).
- Do not stop a useful drug without careful risk–benefit analysis. Good examples are drugs for epilepsy, asthma and thromboembolic disease.
- Although most drugs cross the placenta, few have been shown to be teratogenic.
- Prepregnancy counselling for chronic medical conditions is the gold standard to reduce the risk of harm, by optimising, altering or stopping treatment.
- Consider screening if exposure has occurred.

If a prescription is needed, the following recommendations should be applied:

- Use the smallest effective dose for the shortest possible time.
- Choose a drug for which there is extensive experience in human pregnancy.
- Avoid polypharmacy where possible. The risk of teratogenesis with anticonvulsants increases each time another agent is introduced.

Drugs that result in miscarriage are:

- ergotamine
- misoprostol
- mifepristone
- thrombolytics.

## TERATOGENESIS

About 35% of women take prescribed drug therapy at least once in pregnancy. This proportion is likely to increase as more women with medical problems become pregnant. In the first trimester, 6% of women take prescribed drug therapy (excluding iron and folic acid) and 90% of women take something, whether it is a prescribed preparation or not.

The background incidence of congenital abnormalities is approximately 2%. This relatively high incidence of congenital abnormality makes it difficult to assess drug effect in retrospective cohort studies comparing women who were exposed with women who were not. Moreover, although most drugs do reach the fetus to some extent, teratogenesis remains difficult to predict (for example, warfarin exposure risk is estimated at around 5%). It should also be remembered that animal studies are idiosyncratic and many risks are likely to be species specific, that risks are dose dependent and that negative study results do not guarantee that a drug is safe. However, it is known that some drugs do not cross the placenta (for example, heparin and insulin).

## Effects of drugs on the embryo and fetus

Table 26.5 shows the types of defects that can arise during the first 84 days of gestation.

During the pre-embryonic stage, up to day 17 while the conceptus consists of totipotent cells, there is an 'all or nothing' effect (that is, death and resorption or survival).

TABLE 26.5  **Types of defect arising as a result of a drug effect during the first 84 days of gestation**

| Days | Defect |
|------|--------|
| 12–40 | Limb reduction |
| 24 | Anencephaly |
| 34 | Transposition of great vessels |
| 36 | Cleft lip |
| 42 | Ventricular septal defect, syndactyly |
| 84 | Hypospadia |

As well as requiring caution with drugs being taken during this time, caution is required with drugs taken previously (for example, retinoids are present up to 2 years, methotrexate up to 3 months).

During the embryonic stage, from day 18 to day 55 (organogenesis during weeks 2–8), there is the potential for structural damage and major anatomical defects from irreparable tissue damage. The earlier the exposure, the more marked is the effect. Each organ has a period of maximum sensitivity. Some systems are not complete until well after the embryonic period and are, therefore, at risk much later in gestation (for example, the genital system and the effect of cyproterone acetate on male genitalia).

During the post-embryonic stage, from 8 weeks to term, drugs may affect fetal growth, leading to fetal growth restriction (for example, betablockers) and the continuing differentiation and maturation in organs such as the brain and kidney (for example, angiotensin-converting enzyme inhibitors). Drugs with effects late in gestation may cause subfertility and carcinogenesis (for example, chemotherapy exposure *in utero*). Drugs that have effects if administered shortly before term and labour include pethidine, which leads to neonatal respiratory depression, and nonsteroidal anti-inflammatory drugs, which cause premature closure of the ductus arteriosus.

Particular teratogenic drugs to consider avoiding are 'all the As':

- anticonvulsants
- antibiotics
- anticoagulants
- antimetabolites
- antipsychotics
- androgens
- acne drugs (vitamin A)
- alcohol.

Further sources of information are available in Appendix 4 of the British National Formulary (www.bnf.org) and from the UK Teratology Information Service (www.nyrdtc.nhs.uk/Services/teratology/teratology.html).

### ANTICONVULSANTS

Data show that 90% of women with epilepsy have a normal pregnancy. The slight increase in risk is regardless of anticonvulsant therapy (2.4% no therapy, 3–4% single-agent carbamazepine or phenytoin, 6% valproate, 3% lamotrigine).[1]

Valproate has been repeatedly shown to have the highest risks and it also appears to have a dose-related effect on verbal IQ.[2] Topiramate, gabapentin and levetiracetam currently have no firm information in pregnancy to guide risk assessment. It is known that risk increases with polypharmacy.

Phenytoin is associated with malformations, mainly due to alterations in folate metabolism. The fetal anticonvulsant syndrome is cleft lip and palate, microcephaly, cardiac abnormalities and mental restriction. Carbamazepine and valproate have similar effects to phenytoin but also lead to neural tube defects.

Risk reduction appears to be possible if:

- preconception folic acid, 5 mg once daily, is taken for at least 3 months
- polypharmacy is avoided
- the lowest dose required for control of convulsions is used
- vitamin K is routinely given to mothers from 36 weeks and to babies intramuscularly, to reduce the risk of postpartum haemorrhage and neonatal haemorrhage, respectively, although evidence for a significant effect is lacking.

### ANTIBIOTICS

The particular antibiotics to avoid are the tetracyclines and the sulphonamides.

It has been demonstrated that tetracyclines lead to teratogenesis in animals. They cause permanent discolouration of teeth and impaired bone growth *in utero* and up to the age of 7 years, as they chelate calcium.

Sulphonamides inhibit folate metabolism. Conversion of benzoic acid to folate is inhibited by sulphonamides and conversion from folate to tetrahydrofolate is inhibited by trimethoprim. Sulphonamides displace bilirubin from protein and may cause kernicterus in the neonate. Sulphasalazine is probably safe.

Caution is required with aminoglycosides, quinolones, nitrofurantoin and chloramphenicol. Aminoglycosides are nephrotoxic and cause VIIIth nerve damage (vestibular component). Quinolones in animals may cause permanent arthropathy. Nitrofurantoin may cause neonatal haemolysis and chloramphenicol may cause cardiovascular collapse (grey baby syndrome) if given close to term. Safer alternatives should be used if possible.

Penicillins, cephalosporins and macrolides are considered to be probably safe. Penicillins can be used to treat fetal infection (for example, syphilis) as 70% of the total dose is present in the fetus, although there is a theoretical risk of allergic sensitisation of the fetus. Cephalosporins appear to be safe and macrolides appear to be safe with a small risk of neonatal cholestatic jaundice.

## ANTICOAGULANTS

Heparin is considered to be safe, as both unfractionated and low-molecular-weight heparins are very large and do not cross the placenta. Warfarin is teratogenic between 6–12 weeks of gestation. If the fetus is exposed, the risk of damage appears to be around 5%. It is associated with multiple craniofacial abnormalities (Conradi–Hunnerman syndrome). Warfarin may be used at 12–36 weeks of gestation if absolutely necessary but it can cause fetal haemorrhage if taken close to delivery.

## ANTIMETABOLITES

Most anti-neoplastics have been shown to be teratogenic at some stage. However, information is mainly based on animal studies and small numbers of humans. Most fetuses have multiagent exposure and longer-term effects are not yet known. These drugs are contraindicated during the first trimester and breastfeeding and within 2–3 weeks of delivery. Most have been safely used in the second and third trimester.

## Effects of drugs on the neonate

Most drugs enter breast milk. Therefore, all the principles of prescribing in pregnancy are equally applicable to lactation. In addition, the likelihood of a problem in the neonate is determined by the rate of drug transfer (which is dependent on blood flow, size and lipid solubility), the drug concentration in the milk, the volume of milk taken (hindmilk having a higher fat concentration), the pharmacokinetics of the drug in infants and the drug's inherent toxicity.

There are several types of effects arising from drugs in breast milk:

- harm to the neonate (for example, lithium)
- no effect to the neonate (for example, digoxin)
- hypersensitivity in the neonate (for example, penicillin)
- lactation suppression (for example, bromocriptine)
- reduction in suckling (for example, phenobarbitone).

The drugs to avoid during lactation are cytotoxics, sedatives (benzodiazepines, barbiturates), amiodarone, antibiotics (tetracyclines, metronidazole, chloramphenicol), oral contraception (reduces milk production), theophylline (causes neonatal irritability) and aspirin (Reye's syndrome).

## Fetal pharmacotherapy

In fetal pharmacotherapy, drugs that cross the placenta are deliberately administered via the mother to treat fetal conditions. They have the potential for maternal harm from adverse effects and, thus, present an ethical dilemma. Drugs that are in use include betamethasone (proven to reduce respiratory distress syndrome and intraventricular haemorrhage between 26–32 weeks), corticosteroids (to prevent masculinisation of female fetuses in congenital adrenal hyperplasia), flecainide and amiodarone (to treat fetal tachycardia) and salbutamol (to treat hydrops fetalis due to congenital heart block).

## REFERENCES

1. TOMSON T, HIILESMAA V. Epilepsy in pregnancy. *Br Med J* 2007;335:769–73.

2. ADAB N, KINI U, VINTEN J, AYRES J, BAKER G, CLAYTON-SMITH J, COYLE H *et al.* The longer term outcome of children born to mothers with epilepsy. *J Neurol Neurosurg Psychiatry* 2004;75:1575–83.

CHAPTER 27

# Non-hormonal therapy in obstetrics and gynaecology

*Kevin Hayes*

## Drugs in common use in pregnancy

### ANTIHYPERTENSIVES

Methyldopa is considered to be safe and has been used extensively in pregnancy. It has a centrally acting function as a post-synaptic alpha-2 agonist (reduces sympathetic outflow). It is metabolised to alpha-methyl noradrenaline. Adverse effects include rebound hypertension, depressed mood, flattened cardiotocograph variability, autoimmune haemolytic anaemia (rare), raised prolactin and hepatitis.

The beta blocker labetalol is considered safe and has also been used extensively in human pregnancy. It acts by non-specific alpha and beta blockade and may be used for acute hypertension as an intravenous infusion. It may cause fetal growth restriction with prolonged use. Neonatal hypoglycaemia and bradycardia have rarely been reported.

Nifedipine contains a dihydropyridine group, which blocks inward flux of calcium ions through voltage-gated calcium channels. It acts preferentially on vessels, as opposed to myocardium, and results in vasodilation. It has no antiarrhythmic activity but has a known effect on the uterus and may inhibit premature labour (unlicensed use). Adverse effects are peripheral oedema, headache and flushing.

Hydralazine is used for acute hypertension. It is a potent vasodilator that is metabolised by acetylation. Fast and slow acetylators are genetically determined and an idiosyncratic adverse event of a lupus-like syndrome occurs rarely in slow acetylators.

Magnesium sulphate is proven to be the best prevention and best treatment of fits in severe pre-eclampsia and eclampsia. It stabilises membranes and has a rapid onset of action. It should be maintained for 24 hours post delivery or seizure and levels require monitoring if there is oliguria. Adverse effects in toxicity include hyporeflexia, respiratory depression and cardiorespiratory arrest.

### DRUGS TO AVOID IN PREGNANCY

Angiotensin-converting enzyme inhibitors are associated with congenital malformations – cardiovascular system, skull defects, oligohydramnios and impaired fetal renal function.

Thiazides have been rarely associated with neonatal thrombocytopenia.

## Tocolytic agents

Tocolytic agents are used to abolish unwanted uterine activity, most commonly for preterm labour but also for acute hyperstimulation and external cephalic version.

### PRETERM LABOUR

There is little evidence of benefit to overall outcome for the fetus with blanket tocolysis for preterm labour and not using it is reasonable. Currently the two clinical uses are to achieve 24-hour steroid latency before 34 weeks and where *in utero* transfer is necessary for neonatal care.

Atosiban (oxytocin antagonist) has fewer adverse effects than most other tocolytics but a Cochrane review suggested no overall benefit. It appears to cause no fetal or neonatal harm. Adverse effects are nausea, tachycardia and hypotension.

Nifedipine (unlicensed use) has efficacy at least comparable with magnesium sulphate and ritodrine.

Magnesium sulphate is more commonly used in the USA and needs monitoring for toxicity.

Glyceryl trinitrate patches have no evidence of benefit over ritodrine and adverse effects are headache and, rarely, hypotension.

The use of beta sympathomimetics (salbutamol, ritodrine, terbutaline) is limited by their significant adverse effects: tachycardia, hypotension, pulmonary oedema, hypokalaemia and hyperglycaemia.

Nonsteroidal anti-inflammatory drugs are not recommended.

### EXTERNAL CEPHALIC VERSION

Terbutaline subcutaneously prior to external cephalic version has some evidence of increased procedural success in primigravidae and should only be used for this group.

### EMERGENCY TOCOLYSIS

Terbutaline intravenously has been shown to improve fetal heart-rate patterns and fetal pH in the presence of hyperstimulation (usually with oxytocin) and possibly even without hyperstimulation. Adverse effects are as above for beta sympathomimetics.

## Pain relief in labour

Entonox® (50:50 nitrous oxide/oxygen mix; BOC Healthcare, Manchester, Lancs) is safe and stable and has a rapid onset and offset. It is widely used and is highly effective for many women. Adverse effects are nausea and 'feeling drunk'.

Pethidine intramuscularly is widely used despite having little evidence of effective pain relief. It has a rapid onset and short half-life. Adverse effects are nausea and vomiting, narcosis and respiratory depression in the neonate if administered within 2 hours of delivery.

Morphine, although less widely used, appears to be more effective and as safe. Both pethidine and morphine are micro-opioid receptor agonists.

Combinations of bupivicaine (local anaesthetic) and fentanyl (opiate) in epidural administration provide highly effective pain relief. Adverse effects are hypotension, loss of mobility and a higher risk of assisted delivery.

## Third stage of labour

Active management of the third stage has been shown to reduce the rate of postpartum haemorrhage by around 50%. Most women receive drugs for their third stage.

Syntometrine® (Alliance, Chippenham, Wilts) – ergometrine 500 micrograms/Syntocinon® (Alliance, Chippenham, Wilts) 5 iu – is administered intramuscularly. Ergometrine causes prolonged vasoconstriction and has the adverse effects of nausea and vomiting and hypertension; it is contraindicated in hypertensive pregnancies. Syntocinon is synthetic oxytocin and causes short-term uterine contractions.

Syntocinon (infusion of 40 iu in saline) and ergometrine can also be used singly for the treatment of postpartum haemorrhage.

Misoprostol (prostaglandin $E_1$ analogue) 800 micrograms, administered orally, vaginally or rectally, is highly effective in treating and preventing postpartum haemorrhage. It is stable and cheap and does not need refrigeration. Adverse effects are commonly diarrhoea and nausea and vomiting.

Carboprost (prostaglandin $F_{2\alpha}$ analogue) is effective intramuscularly or intramyometrially as second-line treatment of postpartum haemorrhage. Caution is required in hypertension and carboprost is to be avoided in asthmatics.

## Drugs used in gynaecological practice

### UROGYNAECOLOGY

Detrusor muscle overactivity is commonly treated by drugs with antimuscarinic properties.

Tolterodine and oxybutynin are both muscarinic receptor antagonists (particularly the $M_3$ receptor, although oxybutynin is less selective). Both are effective in reducing symptoms of detrusor muscle overactivity and give improvements in incontinence and irritative symptoms in 60–70% of affected women. Adverse effects are dry mouth, dry eyes, constipation and dizziness. These effects can limit their use but usually habituate over time.

Imipramine is often used as a second-line treatment but may be effective, owing to its antimuscarinic effect.

Trospium chloride, propiverine and desmopressin are also effective for some women.

### STRESS URINARY INCONTINENCE

Duloxetine is a balanced serotonin and noradrenaline reuptake inhibitor. It increases urinary sphincter tone and has been shown to reduce (but not cure) incontinence by about 50%, with improvements in quality of life. Adverse effects are nausea, dizziness and insomnia in 10–20% of women.

## Chemotherapeutic drugs in gynaecological oncology

Chemotherapeutic agents (usually given as an outpatient treatment) interfere with cell division by acting either specifically on a phase of the cell cycle (for example, taxanes are active against cells in $G_2/M$ phases) or non-specifically (for example, alkylating agents, which exert their effects throughout the cell cycle). As chemotherapy has a propensity for actively proliferating cells, cancer cells are more vulnerable than normal cells. However, chemotherapeutic agents do act on normal cells so adverse effects are common. Chemotherapy has a narrow therapeutic index and close monitoring under oncological guidance while on treatment is essential.

### SOME CLASSES OF CYTOTOXIC AGENTS

Antimetabolites interfere with DNA and RNA synthesis (for example, fluorouracil and the folate antagonist methotrexate).

Alkylating agents form covalent bonds with DNA bases (for example, cyclophosphamide, ifosfamide).

Intercalating agents bind to DNA, thus inhibiting its replication (for example, cisplatin, carboplatin).

Antitumour antibiotics act by a complex mechanism leading to the inhibition of DNA synthesis (for example, bleomycin, doxorubicin, etoposide).

There are also drugs that are directed against spindle microtubules, thus inhibiting mitosis (for example, paclitaxel, vincristine).

### COMMON REGIMENS

Ovarian cancer is sensitive to platinum-based regimens and has a response rate of about 70%. Carboplatin with or without paclitaxel may be used neoadjuvantly, adjuvantly or palliatively. More than 50% of women with ovarian cancer will relapse and require further treatment. If more than 6 months have elapsed since initial chemotherapy, the tumour is more likely to be sensitive to carboplatin, which is often given again.

For endometrial cancer, chemotherapy (carboplatin with or without paclitaxel, doxorubicin or cisplatin) has a limited role and it is reserved for recurrent or metastatic disease.

Cervical cancer tumours above stage Ib1 are treated with primary chemoradiation using cisplatin. Additionally, cisplatin combined with radiotherapy has been shown to reduce risk of relapse for those undergoing radiotherapy after surgery (that is, adjunctive therapy for tumours with poor prognostic factors). Cisplatin and methotrexate may be used for metastatic disease but there is a low response rate.

For vulval cancer, fluorouracil with or without cisplatin is used in combination with radiotherapy for patients unfit for surgery or as a sole therapy for symptom control in metastatic disease.

For trophoblastic disease, chemotherapy alone is highly curative. Methotrexate is used for simple trophoblastic disease. Combined etoposide, methotrexate, dactinomycin, cyclophosphamide and vincristine are used for high-risk trophoblastic disease. Both have cure rates around 99%.

### ADVERSE EFFECTS OF CHEMOTHERAPY

Haematological adverse effects are caused by bone marrow suppression, which eventually recovers (nadir around 7–14 days), and include neutropenia, anaemia and thrombocytopenia.

Gastrointestinal adverse effects are caused by loss of epithelial cells. Nausea and vomiting are very common with most agents. Mucositis, especially with methotrexate, resolves spontaneously. Diarrhoea is also common.

Alopecia is commonly and temporarily caused by taxanes (for example, paclitaxel), doxorubicin and etoposide. Carboplatin and cisplatin may more unusually cause temporary hair loss.

Neurological adverse effects are dose related and improve on reducing the dose or stopping treatment. Peripheral neuropathy is commonly seen with paclitaxel and cisplatin. Tinnitus is associated with cisplatin.

Constitutional adverse effects, such as lethargy and anorexia, tend to have cumulative effects but resolve on cessation.

# Hormonal treatment in non-malignant gynaecological conditions

*Michael Marsh*

## Pharmacology of hormones used in gynaecological treatment

### ESTROGENS AND PROGESTOGENS

Natural or synthetic estrogens are compounds that bind to estrogen receptors and exert biological effects characteristic of endogenous estradiol. Progestogens are synthetic versions of progesterone and bind to progesterone receptors, resulting in effects similar to endogenous progesterone.

Female sex hormones have a long history of therapeutic applications. In combination, estrogens and progestogens are used for contraception, menstrual regulation, treatment of endometriosis and postmenopausal hormone replacement therapy (HRT).

Exogenous estrogen used alone, unopposed by progestogen therapy, is of limited use because of its proliferative effects on the uterine endometrium, leading to irregular menstrual bleeding when used in premenopausal women and to endometrial hyperplasia when used alone as HRT.[1] Thus, estrogen-only therapy in gynaecology is restricted to HRT use in women who have undergone hysterectomy. In contrast, progestogens used alone have widespread applications and are used in contraception, menstrual regulation in women suffering from dysfunctional uterine bleeding and menorrhagia and treatment of endometriosis and endometrial hyperplasia. Exogenous progesterone is used in assisted reproduction to provide support for embryo implantation in the luteal phase.

### ENDOGENOUS ESTROGENS

In the reproductive years, the most potent endogenous estrogen is 17-beta-estradiol ($E_2$), followed by estrone ($E_1$). In young women, both are secreted by the ovaries, with a production rate of $E_2$ ranging from 100–600 micrograms/day, varying during the menstrual cycle. Small amounts of $E_1$ derive from aromatisation of androstenedione from the adrenal glands and ovaries. Estriol ($E_3$) is the least potent physiological estrogen and is not a secretory product of the ovary. It is formed by irreversible metabolism of $E_1$.

After the menopause, $E_1$ is the predominant estrogen as ovarian secretion of all estrogens ceases. The residual production of $E_2$ and $E_1$ after the menopause originates from the peripheral aromatisation of circulating androstenedione and $E_2$ and $E_1$ are found in the range of 15 and 45 micrograms/day, respectively. As this aromatisation process occurs in adipose tissue, women who are obese may produce twice as much $E_2$ and $E_1$ as women who are not obese.

### *The estrogen receptor*

Estrogens, through binding to their specific receptor in the target cell, promote development of secondary sexual characteristics in women and stimulate endometrial proliferation, thickening of the vaginal mucosa and maintenance of urogenital tissues. Estrogen receptors are present in many organ systems and demonstrate actions that are not directly related to reproduction, such as maintenance of bone strength, initiation and termination of the pubertal growth spurt and pigmentation of the nipples and genitals.

The estrogen receptor belongs to the steroid receptor superfamily, which comprises the glucocorticoids, vitamin D, thyroid hormone, androgen and retinoid receptors. Estrogen acts through two receptors, alpha and beta. The alpha estrogen receptor is found in endometrium, bone, breast cancer cells, ovarian stroma cells and in the hypothalamus. The expression of the beta estrogen receptor protein has been documented in kidney, brain, bone, heart, lungs, intestinal mucosa, prostate and endothelial cells. The presence of the receptor in a tissue does not predict its role in mediating estrogenic effects. For example, alpha receptors appear to be the chief mediator of estrogen's actions on the skeleton. Osteoblasts express beta receptor but the actions of beta receptor agonists on bone are less clear. Some reports suggest that the effects of estrogen signalling through alpha and beta receptors are in opposition, while other studies suggest that activation of these receptors have similar effects on bone.

Different ligands may differ in their affinity for alpha and beta isoforms of the estrogen receptor. $E_2$ appears to bind equally well to both receptors, whereas $E_1$ and raloxifene bind preferentially to the alpha receptor and $E_3$ and genistein bind preferentially to the beta receptor.

### Estrogen metabolism

Circulating estrogens are metabolised primarily in the liver by conjugation and hydroxylation. Conjugation is catalysed by glucuronyl transferases and by sulphotransferases, whereas hydroxylation is catalysed by the enzymes of the cytochrome P450 complex. The residence time of $E_2$ is prolonged by conversion to $E_1$ and by enterohepatic recirculation of estrogen conjugates excreted in the bile. $E_2$ is rapidly cleared from the circulation with a mean half-life of 1.7 hours. The half-life for $E_1$ and $E_1$ sulphate is about four times longer.

### Effects of estrogen

The physiological effects of estrogens are influenced by sex hormone-binding globulin (SHBG) and albumin production. $E_2$ bound to SHBG is not biologically active. Thyroxine and $E_2$ itself promote SHBG production while androgens, insulin, corticoids, progestogens and growth hormone suppress hepatic SHBG production.

### Pharmacological estrogens

Orally administered natural estrogens are inactivated in the gut and the residual small amount that is absorbed undergoes considerable metabolism in the liver before reaching the circulation. In 1938, it was realised that the addition of an ethinyl group to $E_2$ prevented inactivation and enabled efficient gut absorption. However, the first-pass hepatic effect was still present. Currently, most oral contraceptives contain ethinyl estradiol as the estrogenic component.

Natural estrogen preparations are derived from plant or animal sources and are widely used in HRT. They do not have potent enough effects on the $E_2$ receptor to control the endometrium and menstrual cycle in premenopausal women and are therefore not used in the contraceptive pill. Conjugated equine estrogens contain the sodium salts of the sulphate ester forms of various naturally occurring estrogens derived from the urine of pregnant mares. Micronised estradiol is manufactured by the formation of extremely small particles of drug with a relatively high surface area to improve gastric absorption. $E_2$ valerate, piperazine $E_1$ sulphate and $E_2$ cypionate are conjugated forms that have been modified for better absorption in the gastrointestinal system and are also used in HRT.

### Selective estrogen receptor modulators

Selective estrogen receptor modulators are compounds that interact with estrogen receptors. Selective estrogen receptor modulators were originally thought to be anti-estrogens. However, it is now clear that they contain an admixture of agonist and antagonist activities.

The first selective estrogen receptor modulator, clomiphene citrate, a triphenylethylene, was synthesised in 1956 and is used widely in the treatment of polycystic disease and for ovulation induction. It acts centrally to block the negative feedback of estrogen and to induce a follicle-stimulating hormone surge of anterior pituitary gonadotrophs through positive feedback. In 1984, it was observed that clomiphene citrate attenuated bone loss in the oophorectomised rat, suggesting that it had estrogenic agonist activities on the bone. Clomiphene is a combination of two geometric isomers. The *trans* isomer, enclomiphene, is a partial estrogen whereas the *cis* isomer, zuclomiphene, is a pure estrogen.

Another triphenylethylene, tamoxifen, was subsequently shown to prevent bone loss in the oophorectomised rat. Tamoxifen acts as an estrogen antagonist in the breast but as an agonist in the skeleton and the cardiovascular system. Tamoxifen was not further developed as a bone-sparing agent as it causes endometrial stimulation and endometrial hyperplasia and adenocarcinoma in some women. Tamoxifen is widely used in the management of breast cancer.

Raloxifene is a nonsteroidal benzothiophene that inhibits bone mineral density loss but does not stimulate the endometrium and is an estrogen antagonist for breast tissue. Raloxifene is not a steroid and hence not technically an estrogen but it possesses a phenolic ring – similar to the A ring of estradiol – necessary to obtain lodgement in the ligand-binding cavity of the estrogen receptor. There is no evidence that raloxifene decreases the incidence of nonvertebral fractures, so although raloxifene can be used for the prevention of vertebral fractures in women with osteopenia/osteoporosis, its use is probably not appropriate for women who are at high risk of nonvertebral fractures. Like tamoxifen, raloxifene is used in the management of breast cancer.

## ENDOGENOUS PROGESTERONE

Outside of pregnancy, progesterone is chiefly produced by the corpus luteum, with very small amounts produced by the adrenal cortex and the glial cells of the central nervous system. The production rate of progesterone in the preovulatory phase is less than 1 mg/day, which increases to 20–30 mg/day during the luteal phase. Progesterone is responsible for induction of secretory activity and decidual development in the endometrium in the estrogen-primed uterus. If pregnancy does not occur, withdrawal of progesterone results in menstrual sloughing of the endometrium. Progesterone is needed for the implantation of the fertilised ovum and maintenance of pregnancy. It increases viscosity of cervical mucus, promotes glandular development of the breast and increases basal body temperature. During pregnancy, the placenta eventually becomes the major source of progesterone and

this placental progesterone is believed to inhibit uterine contractions allowing for the maintenance of the gestation until the start of labour.

### Effects of progestogens

Progestogens and progesterone, have a well-established anti-estrogenic effect on the endometrium. In an estrogen-primed endometrium, progestogens downregulate nuclear $E_2$ receptors by inhibiting receptor synthesis and accelerating their turnover, and downregulate the genes required for epithelial growth leading to reduced epidermal growth factor production. Progestogens promote differentiation of glands and stroma, decidualisation and secretory activity of the endometrium, increase blood vessel volume and stimulate secretion of insulin-like growth factor binding protein-1. Progestogens also stimulate 17-hydroxysteroid dehydrogenase production, which converts $E_2$ to the weaker estrogen, $E_1$ sulphate, and induce endometrial sloughing and uterine bleeding.

### Progesterone and progestogen metabolism

Progesterone and progestogens are metabolised primarily by the liver, largely to pregnanetriols and pregnanediols, which are then conjugated in the liver to glucoronides and sulphates. These metabolites are excreted in the bile and may be deconjugated and further metabolised in the gut. There is no significant enterohepatic circulation of progesterone.

### Pharmacological properties of progesterone and progestogens

When first produced pharmaceutically, progesterone was ineffective when given orally, as it is metabolised extensively in the gastrointestinal tract by microorganisms and digestive enzymes. Although micronised progesterone results in more efficient absorption from the gastrointestinal tract, large doses need to be given often to obtain therapeutic serum levels. However, natural progesterone is also available in transvaginal or transrectal suppositories and absorption is sufficient for it to be used as the progestogenic component of HRT regimens.

Progestogens are synthetic preparations with progesterone action that were developed to be orally effective.

These are divided into the 21-carbon steroids derived from 17-alpha-hydroxyprogesterone and the 19-carbon steroids derived from nortestosterone.

The 21-carbon steroids (for example, medroxyprogesterone acetate and dydrogesterone) simulate the profile of progesterone more closely, especially in their effects on the hypothalamic–pituitary system and on carbohydrate and lipid metabolism. Medroxyprogesterone acetate is probably the most widely used compound in this group. It is used in depot preparations for contraception and in oral form for postmenopausal hormone replacement and treatment of endometriosis and menorrhagia.

Progestogens derived from 19-nortestosterone are subdivided into compounds related to norethisterone (estranes) or to levonorgestrel (gonanes). Norethisterone is widely used in oral contraceptives and has androgenic properties and potent progestational activity. Many related progestogens have since been developed, including norethisterone acetate and etynodiol diacetate. However, all are converted *in vivo* to norethisterone before they are active. The gonanes are all derived from norgestrol, made from the addition of a methyl group to norethisterone. Norgestimate is a prodrug, which is metabolised in two steps to the active levonorgestrel. Gestodene and desogestrel are closely related gonanes developed for use in the contraceptive pill and in HRT. An active intermediate metabolite of this conversion, levonorgestrel oxime, is a component of the weekly contraceptive patch. Drospirenone, a new progestogen for oral contraception, is chemically related to spironolactone and demonstrates potent progestational activity, together with antimineral corticoid and antiandrogenic properties.

### Routes of administration of progestogens

A progestogen-containing intrauterine device (the intrauterine system containing levonorgestrel), subcutaneous pellets, transdermal cream, transdermal patch, vaginal suppositories and intramuscular injection of progesterone are all delivery systems in use, although oral administration remains the most common mode of delivery. For HRT, progestogens are added in either a cyclic or continuous fashion to prevent endometrial hyperplasia and endometrial cancer. This is usually accomplished using the oral route, the transdermal patch or the progestogen-containing intrauterine system.

### Adverse effects of progestogens

Common symptoms of progestogens include weight gain, acne, fluid retention, headaches and breast tenderness. Sedation and mood changes reflect progestogenic effects on the central nervous system and may be related to progestogen binding to a membrane receptor of gamma aminobutyric acid in the central nervous system, which is the same receptor site for benzodiazepines and barbiturates.

Many progestogens (particularly 19-carbon compounds) when used alone cause androgenic effects such as acne and hirsutism owing to their similarity to testosterone. However, when combined with ethinyl estradiol in oral contraceptives, the suppression of ovarian androgens and the beneficial effect on SHBG induces an overall antiandrogenic effect in most women. Drospirenone, given its similarity to spironolactone, may be associated with less bloating and weight gain.

### Danazol

Danazol, an isoxazole derivative of ethinyl testosterone, is an orally active, pituitary-gonadotrophin inhibitory agent with androgenic effects but minimal estrogenic and progestational activity. It has the inhibitory effect on the synthesis and/or release of pituitary–gonadotrophic hormones by an effect on the pituitary. Androgen-like effects limit use and include weight gain, acne and seborrhoea. Mild hirsutism, oedema, hair loss and voice change, which may take the form of hoarseness, sore throat or instability or deepening of pitch, may occur and have been reported to persist after cessation of therapy. Clitoral hypertrophy is rare. Flushing, sweating, vaginal dryness and irritation and reduction in breast size occasionally occur and reflect gonadotrophin suppression.

### GONADOTROPHIN-RELEASING HORMONE ANALOGUES

Hypothalamic gonadotrophin-releasing hormone (GnRH) is a decapeptide that is synthesised and released in a pulsatile manner from hypothalamic neurosecretory cells. It stimulates pituitary synthesis and secretion of gonadotrophins and therefore causes increased secretion of gonadal hormones. Synthetic GnRH antagonists inhibit the endogenous hormone from binding to its receptor, inducing a pharmacological hypophysectomy. Nonpulsatile administration of GnRH agonist results in downregulation of GnRH receptors. The exact mechanism of suppression is unclear. Such agonists are used widely for the treatment of endometriosis and other gynaecological conditions when estrogen suppression is required (for example, for the shrinking of fibroids prior to surgery). Use of GnRH agonists is accompanied by an initial gonadotrophin and gonadal hormone surge known as the 'flare' and women will experience a temporary worsening of symptoms in the first 2 weeks of treatment.

GnRH agonists may be given by 3-monthly injection, monthly injection, daily injection and nasal spray. Common adverse effects when GnRH anologues are used without estrogen add-back therapy are the symptoms associated with the menopause, such as hot flushes, night sweats, insomnia, decreased libido, headaches, mood swings, vaginal dryness, change in breast size, acne, muscle pains and poor mood. These symptoms usually disappear soon after treatment ceases.

As in the menopause, bone density falls when GnRH analogues are used without estrogen add-back therapy. The decrease in bone density is about 4–6% during a 6-month course of treatment. Most of the bone lost during treatment regenerates within 6 months of completing treatment. Most lost bone will probably have been regained 18–24 months after completing treatment.

## The management of specific gynaecological conditions with hormonal therapy

### PROGESTOGENS USED ALONE FOR MENORRHAGIA

A variety of cyclical regimens of both 19-carbon and 21-carbon progestogens have been widely used for the treatment of menorrhagia. A Cochrane meta-analysis in 1998 concluded that progestogens administered from day 15 or 19 to day 26 of the cycle offer no advantage over other medical therapies such as danazol, tranexamic acid, nonsteroidal anti-inflammatory drugs and the intrauterine system in the treatment of menorrhagia in women with ovulatory cycles.[2] However, progestogen therapy for 21 days of the cycle results in a significant reduction in menstrual blood loss, although women found the treatment less acceptable than intrauterine levonorgestrel. The 21-day regimen of progestogen may have a role in the short-term treatment of menorrhagia. Progestogenic adverse effects may limit their use. In one randomised controlled trial within the Cochrane meta-analysis, 56% of women taking oral progestogens did not feel 'well' or 'very well' and only 22% elected to continue treatment with oral progestogens after the 3 months of the study.

### THE COMBINED CONTRACEPTIVE PILL AND MENORRHAGIA

The combined contraceptive pill has been widely used for the treatment of menorrhagia for many years and anecdotally appears effective. Surprisingly, a Cochrane analysis in 1997 found only one satisfactory small study, which found no significant difference between groups treated with the combined contraceptive pill, mefenamic acid, low-dose danazol or naproxen.[3] They concluded that the evidence from the one study was not sufficient to adequately assess the effectiveness of the combined contraceptive pill.

### THE INTRAUTERINE SYSTEM AND MENORRHAGIA

The levonorgestrel-releasing intrauterine system (LNG-IUS) appears to be more effective than 21-day cyclical norethisterone as a treatment for heavy menstrual bleeding.[4] Women with an LNG-IUS are more satisfied and willing to continue with treatment but experience more adverse effects, such as intermenstrual bleeding and breast tenderness.

### DANAZOL AND MENORRHAGIA

Danazol appears to be an effective treatment for heavy menstrual bleeding compared to other medical treatments. However, the use of danazol may be limited by its adverse effects, its acceptability to women and the need for long-term treatment. A meta-analysis in 2002 concluded that danazol was more effective than placebo, progestogens, nonsteroidal anti-inflammatory drugs (NSAIDs) and the combined contraceptive pill at reducing menstrual blood loss.[5] Treatment with danazol caused more adverse events than NSAIDs and progestogens. Danazol was also shown to significantly lower the duration of menses when compared with NSAIDs and a progestogen-releasing intrauterine device.

## COMBINED CONTRACEPTIVE PILL AND DYSMENORRHOEA

Combined contraceptive pills with medium-dose estrogen (more than 35 micrograms) and first- or second-generation progestogens appear to be more effective than placebo for pain relief.[6]

While there is some evidence from randomised controlled trials that the combined contraceptive pill with medium-dose estrogen and first- or second-generation progestogens are more effective than placebo, studies are small, of poor quality and all include much higher doses of hormones than those commonly prescribed today. Surprisingly, the efficacy of modern combined oral contraceptives has not been the subject of satisfactory studies.[6]

## HORMONAL TREATMENT OF ENDOMETRIOSIS

Ovarian hormones are required for the establishment or continued presence of endometriosis and it is clear that estrogen is needed to support the growth of ectopic endometrial tissue. The disorder occurs only after the onset of puberty and normally disappears after menopause. Medical therapy for endometriosis aims to relieve pain and bleeding. It is very seldom offered to women wishing pregnancy because treatment may compromise fertility. Long-term or repeated courses of treatment are often required.

### Oral estrogens and progestogens

The contraceptive pill is widely used for treating endometriosis-related pain but the clinical trial evidence for its use is poor.[7] Long cycle use (using the combined pill for 3 months in a row with a week break every 3 months) of the combined contraceptive is common for the relief of pain.

Progestogens have been used for the therapy of endometriosis worldwide for 50 years. Progestogenic adverse effects and irregular bleeding limit their use.

The mechanism of action and the morphological changes induced by progestogens remain unclear,

although high-dosage regimens are likely to act by menstrual-cycle suppression. Progesterone receptors in endometriotic foci are present in a very low concentration or are even absent, and enzyme systems differ widely in eutopic and ectopic endometrial tissue. Progestogens reduce the synthesis of their own receptors, resulting in diminished sensitivity of the implants during long-term treatment.[8]

### Levonorgestrel-releasing intrauterine system

The steady low-level release of levonorgestrel from the coil is likely to have a direct effect on endometriotic deposits through peritoneal fluid, possibly via a haematogenous spread. Three studies, two of which were controlled studies, have shown reduction in pain.

### Danazol

Danazol has been shown to be effective in some studies of mild and moderate endometriosis in the short term. However, the rate of recurrence of endometriosis is high and danazol causes marked weight gain and androgenic adverse effects in up to 25% of women, so its use is now uncommon in the medical management of endometriosis. Although it is still licensed for treatment of endometriosis, there remains insufficient evidence to recommend usage over other treatment methods.

### Gonadotrophin-releasing hormone analogues and add-back therapy

There is good evidence that inducing a medical menopause with nonpulsatile GnRH analogues to downregulate the pituitary will reduce endometriotic deposits and symptoms but the induced bone loss and climacteric symptoms limit their use alone. Add-back therapy, with either estrogens and progestogens or tibolone, appears to prevent climacteric symptoms and reduce the degree of bone loss without apparent reduction in efficacy.[9]

## HORMONE REPLACEMENT THERAPY

The chief role of HRT at present is for the prevention or treatment of climacteric symptoms around the time of the menopause. There is overwhelming evidence that

HRT provides the most effective method of treating climacteric hot flushes, night sweats and vaginal dryness. When hormonal treatment of the menopause was first introduced, estrogen was used alone, but it became clear in the 1970s and 1980s that unopposed estrogen may stimulate endometrial growth and lead to endometrial hyperplasia and a high risk of developing endometrial carcinoma. As a result, progestogens were added to HRT regimes, initially cyclically and later continually in continuous combined regimens, in which progestogens are added to estrogens every day.

### Endometrial cancer and unopposed estrogen use

The relationship between unopposed estrogen use in HRT and endometrial cancer has been clearly established since the 1970s by numerous experimental and epidemiological studies.[10–13] The estimated increase in relative risk for users compared with non-users from a 1995 meta-analysis was reported as 2.3 (95% CI 2.1–2.5), with a greater relative risk associated with prolonged duration of use (9.5 for 10 or more years).[14] The incidence of endometrial hyperplasia is increased in postmenopausal women on unopposed estrogen therapy, with an incidence of about 15–20% per year.[12]

### Estrogen and progestogen use

Histological changes produced by progestogens are dose- and duration-dependent. In a 28-day estrogen regimen, progestogen supplementation for less than 10 days/month is associated with increased risk of endometrial abnormalities compared to non-users, while the use of a progestogen for 10–12 days or more day/month, depending on its potency and half-life, removes the excess risk. The currently recommended duration of progestogens to protect the endometrium is 12–14 days each month.

Long-cycle HRT regimens, in which progestogens are added to continuous estrogens every 2 or 3 months, have been shown to be associated with an increased risk of endometrial hyperplasia. Such regimens should be used with caution and the endometrium should be carefully monitored during treatment. It is not known whether long-cycle therapy elevates the risk of endometrial carcinoma after treatment is stopped, as occurs with unopposed estrogen.

It is probable that most commercially available sequential HRT preparations do not cause any clinically significant rise in the risk of endometrial carcinoma.[15] However, many studies are not placebo controlled and are of short duration. Longer-term studies of sequential HRT using endometrial cancer as the endpoint have produced conflicting results. Some do not demonstrate an increase in risk whereas others show an increase in risk after 5 years of use.[16] In contrast to the studies of sequential therapy, where current data suggest no effect on endometrial cancer risk, or a very slight increase, continuous combined HRT in which estrogens and progestogens are both given daily appears to reduce the risk.[17]

### Estrogen therapy: routes of administration and dosage

Exogenous estrogens can be prescribed orally or parenterally. Currently available parenteral methods of delivery include transdermal patches, vaginal creams, pessaries or rings and subcutaneous implantation.

Estradiol transdermal patches contain $E_2$ either dissolved in alcohol within a thin, clear, circular multilayered patch with an outer impermeable membrane or within a solid matrix. The latter form of patch adheres best and is now most commonly used. Patches are available that must be changed twice or once a week. The most troublesome problem is skin reactions, which lead to discontinuation of this method in approximately 5% of women. A transdermal method of delivery for progestogen in a solid matrix patch is available.

Crystalline implants containing $E_2$ in a cholesterol base are inserted into the subcutaneous fat of the abdominal wall or buttock under local anaesthesia, a procedure that causes little discomfort and that takes approximately 5 minutes. Implants need to be repeated every 3–6 months. There is significant tachyphylaxis in some women, leading to women requesting further implantation at ever-decreasing intervals. There is also concern about the long-lasting effects of $E_2$ implants on the endometrium after implant therapy has been withdrawn and about the effect of ceasing implant treatment on symptoms. The duration of endometrial stimulation after the last implantation can be prolonged up to 43 months. Therefore, cyclical progestogens should be given until withdrawal bleeding has not occurred for 3 consecutive months.

### Long-term risks and benefits

Postmenopausal women who use exogenous estrogens are at an increased risk for venous thromboembolism, partly through a reduction in antithrombin III.[18] HRT has also been associated with an increased risk of gall bladder disease, stroke and breast cancer, particularly with long-term therapy.[19] The actual risk of these conditions for an individual is small.[17,20]

HRT is a well-established method for the treatment and prevention of osteoporosis whose effects, beneficial or not, have been widely studied. However, HRT use for the treatment or prevention of osteoporosis has declined as a result of women's concern about breast cancer and following the publication of studies that failed to show an effect of HRT on cardiovascular disease risk.[17,20]

### The use of progestogens alone

Progestogens are effective in the treatment of hot flushes and an efficacy better than placebo has been noted using oral norethisterone, intramuscular or oral medroxyprogesterone acetate and oral megestrol acetate. There is no consistent evidence of an effect of progestogens on other symptoms of the menopause, nor of significant metabolism to estrogenic substances. Some data suggest that certain progestogens (for example, norethisterone 5–10 mg/day) may preserve bone density.

### Tibolone

Tibolone is a synthetic steroid that has estrogenic, progestogenic and androgenic properties and is used orally as an alternative to estrogen/progestogen HRT. Structurally it is related to 19-nortestosterone. Tibolone is metabolised predominantly to three other steroid molecules; a delta-4-isomer, 3-alpha-hydroxymetabolite and 3-beta-hydroxymetabolite. In the endometrium, the delta-4-isomer predominates and, because it has a progestogenic effect, the endometrium atrophies. As there is no stimulation of the endometrium, there is no withdrawal bleeding. Tibolone is therefore a suitable alternative to continuous combined HRT and it has many comparable effects to HRT in the relief of menopausal symptoms and prevention of bone loss.[21]

Adverse effects reflect the androgenic and progestogenic activity of the molecule and include weight change, ankle swelling, dizziness, headache, vaginal bleeding, gastrointestinal symptoms, some increased facial hair, depression and joint pains.

### REFERENCES

1. WHITEHEAD M I, TOWNSEND P T, PRYSE-DAVIES J, RYDER TA, KING RJB. Effects of estrogens and progestins on the biochemistry and morphology of the postmenopausal endometrium. *New Engl J Med* 1981;305:1599–605.

2. LETHABY A, IRVINE G, CAMERON I. Cyclical progestogens for heavy menstrual bleeding. *Cochrane Database Syst Rev* 1998;(4):CD001016.

3. IYER V, FARQUHAR C, JEPSON R. Oral contraceptive pills for heavy menstrual bleeding. *Cochrane Database Syst Rev* 1997;(3):CD000154.

4. LETHABY A E, COOKE I, REES M. Progesterone or progestogen-releasing intrauterine systems for heavy menstrual bleeding. *Cochrane Database Syst Rev* 2000;(2):CD002126.

5. BEAUMONT H, AUGOOD C, DUCKITT K, LETHABY A. Danazol for heavy menstrual bleeding. *Cochrane Database Syst Rev* 2002;(2):CD001017.

6. PROCTOR M L, ROBERTS H, FARQUHAR C M. Combined oral contraceptive pill (OCP) as treatment for primary dysmenorrhoea. *Cochrane Database Syst Rev* 2001(4): CD002120.

7. DAVIS L, KENNEDY SS, MOORE J, PRENTICE A. Modern combined oral contraceptives for pain associated with endometriosis. *Cochrane Database Syst Rev* 2007;(3):CD001019.

8. SCHWEPPE K W. Drug treatment of endometriosis. *Contemporary Clinical Gynecology and Obstetrics* 2001;2:167–77.

9. SAGSVEEN M, FARMER J E, PRENTICE A, Breeze A. Gonadotrophin-releasing hormone analogues for endometriosis: bone mineral density. *Cochrane Database Syst Rev* 2003;(4):CD001297.

10. BERAL V, BANKS E, REEVES G. Evidence from randomised trials on the long-term effects of hormone replacement therapy. *Lancet* 2002;360:942–4.

11. BERAL V, BANKS E, REEVES G, APPLEBY P. Use of HRT and the subsequent risk of cancer. *J Epidemiol Biostat* 1999;4:191–210.

12. LETHABY A, FARQUHAR C, SARKIS A, *et al*. Hormone replacement therapy in postmenopausal women: endometrial hyperplasia and irregular bleeding. *Cochrane Database Syst Rev* 2000;(2):CD000402 .

13. BRINTON LA, HOOVER RN. Estrogen replacement therapy and endometrial cancer risk: unresolved issues. The Endometrial Cancer Collaborative Group. *Obstet Gynecol* 1993;81:265–71.

14. GRADY D, GEBRETSADIK T, KERLIKOWSKE K, ERNSTER V, PETITTI D. Hormone replacement therapy and endometrial cancer risk: a meta-analysis. *Obstet Gynecol* 1995;85:304–13.

15. The Writing Group for the PEPI Trial. Effects of hormone replacement therapy on endometrial histology in postmenopausal women. The Postmenopausal Estrogen/ Progestin Interventions (PEPI) Trial. *JAMA* 1996;275:370–5.

16. BERESFORD SA, WEISS NS, VOIGT LF, McKNIGHT B. Risk of endometrial cancer in relation to use of oestrogen combined with cyclic progestagen therapy in postmenopausal women. *Lancet* 1997;349:458–61.

17. ROSSOUW JE, ANDERSON GL, PRENTICE RL, LaCROIX AZ, KOOPERBERG C, STEFANICK ML, *et al*. Risks and benefits of estrogen plus progestin in healthy postmenopausal women: principal results from the Women's Health Initiative randomized controlled trial. *JAMA* 2002;288:321–33.

18. DALY E, VESSEY MP, HAWKINS MM, CARSON JL, GOUGH P, MARSH S. Risk of venous thromboembolism in users of hormone replacement therapy. *Lancet* 1996;348:977–80.

19. COLDITZ GA, HANKINSON SE, HUNTER DJ, *et al*. The use of estrogens and progestins and the risk of breast cancer in postmenopausal women. *New Engl J Med* 1995;332:1589–93.

20. ANDERSON GL, LIMACHER M, ASSAF AR, BASSFORD T, BERESFORD SA, BLACK H, *et al*. Effects of conjugated equine estrogen in postmenopausal women with hysterectomy: the Women's Health Initiative randomized controlled trial. *JAMA* 2004;291:1701–12.

21. RYMER J, CHAPMAN MG, FOGELMAN I. Effect of tibolone on postmenopausal bone loss. *Osteoporosis Int* 1994;4:314–17.

# Sample questions relating to pharmacokinetics, pharmacodynamics and teratogenesis

## EXTENDED MATCHING QUESTIONS

### Questions 1–9

■ *These questions relate to drugs with agonistic and antagonistic actions on receptors. For each item below, select the **single** best option from the list of options (A–M). Each option may be used once, more than once or not at all.*

OPTIONS

▷ A  Salbutamol
▷ B  Methyldopa
▷ C  Phenylephrine
▷ D  Pilocarpine
▷ E  Diazepam
▷ F  Cabergoline
▷ G  Atenolol
▷ H  Labetalol
▷ I  Doxazosin
▷ J  Tolterodine
▷ K  Ranitidine
▷ L  Cyproterone acetate
▷ M  Metoclopramide

1 ▶ Acts on histamine antagonist

2 ▶ Acts on testosterone receptors

3 ▶ Is a dopamine agonist

4 ▶ Is a dopamine antagonist

5 ▶ Is a muscarinic agonist

6 ▶ Is a muscarinic antagonist

7 ▶ Is a $\beta$1 adrenergic antagonist

8 ▶ Is a $\beta$1 and $\beta$2 agonist

9 ▶ Is an $\alpha$2 agonist

### Questions 10–19

■ *These questions relate to the use of antibiotics in pregnancy. For each item below, select the **single** best option from the list of options (A–I). Each option may be used once, more than once or not at all.*

OPTIONS

▷ A  Aminoglycosides
▷ B  Cephalosporins
▷ C  Chloramphenicol
▷ D  Macrolides
▷ E  Nitrofurantoin
▷ F  Penicillins
▷ G  Quinolones
▷ H  Sulphonamides
▷ I  Tetracyclines

10 ▶ Can cause fetal cardiovascular collapse

11 ▶ Can cause neonatal haemolysis

12 ▶ Can cause neonatal jaundice

13 ▶ Can treat fetal syphilis

14 ▶ Cause impaired bone growth *in utero*

15 ▶ Cause permanent discolouration of teeth

16 ▶ Cause VIIIth cranial nerve palsy

17 ▶ Cause neonatal kernicterus

18 ▶ Inhibit folate metabolism

19 ▶ Are nephrotoxic

## Questions 20–27

■ *These questions relate to the use of drugs in pregnancy. For each item below, select the **single** best option from the list of options (A–O). Each option may be used once, more than once or not at all.*

OPTIONS

▷ **A** Angiotensin-converting enzyme inhibitors
▷ **B** Alpha blockers
▷ **C** Beta blockers
▷ **D** Nitrofurantoin
▷ **E** Carbamazepine
▷ **F** Carbimazole
▷ **G** Tetracyclines
▷ **H** Dopamine agonists
▷ **I** Low-molecular-weight heparin
▷ **J** Aspirin
▷ **K** Paracetamol
▷ **L** Pethidine
▷ **M** Retinoids
▷ **N** Thyroxine
▷ **O** Warfarin

**20** ▶ Causes impaired bone growth

**21** ▶ Causes Reye syndrome

**22** ▶ Causes fetal and neonatal renal dysfunction

**23** ▶ Causes fetal head growth restriction

**24** ▶ Causes craniofacial abnormalities

**25** ▶ Causes neonatal haemolysis

**26** ▶ Causes intracerebral bleeding

**27** ▶ Causes fetal growth restriction

## MULTIPLE CHOICE QUESTIONS

**28** ▶ A drug's absorption rate is increased by:

**A** ▷ lipid solubility
**B** ▷ high polarity
**C** ▷ attaching to a specific carrier
**D** ▷ accelerating gastric emptying
**E** ▷ rectal rather than oral administration

**29** ▶ Regarding renal clearance:

**A** ▷ Large drugs are not renally excreted
**B** ▷ Protein-bound drugs are poorly excreted
**C** ▷ Excretion is passive in the proximal convoluted tubule
**D** ▷ Excretion is active in the descending loops of Henle
**E** ▷ Acidic drugs use cation transporters

**30** ▶ Regarding kidney excretion:

**A** ▷ Polar drugs are distributed over a large volume
**B** ▷ Polar drugs are easily cleared by the kidney
**C** ▷ Albumin-bound drugs are easily cleared
**D** ▷ Acidic drugs are not secreted into the proximal tubule
**E** ▷ Tubular reabsorption rates are the same for all drugs

**31** ▶ Regarding drug pharmacokinetics:

**A** ▷ There is an increase in volume of the third space
**B** ▷ There is an increase in serum concentration of drugs
**C** ▷ There is an increase in clearance of drugs
**D** ▷ Liver metabolism is increased
**E** ▷ Fat-soluble drugs are more affected by pregnancy changes

**32** ▶ Regarding drug interactions:

**A** ▷ Enzyme inducers cause an increase in serum concentration of other drugs
**B** ▷ Enzyme inhibitors increase the risk of drug toxicity
**C** ▷ Phenytoin is an enzyme inducer
**D** ▷ Sulphonamides are an enzyme inducer
**E** ▷ Ampicillin increases the effects of oral estrogens

**33 ▶** Regarding the effects of drugs on enzyme expression:

**A** ▷ Smoking decreases enzyme induction
**B** ▷ Alcohol decreases enzyme induction
**C** ▷ Enzyme induction is usually due to a decrease in enzyme breakdown
**D** ▷ Enzyme inhibition can increase the action of other drugs
**E** ▷ Phenytoin leads to reduced efficiency of warfarin

**34 ▶** Regarding drug prescription in relation to pregnancy and lactation:

**A** ▷ All women of reproductive age might be pregnant
**B** ▷ Drugs should be avoided in the first trimester if possible
**C** ▷ Known teratogenic anticonvulsant drugs should be stopped in pregnancy
**D** ▷ Most drugs cross the placenta
**E** ▷ Large doses should be used for the shortest possible time

**35 ▶** Regarding prenatal exposure to a teratogen:

**A** ▷ Up to day 17, any teratogenic effect results in miscarriage
**B** ▷ The earlier the exposure, the more marked the effect
**C** ▷ All organs are sensitive for the same period of time
**D** ▷ There is no risk of teratogenicity after week 8
**E** ▷ Anencephaly is most likely to occur with exposure to tetratogens around day 24

**36 ▶** Miscarriage can be caused by:

**A** ▷ ergotamine
**B** ▷ gabapentin
**C** ▷ mifepristone
**D** ▷ thrombolytics
**E** ▷ carbamazepine

**37 ▶** Regarding the use of anticonvulsants:

**A** ▷ Risks of teratogenicity decrease if folic acid is given at the start of pregnancy
**B** ▷ Women who have not had a fit for more than a year should stop taking them
**C** ▷ Polypharmacy increases the risks of teratogenicity
**D** ▷ Sodium valproate is the most teratogenic anticonvulsant
**E** ▷ Phenytoin has dose-related effect on verbal IQ

**38 ▶** Phenytoin is associated with:

**A** ▷ cleft lip/palate
**B** ▷ microcephaly
**C** ▷ cardiac abnormalities
**D** ▷ mental retardation
**E** ▷ neural tube defects

**39 ▶** Antibiotics contraindicated in pregnancy are:

**A** ▷ macrolides
**B** ▷ penicillins
**C** ▷ quinolones
**D** ▷ sulphonamides
**E** ▷ tetracyclines

**40 ▶** Antibiotics used with caution in pregnancy are:

**A** ▷ macrolides
**B** ▷ cephalosporins
**C** ▷ quinolones
**D** ▷ nitrofurantoin
**E** ▷ aminoglycosides

**41 ▶** Regarding the use of anticonvulsants in pregnancy:

**A** ▷ Of the anticonvulsants sodium valproate has the highest risk of teratogenesis
**B** ▷ Carbamazepine causes neural tube defects
**C** ▷ Folic acid should always be given as well
**D** ▷ There is a five-fold increase in fetal malformations
**E** ▷ Teratogenicity is a more important consideration than good seizure control

**42 ▶** Regarding the use of anticoagulants in pregnancy:

**A** ▷ Warfarin causes nasal hypoplasia in the second trimester
**B** ▷ Heparin use in the first trimester causes chondroplasia
**C** ▷ Warfarin may cause major haemorrhage towards the end of pregnancy
**D** ▷ There are no common fetal abnormalities with the use of heparin in pregnancy
**E** ▷ Warfarin must be exchanged for heparin by week 8

# Sample questions relating to non-hormonal therapy in obstetrics and gynaecology

## EXTENDED MATCHING QUESTIONS

### Questions 1–10

■ *These questions relate to antihypertensives in pregnancy. For each item below, select the **single** best option from the list of options (A–G). Each option may be used once, more than once or not at all.*

OPTIONS

▷ **A** Angiotensin-converting enzyme inhibitors
▷ **B** Beta blockers
▷ **C** Hydralazine
▷ **D** Magnesium sulphate
▷ **E** Methyldopa
▷ **F** Nifedipine
▷ **G** Thiazides

1 ▶ Causes skull defects

2 ▶ Causes neonatal thrombocytopenia

3 ▶ Acts centrally

4 ▶ Causes depression

5 ▶ Causes decreased variability on cardiotocograph

6 ▶ Causes fetal growth restriction

7 ▶ Causes neonatal hypoglycaemia

8 ▶ Is a calcium channel blocker

9 ▶ Is a potent vasodilator

10 ▶ Causes respiratory depression

### Questions 11–15

■ *These questions relate to tocolytics. For each item below, select the **single** best option from the list of options (A–G). Each option may be used once, more than once or not at all.*

OPTIONS

▷ **A** Atosiban
▷ **B** Beta mimetics
▷ **C** Glyceryl trinitrate patches
▷ **D** Magnesium sulphate
▷ **E** Nifedipine
▷ **F** Atenolol
▷ **G** Vasopressin

11 ▶ Is used prior to external cephalic version

12 ▶ Is an oxytocin antagonist

13 ▶ Needs toxicity measurements taken

14 ▶ Has the least adverse effects

15 ▶ Has the most significant adverse effects

### Questions 16–22

■ *These questions relate to drugs are given to minimise the risk of postpartum haemorrhage. For each item below, select the single best option from the list of options (A–E). Each option may be used once, more than once or not at all.*

OPTIONS

▷ **A** Carboprost
▷ **B** Ergometrine
▷ **C** Misoprostol
▷ **D** Syntocinon
▷ **E** Syntometrine

16 ▶ Can be given via several routes

17 ▶ Is a prostaglandin $F_{2\alpha}$ analogue

18 ▶ Causes prolonged vasoconstriction

19 ▶ Causes short-term uterine contractions

20 ▶ Can cause diarrhoea

21 ▶ Is contraindicated in asthmatics

**22** ▶ Is contraindicated in hypertensive patients

### Questions 23–30

■ *These questions relate to chemotherapeutic drugs. For each item below, select the **single** best option from the list of options (A–F). Each option may be used once, more than once or not at all.*

OPTIONS

▷ **A** Fluorouracil
▷ **B** Cisplatin
▷ **C** Cyclophosphamide
▷ **D** Doxorubicin
▷ **E** Methotrexate
▷ **F** Paclitaxel

**23** ▶ Forms covalent bonds with DNA bases, thus preventing separation during replication

**24** ▶ Has an effect on both RNA and DNA

**25** ▶ Inhibits mitosis by stabilising tubulin in spindle microtubules

**26** ▶ Is a folate antagonist

**27** ▶ Is a platinum compound

**28** ▶ Is an immunosuppressant

**29** ▶ Is an antibiotic

**30** ▶ Is selective at only binding to tumour DNA

**31** ▶ Methyldopa:

    **A** ▷ is safe in pregnancy
    **B** ▷ acts centrally
    **C** ▷ has no effect on sympathetic outflow
    **D** ▷ causes depression
    **E** ▷ causes a drop in baseline on cardiotocograph

**32** ▶ Nifedipine:

    **A** ▷ is a calcium channel blocker
    **B** ▷ is licensed in pregnancy
    **C** ▷ is a tocolytic
    **D** ▷ causes peripheral oedema
    **E** ▷ causes arrhythmia

**33** ▶ Regarding intravenous antihypertensives:

    **A** ▷ Hydralazine acts centrally
    **B** ▷ Hydralazine is known to cause lupus-like events
    **C** ▷ Magnesium sulphate is a membrane stabiliser
    **D** ▷ Magnesium sulphate is the best antihypertensive at reducing eclamptic fits
    **E** ▷ Magnesium sulphate causes cardiorespiratory arrest

**34** ▶ Drugs to treat detrusor overactivity:

    **A** ▷ include antimuscarinics
    **B** ▷ include desmopressin
    **C** ▷ include duloxetine
    **D** ▷ cause a dry mouth
    **E** ▷ cause diarrhoea

**35** ▶ Regarding chemotheraputic drugs used in gynaecological oncology:

    **A** ▷ Platinum agents are used in ovarian cancer
    **B** ▷ Cisplatin is used in cervical cancer
    **C** ▷ Methotrexate has a use in metastatic cervical cancer
    **D** ▷ Folate antagonists are used in vulval cancer
    **E** ▷ Methotrexate alone is used in high-risk trophoblastic disease

## Sample questions relating to hormonal treatment in non-malignant gynaecological conditions

### MULTIPLE CHOICE QUESTIONS

1 ▶ Regarding estrogens:

   A ▷ During the childbearing years, estradiol is the most potent estrogen

   B ▷ After the menopause, estriol is the most abundant estrogen

   C ▷ After the menopause, the ovaries stop producing estrogens completely

   D ▷ Estrogens terminate the pubertal growth spurt in women

   E ▷ The hypothalamus and the heart contain the same type of estrogen receptor

2 ▶ Regarding pharmacological estrogens:

   A ▷ Pharmacological estrogens contain an ethinyl group to prevent first-pass metabolism

   B ▷ Pharmacological estrogens are usually estradiols

   C ▷ Plant estrogens are used in the combined oral contraceptive

   D ▷ Clomiphene citrate acts by replicating the actions of estrogen

   E ▷ Tamoxifen is an estrogen antagonist in the breast but an agonist in the skeleton

3 ▶ Regarding endogenous progesterone:

   A ▷ Outside of pregnancy, progesterone is mainly produced by the adrenal cortex

   B ▷ Progesterone production is at its peak during the luteal phase

   C ▷ Progesterone causes an increase in body temperature

   D ▷ Progesterone is responsible for decidual development

   E ▷ Progesterone is an antagonistic estrogen on the uterus

4 ▶ Regarding pharmacological progestogens:

   A ▷ Large doses need to be given orally

   B ▷ Medroxyprogesterone acetate is a 19-carbon steroid

   C ▷ Medroxyprogesterone acetate is used for the treatment of endometriosis

   D ▷ Norethisterone has androgenic properties

   E ▷ In hormone replacement therapy, progesterone is given at constant doses

5 ▶ Adverse effects of progesterone treatment are:

   A ▷ loss of libido

   B ▷ acne

   C ▷ mood swings

   D ▷ insomnia

   E ▷ hirsutism

6 ▶ Gonadotrophin-releasing hormone analogues:

   A ▷ are used for oestrogen suppression

   B ▷ when used, may cause a worsening of symptoms before improvement

   C ▷ are well known to cause insomnia

   D ▷ produce long-lasting adverse effects

   E ▷ have no effect on bone density

7 ▶ Regarding hormone replacement therapy:

   A ▷ Progesterone produces a dose-dependent histological change

   B ▷ Progesterone must be used for at least 7 days a month to reduce the risk of endometrial cancer

   C ▷ Transdermal patches use estradiol

   D ▷ Estrogen levels should be checked prior to each subcutaneous insertion of an implant, regardless of the patient's symptoms

   E ▷ Tibolone should not be given unopposed

8 ▶ Regarding hormone replacement therapy:

   A ▷ The risk of deep vein thrombosis is increased

   B ▷ The therapy is a well-known treatment for osteoporosis

   C ▷ If unopposed estrogen is used, there is a relative risk of endometrial cancer of 95

   D ▷ Tibolone is an estrogen and progesterone preparation

   E ▷ Tibolone produces a withdrawal bleed

# Physiology

# CHAPTER 29

# Female reproductive physiology

*Helen Mason*

## Introduction

The structure of the female reproductive organs and the cycles that control adult reproductive function are designed to bring about a number of important processes that permit fertility. These range from storage of sufficient ova for the lifetime, sequential follicular growth and regular spontaneous ovulation, to fertilisation, preparation of the endometrium of the uterus and support of the fertilised oocyte by the corpus luteum prior to implantation.

## Storage of sufficient ova for a lifetime

During embryonic life, the primordial germ cells migrate from the hindgut into the tissue that will develop into the gonad. In the absence of the *SRY* gene, the gonad develops into an ovary and the germ cells become oogonia. The small number of oogonia that initially populate the ovary is increased dramatically by rapid mitosis until several million oogonia are present. Each oogonium is surrounded by cells that differentiate from the surrounding stroma to become granulosa cells and the whole structure is now a primordial follicle. The oocyte enters the first meiotic division at this time but does not complete it. These follicles are stored in the outer cortical layer of the ovary and many are lost through atresia from the second trimester onwards. By puberty, the numbers are reduced to less than one million.

## Sequential growth of follicles

Following pubertal activation of the hypothalamus and pituitary, the follicles in the ovary become activated. It is clear that follicle-stimulating hormone (FSH) is not required for the very earliest stages of follicle growth as women who have inactivating defects in the FSH receptor are still able to grow small follicles. The primordial follicles grow by divisions of the granulosa cells such that the oocyte is contained within a ball of growing cells. These cells then produce a non-cellular barrier around their outsides, a basal lamina, which subsequently acts as a protective layer for the oocyte. External to this, a second layer of cells differentiates from the stroma and becomes the theca layer. It is within the theca layer that the capillaries, which will provide nutrients for the growing follicle, reside. The theca layer is the only layer that is vascular; the inner granulosa layer remains avascular.

It is thought that follicles grow for approximately 80 days until they reach the size at which they can release the oocyte (Figure 29.1). There is continual loss of follicles by death during this process so that only a few follicles reach the size at which they can respond to the hormonal changes in the menstrual cycle. Once initiated, follicles take approximately 65 days to reach the size at which they can be recruited into a menstrual cycle. Follicle diameter increases by 1000-fold, from approximately 0.02 mm to 20–50 mm, by the time the single selected follicle is at the pre-ovulatory stage. The follicle reaches the antral phase (Figure 29.2), the oocyte is displaced to one side and the granulosa cells surround a fluid-filled central cavity called the antrum. A subset of granulosa

FIGURE 29.1 **The main stages of follicle growth**

FIGURE 29.2 **Cross-section through an antral or Graafian, follicle**

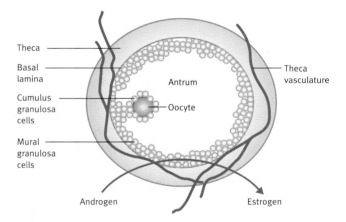

cells differentiates and surrounds the oocyte. These cells are called cumulus cells and their role is protective and nourishing. The granulosa cells against the follicle wall, the basal lamina, are called mural cells.

## Selection of a single follicle and oocyte

Folliculogenesis is defined as growth of the follicles from the earliest resting phases through to ovulation. Only the latter stages of this process are dependent on the hormonal changes of the menstrual cycle. The granulosa cells develop receptors for FSH and the theca cells develop receptors for luteinising hormone (LH). Once follicles develop an antrum, they are dependent on FSH for further growth.

The ovarian steroids are produced in the follicle by sequential loss of carbon atoms from cholesterol (Figure

29.3). LH drives the conversion of cholesterol to androgen by the theca layer. Androgens act as the precursor for estradiol synthesis and FSH primarily drives the conversion of androgen diffusing across the basement membrane to estradiol, a reaction that is catalysed by the enzyme aromatase in the granulosa cells. Both theca and granulosa cells can convert cholesterol into progesterone but only theca cells express *CYP 17*, which encodes for the enzymes necessary for androgen production, 17-alpha-hydroxylase and 17,20-lyase, and only granulosa cells contain aromatase. Therefore, both cell types are essential for the production of all steroids. This is known as the two-cell two-gonadotrophin theory. It is the cyclical changes in the peptide hormones and the steroids subsequently produced by the follicles that bring about the menstrual cycle and permit selection of a single ovulatory follicle.

Assuming that pregnancy did not occur in the previous cycle, the cells in the corpus luteum will die 14 days after ovulation. Death of the cells results in a fall in progesterone and estrogen and subsequent shedding of the endometrium (Figure 29.4). At the beginning of the cycle (day 1) there are from four to six antral follicles of size 2–4 mm in the ovary. As the corpus luteum dies, the fall in steroids results in removal of negative feedback at the hypothalamus and pituitary and this causes a specific rise in FSH (Figure 29.5 A). Although both LH and FSH are produced by the pituitary gonadotrophs, it is only FSH that rises at this time. FSH levels remain elevated for approximately 3 days: this is known as the intercycle rise in FSH. It is this rise in FSH that is primarily responsible for selection of the dominant follicle. One follicle has the correct qualities, because of FSH receptor numbers, intracellular cyclic adenosine monophosphate levels or granulosa cell number, and this follicle rapidly increases in size in response. As the number of granulosa cells in the follicle increases exponentially, their products, namely inhibin and estradiol, rise in the serum. This reinstates the negative feedback and FSH levels fall (Figures 29.4 and 29.5 B).

The action of FSH on the dominant or selected follicle induces LH receptors on the granulosa cells at this time. No other follicle acquires granulosa cell LH receptors. This means that this follicle can survive the fall in FSH whereas the other small follicles in the cohort, which are FSH dependent, will die by atresia.

Across the follicular phase, the level of LH gradually increases. The dominant follicle grows from 4 mm to

**FIGURE 29.3  Ovarian steroid production**

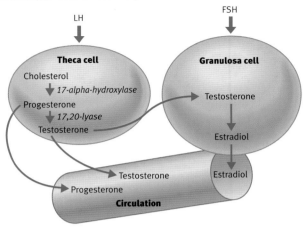

FSH = follicle-stimulating hormone | LH = luteinising hormone

20 mm with an accompanying considerable increase in granulosa cell number. As each cell is converting androgen from the theca cells into estrogen by the action of aromatase, the serum concentration of estradiol increases rapidly. Once the level has been above 300 nmol/l for 2–3 days, the negative feedback switches to positive. This causes a rapid and massive release of LH from the pituitary, known as the LH surge (Figures 29.4 and 29.5 C).

## Regular spontaneous ovulation

The LH surge is responsible for the cascade of events leading to ovulation. The capillaries in the theca become leaky, leading to increased fluid pressure in the antrum. The pressure helps to assist the follicle in protruding from the surface of the ovary at the apex and the follicle wall becomes thin by stretching. Finally, a cascade of locally made enzymes breaks down the follicle wall and the oocyte and its surrounding cumulus cells are extruded because of the intrafollicular pressure.

The oocyte–cell complex is collected by the fimbrial end of the uterine tube, which is mobile and able to detect the oocyte, probably by a process of chemoattraction. The follicle that is left behind collapses, the basal lamina breaks down and the blood vessels invade the centre of the follicle to form a clot. The theca and granulosa layers are disrupted and there is a dramatic fall in steroid production directly after the release of the oocyte. The corpus luteum then forms from the involuted layers of the follicle and steroid production resumes in earnest, with estradiol and progesterone reaching a peak approximately 1 week after ovulation (Figures 29.4 and 29.5 D). The corpus luteum is the only source of significant levels of progesterone during the cycle, making this the ideal marker of ovulation.

**FIGURE 29.4  Changes in principal hormones during the menstrual cycle and the accompanying changes in the follicle**

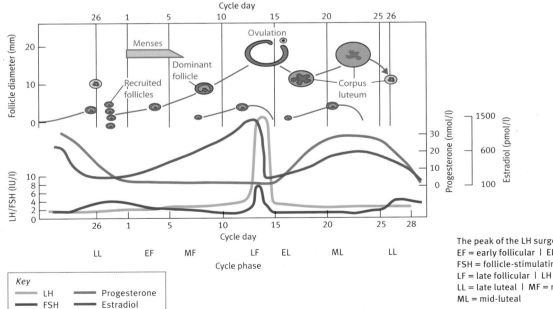

The peak of the LH surge is >50 IU/l.
EF = early follicular | EL = early luteal |
FSH = follicle-stimulating hormone |
LF = late follicular | LH = luteinising hormone |
LL = late luteal | MF = mid-follicular |
ML = mid-luteal

FIGURE 29.5 **Hypothalamic–pituitary–ovarian feedback through the menstrual cycle**

**A** Late luteal/early follicular phase

P −ve / LH FSH

P declines and selectively raises FSH
**Intercycle rise**

**B** Mid-follicular phase

$E_2$ −ve / LH FSH

$E_2$ increases, leading to negative feedback
**FSH falls**

**C** Mid-cycle

$E_2$ +ve / LH FSH

2 days of $E_2$ >300 pmol/l leads to positive feedback
**LH surge**

**D** Mid-luteal phase

P −ve / LH FSH

High P leads to negative feedback
**Low LH/FSH P overcomes $E_2$**

*Key*

Hypothalamus

Pituitary gland

Ovary with growing follicles (black) or corpus luteum (red)

Direction of hormone action

$E_2$ = estradiol | FSH = follicle-stimulating hormone | LH = luteinising hormone | P = progesterone

## Correct number of chromosomes in the oocyte

In addition to its effects on the follicle, the LH surge also has an important effect on the oocyte in that it causes the oocyte to complete the first meiotic division. This would normally result in the production of two cells but the oocyte needs to remain as a large cell, as it has to provide for the early divisions of the blastocyst. To retain maximum cytoplasm, the second set of chromosomes produced at this time is parcelled into a package known as the first polar body. These chromosomes take no further part in the function of the oocyte. The second meiotic division is commenced and, like the first meiotic division, is not completed.

## Transport of oocyte to uterus

The oocyte is passed along the tube by the combined action of peristalsis and cilia. The cells lining the tubes are of two types and are steroid sensitive. In response to estradiol production by the dominant follicle, the ciliated cells produce the cilia on the surface and the glandular cells secrete products that are designed to support the oocyte and provide an environment for sperm capacitation. Fertilisation normally occurs in the ampulla of the tube. Once the oocyte has passed into the uterus, the level of progesterone increases and this causes the cilia to retract and the glandular cells to shorten. This means that, even if a second oocyte were to be released, it would be unable to pass along the tube.

## Fertilisation

Fertilisation causes a number of changes in the oocyte. The penetrating spermatozoon causes the oocyte to complete the second meiotic division. The second set of chromosomes is packaged into the second polar body. This leaves a haploid cell, which can combine with the nucleus of the sperm head. Penetration of the sperm head results in the movement of a specialised set of cellular contents, cortical granules, within the oocyte cytoplasm. The cortical granules migrate to the outer edge of the oocyte and release their contents. This results in a hardening of the oocyte membrane that precludes entry by a second spermatozoon and prevents polyspermy. Soon after fertilisation, the fertilised oocyte undergoes mitotic cell division to produce the blastocyst. Cells in the blastocyst then begin to produce human chorionic gonadotrophin, which acts on the LH receptors of the corpus luteum and prevents its demise.

## Cyclical changes in the uterus, vagina and cervix

Production of ovarian steroids is not only vital for the growing follicle but is also necessary to bring about cyclical changes in the uterus, vagina and cervix, all of which are designed to facilitate transport and implantation of the dividing blastocyst.

### UTERUS

The myometrium of the uterus is covered by a layer of endometrial cells. Within this endometrial layer there are also glandular cells and vessels supplied by the uterine and, subsequently, the radial arteries. Following menstruation, the myometrium is covered by a basal layer of the endometrium. Under the stimulation of estrogen, these cells divide rapidly; this is known as the proliferative phase and corresponds to the follicular phase of the ovary. At the same time as the endometrial cells are undergoing rapid divisions, the glandular cells grow and expand to make glands and there is new growth of blood vessels. The actions of estrogen induce progesterone receptors on the endometrial cells so that after ovulation the cells can respond to the rising levels of progesterone being made by the corpus luteum. Two or three days after ovulation, progesterone causes the rapid rate of cell division to reduce and, although the thickness of the endometrium continues to increase, this occurs mainly by oedema. Contributing to this oedema are the increased number of vessels, which become spiral, to accommodate maximum vascularity in a minimum space, and which become increasingly permeable. At the same time, the glands distend and increase in tortuosity to give the maximum surface area on which to produce their product (glycoproteins), which are secreted on to the surface. For this reason, this is known as the secretory phase, corresponding to the luteal phase in the ovary. The endometrium will now have reached approximately

6 mm in thickness. It is the responsiveness to steroids, estrogen in particular, that makes measurement of endometrial thickness a good indicator of the degree of estrogenisation of a woman.

Progesterone also has an effect on the myometrial wall of the uterus. This undergoes continual small contractions in response to estrogen and, during the luteal phase, these are suppressed by progesterone, presumably to increase the chances of implantation. If fertilisation does not occur, the corpus luteum will die and the level of steroids will fall. In response to steroid withdrawal, prostaglandins are released by the endometrial cells. These cause a temporary constriction of the spiral arterioles, which later dilate and begin to bleed. The ensuing hypoxia in the surrounding tissues causes necrosis and as the cells break down they release proteolytic enzymes, which accelerate this process. The outer layer of the endometrium is thus shed with 50% being lost within the first 24 hours. Normal menstrual flow is difficult to measure in practice but is considered to be anything up to 80 ml. All but the basal layer is shed and this layer recommences division in response to rising estradiol in the next cycle.

### VAGINA AND CERVIX

The vagina is lined by stratified, nonkeratinised squamous epithelium. The layers divide continually and are shed creating a downward movement of cells. This downflow is added to by cervical secretions and transudation from the vaginal epithelium. It is designed to decrease the chances of opportunistic infection. The secretions in the vagina change with the cycle and are generally acidic, thus providing an antimicrobial action.

During the follicular phase, there is an increase in vascularity of the cervix, which results in oedema. The mucus becomes watery as a result and the composition changes such that the glycoproteins contained within it align to form microscopic channels. These channels are designed to facilitate the passage of spermatozoa through the cervix. After ovulation, under the influence of progesterone, the oedema reduces, the mucus becomes thicker and the glycoproteins now form a mesh. This acts as a potential barrier to spermatozoa and is one of the mechanisms of action of the progesterone-only oral contraceptive.

# Male reproductive physiology and the fertilisation process

*Helen Mason*

## Introduction

In terms of reproduction, the main requirement for the male is to deliver a package of chromosomes to the oocyte. The male reproductive tract is designed to facilitate every step of this process.

## Gross anatomy

The gross anatomy of the male reproductive tract is shown in Figure 30.1. The structure is designed to have a combined outlet for the ureter and vas deferens through the urethra and to provide a site for sperm production that is protective and yet in close proximity to this outlet. The glands contribute to seminal fluid, which is important for preservation and transport of the spermatozoa.

## The internal structure of the testes

The testes are oval structures of 3.3–5.5 cm in length and 2–3 cm wide giving a normal volume of 15–30 ml. Testicular volume is important as any reduction in the mass of tissue producing spermatozoa may result in a reduced sperm count. The volume is measured by means of an orchidometer. The testes lie in the scrotal sac outside the body cavity. The reason for this is that spermatogenesis requires a temperature that is 1.5–2 degrees C below core body temperature in order to proceed. It is common to find reduced sperm counts in men whose testes are overheated for significant periods of the day (for example, long-distance lorry drivers). The testes are very vascular and well innervated.

One of the main adaptations to improve the chances of fertilisation is to produce spermatozoa in very large numbers and much of the structure of the testes is designed to facilitate this. Internally, the testes are divided into a number of lobules, each of which is filled with coiled seminiferous tubules: these tubules make up 90% of the internal structure. The seminiferous tubule is the site of sperm production and the immense coiling permits the largest surface area to be contained in the smallest volume. The tubules lead to an area on one side called the rete. Here, the contents of many tubules are mixed and the number of tubes gradually reduces as they join together in the rete to become a single tube in the epididymis. The epididymis acts as a storage and maturation area and leads to the outlet to the penis, the vas deferens.

The tubules are lined with columnar endothelial Sertoli cells between which spermatogenesis takes place. The space between adjacent tubules is filled with blood and lymphatic vessels, Leydig cells and interstitial fluid. On the basement membrane between each pair of adjacent cells lie the gamete progenitor cells, the spermatogonia, which are equivalent to the oogonia in the ovary. Similarly to the oogonia, the spermatogonia are laid down during fetal life; however, in contrast to the oogonia, new progenitor cells will be made throughout reproductive life to give an inexhaustible supply.

FIGURE 30.1 **Anatomy of the male reproductive tract and fine structure of the rete, epididymis and vas deferens**

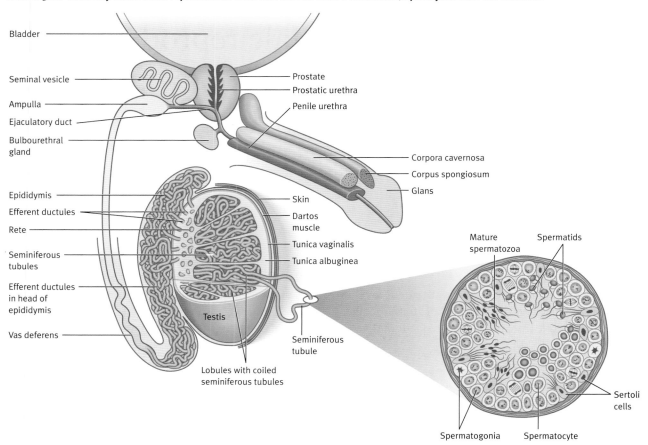

As in the ovary, the basement membrane provides protection from blood borne contaminants and encloses an avascular region. The passage of hormones and nutrients necessary for the energy-demanding process of spermatogenesis, therefore, all occurs via the interstitial fluid. The volume of interstitial fluid within the testes is very high; such a volume would be considered oedemic in any other tissue. In addition to the basal lamina, there is also a second protective barrier in the testes, called the tight junction.

## Spermatogenesis

The changes in cell morphology during the development of spermatogonia into a mature spermatozoon are illustrated in Figure 30.2 A. Spermatogonia lie on the basement membrane of the seminiferous epithelium. Following puberty, as gonadotrophins rise, every 16 days there is a wave of mitotic division of the spermatogonia into primary spermatocytes or daughter spermatogonia. The daughter spermatogonia remain on the basal lamina and keep the pool replenished whereas the primary spermatocytes are committed to starting development into spermatozoa. The primary spermatocytes still possess a diploid number of chromosomes. These cells must divide meiotically to form secondary spermatocytes possessing 23 chromosomes. Just before meiosis, the tight junction between the Sertoli cells parts and allows the spermatocytes to move from the basal (outside) to the adluminal (inside) compartment, then closes again. These tight junctions prevent molecules and cells passing into the intercellular spaces. This means that all molecules passing to the spermatocytes must pass through the blood–

FIGURE 30.2 **Spermatogenesis and spermiogenesis**

**A** The cell stages of spermatogenesis

**(a)** Spermatogonia | **(b)** primary spermatocytes | **(c)** secondary spermatocytes | **(d)** spermatids | **(e)** spermatozoon

**B** Spermiogenesis

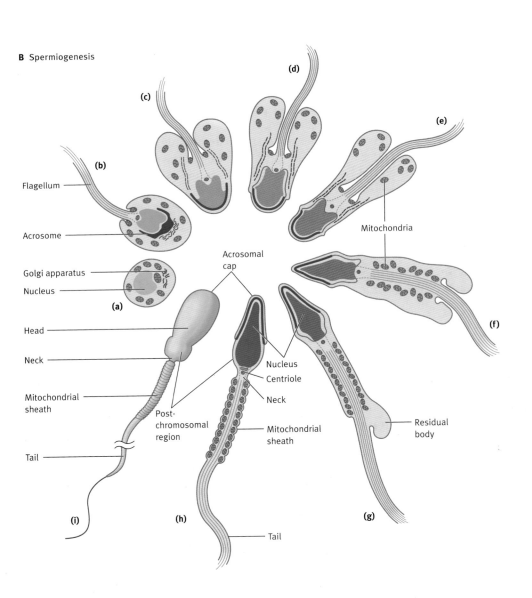

(a) Round secondary; (b) the flagellum starts to grow; (c), (d) and (e) at the spermatid stage, the acrosome moves to the head of the cell, the cellular contents move behind the nucleus and the cell elongates; (f) mitochondria align with the mid-piece; (g) remaining cellular content enters the residual body, which is reabsorbed into Sertoli cells; (h) and (i) fully formed spermatozoa in section and in three dimensions, respectively.

testes barrier or be secreted into the adluminal space by the Sertoli cells. Note that once meiosis has taken place, the haploid germ cells are 'foreign', so the blood–testes barrier isolates the germ cells from the rest of the body (including circulation) and protects them from attack by the immune system. In addition, it allows the haploid germ cell to exist within the adluminal compartment in a different and unique ionic microenvironment, with especially high levels of certain amino acids, peptides, steroids and sugars that are required for germ cell production.

Two meiotic divisions occur with doubling of the chromosomes in between to give first two secondary spermatocytes and then four spermatids, each containing 23Y or 23X. This results in a great reduction in cytoplasmic volume and each spermatozoon containing half of the DNA of its parent. At this point, the genetic constitution of each spermatozoon will also be different, as crossing over has occurred during meiosis. In order to retain access to all DNA for all cells, the new secondary spermatocytes and spermatids remain connected by a syncytium, a membrane that encompasses the four spermatozoa. This breaks when the spermatozoa leave the space between the Sertoli cells.

At this point, the spermatozoon is still a rounded cell and it must undergo the most remarkable cellular transformation to give the elongated spermatozoon. This process is known as spermiogenesis and it involves the elongation of the head, production of a tail and midpiece and the removal of the vast majority of the remaining cytoplasm, which is absorbed into the Sertoli cells (Figure 30.2B). All of these processes occur within the seminiferous epithelium, in the spaces between the Sertoli cells. After each division, the germ cells move toward the lumen of the tubule, so that eventually the spermatids are embedded in the apical region of the Sertoli cells, from where they are extruded into the lumen. This cyclical process is completed in 64 days. In addition, there are waves of development occurring every 16 days, longitudinally along the tubule, so that at a given site there are more mature stages in front and less mature stages behind. This ensures a continual supply of spermatozoa leaving the tubules and entering the rete. At each stage, the germ cells need different agents for their maintenance and development. These factors are all produced by Sertoli cells.

The spermatozoa, having reached the lumen of the seminiferous tubules, pass into a common area (the rete), where all the tubules open out. From there they pass into the ductus epididymis. The epididymis is a tube of 5 m in length, again highly coiled. Passage of spermatozoa through the epididymis takes 8–14 days. Its structure can be divided into three parts: caput, corpus and cauda (head, body and tail). In the epididymis, fluid is reduced, motility gained and maturation advanced. The spermatozoa become progressively motile; this means they can move forward. This is the final stage of maturation of the spermatozoa. In addition to gaining motility, it is possible that other maturational processes occur in the epididymis. It is for this reason that, in men with a blockage in the vas deferens, it is the preferred site of aspiration of spermatozoa to be used for intracytoplasmic sperm injection. Round spermatids aspirated from the seminiferous tubule have, however, also been shown to be capable of fertilisation by this method.

The spermatozoa are mainly stored in the epididymis, but also in the ampulla of the vas deferens. The spermatozoa are stored in epididymal fluid but, at ejaculation, secretions from the accessory sex glands are added to form seminal fluid and the latter make up a large percentage of the total volume. These secretory glands are the seminal vesicles, the prostate and the bulbourethral gland.

## Steroidogenesis

The two functions of the testes, spermatogenesis and steroidogenesis, are controlled by luteinising hormone (LH) and follicle-stimulating hormone (FSH) released in a pulsatile manner from the anterior pituitary as for the female. Only the feedback mechanism differs between the male and female, in that progesterone and estradiol act alternately and cyclically in the female and testosterone and estradiol provide constant feedback in the male.

### ANDROGEN SYNTHESIS

This occurs mainly in the interstitial Leydig cells and is predominantly under the control of LH. All of the steroids in these synthetic pathways leak out in small amounts into the circulation but the main circulating androgen is testosterone. Once in the circulation, the testosterone can be either aromatised to estrone and estradiol in skin and adipose tissue or reduced by 5-alpha-reductase in peripheral target tissues to the more active dihydrotestosterone.

Within the testes, testosterone is aromatised to estradiol by the Sertoli cells under the control of FSH. In this sense, Leydig cells are equivalent to theca cells and Sertoli cells are equivalent to granulosa cells. LH acts on the Leydig cells to stimulate the production of testosterone via cyclic adenosine monophosphate. FSH can only act on Sertoli cells. The Sertoli cells produce over 50 protein substances, which are required for spermatogenesis and secreted into the intercellular gap. Testicular steroidogenesis is outlined in Figure 30.3.

Testosterone secretion by the Leydig cells in the fetal testes is under the control of human chorionic gonadotrophin (hCG) in early pregnancy and extends over the period of sexual differentiation when fetal testosterone levels are at their highest *in utero*. hCG is LH-like in action and acts on LH receptors present on the Leydig cells in the fetal testes. The level of testosterone then falls until adrenarche and puberty.

## Hormonal control of spermatogenesis

Normal spermatogenesis requires the presence of testosterone and FSH, which act together synergistically. There are androgen and FSH receptors on Sertoli cells.

FIGURE 30.3 **Testicular steroidogenesis**

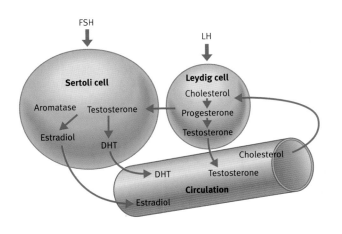

DHT = dihydrotestosterone | FSH = follicle-stimulating hormone | LH = luteinising hormone

The situation can be compared to the two-cell two-gonadotrophin system in the ovarian follicle. Sertoli cells are the site of conversion of testosterone to estradiol by aromatase: estradiol is important for the negative feedback control of the gonadotrophins and has an inhibitory modulating effect on testosterone production by Leydig cells; there are estrogen receptors present on Leydig cells. Sertoli cells also make androgen-binding protein, which acts to concentrate testosterone within the seminal tubules and thus increase its availability at the time and site where it is required. No such protein is present in the follicle. Spermatogenesis cannot proceed without FSH and testosterone, and testosterone is also essential for maintenance of the prostate, seminal vesicles, ampulla and bulbourethral glands.

## Control of gonadotrophin secretion in the male

LH and FSH release are controlled separately, which is not seen so clearly in the female. Testosterone and dihydrotestosterone exert a negative feedback effect on LH release at the hypothalamic level by inhibiting gonadotrophin-releasing hormone (GnRH) release. They also act at the pituitary level reducing its sensitivity toward GnRH. Testosterone also inhibits FSH release but is five times less effective than on LH. Estrogen exerts a negative feedback effect on FSH release at both the hypothalamic level and also at the pituitary level, decreasing the pituitary gland's sensitivity towards GnRH. Estrogen also inhibits LH release but less potently than its effect on FSH release.

## Transport of spermatozoa

The comparative distance that must be travelled by the mature spermatozoa collecting in the epididymis to reach the oocyte in the uterine tube is great and it is a journey that very few will survive. Mature spermatozoa are a few micrometres in length ($10^{-6}$ m) and they must pass through the combined length of the male and female reproductive tract (30–40 cm). Emission of spermatozoa requires erection and ejaculation. Somatic and autonomic efferents to the genitalia can be stimulated psychogenically or by tactile stimulation. The afferent limb of the reflex is carried by the internal pudendal nerves and three efferent outflows influence erection: the parasympathetic pelvic nerve (stimulatory), the sympathetic hypogastric nerve (inhibitory and some stimulatory fibres) and the somatic pudendal nerve (stimulatory). Erection occurs owing to an inflow of blood primarily into the corpus cavernosum under the influence of vasodilator agents such as vasoactive intestinal peptide and nitric oxide. Blood is prevented from leaving, thus causing increased pressure. The pressure in the corpus spongiosum does not increase as much so as to prevent occlusion of the urethra.

Ejaculation consists of coordinated contractions of the vas deferens, the seminal vesicles and the prostate and bulbourethral glands. The ejaculated semen is made up of spermatozoa and seminal plasma. Movement of the spermatozoa into the pelvic urethra, expulsion of the glandular secretions making seminal plasma into the pelvic urethra and ejaculation are controlled by the sympathetic system together with a striated muscle component. Movement of semen into the bladder is prevented by contraction of the urethral sphincter. Ejaculation is partially fractionated, in that most of the spermatozoa are ejaculated in the first half of the fluid.

Three hundred million spermatozoa are produced each day and there are 40–100 million/ml in the ejaculate, of which 99.9% are lost. Thus, in a normal ejaculate volume of 3–5 ml, of the 120 million spermatozoa present, only 120 000 will have a chance of fertilising the oocyte. A sperm count of less than 20 million/ml is considered oligozoospermic and, in these cases, the quality is often poor also. Teratozoospermia is the condition where more than 70% of spermatozoa are abnormal in form.

The ejaculate coagulates within 1 minute of entry into the vagina and then gradually reliquifies after about 20 minutes. This forms a temporary reservoir of spermatozoa and also prevents loss from the vagina. The pH of vaginal secretions is between pH 3 and 4 and the motility of spermatozoa is inhibited by an acidic pH. The ejaculate raises the pH to 7.2; this is one of the functions of seminal fluid.

The cervix, with a narrow lumen and convoluted folds in its walls, is a barrier to spermatozoa. In addition, it is normally occluded by viscous impenetrable mucus. At the time of ovulation, however, under the influence of estrogen, the mucus becomes thinner as the water content rises and the protein content is reduced. Glycoprotein molecules within the mucus arrange themselves in parallel micelles (aggregations) and spermatozoa can swim along the channels formed between them. The micelles vibrate and help to propel the spermatozoa along, especially those whose tail-beat frequency coincides with the micelle vibration frequency; this will favour the healthy motile spermatozoa. Many of the spermatozoa are not orientated correctly to pass along the channels and so form a reservoir, protected from the phagocytosis that can occur in the uterine lumen. Many of the spermatozoa are destroyed in their passage along the uterus by leucocytes. The uterotubal junction is another site of accumulation of spermatozoa and is therefore another reservoir. Entry occurs spasmodically and only motile spermatozoa can pass into the tubes. By having these barrier-forming reservoirs, a continuous supply of small numbers of spermatozoa can be ensured over a period of time, which maximises the chance of an oocyte being fertilised.

Spermatozoa appear in the oviducts a few minutes after ejaculation; since spermatozoa travel at less than 8 mm/minute, the movement must be mainly due to propulsive contractions of the female tract. At the same time, pressure in the uterus falls sharply on female orgasm and therefore 'suction' of the spermatozoa from the vagina into the uterus may occur.

The events that occur during fertilisation can be divided into a number of distinct steps. Capacitation involves biochemical alteration of the sperm plasma membrane that initiates hyperactivated motility known as 'whiplash movement'. Capacitation occurs in the presence of uterine or uterine tube fluid and before contact with the oocyte. The factor that induces capacitation is unknown. It is the whiplash movement of the tail that endows the spermatozoa with the velocity required to reach the oocyte. This usually occurs in the ampulla of the tube. Capacitation alters the surface of the sperm head and makes it more responsive to signals in the immediate area of the oocyte.

## Fertilisation and establishment of early pregnancy

The fertilisation process, from when a spermatozoon starts to respond to the oocyte's signal to when spermatozoon–oocyte fusion occurs, is shown in Figure 30.4. Once the spermatozoon has undergone capacitation and penetrated the outer layer of remaining cumulus cells, it reaches the zona pellucida, a non-cellular barrier secreted by the oocyte early in folliculogenesis. The spermatozoon is attracted to the oocyte by a combination of chemotactic agents and an increasing temperature gradient and passes between the cells of the corona radiata, which is composed of differentiated cumulus cells (Figure 30.4 A and B). The equatorial region of the sperm head binds to the zona pellucida and the acrosome reaction is initiated, which fuses the outer acrosomal membrane and the plasma membrane of the sperm head beneath it and forms pores through which hydrolytic enzymes are released. Eventually, the porous membrane breaks away and exposes the inner acrosomal membrane (Figure 30.4 C and D). The hyperactivated motility gener-

ates the forward thrust necessary to penetrate the zona pellucida, and the spermatozoon moves into the perivitelline space (the space around the oocyte) by a process of proteolysis and forms a slit (Figure 30.4 E). The spermatozoon fuses with the oocyte's plasma membrane, causing a series of calcium waves within the oocyte that lead to completion of the oocyte's second meiotic division and the second set of chromosomes is packaged into the extruded second polar body within the oocyte. The sperm head is taken up into the oocyte's cytoplasm by a process similar to phagocytosis, leaving the majority of the tail behind (Figure 30.4 F).

The calcium waves arising from the fusion also cause migration of the cortical granules to the periphery of the oocyte. These fuse with the zona pellucida and release their contents, changing the nature of the plasma membrane of the oocyte and making it impenetrable to other spermatozoa, thus preventing polyspermy. The spermatozoon's and oocyte's nuclei come together, the nuclear membranes break down and the chromosomes mingle and come together on a common spindle, thus recreating a diploid cell. Fertilisation is only complete when there is a mitotic division and two cells are formed. The spermatozoon contributes only DNA and some of the cellular machinery required for cell division; the oocyte contributes the cytoplasm and, hence, the organelles, including mitochondria and the cell membrane. The fertilised oocyte is now called a zygote.

The zygote remains in the tube for a few days and then passes through the isthmus into the uterus aided by uterine-tube cilia. The initial cell divisions result in a reduction in the volume of each cell or blastomere. At around the 8–16-cell stage, the blastocyst begins to change its morphology and become a morula. At this stage, the cell mass becomes polarised and two distinctive cell types become visible: the outer trophoblast cells and the inner cell mass. The trophoblast cells will develop into the chorion, which contributes the fetal part of the placenta, and the inner cell mass develops into the embryo. It is important at this time for the conceptus to signal its presence and to prevent the demise of the corpus luteum, which would result in the shedding of the endometrium. This is achieved by production of beta-hCG by the syncytiotrophoblast; beta-hCG interacts with LH receptors on the corpus luteum and prevents luteolysis. At this time, the conceptus establishes attachment to the uterine wall

FIGURE 30.4  **The fertilisation process**

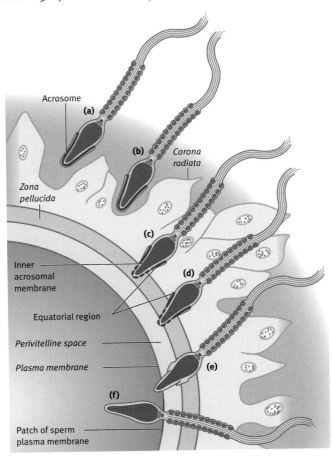

Acrosome

**(a)**

**(b)**    *Corona radiata*

*Zona pellucida*

**(c)**

Inner acrosomal membrane

**(d)**

Equatorial region

*Perivitelline space*

*Plasma membrane*    **(e)**

**(f)**

Patch of sperm plasma membrane

**(a)** Attraction to the oocyte; **(b)** Penetration of the corona radiata; **(c)** Binding to the zona pellucida; **(d)** Proteolysis of the zona pellucida; **(e)** Fusion with the oocyte's plasma membrane; **(f)** Entry of the spermatozoon. | Female elements in italics and begins the process of implantation. During the next few weeks, the cells differentiate and the body plan is laid down. The conceptus signals its presence through the epithelial cells of the endometrium to the underlying stromal tissue and begins the process of decidualisation and production of the placenta.

CHAPTER 31

# Physiology of pregnancy

*Asma Khalil*

## Introduction

In pregnancy, changes occur that are designed to meet the demands of the mother and the developing fetus and the birth process. These changes may occur at different stages in pregnancy. The study of these changes, which may occur at different stages in pregnancy, is elemental in understanding normal and high-risk pregnancy.

FIGURE 31.1 **Maternal intravascular volume changes**

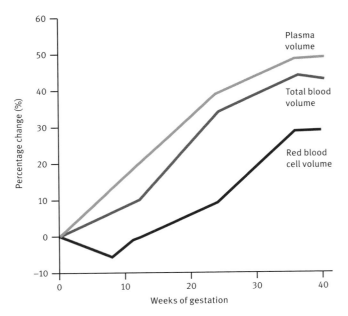

## Cardiovascular system

Cardiac output increases by approximately 40% in pregnancy, from 4.5 l/minute to approximately 6 l/minute. This rise starts early in pregnancy but reaches a plateau by 24–30 weeks. Early in pregnancy, this extra output goes mainly to the skin and breasts, but at term the extra 1.5 l/minute is distributed as follows: uterus (400 ml/minute), kidneys (300 ml/minute), skin (500 ml/minute) and the gastrointestinal tract, breasts and other organs (300 ml/minute). After delivery, cardiac output falls; most of this fall occurs in the first 6 weeks but it may take several months before prepregnancy levels are reached again. The changes in blood volumes in pregnancy are illustrated in Figure 31.1 and the cardiovascular changes are summarised in Table 31.1 and Figure 31.2. Stroke volume increases in pregnancy. Heart rate also increases (by approximately 10%, from 80 to 90 beats/minute). Peripheral vascular resistance is reduced in pregnancy, probably as a result of the relaxant effect of progesterone on arterial smooth muscle. Several other factors, such as an increase in nitric oxide, prostaglandin-$I_2$ and a decline in asymmetrical dimethyl arginine may also play a role in the vasodilation of pregnancy.

Overall, from 8 to 36 weeks, systolic blood pressure falls by approximately 5 mmHg and diastolic blood pressure by around 10 mmHg. Blood pressure reaches its nadir at approximately 24 weeks, rising again as term approaches, often reaching nonpregnant values by 40 weeks. If a pregnant woman in the third trimester lies supine, the gravid uterus may compress the inferior vena cava against her spine, impeding venous return and leading to a fall in cardiac output. She may experience a

TABLE 31.1 **Cardiovascular changes in pregnancy**

| Parameter | Change in pregnancy |
|---|---|
| Blood volume | 30% increase |
| Plasma volume | 45% increase |
| Red blood cell volume | 20–30% increase |
| Cardiac output | 40% increase |
| Stroke volume | 30% increase |
| Heart rate | 10% increase |
| Systolic blood pressure | 5 mmHg decrease |
| Diastolic blood pressure | 10 mmHg decrease |
| Peripheral resistance | Decrease |
| Oxygen consumption | 30–50 ml/minute increase |
| $PCO_2$ | Decrease to 4.1 kPa31 |

FIGURE 31.2 **Maternal cardiovascular changes**

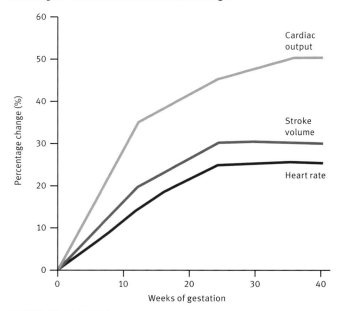

Anaestheia UK, www.frca.co.uk

marked fall in blood pressure and may feel faint, dizzy and nauseous. This is known as supine hypotensive syndrome; it is quickly relieved if the woman moves to the lateral position.

### ELECTROCARDIOGRAPHIC CHANGES

The increase in cardiac output in pregnancy causes hypertrophy and dilation of the left ventricle and atrium. However, there is no change in contractility. As a result of the upward displacement of the diaphragm by the enlarging uterus, the axis of the heart is shifted anteriorly and to the left. These changes explain the typical features of the electrocardiogram in pregnancy: heart rate 10–15% faster than normal; left axis deviation by approximately 15 degrees; inverted T wave in lead III; a Q wave in leads III and aVF.

## Respiratory system

Ventilation increases by approximately 40% owing to stimulation of the respiratory centre by progesterone both directly and indirectly (by increasing the sensitivity of the respiratory centre to carbon dioxide). This rise

begins in the first trimester and the increased ventilation results in a mild fall in $PCO_2$ to 4.1 kPa and increase in $PCO_2$ to 14 kPa during the third trimester. Towards term, $PCO_2$ falls a little again to 13.5 kPa, as the increased cardiac output is unable to compensate for the increase in oxygen consumption. The mild decrease in $PCO_2$ leads to a slightly alkaline pH. In response, there is an increase in bicarbonate excretion by the kidney, leading to a fall in bicarbonate levels to approximately 19–20 mEq/l. This is associated with a fall in sodium levels and in osmolarity (by 10 mmol/l). The changes in maternal respiration are illustrated in Figures 31.3 and 31.4.

Progesterone also relaxes bronchial smooth muscle; the calibre of the tracheobronchial tree increases and resistance falls. During pregnancy, breathing is more diaphragmatic than thoracic. Tidal volume increases by approximately 40% but there is no change in the respiratory rate. The residual volume (the volume of gas that remains at the end of forced expiration, which is normally 1500 ml in the nonpregnant state) decreases by 200 ml, leading to a reduction in expiratory reserve volume and inspiratory reserve volume. Total lung capacity (5 l in the nonpregnant individual) decreases by 200 ml. However, there is no change in the forced expiratory volume or peak flow rate.

FIGURE 31.3  **Maternal respiratory changes**

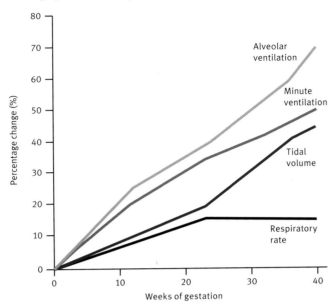

Anaestheia UK, www.frca.co.uk

FIGURE 31.4  **Differences in lung volumes between pregnant and nonpregnant women**

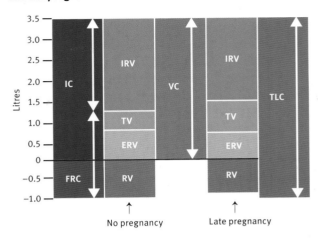

ERV = expiratory reserve volume | FRC = functional reserve capacity |
IC = inspiratory capacity | IRV = inspiratory reserve volume |
RV = residual volume | TLC = total lung capacity | TV = tidal volume |
VC = vital capacity

University of Utah, http://library.med.utah.edu

Vital capacity (the volume of gas that can be inhaled from forced expiration to forced inspiration) is unchanged at about 3.5 l as the reduction in the expiratory reserve and inspiratory volumes are compensated for by the increase in tidal volume. Lung compliance is unaffected, but chest compliance is reduced, especially if the woman is in the lithotomy position. Seventy percent of pregnant women experience subjective dyspnoea. Oxygen consumption increases by 50 ml/minute at term. This increased demand comes from the fetus (20 ml/minute), increased cardiac output (6 ml/minute), increase in renal work (6 ml/minute) and increase in metabolic rate (18 ml/minute). During pregnancy, the increase in ventilation is greater than the increase in oxygen consumption. In pregnancy, there is also an increased risk of pulmonary embolism (see below).

## Urinary system

In pregnancy, the kidneys increase in size by approximately 1 cm. The ureters dilate, partly from the effect of progesterone on the smooth muscle in their walls and partly from obstruction caused by pressure from the growing uterus. As a result, women are more prone to urinary tract infections in pregnancy and, if they have a urinary tract infection, are more likely to develop pyelonephritis. Both renal blood flow and glomerular filtration rate increase in pregnancy. These rises start in the first trimester and, by term, both are 50–60% higher than before pregnancy, the glomerular filtration rate reaching 140–170 ml/minute.

As a result of these changes, the urea level in pregnancy falls from 4.3 to 3.1 mmol/l and serum creatinine falls from 73 to 47 micromol/l. Urate and bicarbonate levels also fall. In pregnancy, there is mild glycosuria and proteinuria. Plasma osmolality decreases because of the combined effect of increased progesterone and changes in the renin–angiotensin–aldosterone pathway.

## Gastrointestinal tract

The nausea and vomiting that commonly occur in early pregnancy are largely explained by increasing levels of human chorionic gonadotrophin and/or progesterone. Gastrointestinal tone and motility are reduced by the high levels of progesterone, leading to delayed gastric emptying, particularly during labour. Progesterone also relaxes the oesophageal sphincter, which means that acid reflux is common; at term, 81% of pregnant women complain of heartburn. More importantly, these changes make pregnant women more prone to aspiration of gastric contents, particularly during induction of general anaesthesia. Furthermore, because gastric contents are more acidic in pregnancy, if aspiration occurs, the resulting pneumonitis (Mendelson syndrome) may be severe and even fatal. Some of the dyspepsia in pregnancy can also be explained by reduced motility of the gallbladder, again most likely due to the effects of progesterone.

Small and large bowel motility is decreased. Stools become firmer as transit time is longer, allowing more time in the colon for reabsorption of water. Consequently, constipation is a common problem in pregnancy.

### CHANGES AFFECTING THE LIVER

In pregnancy, plasma alkaline phosphatase increases up to three times the normal level, because it is also produced by the placenta. Gallbladder contractility decreases as cholecystokinin secretion falls. As a result, pregnant women are more prone to develop gallstones during pregnancy.

Obstetric cholestasis is a pregnancy-specific hepatic condition, characterised by itching in pregnancy and accompanied by raised liver transaminases and bile acids. This condition is associated with an increased risk of intrauterine fetal death and fetal distress in labour. One hypothesis proposes that obstetric cholestasis is caused by an interaction between inherited and acquired abnormalities in bile acid transport. Women who experience obstetric cholestasis in pregnancy may have a similar reaction to the combined oral contraceptive pill.

## Haematological system

In pregnancy, plasma volume expands by around 45% (from 2600 ml to 3800 ml). This expansion begins early in pregnancy (around 6–8 weeks of gestation) and reaches a peak at 32 weeks. Red cell mass increases steadily until term (from 1400 ml to 1700 ml), reaching a maximum of 20–30% above nonpregnant levels. This increase in erythropoiesis is probably mainly explained by an increase in erythropoietin and, to a lesser extent, by an increase in human placental lactogen. Because the rise in plasma volume is proportionately greater than the rise in red cell mass, haemoglobin concentration and haematocrit fall, averaging approximately 11.5 g/100 ml and 34%, respectively, by 30 weeks. This dilution of haemoglobin and haematocrit levels in pregnancy is known as 'physiological anaemia' and is most marked at 32 weeks of gestation. The definition of anaemia must therefore be changed during pregnancy.

Other permanent elements in the blood are changed to a lesser extent in pregnancy. There is a modest rise in leucocyte count, although in the weeks after delivery the count may reach as high as 25 000 leucocytes/mm$^3$. This rise is primarily in neutrophils.

The effect of pregnancy on the platelet count is debated, but in some women there may be a modest decline by term, perhaps by as much as 25%. This fall is believed to be due to increased destruction of platelets not caused by immune factors and is termed gestational thrombocytopenia. Platelet size increases, indicating less mature platelets in the circulation.

### IRON METABOLISM

Iron demand increases in pregnancy; the total extra requirement is around 1000 mg (500 mg for the increased red cell mass, 300 mg to meet the needs of the fetus and placenta and 200 mg to cover the obligatory excretion of iron). The extra requirement comes to approximately 4 mg/day (increased from 2.8 mg/day in a nonpregnant woman to 6.6 mg/day by the end of pregnancy).

In pregnancy, iron absorption is increased, owing to erythroid hyperplasia. Absorption is dependent on iron stores (represented by ferritin levels and iron binding saturation) and the amount of iron in the diet (including any supplements), but only 10–20% of ingested iron is absorbed. Absorption increases in the second and third trimesters, when the need is greatest, but may still not meet the needs of pregnancy and the puerperium. Consequently, iron deficiency anaemia is the most common haematological problem in pregnancy, with symptoms of dyspnoea, tiredness and occasionally faintness. Investigations usually reveal serum iron below 12 mmol/l and saturation of the total iron-binding capacity less than 15%. Thalassaemia trait may have a similar presentation to iron deficiency anaemia, so this possibility must be considered and excluded. Fortunately, maternal iron deficiency does not appear to reduce iron transport to the fetus.

## HAEMOSTASIS IN PREGNANCY

Pregnancy is known to be a hypercoagulable state. This is due to an increase in coagulation factors and a decrease in fibrinolytic activity, changes that can be demonstrated from the third month of pregnancy. The concentrations of most of the coagulation factors (VII, VIII, X) increase in pregnancy, but factors XI and XIII do not. The rise in fibrinogen levels leads to an accelerated erythrocyte sedimentation rate, which, in late pregnancy, reaches double nonpregnant levels.

Routine coagulation screening in pregnancy is essentially normal; the activated partial thromboplastin time is unchanged or slightly shortened and the bleeding and clotting times are unaffected. Levels of antithrombin III (the main physiological inhibitor of thrombin and factor Xa) change little although, as plasma volume expands, production is increased to maintain this normal concentration. The activity of the fibrinolytic system remains low in pregnancy and labour, but returns to normal within 1 hour of delivery of the placenta. During the third stage of labour, myometrial contraction and increased coagulability of the blood combine to stop bleeding after delivery of the placenta.

## Implications of maternal physiological changes on therapeutic drug administration

Absorption of drugs from the gastrointestinal tract may be impaired by gastric stasis, poor gut motility and, for some drugs, lower gastric pH. The increase in plasma volume means that the volume of distribution of the drug increases, so concentrations may be lower than expected. This is particularly important in women taking anticonvulsant drugs or thyroxine. Because of the increased glomerular filtration rate, excretion of drugs that are mainly excreted by the kidneys will be accelerated. These changes often require doses of a drug given during pregnancy to be adjusted.

## Physiology of lactation

Development of human breasts takes place around the time of puberty (that is, prior to pregnancy). From then on, the adult breasts require surprisingly little hormonal stimulation to begin milk secretion: 14 days' exposure to estrogen followed by stimulation of prolactin secretion may be enough to establish milk production; this has been used to encourage lactation in women who wish to breastfeed an adopted baby. Prolactin is a long-chain polypeptide hormone and is essential for successful lactation. In early pregnancy, there is hyperplasia of the alveolar cells and lactiferous ducts, which is followed in later pregnancy by alveolar cell hypertrophy and the initiation of secretion. These changes are stimulated by the increased levels of prolactin and human placental lactogen. During pregnancy, the high levels of estrogen and progesterone hold this process in check and full milk production is achieved only after delivery, when progesterone and estrogen levels fall rapidly. Similarly, women who take estrogen while breastfeeding (for example, in the combined oral contraceptive pill) will find that milk production is decreased.

After delivery, the colostrum (or early milk) has a high concentration of protein relative to the concentration of lactose. However, over the following 3 days or so, the concentration of lactose increases sharply and the concentration of protein falls. However, the main reason for this fall in protein concentration is actually dilution. In order to maintain ionic equilibrium, water is drawn into the breast, causing an increase in milk volume while the total amount of protein in the milk remains unchanged.

Milk production averages 500–1000 ml/day and is highly dependent on continued suckling, which causes release of both prolactin and oxytocin. In women who do not suckle, milk production gradually falls and may persist for 3–4 weeks postpartum. In breastfeeding mothers, equilibrium is reached after around 3 weeks whereby milk production is tailored to the amount taken by the baby. Interestingly, mothers who are breastfeeding twins produce twice as much milk. A breastfeeding woman requires 2950 kcal/day. The recommended daily calorie intake is 2700 kcal (2200 kcal for the nonlactating nonpregnant requirement plus 500 kcal towards the energy requirement of the milk); an extra 250 kcal/day required for milk should come from maternal fat stores laid down during pregnancy.

The suckling stimulus sends afferent impulses to the hypothalamus that lead to a surge of prolactin release. This surge reaches a peak around 30 minutes after the baby

TABLE 31.2 **Constituents of breast milk**

| Constituent | Content/100 ml |
| --- | --- |
| ENERGY | 75 kcal |
| PROTEIN | 1.1 g |
| Casein | 40 (% of protein) |
| Whey protein | 60 (% of protein) |
| LACTOSE | 6.8 g |
| FAT | 4.5 g |
| SODIUM | 7 mmol |
| CHLORIDE | 11 mmol |

This table was published in Lactation. Howie P. In *Turnbull's Obstetrics*. 3rd ed. Edinburgh: Churchill Livingstone. Copyright Elsevier; 2001.

is put to the breast and gradually declines to basal levels by 120 minutes. The control of prolactin release from the anterior pituitary is primarily via prolactin inhibitory factors from the hypothalamus that are secreted into the pituitary portal blood system. The most important prolactin inhibitory factor is dopamine. In fact, dopamine agonists, such as bromocriptine and cabergoline, can be used in the early puerperium to suppress milk production in women who do not wish to breastfeed. Conversely, dopamine antagonists such as metoclopramide increase prolactin levels and are sometimes used in breastfeeding women to stimulate milk production. Thyrotrophin-releasing hormone may also play a role in stimulating prolactin production. After the sixth week postpartum, both basal prolactin levels and the peak level following suckling gradually decline; the greater the frequency and duration of suckling, the slower the decline.

Suckling also stimulates oxytocin release. The afferent impulses trigger the synthesis of this octapeptide hormone from specialised neurons in the supraoptic and paraventricular nuclei of the hypothalamus and its release from the posterior pituitary gland. This neuroendocrine reflex can also be initiated by the mother hearing her baby cry or even thinking about breastfeeding. In this way, the release of oxytocin, which typically occurs in short 1 minute bursts, may begin even before the baby is put to the breast. Oxytocin binds to specific receptors on the myoepithelial cells, which surround the alveolar (milk-producing) cells in the breasts and are longitudi-

nally arranged in the walls of the milk ducts. Contraction of the myoepithelial cells forces the milk into the ducts; contraction of the longitudinally arranged cells in the duct walls causes the ducts to dilate and allows milk to flow more easily towards the nipple. Both prolactin and oxytocin are necessary for successful breastfeeding; in general terms, prolactin stimulates the production of milk while oxytocin stimulates its ejection (or let down).

Table 31.2 shows the typical composition of breast milk. The composition varies from woman to woman, over time in an individual woman and even differs between the beginning and end of the same feed. The most important factor, however, is the time since the birth, suggesting that the milk is adapted in a very sensitive way to the changing needs of the baby. Thus, any statements about the composition of human breast milk are averages; these are the basis for the composition of artificial feeds.

The main carbohydrate in human milk is lactose. In the baby's intestine, it is broken down by the enzyme lactase into galactose and glucose. Of the protein in human milk, 40% is casein, compared with 80% of cow's milk. Other proteins include immunoglobulins and lactoferrin. Triglycerides are the main fat found in milk and are its most variable component, which means that the estimated energy content of 75 kcal/100 ml is only an approximation. Fat also carries the fat-soluble vitamins A, D, E and K. Vitamin D deficiency can lead to rickets while vitamin K deficiency can lead to haemorrhagic disease of the newborn. A comparison of the daily vitamin requirements in nonpregnant, pregnant and lactating women is shown in Table 31.3 and the micronutrient supplementation regimen is illustrated in Figure 31.5.

Compared with cow's milk, human milk has approximately one-third the concentrations of sodium and chloride. This is advantageous in babies with diarrhoea because a high solute load can exacerbate diarrhoea. There is little iron in breast milk.

## IMMUNITY GAINED FROM BREAST MILK

The major immunoglobulin (Ig) in breast milk is IgA, with smaller amounts of IgM and IgG. The IgA in breast milk is poorly absorbed so most stays in the baby's intestinal tract, where it protects against infection. This is obviously particularly important in areas where there is poor access to clean water: in many developing countries, diarrhoea is

TABLE 31.3  **Daily vitamin requirements in nonpregnant, pregnant and lactating women**

| Vitamin | Nonpregnant | Pregnant | Lactating |
|---|---|---|---|
| A (microgram) | 800 | 1000 | 1200 |
| $B_1$ (mg) | 1 | 1.3 | 1.3 |
| $B_2$ (mg) | 1.5 | 1.8 | 2 |
| Niacin (mg) | 15 | 20 | 20 |
| Pantothenic acid (mg) | 5 | 10 | 10 |
| $B_6$ (mg) | 2 | 2.5 | 2.5 |
| Folic acid (microgram) | 200 | 500 | 400 |
| $B_{12}$ (mg) | 2 | 3 | 3 |
| C (mg) | 30 | 60 | 80 |
| D (microgram) | 10 | 10 | 10 |
| E (mg) | 10 | 12 | 11 |
| K | 90 mg | 90 mg | 90 mg |

one of the major causes of infant mortality. When a mother encounters a specific pathogen in her own gastrointestinal tract, plasma cells migrate from her gut to her breast where they release a specific IgA against that pathogen into the milk, thus protecting her baby. Clearly, the presence of immunoglobulin, as well as other anti-infective agents such as lysozyme and lactoferrin, is a major advantage of breast milk over artificial formula feed.

### CONTRACEPTIVE EFFECT OF BREASTFEEDING

If a woman conceives during lactation, the rapidly rising levels of estrogen and progesterone will suppress milk production, despite the effects of the baby's suckling. High prolactin levels during breastfeeding tend to suppress ovulation and therefore cause amenorrhoea. However, this is not a reliable form of contraception; at the end of a year of exclusive breastfeeding, 10% of women who do not use another form of contraception will have fallen pregnant. Nevertheless, it is estimated that, in developing countries, breastfeeding prevents more pregnancies than all other forms of contraception combined.

FIGURE 31.5  **Micronutrient supplements for pregnant women**

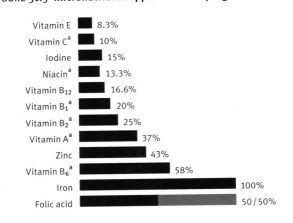

- Vitamin E — 8.3%
- Vitamin C[a] — 10%
- Iodine — 15%
- Niacin[a] — 13.3%
- Vitamin $B_{12}$ — 16.6%
- Vitamin $B_1$[a] — 20%
- Vitamin $B_2$[a] — 25%
- Vitamin A[a] — 37%
- Zinc — 43%
- Vitamin $B_6$[a] — 58%
- Iron — 100%
- Folic acid — 50/50%

■ Recommended additional intake

■ Safety supplement from 4 weeks before to 12 weeks after conception

[a] Vitamins to be taken from 4 months of pregnancy onwards.

Schwarz Pharma, www.ferro-info.com.

## The onset of labour, myometrial contractility and cervical dilatation

The precise mechanism of the onset and maintenance of labour is still poorly understood. During pregnancy, myometrial quiescence is maintained by pro-pregnancy factors, the most important of which is probably progesterone. The fact that this quiescence is maintained despite the extreme stretching of the myometrial fibres and their tendency to contract when stretched is remarkable. Progesterone suppresses the formation of myometrial gap junctions and the effect of interleukin 8 (which causes cervical ripening). It also decreases uterine sensitivity to oxytocin. Antiprogesterones such as mifepristone cause cervical ripening and increase myometrial contractility. Catecholamines and relaxin may also play a role in the maintenance of uterine quiescence.

During the third trimester, maternal estrogen and corticotrophin-releasing hormone (CRH) gradually rise. Estradiol increases the concentration of oxytocin receptors in the myometrium and also increases oxytocin synthesis in the uterus. CRH increases prostaglandin synthesis and may stimulate myometrial contractility. The concentration of myometrial gap junctions increases as labour approaches; these are small communicating channels between adjacent myometrial cells that allow the transmission of electrical and chemical signals, thus promoting coordinated contraction. Estrogen promotes the formation of gap junctions. CRH also promotes an inflammatory-type mechanism by increasing the expression of inflammatory cytokines, such as interleukin 1$\beta$ and interleukin 8, and cyclooxygenase type II (COX-2).

These gradual changes accumulate during the third trimester but it is not clear what event actually triggers the onset of labour. In some species (such as sheep), an abrupt withdrawal of progesterone immediately precedes the onset of labour. For many years, investigators were convinced that the same must be true in humans, but it now seems certain that this is not the case. It is possible that there is a 'functional withdrawal' of progesterone, perhaps because it happens only locally within the fetal membranes or perhaps because, close to term, the dominant progesterone receptor within the uterus changes from type 1 to type 2.

Nitric oxide does not seem to play a significant role in the onset of labour. Neither does oxytocin; there is no significant rise in maternal oxytocin concentration immediately prior to labour (or indeed during labour). However, there is a marked increase in oxytocin receptors in the myometrium as term approaches so it seems certain that oxytocin plays an important role in labour, probably in combination with prostaglandins. Nevertheless, it does not seem to be the trigger for its onset. The fetus also secretes some oxytocin (the concentration in the umbilical artery is twice that in the umbilical vein) but it is not certain if this plays a role in labour. It is possible that the fetus triggers labour through increased cortisol release, which can stimulate placental CRH synthesis.

There is a rapid rise in the activity of COX-2 and other inflammatory cytokines at the onset of labour, leading some to compare labour to an inflammatory process. Increased COX-2 activity leads to an increase in prostaglandin synthesis; the amnion and chorion secrete primarily prostaglandin-$E_2$ while the decidua favours prostaglandin-$F_{2\alpha}$. Prostaglandin synthase inhibitors such as indometacin may thus be used in the management of preterm labour.

Prostaglandins act on the myometrium in the uterine body to cause contractions. Towards the end of pregnancy and in early labour, under the influence of prostaglandins and interleukin 8 (and perhaps in combination with relaxin and estrogen), neutrophils are attracted into the cervix where they release collagenase. This leads to gradual proteolysis of the collagen fibres in the cervix, making it softer and more stretchy; this process is known as cervical ripening.

Contraction of the myometrium results from the interaction of actin and myosin. This interaction is controlled by a calcium-modulated protein kinase. Communication between myometrial cells through gap junctions facilitates coordinated contraction of the uterus. Drugs that reduce available calcium, such as beta agonists (for example, ritodrine, salbutamol), thus cause uterine relaxation. Similarly, magnesium sulphate, which inhibits calcium influx into myometrial cells, inhibits the action of myosin-light-chain kinase, thus causing uterine relaxation. Calcium channel blockers also inhibit calcium influx through the cell membrane and are used for tocolysis. It seems that, once labour has started, there are multiple feedback mechanisms that further increase prostaglandin and cytokine activity; this process is currently poorly understood.

## The third stage of labour

The third stage of labour is the time from delivery of the baby until delivery of the placenta and membranes. Soon after delivery of the baby, the uterus has a strong and sustained contraction. This reduces the surface area of the placental bed, thus shearing off the placenta. The placenta and membranes are usually delivered soon after. This contraction also helps to control bleeding from the vessels of the placental bed. It is likely that prostaglandins such as prostaglandin-$F_{2\alpha}$ play a major role here; certainly, oxytocin levels do not change significantly during this time. This effect can be mimicked by the administration of synthetic prostaglandins (carboprost or misoprostol) to control postpartum haemorrhage.

## Uterine involution

Immediately after delivery of the placenta, the uterus weighs around 900 g. By 7 days postpartum, it will weigh half that and by 6 weeks it will have almost returned to its prepregnancy size and weight of around 100 g. Uterine water, weight, muscle, protein and collagen all decrease in the same proportions during this time; these changes are likely to result from the rapid withdrawal of placental hormones after delivery.

Three days postpartum, the superficial layer of the decidua becomes necrotic and is shed with the lochia. Within 1 week, the uterine cavity has a new endometrial layer, with the exception of the placental bed; this takes around 3 weeks to establish an endometrial cover. The lochia gradually decreases over 3–6 weeks, changing in turn from red (lochia rubra) to pink (lochia serosa) to yellowish white (lochia alba).

**FURTHER READING**

BURROW G, FERRIS T. *Medical Complications During Pregnancy.* 4th ed. Philadelphia: Saunders; 1984.

CHAMBERLAIN G, PIPKIN F B. *Clinical Physiology in Obstetrics.* 3rd ed. Oxford: Blackwell Science; 1998.

COUSTAN D R. Maternal physiology. In: Coustan D R, Haning R V, Singer D B, editors. *Human Reproduction: Growth and Development.* Boston: Little, Brown; 1995. p. 161–81.

CRUIKSHANK D P, HAYS P M. Maternal physiology in pregnancy. In: Gabbe S G, Niebyl J R, Simpson J L, editors. *Obstetrics: Normal and Problem Pregnancies.* 2nd ed. New York: Churchill Livingstone; 1991. p. 125–46.

CUNNINGHAM F G, MacDONALD P C, GANT N F, LEVENO K J, GILSTRAP L C. Maternal adaptations to pregnancy. In: *Williams Obstetrics.* 19th ed. Norwalk: Appleton and Lange; 1989. p. 209–46.

DE SWIET M, POSTON L, WILLIAMS D. Physiology. In: de Swiet M, Chamberlain G, Bennett P, editors. *Basic Science in Obstetrics and Gynaecology, A textbook for MRCOG part 1.* 3rd ed. Edinburgh: Churchill Livingstone; 2002. p. 173–231.

DE SWIET M. *Medical Disorders in Obstetric Practice.* 4th ed. Oxford: Blackwell Publishing; 2002.

HUNTER S, ROBSON S C. Adaptation of the maternal heart in pregnancy. *Br Heart J* 1992;68:540–3.

NELSON-PIERCY C. *Obstetric Medicine.* 3rd ed. Abingdon: Informa Healthcare UK; 2006.

WILLIAMS D J. Physiology of healthy pregnancy. In: Warrell D A, Cox T M, Firth J D, editors. *Oxford Textbook of Medicine.* 4th ed. Oxford: Oxford University Press; 2003. p. 383–5.

CHAPTER 32

# Fetal physiology

*Aris T Papageorghiou*

## Fetal cardiovascular physiology

The fetal cardiovascular system develops early in fetal life, with blood circulation established by week 4. In this section, the heart and vessels are considered separately, but it is important to realise that development of these structures is synchronous.

### THE FETAL HEART

#### Cardiac output

In the adult circulation, the circulatory system is in series and there are no shunts. Therefore, stroke volume of the right ventricle equals that of the left ventricle and cardiac output can be defined in terms of the volume of blood ejected by one ventricle (by convention the left) in 1 minute. This can be described by the equation:

Cardiac output = Stroke volume × Heart rate

In the fetus, there is shunting of blood through the ductus venosus, foramen ovale and ductus arteriosus (see fetal circulation below). As a result, the stroke volume of the fetal right ventricle is not equal to the stroke volume of the left ventricle: in fact about two-thirds of blood returns to the right ventricle and one-third to the left ventricle. Therefore, cardiac output in the fetus is measured as the total output of both ventricles, termed the combined ventricular output.

#### Myocardial function

The myocardium grows by cell division (hyperplasia) until birth and by cell enlargement (hypertrophy) after birth. Fetal heart myocytes have a much smaller amount of contractile tissue (30%) than in the adult (60%). Furthermore, fetal myofibrils are fewer in number and not arranged as parallel fibres but more randomly. Finally the fetal heart is less compliant (more stiff) than in the adult owing to the constraining effects of the lungs and chest wall in the absence of air. Owing to these factors, the fetal stroke volume is maximal with little functional reserve. The fetal heart has limited capacity to increase stroke volume. The principal way that cardiac output in the fetus is increased is, therefore, by an increase in heart rate.

#### Cardiac metabolism

In the adult heart, long-chain fatty acids are the main source of fuel, with glucose and lactate being minor fuels that are usually only used during hypoxia. In contrast, the fetal heart lacks the enzyme responsible for transport of fatty acids into mitochondria, which means that lactate and carbohydrates are the primary fuel.

#### Fetal heart rate

The fetal heart rate (FHR) is determined by depolarisation of the sinoatrial node, which is under sympathetic influence and inhibited by vagal (parasympathetic) stimulation. Vagal tone exerts the major influence, causing a fall in heart rate while sympathetic activity causes a rise in heart rate and myocardial contractility. Other factors influencing the heart rate include hormonal factors (epinephrine and norepinephrine released from the adrenal medulla), drugs and temperature. Finally, baroreceptors in the aortic arch and chemoreceptors are

467

sensitive to changes in blood pressure and partial oxygen pressures, respectively, and mediate heart rate via the autonomic nervous system.

The FHR decreases with advancing gestation, a reflection of the maturing parasympathetic nervous system. The parasympathetic control also influences beat-to-beat variability via its interaction with the sympathetic system (a constant 'push and pull') and also changing vagal impulses. As these FHR patterns are controlled by the parasympathetic and sympathetic nervous systems, the FHR is a reflection of the status of the fetal brain stem's medulla oblongata. Pathological events, such as fetal hypoxia, that affect these nerve fibre impulses can therefore be observed in FHR patterns. Other influences, such as the fetal sleep and wake states and drugs may also have effects.

### Baseline FHR

After the early first trimester, the normal baseline FHR decreases with gestational age. At term, the normal FHR is 110–150 beats/minute.

Fetal tachycardia (at least 160 beats per minute for 10 minutes) can be normal at earlier gestation. Depending on the cause, it is usually mediated via catecholamine release, sympathetic nervous system stimulation or lack of parasympathetic stimulation. Common causes are fetal hypoxia (where it is accompanied by an evolving picture of loss of beat-to-beat variability and late decelerations), maternal pyrexia, chorioamnionitis, tocolysis using beta-sympathomimetic drugs or fetal heart rhythm abnormalities.

Bradycardia is defined as a heart rate of less than 110 beats/minute lasting 10 minutes or longer. Occasionally this can be the normal heart rate of the fetus, when it is an isolated abnormality with normal beat-to-beat variability and accelerations. If the bradycardia occurs with previously normal heart rate, it is usually the response to fetal hypoxia, in particular if the heart rate is below 100 beats/minute. Possible causes include cord compression, placental abruption, maternal hypotension or uterine hyperstimulation. Fetal heart block is a rare cause of persistent fetal bradycardia.

### Beat-to-beat variability

The interval between successive fetal heart beats varies in normal circumstances. This beat-to-beat variability is defined as fluctuation in the FHR of at least two cycles per minute and it increases with gestational age. Beat-to-beat variability is divided into long-term variability (LTV) and short-term variability (STV). In clinical interpretation these two are usually reported together, but computerised cardiotocography (CTG) and fetal electrocardiogram (ECG) can measure LTV and STV separately. The LTV measures the oscillations or fluctuations of the heart rate within its baseline range (excluding accelerations or decelerations) and it is measured in cycles/minute. STV is measured in milliseconds and measures the R–R interval between two consecutive QRS complexes on the fetal ECG. Although modern external ultrasound devices use standard CTG to give a close approximation, STV can only be correctly measured using a scalp electrode. The STV therefore reflects the change in the FHR from one beat to the next and is the cause of the rapidly changing display in FHR when using fetal scalp electrode monitoring.

In the absence of any input from the autonomic nervous system, the fetal heart will beat at 110–150 beats/minute without variability. It is the constant modulation of this basal heart rate by the autonomic nervous system that produces the characteristic pattern of beat-to-beat variability. This is usually ascribed to the opposing actions of the sympathetic nervous system causing an increase and the parasympathetic causing a decrease in the FHR, but it may also be caused by repeated, short-lived parasympathetic impulses. Absent or reduced variability may simply be due to preterm gestation, but other causes include the fetal sleep cycle, fetal metabolic acidosis, drugs (central nervous system depressants such as magnesium sulphate, morphine or alcohol) or pre-existing neurologic abnormality.

### Fetal heart accelerations

Fetal heart accelerations are defined as an increase of 15 beats/minute for at least 15 seconds. Accelerations are rarely seen in the presence of fetal hypoxia. Conversely, the absence of accelerations for more than 80 minutes correlates with increased neonatal morbidity. Accelerations are usually caused by fetal movements or stimulation, (for example, vibroacoustic). Accelerations are thought to occur from direct sympathetic stimulation; repeated accelerations during uterine contractions may be due to mild umbilical vein compression leading to systemic hypotension, which triggers acceleration of FHR.

## Fetal heart decelerations

Fetal heart decelerations are defined as a decrease of 15 beats/minute for at least 15 seconds. Decelerations are subclassified into early, variable and late decelerations. Early decelerations occur during uterine contractions. Fetal head compression leads to a transient reduction in fetal cerebral blood flow, hypoxia, hypercapna and hypertension. Triggering of baroreceptors causes parasympathetic stimulation resulting in a reduction in heart rate.

Variable decelerations occur without a regular pattern in terms of relation with uterine contractions, duration and depth. They are thought to be caused by umbilical cord compression or stretching. The differential compression of umbilical vein and artery may be responsible for the variable appearance of the decelerations. Umbilical vein compression causes a transient reduction of venous return to the heart and reduction in blood pressure. Carotid body baroreceptors are triggered and stimulation of the sympathetic nervous system causes fetal tachycardia. Umbilical artery compression causes an increase in systemic vascular resistance and a rise in blood pressure, and baroreceptor-mediated parasympathetic stimulation causes fetal bradycardia. The frequently observed picture of an FHR deceleration with acceleration before and after its occurrence can be explained by the gradual compression of umbilical vein and then umbilical vein and artery, followed by a gradual release in reverse order. As the depth of variable decelerations is a reflection of baroreceptor stimulation rather than hypoxaemia, fetal wellbeing should be assessed based on the baseline rate, variability and presence of accelerations.

Late decelerations usually begin before the peak of the contraction and are defined as decelerations where the nadir of the deceleration is after the peak of the contraction. They usually have a slow recovery phase. During uterine contractions, the blood supply in the placental intervillous spaces temporarily stops. This means that gas exchange also ceases temporarily and, if there is reduced fetal reserve or uterine overactivity, this leads to a reduction in oxygen absorption (leading to hypoxaemia) and accumulation of lactic acid and carbon dioxide (and therefore acidosis). Hypoxaemia causes chemoreceptor stimulation and results in parasympathetic slowing of FHR. In addition, fetal myocardial hypoxia leads to inability of the myocardium to respond and to further

bradycardia. This inability of the fetal heart to respond to autonomic nervous system stimulation often leads to a concomitant reduction in variability.

## TRANSITIONAL EVENTS AT BIRTH

After birth, there is loss of the placental circulation and shunts between the pulmonary and systemic circulations. The cardiac output can then be measured as in the adult. There is a rapid change in the function of the myocardium, with an increase in myocardial contractility. During the first weeks, there is a preferential increase in left rather than right ventricular mass. In the myocardium, there is a switch from lactate and carbohydrate metabolism to using free fatty acids as the preferred fuel.

## Fetal circulation

An important prerequisite for the understanding of fetal cardiovascular function is the fetal circulation and the differences with postnatal function. Unlike the adult heart, the four chambers of the fetal heart are arranged as a parallel system where the output of the right and left ventricles mix. This is due to shunts that normally close at birth. There are three such shunts, which are illustrated in Figures 32.1 and 32.2:

- **ductus venosus:** directs blood to the inferior vena cava
- **foramen ovale:** allows blood to pass from the right to the left atrium
- **ductus arteriosus:** connects the pulmonary artery to the aorta. It carries the output of the right ventricle owing to the higher pressure of the pulmonary compared with the systemic circulation.

Before birth, the pulmonary circuit is at high resistance, mainly becasue of compression of the pulmonary capillaries by the collapsed lung, the smooth muscle layer of the pulmonary arteries and the vasoconstrictive effects of low fetal partial pressure of oxygen ($PO_2$). At the same time, the systemic circulation is at low resistance to blood flow, owing to the large placental bed. The presence of shunts, high pulmonary resistance and low systemic resistance allows blood to be diverted from the lungs to the placenta.

FIGURE 32.1 **Main characteristics of the fetal circulation showing the fetal shunts**

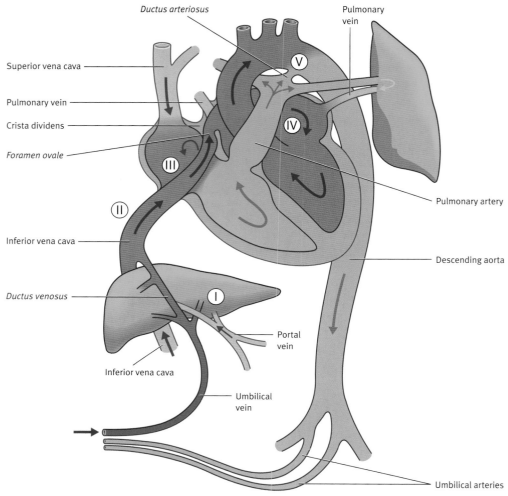

Red = fully oxygenated blood | blue = deoxygenated blood | red/blue = mixed blood | Shunts in italic

Source: Murphy PJ. The fetal circulation. *Continuing Education in Anaesthesia, Critical Care & Pain* 2005;5:107–12.

An important feature of the fetal circulation is that, although there is mixing of oxygenated and deoxygenated blood, this does not result in homogenous semi-oxygenated blood. Rather, preferential streaming of oxygenated blood occurs from the umbilical vein via the ductus venosus and foramen ovale into the left ventricle and proximal aorta, allowing highly oxygenated blood to reach the coronary and carotid arteries. Deoxygenated blood enters the right atrium from the inferior and superior vena cava, through the tricuspid valve into the right ventricle, pulmonary trunk and ductus arteriosus, entering the descending aorta and the umbilical arteries. The physiology of the three fetal shunts allows this preferential streaming of blood.

### DUCTUS VENOSUS

The ductus venosus connects the umbilical vein to the inferior vena cava (IVC) at the inlet to the heart. The ductus venosus has a small diameter (0.5 mm at mid-

FIGURE 32.2 **Comparison of fetal and adult circulatory systems**

**A** Fetal (parallel)

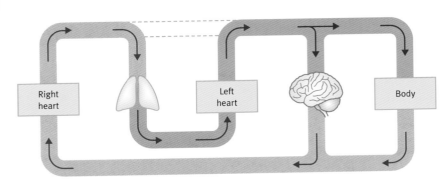

**B** Adult (series)

*Adapted with permission from*: Blackburn ST. *Maternal, Fetal and Neonatal Physiology*. 2nd ed. St Louis: Saunders; 2003.

gestation to about 2 mm at later gestation) and this narrowing causes an acceleration in blood velocity. This high-velocity blood flow allows preferential streaming of the oxygenated blood coming from the ductus venosus and via the IVC by exerting pressure on the flap-valve of the foramen ovale. About 30% of the umbilical blood is shunted through the ductus venosus at midgestation and this drops to about 20% at 30–40 weeks. This is likely to be because of the development of the fetal liver at later gestations requiring a larger proportion of the umbilical venous blood.

### FORAMEN OVALE

The foramen ovale is a communication between right and left atria and is formed by the overlap of the septum secundum over the septum primum, producing a flap-valve. The higher pressure in the right atrium ensures that the valve is maintained open and allows a right-to-left flow of blood. Blood enters the right atrium from the IVC. Within the IVC, blood flow is not uniform, with the highly oxygenated blood that originated from the umbilical vein flowing anteriorly and to the left within the IVC. As blood enters the atrium from the IVC, it is divided into two streams by the free edge of the atrial septum (the crista dividens). The high-velocity oxygenated blood is shunted towards the left, through the foramen ovale and into the left atrium. The lower velocity, less oxygenated blood is shunted towards the right, mixing with blood from the superior vena cava and coronary sinus.

The net result of this is that blood in the left ventricle is more highly oxygenated than in the right ventricle. The highly oxygenated blood in the left ventricle is pumped into the ascending aorta and 90% of it flows into

471

the coronary arteries, left carotid and subclavian arteries; the remaining 10% flows via the aortic arch and into the descending aorta, mixing with blood from the ductus arteriosus.

## DUCTUS ARTERIOSUS

The ductus arteriosus connects the pulmonary trunk to the descending aorta. This allows blood to bypass the immature lungs. After right ventricular contraction, blood flows mainly through this vessel and into the descending aorta, with about 13% of the combined cardiac output entering the pulmonary circulation, to support lung development. After 30 weeks, the proportion of blood flow to the lungs increases to about 20% of the combined cardiac output. The patency of the ductus arteriosus is maintained by the vasodilator effects of prostaglandins ($PGE_1$ and $PGE_2$) and prostacyclin ($PGI_2$) and reduced fetal oxygen tension.

## FETOPLACENTAL CIRCULATION

Blood flow from the fetus to the placenta is via the umbilical arteries and this represents about 33% of the combined ventricular output at 20 weeks of gestation and about 20% after 32 weeks. With increasing fetal growth, the absolute volume of umbilical blood flow increases throughout gestation, but it is lowest at 41 weeks if normalised for fetal weight. The resistance to blood flow through the placental vascular bed has no neural regulation and catecholamines have little effect.

## CONTROL OF FETAL CIRCULATION

The control of the fetal circulation is complex and poorly understood. The peripheral circulation of the fetus is under a tonic adrenergic influence (predominantly vasoconstriction), probably mediated by circulating catecholamines and in particular by norepinephrine. Other factors such as arginine vasopressin, the renin–angiotensin system and prostaglandins also have a role. Baroreceptors in the aortic arch and carotid arteries are sensitive to changes in arterial blood pressure. Chemoreceptors that are sensitive to changes in the oxygen content ensure that, during hypoxaemia, the blood flow increases to the brain, myocardium and adrenals and decreases to the lungs and lower body. This phenomenon

of arterial redistribution is used in clinical practice in the monitoring of fetal growth restriction.

## MEETING FETAL OXYGEN NEEDS

The mixing of oxygenated and deoxygenated blood in the fetal circulation means that oxygen content is lower in the fetus than in postnatal life. The mechanisms to ensure adequate oxygen delivery are:

- preferential delivery of oxygen-rich blood to the myocardium and brain by presence of shunts
- preferential shunting of oxygen-poor blood to the placenta for oxygenation
- high heart rate
- fetal haemoglobin, which results in oxygen binding even at a low $PO_2$, which results in high saturation, even at low oxygen tensions.

## TRANSITIONAL EVENTS AT BIRTH

Shortly after birth, the low-resistance placental circulation is lost. This loss of blood flow through the placenta means that the systemic resistance is approximately doubled and pressures in the aorta, left ventricle and left atrium increase. At the same time, with the first breath of air there is lung expansion, vasodilation in the pulmonary vascular bed due to higher oxygen tension and a fall in the pulmonary vascular resistance.

The changes in the relative pressures between pulmonary and systemic systems mean that there is a change from the parallel (fetal) system with placental respiration to a neonatal circulatory system in series with pulmonary respiration.

The fall in pulmonary and rise in systemic pressures cause a massive reduction in blood flow through the ductus arteriosus. The ductus arteriosus then closes spontaneously, on average 2 days after birth, most likely because of the increase in oxygen tension. Failure of the closure of the ductus arteriosus can lead to the common problem of 'patent ductus arteriosus' in the postnatal period and this is more common in premature infants or those with low oxygen tensions from continuing hypoxia. The ductus arteriosus is sensitive to the influence of prostaglandin $E_2$, which maintains the patency of the vessel. Administration of prostaglandin synthase inhibitors

TABLE 32.1 **Stages of fetal lung development**

| Stage | Time period | Developmental events |
|---|---|---|
| Embryonic | Conception to 7 weeks of gestation | Formation of main bronchi and bronchopulmonary segments |
| Pseudoglandular | 7–17 weeks | Branching of airways and blood vessels, forming the conducting airways of the lung |
| Canalicular | 17–27 weeks | Formation of the acini, the gas-exchanging parts of the lung |
| Saccular | 28–36 weeks | Enlargement of peripheral airways, thinning of the airway walls to form terminal sacs |
| Alveolar | 36 weeks of gestation to 2 years post-birth | Formation of definitive alveoli |

(such as indometacin) can be used postnatally in cases of patent ductus arteriosus for therapeutic purposes, but can cause severe constriction of the ductus arteriosus antenatally if administered during the third trimester.

The ductus venosus usually closes 1–3 weeks after birth in term infants. Unlike closure of the ductus arteriosus, it is thought that in the ductus venosus this is mechanical. Finally, there is functional closure of the flap-like opening of the foramen ovale due to the increase in left atrial pressure. Anatomical closure of the septum primum and septum secundum occurs in the majority of cases by the age of 1 year. Persistent patent foramen ovale can lead to paradoxical embolic events in later life.

## Fetal respiratory physiology

Normal fetal lung development depends on normal anatomical development, fetal breathing movements, absorption of lung fluid at birth and surfactant production.

### ANATOMICAL DEVELOPMENT

Lung development occurs in five stages, which are described below and in Table 32.1.

The embryonic phase is characterised by an outpouching of the ventral wall of the foregut. This is separated from the oesophagus by a septum and the lung bud divides into the two main bronchi and subsequently subdivides into the tracheobronchial tree. Pulmonary arteries, which develop from the sixth aortic arches, develop alongside these airways.

During the pseudoglandular phase, there is continued branching of both airways and blood vessels. By 16–17 weeks of gestation, this branching is complete and the total number of pre-acinar airways will not change further.

During the canalicular stage, the acinar structures are formed. These will give rise to the gas-exchanging structures of the lung and contain the terminal bronchioles, alveolar ducts and primitive alveoli.

The saccular phase is characterised by enlargement of the peripheral airways and thinning of the airway walls to form a large number of terminal sacs. This allows a large increase in the surface area of the lung.

The formation of definitive alveoli marks the alveolar stage, which continues well into the postnatal period. About 1000 alveoli will form per acinus.

### FETAL BREATHING MOVEMENTS

Fetal breathing movements occur from the end of the first trimester and increase in frequency and strength with gestation. It is thought that fetal breathing movements regulate lung growth by lung fluid regulation and lung cell growth. The importance of fetal breathing movements has been demonstrated in animal experiments, which have shown that ablation of the phrenic nerve, which innervates the diaphragm, leads to lung hypoplasia. Fetal breathing movements increase after a maternal meal, maternal glucose administration and conditions of acidosis. They are decreased by fetal hypoxia, maternal consumption of alcohol and sedative drugs.

## LUNG FLUID

Lung fluid is mainly formed from secretions of alveolar epithelial cells and this begins at the canalicular stage of development. Fluid is swallowed or released into the amniotic fluid but lung fluid only contributes a small amount to amniotic fluid volume. Lung fluid is essential for normal lung development and lung hypoplasia can result if lung fluid is decreased or there is an absence of amniotic fluid.

## SURFACTANT

Surfactant is a lipoprotein produced by type II pneumocytes. About 90% is made of lipids, with two-thirds of this being dipalmitoylphosphatidylcholine (DPPC). The remaining 10% of surfactant is made of proteins, including surfactant proteins A–D. Surfactant has a major role in pulmonary function. Its main functions include reducing the surface tension part of elastic recoil, thus increasing pulmonary compliance and allowing normal inflation. The same mechanism prevents lung collapse at the end of expiration. The surface tension is mainly regulated by DPPC, with surfactant protein B and surfactant protein C allowing surfactant spread over the alveolar surfaces. Surfactant protein A and surfactant protein D have pathogen-recognising functions and aid innate immunity.

Glucocorticoids, such as betamethasone and dexamethasone, allow accelerated surfactant synthesis and lung maturation. Other factors that have been shown to stimulate lung maturity are thyroid hormones, prolactin and catecholamines. Delayed lung maturation is seen in maternal diabetes and it is unclear whether this is an effect of insulin administration or hyperglycaemia. Androgens also delay lung maturation, which may explain why male infants are more likely to develop respiratory distress than female infants of similar gestational age.

## TRANSITIONAL EVENTS AT BIRTH

Even before the onset of labour, lung fluid secretion falls and reabsorption of fluid from the alveolar spaces begins. With the first breath of air into the lungs, an air/liquid interface is created and surfactant facilitates the formation of the alveolar lining. The pulmonary fluid continues to be replaced by air and most has been actively absorbed (across the alveolar wall into capillaries and lymphatics) within 2 hours of breathing. The transition from fetal breathing movements to normal ventilation is triggered by a series of tactile and thermal stimuli. The first breaths are important in inflating the fluid-filled lungs. These initial inflation breaths generate pressures that are 10–15 times greater than that needed for subsequent breathing. Once the alveoli are aerated, breathing requires minimal negative intrathoracic pressure to maintain a normal tidal volume and alveolar surface tension is stabilised by the surfactant released by distension and ventilation of the lungs.

# Fetal haematology

Fetal haematopoiesis occurs in three overlapping periods:

- **mesoblastic period:** in the yolk sac, from 14 days to 12 weeks
- **hepatic period:** from 6 weeks and peaking from 10 to 18 weeks, when it is the main source of fetal haematopoiesis
- **myeloid period:** from 8 weeks through to the adult period. Blood cells develop from stem cells, which first appear in the yolk sac but migrate to these fetal tissues where they give rise to primitive cells in the first instance, followed by definitive cells.

## FORMATION OF FETAL BLOOD CELLS

Fetal red blood cell formation occurs independently of the mother and is controlled endogenously. While primitive cells contain embryonic haemoglobin, which is not controlled by erythropoietin (EPO), definitive red blood cells containing mainly fetal haemoglobin (HbF) are regulated by EPO. Fetal EPO, produced initially from the liver and then the kidneys, increases from 20 weeks onwards and increased EPO production occurs in hypoxic conditions such as placental insufficiency and severe maternal anaemia. Fetal white blood cell formation begins at 6 weeks in the liver but they are also produced in the spleen, thymus and lymphatic system. Circulating granulocytes increase rapidly in the third trimester and at birth they are equal to or greater than

FIGURE 32.3 **Oxygen dissociation curves for fetal and adult blood**

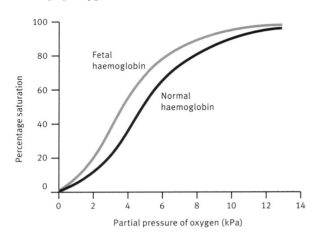

found in adults. Platelet production begins in the yolk sac at 6 weeks and in the liver from 8 weeks.

## FETAL HAEMOGLOBIN

Adult haemoglobin (Hb) is made of two alpha (or alpha-like) and two beta (or beta-like) globulin chains. During development, embryonic haemoglobins (HbGower 1, HbGower 2, HbPortland) are replaced from 10 weeks by HbF, which consists of two alpha and two gamma chains. This is the predominant haemoglobin from 10 weeks and peaks at over 90% of haemoglobin at 32 weeks, declines to 60–80% of haemoglobin at birth and is present until 3–6 months postnatally. Adult haemoglobin (HbA) is present from 10 weeks of gestation in small amounts and increases rapidly in the third trimester. The switch from HbF to HbA as the predominant haemoglobin occurs between birth and 12 weeks of postnatal life.

### Oxygen affinity of fetal haemoglobin

All forms of haemoglobin bind oxygen but the affinity with which this occurs varies. An important feature of HbF is that it binds oxygen with greater affinity than HbA. This is because HbA binds with 2,3-diphosphoglycerate (2,3-DPG) reducing its oxygen affinity, while HbF does not bind 2,3-DPG. The differences in affinity between HbA and HbF can be shown graphically using the oxygen saturation curve (Figure 32.3). The value of $P_{50}$ is the partial pressure of oxygen at which Hb is 50%

saturated: the lower the $P_{50}$, the greater the affinity for oxygen. The value of $P_{50}$ for HbF is 3.6 kPa, whereas for HbA $P_{50}$ is about 4.8 kPa. The oxygen saturation curve is therefore shifted to the left for HbF when compared with HbA. This greater affinity of HbF allows oxygen transfer across the placenta. Although this also reduces the ability to release oxygen to the tissues, fetal tissue acid–base balance aids oxygen delivery.

### Acid elution of fetal haemoglobin and the Kleihauer test

HbF is more resistant to alkali denaturation and acid elution than HbA and this forms the basis of the Kleihauer test. In this test, a maternal blood smear is prepared and an acid bath removes HbA. Staining of HbF allows pink-stained fetal cells to be seen on microscopy, while HbA-containing maternal cells appear as pale 'ghost cells'. A simple count allows estimation of the amount of fetal blood in the maternal circulation, as may occur after a fetal–maternal haemorrhage.

Persistence of maternally derived HbF in the maternal blood cells, as can occur in haemoglobinopathies, needs to be taken into account to avoid false interpretation. Postnatally the ability of the Kleihauer test to assess fetal red cells in the maternal circulation will depend on the persistence of the cells. If the mother and fetus are ABO, incompatible fetal red blood cells may be eliminated from the maternal bloodstream very quickly and a Kleihauer test should be performed as soon as possible in these circumstances.

### FETAL IMMUNE DEVELOPMENT

Precursors of the immune system develop in the embryonic yolk sac and migrate to the liver, spleen, bone marrow and thymus. Lymphoid stem cells give rise to B lymphocytes (from the liver) and T cells (from the thymus). B cells appear in peripheral blood from 12 weeks and mature T cells from 14 weeks. Although immunoglobulin synthesis begins at 12 weeks of gestation, production remains low throughout fetal life and the rise in immunoglobulin (Ig) G seen in the second trimester is caused by placental transfer of maternal IgG. As IgM does not cross the placental barrier, any increase in IgM is fetal in origin and may be due to intrauterine infection. Although neutrophils and macrophages can be isolated from 14 weeks, their levels in fetal peripheral blood remain low until the last trimester. From 32 weeks, the function of the immune system rapidly approaches that of a term infant, whereas before this time the system is largely immature, an important aspect of care of the preterm infant.

## TRANSITIONAL EVENTS AT BIRTH

The neonatal blood parameters change depending on the degree of placental transfusion. Late clamping of the cord and holding the newborn below the level of the placenta results in a significant increase in blood volume and red blood cell mass. Whether this is of benefit is controversial. In preterm infants it has been suggested that hyperbilirubinaemia may result from excessive placental transfusion; however, hypovolaemia may result if immediate clamping occurs. Haemoglobin levels in newborns are usually around 16.5–17.5 g/dl with a haematocrit of around 53% and mean white blood cell counts are

TABLE 32.2 **Functional development of the fetal gastrointestinal system**

| Development | Gestational age (weeks) |
|---|---|
| **SUCKING AND SWALLOWING** | |
| Swallowing | 10–14 |
| Immature suck–swallow | 33–36 |
| **STOMACH** | |
| Motility and secretion | 20 |
| **PANCREAS** | |
| Zymogen granules | 20 |
| **LIVER** | |
| Bile metabolism | 11 |
| Bile secretion | 22 |
| **SMALL INTESTINE** | |
| Active transport of amino acids | 14 |
| Glucose transport | 18 |
| Fatty acid absorption | 24 |

*Adapted with permission from:* Blackburn ST. *Maternal, Fetal and Neonatal Physiology.* 2nd ed. St Louis: Saunders; 2003.

$15\,000/mm^3$. Red blood cell and white blood cell counts increase in the initial hours after birth before decreasing by day 4–7. Platelet counts are similar to adult values but increase throughout the first month of postnatal life. Platelet activity is reduced in the neonate and the risk of bleeding and coagulopathy is increased, particularly in preterm infants. This is compounded by the low levels of vitamin K-dependent clotting factors.

# Fetal renal physiology

Functionally, urine production begins at 9–10 weeks and reabsorption in the loop of Henle begins by 12 weeks. Unlike the adult (where about 20% of cardiac output reaches the kidneys), only 2–3% of fetal cardiac output goes to the kidneys; fetal fluid and electrolyte balance is mainly under the control of the placenta rather than the kidney. Urine production is present and after 18 weeks fetal urine is the major contributor to amniotic fluid, while before 16 weeks most amniotic fluid is produced by the fetal skin and placenta. Therefore, reduced urine production from midgestation is an important cause of reduced amniotic fluid volume and can be seen in fetal growth restriction.

The fetal kidney has limited ability in concentrating urine and fetal urine is hypotonic. The ability to concentrate urine increases with fetal renal maturation and advancing gestation. Although the number of nephrons is similar to the adult from about 34 weeks of gestation, their functional maturity is not established until postnatal life. Preterm infants are therefore less able to maintain fluid and electrolyte balance.

## TRANSITIONAL EVENTS AT BIRTH

After birth, there is a dramatic increase in renal blood flow to the kidney, increasing from 2–3% of combined ventricular output in the fetus to about 10% of cardiac output at age 4 days. With renal blood flow, glomerular filtration rate also increases at birth and this continues with a doubling by 2 weeks of neonatal life.

# Gastrointestinal physiology

Although nutrition is provided by the placenta, functional development of the gut during fetal life begins early in gestation and swallowing movements are seen from 12 weeks. The rate of swallowing increases with age and reaches 250 ml/day at term, making swallowing an important aspect of amniotic fluid volume regulation. Intestinal villi start developing from 7 weeks of gestation and by 20 weeks these are well developed. Peristaltic motility develops gradually and is mature by the third trimester; intestinal absorptive processes are only partially available before 26 weeks of gestation. The fetal liver is mainly a haemopoietic organ during intrauterine life and functionally it is the placenta that handles metabolic processes. Liver and pancreatic secretions develop early in gestation. Although the nutritional value of amniotic fluid and cells are in doubt, these enzymes are thought to play a role in preventing bowel obstruction due to cellular debris. Functional development of the gastrointestinal tract is summarised in Table 32.2.

## MECONIUM

Meconium is composed of water (about 75%), intestinal secretions, squamous cells, lanugo hair, bile pigments (responsible for the green colour), pancreatic enzymes and blood. It appears from about 10–12 weeks of gestation and slowly moves into the colon by 16 weeks. Meconium passage is a normal developmental event and 98% of newborns pass meconium in the first 48 hours after birth.

Although the relationship between fetal hypoxia and increased intestinal peristalsis has been considered for many years, the precise mechanism of how stress or hypoxia results in meconium passage is unclear. The effects of meconium depend on the concentration of meconium, duration of exposure and the presence of associated stress factors (for example, hypoxia and infection).

Meconium-stained amniotic fluid is present in about 12% of all deliveries but its incidence increases with gestational age and it is present in 30% of post-term pregnancies. Meconium aspiration syndrome occurs in about 5% of infants with meconium-stained amniotic fluid. It is dependent on the presence of both meconium and fetal hypoxia and is thought to be caused by gasping actions of the fetus causing aspiration of meconium into the lungs. This causes a combination of mechanical blockage of small airways and production of chemical pneumonitis by the inhaled meconium particles. In addition, meconium directly inhibits pulmonary function by displacing surfactant and inhibiting its function and promotes lung tissue inflammation by activating neutrophils and macrophages. If postnatal hypoxia continues, meconium contributes to pulmonary vasospasm, hypertrophy of the pulmonary musculature and pulmonary hypertension.

## TRANSITIONAL EVENTS AT BIRTH

Gut maturation continues postnatally and is partly under the influence of gastrointestinal hormones and neuropeptides. A major stimulus for their release is commencement of enteral feeding and human milk, which is rich in trophic factors and antibodies, is the preferred feeding option.

# Fetal skin physiology

Skin is permeable to water until midpregnancy, with a net loss of water across the skin by transudation. Initially, the water content of skin is close to 100% but this begins to decrease from 20 weeks owing to keratinisation in the epidermis and an increase in connective tissue and vernix caseosa. This thin fatty film forms from 17 weeks and is made up of sebaceous gland secretions and desquamated skin cells. Although this film prevents loss of water and electrolytes, the fetal skin continues to contribute to amniotic fluid production.

# Fetal neurological system

The fetal central nervous system is one of the earliest systems to begin development but also the latest to mature. Lower level structures, including the basal ganglia, thalamus, midbrain and brainstem form first, while the cerebrum and cerebellum form later. Neuronal proliferation, migration, organisation and myelination are overlapping processes that continue throughout fetal life into the postnatal period: in particular, glial proliferation remains active throughout childhood.

Neurons proliferate from 8–20 weeks of gestation, with the most active period from 12–16 weeks. Neurons begin migration from the periventricular germinal areas from 8 weeks, in a radial fashion into areas where grey matter is established. By 20 weeks, the cortex has acquired the majority of neurons, while, in the cerebellum, proliferation and migration continue until 1 year postnatally. Organisation, including synapse formation, begins at 12 weeks of gestation and peaks in the last trimester of pregnancy. Alignment and orientation of cortical neurons continues well into the postnatal period.

Myelinisation begins in midgestation (around 24 weeks), peaks at birth and, especially in the corpus callosum, continues throughout childhood. Biochemical activity in the fetal brain is evident from 16 weeks. Spontaneous electroencephalographic activity appears at around 20 weeks and becomes synchronised at 26 weeks, while wake/sleep cycles are seen from 30 weeks.

### PERIPHERAL NERVOUS SYSTEM

Derived from cells of the neural crest, ganglia appear at 4–5 weeks of gestation. Nerve fibres grow from the spinal plate and form the ventral root (motor fibres) and dorsal root (sensory fibres).

Motor movements depend not only on innervation but also intact muscle cells; body movements appear from 7 weeks and limb movements from 9 weeks of gestation. Motor movements become more coordinated as gestation advances and complex movements are seen in the third trimester. Maternal perception of movements occurs from around 16 weeks in multiparous women but may be as late as 24 weeks in the first pregnancy. There is a steady increase in movements, but a gradual reduction near term is common, most likely owing to reduced space within the uterus. A marked reduction in the quality or frequency of movements experienced by the mother can reflect fetal hypoxia (as in fetal growth restriction) or fetal anaemia (as in rhesus disease).

The earliest sensory abilities are touch sensation and afferent synapses develop from 10 weeks. However, spinothalamic connections do not occur until midgestation and myelination not until 30 weeks. The development of smell, taste, hearing and vision all begin at about 23–26 weeks.

### FETAL PAIN

Although nociceptors first appear at 10 weeks of gestation in the fetus, their presence alone is not sufficient for the fetus to experience pain – electrical activity also has to be conducted from the nociceptors via the spinal cord to the brain.

Although the fetus may display a physiological stress response to painful stimuli (activation of the fetal hypothalamic–pituitary–adrenal axis) from around 19 weeks and the cortex is thought to be able to process sensory input from 24 weeks, controversy remains as to whether the fetus can perceive noxious stimuli at the cortical level as painful. Using activation of the hypothalamic pituitary–adrenal axis as a surrogate indicator of fetal pain has limitations. Pain perception during fetal (or indeed neonatal) development does not engage the same structures involved in pain processing as those used by human adults and this supports the argument that the fetus does not feel pain until late gestation.

### TRANSITIONAL EVENTS

The main transitional event in nervous system activity is during the change from the intrauterine to the extra-uterine environment. The nervous system continues to

FIGURE 32.4 **Summary of fluid flow in to and out of the amniotic space in late gestation**

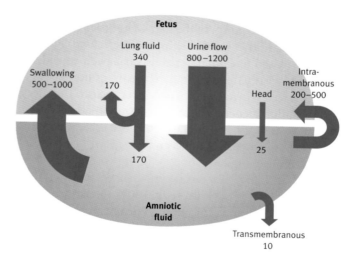

Arrow sizes are proportional to the flow rate | All measurements are in ml/day

mature, but requires adaptation to independent breathing, oral nutrition, thermoregulation by the autonomic nervous system, movements against gravitational effects and adaptation to sensory stimuli by the motor and sensory systems.

## Physiology of amniotic fluid

Amniotic fluid has protective, thermoregulatory and nutritive effects and allows movements and growth of the fetus. The amount of amniotic fluid is about 50 ml at 12 weeks and 150 ml at 16 weeks. It then increases by roughly 50 ml/week until 34 weeks (about 1000 ml) before a decrease to about 500 ml at term.

### PRODUCTION AND REMOVAL

There are six areas where exchange of amniotic fluid occurs: the fetal renal system production, lung, skin, gastrointestinal tract, across the uterine wall and across the placenta/membranes and umbilical cord. Amniotic fluid production is initially from the amniotic membrane and transfer via the fetal skin occurs before keratinisation begins at 20 weeks. In the second trimester, the two primary sources of amniotic fluid are fetal urine and lung liquid. Fetal urine is the main contributor of amniotic fluid at this stage, with reduced production owing to

urinary tract abnormalities leading to oligohydramnios, which is not usually evident before 16 weeks.

Amniotic fluid removal is caused by fetal swallowing and absorption into fetal blood across the surface of the placenta. Passive exchanges across the fetal skin and umbilical cord and via the transmembranous pathway (across the uterine wall) are not significant during the latter half of gestation (Figure 32.4).

### COMPOSITION

Over 98% of amniotic fluid is water. Minerals (mainly sodium, potassium, chloride), carbohydrates (glucose, fructose), proteins (albumin and globulins), lipids (cholesterol, lecithin), hormones, enzymes (mainly alkaline phosphatase) and suspended materials (bile pigments, skin debris, vernix caseosa, lanugo hair) make up the remainder. The composition varies with gestational age; as fetal urine production begins to contribute to amniotic fluid, the osmolarity decreases slightly compared with fetal blood. After keratinisation of the fetal skin, amniotic fluid osmolarity decreases further. The osmolarity of the amniotic fluid decreases with advancing gestation, owing to the contribution of hypotonic fetal urine, and sodium as well as chloride levels decrease with improving fetal kidney function. Amniotic fluid is thought to have antibacterial properties, mainly due to the presence of lysozymes and peroxidase.

### FURTHER READING

BLACKBURN ST. *Maternal Fetal and Neonatal Physiology*. 3rd ed. St Louis: Saunders; 2007.

MOORE KL, PERSAUD TVN. *The Developing Human: Clinically Oriented Embryology*. 8th ed. St Louis: Saunders; 2007.

Royal College of Obstetricians and Gynaecologists. *Fetal Awareness – Review of Research and Recommendations for Practice. Report of a Working Party*. London: RCOG; 2010.

## Sample questions relating to female and male reproductive physiology and the fertilisation process

### MULTIPLE CHOICE QUESTIONS

1 ▶ During female fetal reproductive development:

   A ▷ Oogonia develop from germ cells
   B ▷ The number of oogonia entering the fetal gonad is the number of oocytes that a female will have
   C ▷ The oocyte completes the first meiotic division
   D ▷ The oocytes are stored in the medulla of the ovary
   E ▷ Oocytes are lost from the first trimester onwards

2 ▶ During the process of follicle growth:

   A ▷ Follicle-stimulating hormone is required to begin growth
   B ▷ Follicles grow by increasing fluid in the oocyte
   C ▷ Capillaries for follicular growth form in the granulosa layer
   D ▷ The follicle grows for 45 days from initiation to selection
   E ▷ An antral follicle contains a fluid-filled cavity within the oocyte

3 ▶ Regarding follicular selection:

   A ▷ Follicle-stimulating hormone is required for follicular growth from the antral stage onwards only
   B ▷ Estrogen is formed in the thecal cells
   C ▷ As the corpus luteum of the previous cycle fails, there is a fall in follicle-stimulating hormone
   D ▷ As the follicle's granulosa cells increase, serum inhibin increases
   E ▷ Follicle-stimulating hormone causes the granulosa cells to develop luteinising hormone receptors

4 ▶ During ovulation:

   A ▷ The antral pressure rises prior to ovulation
   B ▷ There is a rise in steroid production directly after ovulation
   C ▷ Luteinising hormone causes the first meiotic division to be completed
   D ▷ After moving into the fallopian tube, the oocyte completes the second meiotic division
   E ▷ Estradiol causes the cilia in the fallopian tube to be produced

5 ▶ Regarding the uterus:

   A ▷ During the follicular phase, the endometrial cells divide
   B ▷ The glands multiply in number in the proliferative phase
   C ▷ After ovulation, the endometrial layer thickens by further hyperplasia
   D ▷ Prostaglandins cause constriction of the spiral arterioles
   E ▷ Necrosis of the endometrial layer is initially due to hypoxia

6 ▶ Regarding the development of the vagina and cervix:

   A ▷ The vagina is lined with keratinised squamous epithelium
   B ▷ Cell shedding from the vagina helps to inhibit infection
   C ▷ The vagina is always acidic
   D ▷ The cervix becomes more oedematous during the follicular phase
   E ▷ Glycoproteins form channels in the cervical mucus to assist fertilisation

7 ▶ Regarding the testes:

   A ▷ The normal volume of each testis is 30–40 ml
   B ▷ The seminiferous tubules are the sites of sperm storage
   C ▷ Spermatogenesis takes place in Sertoli cells
   D ▷ Spermatogonia are only laid down in fetal life
   E ▷ There is good blood flow through the basal lamina to the Sertoli cells

**8 ▶** Regarding spermatogenesis:

**A** ▷ There is a wave of mitotic division of spermatogonia every 28 days

**B** ▷ Daughter spermatogonia are to become spermatozoa

**C** ▷ Primary spermatocytes have 23 chromosomes

**D** ▷ Each spermatocyte gives four spermatids

**E** ▷ Normal spermatogenesis requires the presence of testosterone and follicle-stimulating hormone

**9 ▶** Regarding spermatogenesis:

**A** ▷ Each meiotic division moves the spermatids towards the lumen of the seminiferous tubule

**B** ▷ The process of spermatogenesis takes 80 days

**C** ▷ The tubules all open in the rete

**D** ▷ The epididymis is 5 m long

**E** ▷ Spermatozoa for intracytoplasmic sperm injection are removed from the rete

**10 ▶** Regarding androgen synthesis in males:

**A** ▷ The process occurs mainly in the Leydig cells

**B** ▷ The process is under the control of follicle-stimulating hormone

**C** ▷ Testosterone is converted to estradiol in the Sertoli cells

**D** ▷ In the male fetus, testosterone production is under the control of human chorionic gonadotrophin

**E** ▷ The level of testosterone falls in the male from fetal life until adrenarche

**11 ▶** Regarding the deposition of sperm in the female genital tract:

**A** ▷ Only the parasympathetic pelvic nerves influence erection

**B** ▷ Blood flow mainly into the corpus spongiosum causes an erection

**C** ▷ The vas deferens contacts

**D** ▷ About 120 million spermatozoa are normally deposited

**E** ▷ The ejaculate coagulates within 1 minute of entry into the vagina

**12 ▶** The following statements regarding fertilisation and the oocyte are correct:

**A** ▷ The oocyte completes the second meiotic division

**B** ▷ The first polar body is formed

**C** ▷ The cortical granules release their contents to prevent polyspermy

**D** ▷ There is a further meiotic cell division

**E** ▷ Blastocyst cells begin to produce human chorionic gonadotrophin

## Sample questions relating to physiology of pregnancy

### MULTIPLE CHOICE QUESTIONS

**1 ▶** Regarding maternal cardiac output in pregnancy:

**A** ▷ Cardiac output increases by 25%

**B** ▷ Cardiac output continues to rise until term

**C** ▷ Increase occurs by increasing the heart rate only

**D** ▷ The breasts receive much of the early extra cardiac output

**E** ▷ At term, the skin receives 500 ml per minute (18% of cardiac output)

**2 ▶** Regarding maternal cardiovascular physiology in pregnancy:

**A** ▷ Peripheral vascular resistance is reduced in pregnancy

**B** ▷ Blood pressure falls to its lowest at week 20

**C** ▷ The diastolic blood pressure falls by 10 mmHg

**D** ▷ Maternal electrocardiogram shows left axis deviation

**E** ▷ Maternal electrocardiogram shows Q waves in lead II

**3 ▶** Regarding maternal cardiovascular physiology in pregnancy:

**A** ▷ Blood volume increases by 30%

**B** ▷ Plasma volume increase by 30%

**C** ▷ Stroke volume increases by 25%

**D** ▷ The heart rate increases by 20%

**E** ▷ There is left ventricular hypertrophy

**4 ▶** Regarding the maternal respiratory system in pregnancy:

**A** ▷ Progesterone increases ventilation
**B** ▷ Ventilation increases by 25%
**C** ▷ $PCO_2$ falls during pregnancy
**D** ▷ There is a decrease in the calibre of the tracheobronchial tree
**E** ▷ Respiratory rate increases

**5 ▶** Regarding the maternal respiratory system in pregnancy:

**A** ▷ Breathing becomes increasingly thoracic
**B** ▷ Tidal volume doubles
**C** ▷ Forced expiratory volume increases
**D** ▷ Dyspnoea is experienced in 70% of cases
**E** ▷ 40% of increased oxygen consumption is for the fetus

**6 ▶** During pregnancy:

**A** ▷ The kidneys increase in size
**B** ▷ The ureters dilate owing to the size of the uterus only
**C** ▷ Renal blood flow doubles
**D** ▷ The glomerular filtration rate increases by 50%
**E** ▷ There is increased excretion of bicarbonate

**7 ▶** Regarding the maternal gastrointestinal tract and nutrition in pregnancy:

**A** ▷ Progesterone increases gastric emptying
**B** ▷ 80% of women suffer from acid reflux
**C** ▷ Gastric contents are more acidic
**D** ▷ Gallbladder emptying is increased
**E** ▷ Women with obstetric cholestasis are more likely to have fetal distress in labour

**8 ▶** Lactating women require higher amounts than pregnant women of:

**A** ▷ vitamin A
**B** ▷ vitamin $B_2$
**C** ▷ vitamin C
**D** ▷ vitamin E
**E** ▷ vitamin K

**9 ▶** Regarding haematological system changes in concert with cardiovascular adaptations:

**A** ▷ The plasma volume expands by 30%
**B** ▷ Red cell mass increases until week 32
**C** ▷ Physiological anaemia is at its worst at week 28
**D** ▷ Platelets decrease in size in pregnancy
**E** ▷ White cell count increases predominantly owing to neutrophils

**10 ▶** Regarding changes in the haematological system in pregnancy:

**A** ▷ The pregnant woman requires an extra 600 mg of iron per day
**B** ▷ Iron absorption is increased owing to decreased gastric motility
**C** ▷ Fibrinolytic activity increases during pregnancy
**D** ▷ Concentrations of factor XI increase in pregnancy
**E** ▷ The activity of the fibrinolytic system returns to normal 6 weeks post delivery

**11 ▶** Regarding lactation:

**A** ▷ The alveolar cells undergo hyperplasia in the third trimester
**B** ▷ Human placental lactogen causes lactiferous duct hyperplasia
**C** ▷ High pregnancy levels of progesterone prevent milk production
**D** ▷ The combined oral contraceptive taken during breastfeeding has no effect on milk production
**E** ▷ Colostrum has high concentrations of lactose

**12 ▶** Regarding lactation:

**A** ▷ The amount of protein in milk decreases with time
**B** ▷ Suckling produces oxytocin
**C** ▷ Milk production doubles in twin-feeding mothers
**D** ▷ Extra energy for breast milk production is achieved from greater consumption of food
**E** ▷ Breast milk is the same in all women

**13 ▶** Regarding lactation:

**A** ▷ Prolactin is released from the hypothalamus
**B** ▷ Prolactin surges immediately after suckling begins
**C** ▷ Dopamine suppresses milk production
**D** ▷ Metoclopramide suppresses milk production
**E** ▷ Prolactin levels naturally decrease 28 days after delivery

**14 ▶** Oxytocin:

A ▷ release is stimulated by suckling

B ▷ is released by the anterior pituitary

C ▷ is released if the mother hears the baby crying

D ▷ acts on myoepithelial cells

E ▷ is central to milk production

**15 ▶** Breast milk:

A ▷ has galactose as its main carbohydrate

B ▷ contains more casein than cow's milk

C ▷ carries vitamin E

D ▷ contains high amounts of IgA

E ▷ contains high prolactin levels to suppress ovulation

**16 ▶** Regarding the third stage of labour and uterine involution:

A ▷ There are multiple uterine contractions after delivery of the baby

B ▷ Oxytocin levels increase dramatically during the third stage of labour

C ▷ The uterus halves its weight in the first 7 days post delivery

D ▷ The decidua is shed over the first 6 weeks post delivery

E ▷ Lochia alba is yellow

**17 ▶** During human parturition:

A ▷ Progesterone suppresses the formation of myometrial gap junctions

B ▷ Estradiol increases the oxytocin receptors in the myometrium

C ▷ Oxytocin release is increased prior to labour

D ▷ The fetus releases oxytocin

E ▷ The decidua releases prostaglandin 2

**18 ▶** During human parturition:

A ▷ Neutrophils destroy collagen fibres in the cervix

B ▷ Increasing numbers of myometrial gap junctions increases contraction strength

C ▷ Magnesium sulphate causes uterine relaxation

D ▷ Salbutamol causes uterine relaxation by inhibiting calcium influx into myometrial cells

E ▷ Commencement of labour increases prostaglandin release

## Sample questions relating to fetal physiology

### MULTIPLE CHOICE QUESTIONS

**1 ▶** In fetal cardiovascular physiology:

A ▷ Blood circulation is established in week 5

B ▷ In the fetus, it is the total ventricular output that is important

C ▷ The heart grows by hyperplasia during fetal life

D ▷ The fetus has a large stroke volume reserve

E ▷ Fatty acids are the main cardiac fuel

**2 ▶** In the normal regulation of the fetal heart rate:

A ▷ Sympathetic influence is via the sinoatrial node

B ▷ The adrenal medulla plays no role in fetal heart rate

C ▷ Baroreceptors act through the autonomic nervous system in response to blood pressure

D ▷ The fetal heart rate increases with gestation

E ▷ The variability of the fetal heart is a direct indication of the status of the fetal brain stem's medulla oblongata

**3 ▶** Regarding abnormal fetal heart rates:

A ▷ Tachycardia can be caused by the use of beta-sympathomimetic tocolytics

B ▷ Tachycardia can be caused by fetal hypoxia

C ▷ Bradycardia can be caused by fetal hypoxia

D ▷ A baseline rate of less than 110 beats per minute can be normal

E ▷ Fetal heart block is a common cause of bradycardia

**4 ▶** Regarding fetal heart rate variability:

A ▷ It is defined as fluctuation in the fetal heart rate of at least two cycles per minute

B ▷ It remains stable regardless of gestation

C ▷ Short-term variation measures the time between two T waves on the fetal electrocardiogram

D ▷ The autonomic not the sympathetic nervous system is the cause for variability

E ▷ Magnesium sulphate may cause a decrease in the fetal heart variability

**5 ▶** Regarding the fetal heart:

A ▷ Accelerations are rare in fetal hypoxia
B ▷ The loss of accelerations for more than 1 hour correlates with increase neonatal morbidity
C ▷ Early decelerations are due to baroreceptor activation
D ▷ Late decelerations begin before the peak of the contractions
E ▷ Late decelerations are due to chemoreceptor stimulation and inhibition of the sympathetic nervous system

**6 ▶** Regarding variable fetal heart decelerations:

A ▷ Decelerations are variable in terms of relation with uterine contractions, duration and depth
B ▷ Decelerations are due to gradual cord compression
C ▷ Umbilical vein compression causes fetal bradycardia
D ▷ Umbilical artery compression causes a drop in fetal blood pressure
E ▷ The depth of the deceleration is an indication of hypoxaemia

**7 ▶** With reference to the fetal circulation:

A ▷ The ductus venosus directs blood to the superior vena cava
B ▷ The ductus arteriosus connects the pulmonary artery to the aorta
C ▷ Little blood passes to the lungs
D ▷ Mixing of oxygenated and deoxygenated blood causes mixed blood to flow around the fetus
E ▷ Deoxygenated blood enters the ascending aorta

**8 ▶** Regarding changes to the fetal circulation at birth:

A ▷ The fetal systemic resistance doubles
B ▷ The pulmonary vascular resistance falls with the first breath
C ▷ The ductus arteriosus closes and seals within 2 days of delivery
D ▷ The ductus venosus closes chemically with prostaglandin
E ▷ The foramen ovale seals closed immediately

**9 ▶** During development of the fetal respiratory system:

A ▷ The main bronchi develop by week 7
B ▷ Airway branching is complete by week 17
C ▷ The acini develop by week 24
D ▷ Formation of terminal sacs is complete by week 36
E ▷ Alveolar development is complete by term

**10 ▶** Fetal breathing movements:

A ▷ begin in the first trimester
B ▷ increase in fetal hypoxia
C ▷ increase after maternal eating
D ▷ do not play a role in lung growth
E ▷ cause lung hyperplasia when excessive

**11 ▶** In fetal and neonatal respiratory physiology:

A ▷ Fetal lung fluid is mainly swallowed amniotic fluid
B ▷ Steroids increase surfactant synthesis
C ▷ Maternal diabetes increases lung maturation
D ▷ Androgens increase fetal lung maturation
E ▷ Labour commences fetal lung fluid reabsorption

**12 ▶** In fetal haematopoiesis:

A ▷ The liver is the main source of fetal blood cells until week 24
B ▷ Fetal white cells are formed in the liver
C ▷ Mature T cells appear in the fetus from week 14
D ▷ IgM is of maternal origin
E ▷ The immune system is fully functioning by week 24

**13 ▶** Regarding the physiology of the fetal kidneys and skin:

A ▷ Fetal urine production begins at week 12
B ▷ Fetal urine is isotonic
C ▷ The kidneys receive 20% of cardiac output
D ▷ Fetal skin is permeable to water
E ▷ Fetal skin contributes to amniotic fluid production

**14 ▶** In fetal brain development:

A ▷ Neurons proliferate until week 20
B ▷ Neurons have completely migrated to the cerebellum by term
C ▷ The peripheral nervous system ganglia are derived from cells of the neural crest
D ▷ Fetal movements begin at week 7
E ▷ Fetuses do not feel pain until week 24

**15 ▶** The fetal baseline heart rate:

**A** ▷ is determined by the sinoatrial node
**B** ▷ is strongly influenced by the sympathetic tone
**C** ▷ decreases with advancing gestation
**D** ▷ is unaffected by catecholamine release
**E** ▷ variability is reduced by alcohol

**16 ▶** In the fetal circulation:

**A** ▷ Homogenously semioxygenated blood circulates through the fetal arteries
**B** ▷ The ductus arteriosus connects the umbilical vein to the inferior vena cava
**C** ▷ Blood flow across the foramen ovale is from right to left
**D** ▷ The patency of the ductus arteriosus is maintained by the vasodilator effects of prostaglandins
**E** ▷ There is a rise in pulmonary pressure at birth

**17 ▶** During development of the fetal lungs:

**A** ▷ Fetal breathing movements begin at about week 32
**B** ▷ Surfactant is produced by type II pneumocytes
**C** ▷ Surfactant is a lipoprotein of which 90% is made of protein
**D** ▷ The saccular phase continues well into the postnatal period
**E** ▷ Initial inflation breaths at birth generate lower pressures than those needed for subsequent breathing

**18 ▶** Fetal haemoglobin:

**A** ▷ consists of two alpha and two delta chains
**B** ▷ is the predominant haemoglobin during fetal life
**C** ▷ is replaced by adult haemoglobin as the predominant haemoglobin during the last trimester
**D** ▷ binds oxygen with lower affinity than adult haemoglobin
**E** ▷ can persist in the adult in haemoglobinopathies

**19 ▶** Amniotic fluid volume:

**A** ▷ measures about 200 ml at week 12
**B** ▷ is mainly produced by fetal urine at week 10
**C** ▷ osmolarity increases with advancing gestation as the fetal kidneys mature
**D** ▷ is meconium stained in about 30% of post-term pregnancies
**E** ▷ is essential for pulmonary development

# 13

# Statistics and Epidemiology

# CHAPTER 33

# Basic statistics

*Fiona Broughton Pipkin*

*Statistics are like bikinis – they give you an idea, but hide what is important.* ANONYMOUS

## Introduction

Statistics should be tools, not tyrants. This chapter sets out to describe, as simply as possible, the statistical concepts needed for the MRCOG Part 1 examination. This exam is designed to test understanding, not the ability to carry out complex mathematical procedures. There are a number of examples to try that, if answered correctly, will demonstrate a basic understanding of the concept.

## Descriptive statistics

### SCALES

Data can be described using three different kinds of scale:

- **Nominal**: a naming scale (for example, eye colour: blue, green, brown, black).
- **Ordinal**: an ordering scale (for example, winner: second, third, fourth).
- **Interval**: a scale in which the interval between any two neighbouring points is the same as that between any other two neighbouring points (for example, temperature, °C: 1, 2, 3, 4, 5 or 5, 10, 15, 20). Values can be below zero.
- **Ratio**: an interval scale with a fixed zero (for example, height, weight).

Data measured on interval and ratio scales are sometimes called parametric data, while data expressed on nominal and ordinal scales are called non-parametric. 'Parametric' in this context means that the data set has a normal distribution.

### CONCEPTS OF MEASUREMENT

There are four main points to bear in mind when making a measurement:

- **Accuracy**: a measurement is accurate if it matches exactly an accepted standard.
- **Precision**: a precise measurement is one that has a small random error of estimation.
- **Reliability**: a reliable measurement is one that can be repeated with minimal variation.
- **Validity**: a valid measurement gives genuine information about that which is being measured.

## Summarising data

### CENTRAL TENDENCY AND SCATTER

Most sets of data are samples from populations. Using descriptive statistics, the main measurable characteristics of a sample, in terms of its central tendency (mode or modal group, median, mean [average]) and the scatter in the sample (range, standard deviation, standard error of the mean) can be summarised.

Figure 33.1 is a frequency histogram of population data and shows that they approximate to what is called a normal (Gaussian) distribution. Normal distributions have a single peak, so are known as 'unimodal'. In a

FIGURE 33.1 **Frequency histogram of the data in Table 33.1**

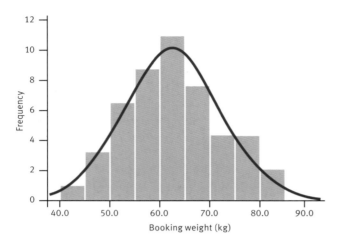

TABLE 33.1 **Ranked booking weights and weight groups for a random sample of 45 primigravidae**

| Ranked data (kg) | Grouped data | |
| --- | --- | --- |
| | Weight range (kg) | Number |
| 42, 46, 46, 49, 50, 50, 51, 53, 54, 54, 55, 56, 56, 56, 57, 58, 59, 59, 60, 60, 61, 61, 62, 62, 62, 63, 64, 64, 65, 66, 67, 67, 68, 68, 69, 70, 70, 72, 74, 75, 76, 77, 78, 80, 84 | 38–42 | 1 |
| | 43–47 | 2 |
| | 48–52 | 4 |
| | 53–57 | 8 |
| | 58–62 | 10 |
| | 63–67 | 7 |
| | 68–72 | 6 |
| | 73–77 | 4 |
| | 78–82 | 2 |
| | 83–87 | 1 |

perfect normal distribution, there would be equal numbers of observations to the left and right of the midpoint of the horizontal axis and they would be symmetrical about the peak. Therefore, the mode, median and mean would be the same. The normal curve is characterised by its mean and standard deviation.

### Assessing normality

An assumption that data are normally distributed underlies many of the commonly used statistical techniques. Therefore, statisticians need to be able to assess whether the data in a sample do indeed follow a normal distribution. Two common ways of doing this are the Shapiro–Wilk test and the Kolmogorov–Smirnov test. Running the Shapiro–Wilk test on the data set in Table 33.1 gives $P = 0.978$, (an explanation of $P$ is given later in this chapter), showing that the data do not deviate significantly from a normal distribution.

Incidentally, it is possible for a distribution to be symmetrical but not normal; this can happen if the distribution is very widely distributed around the mean (i.e. flat) or very closely grouped around it, so the distribution is tall and thin. The 'peakedness' of distributions, both normal and non-normal, can be measured by calculating the kurtosis.

### Range

Range is the spread of data in a sample. In Table 33.1, the range is 42–84 kg. The range is especially unhelpful when a data set is skewed.

### Mode or modal group

The mode is the value that occurs most frequently in a data set. The modal group is the interval on a frequency histogram within which the greatest number of observations fall. In Figure 33.1, the modal group is 58–62 kg.

It is worth remembering that some data will have two or more peaks in their distribution. Always look critically at a frequency histogram to see whether there is evidence for a multimodal distribution.

### Median

The median is the middle value in a ranked data set. The median is much less influenced by skewed data sets than the mean.

## EXAMPLE 1

▷ Find the median of 5, 1, 8, 3, 4:

- First sort the measurements (put them in order): 1, 3, 4, 5, 8.

- The median is the $(n+1)/2$th value in the set, where $n$ is the number of observations.

- In this set, the median is the third value, i.e. 4 (not 3).

## EXAMPLE 2

Where $n$ is an even number, take the average of the two middle numbers.

▷ Find the median of 5, 1, 10, 8, 4, 3:

- First rank the measurements: 1, 3, 4, 5, 8, 10.

- The median is then the $(n+1)/2$th value in the set, that is, the average of the third and fourth values, i.e. 4.5.

## Mean

The mean is the statistician's term for an average ($\bar{x}$).

- Mean $(\bar{x}) = \dfrac{\sum x}{n}$

- where $\sum$ = 'the sum of', $x$ = each individual observation and $n$ = the number of observations.

## EXAMPLE 3

▷ Consider a data set of six families with 4, 2, 1, 3, 2 and 3 children:

- $\bar{x} = \dfrac{\sum 4+2+1+3+2+3}{6} = 2.5$

## QUANTIFYING VARIABILITY (SCATTER) IN A NORMAL DISTRIBUTION

### Variance

By itself, variability is not very helpful in describing the 'average' family, as the same mean as for example 3 could have been arrived at if the families had had 2, 2, 2, 3, 3 and 3 children. To illustrate the differences in the data, an estimate of the scatter in the sample is needed. Variance is the average amount by which any individual measurement differs from the mean.

- Variance $(s^2) = \dfrac{\sum (x-\bar{x})^2}{(n-1)}$

### Standard deviation

Standard deviation ($s$ or SD) is the square root of the variance (in original units). It is used because some of the differences will be positive, and some negative and, if the squaring were not carried out when calculating the variance, some differences would cancel others out, which would be logically useless. The standard deviation gives information about the scatter in a sample.

Standard deviation $(s) = \sqrt{\text{variance}}$

Statisticians describe the population mean and standard deviation as $\mu$ and $\sigma$, respectively. This is different from the sample mean ($\bar{x}$) and standard deviation ($s$).

When data from a population can be described by a normal curve:

- The area covered by $\pm 1\sigma$ from $\mu = 68\%$. This means that 32% of the area lies more than $\pm 1\sigma$ away from the mean. Because the distribution is symmetrical, 16% lies to the left of $\mu$ and 16% to the right of it.

- The area covered by $\pm 2\sigma$ from $\mu = 95\%$. Thus 5% lie outside this range, with 2.5% in each 'tail'.

- The area covered by $\pm 3\sigma$ from $\mu = 99.8\%$. What proportion lies outside this range?

FIGURE 33.2 **The normal distribution curve**

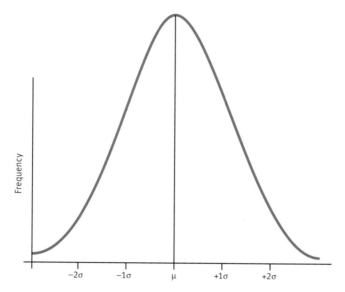

In a normally distributed sample with 30 or more observations ($n \geq 30$), the same approximations can be used for the sample mean ($\bar{x}$) and standard deviation ($s$).

In Figure 33.2, any position on the $x$ axis can be described by how many standard deviations (the distance) it is away from the mean, on either side. This distance is known as the normal ($z$) score or standard normal deviate. All statistical textbooks have tables of $z$ scores.

## Coefficient of variation

The coefficient of variation expresses the standard deviation as a percentage of the mean.

- Coefficient of variation (COV) $= \dfrac{s}{\bar{x}} \times 100$

This is useful, for example, in quantifying the reliability of repeated measurements, since it puts the standard deviation in the context of the mean.

## Standard error of the mean

The standard error of the mean (SEM) gives information on how close a sample mean is to the population mean. If several samples from a population were taken, each sample would have its own mean and variance and only by chance would the sample mean be the same as the

population mean. In a normally distributed population, these sample means would themselves have a normal distribution. Calculating the mean of those sample means would usually give a better idea of the true population mean, so the variability of this distribution of sample means is assessed by calculating their standard deviation. This is known as the SEM. The smaller the SEM is, the closer the sample mean lies to the population mean. It is derived from the standard deviation ($s$) and the sample size ($n$).

- SEM $= \dfrac{s}{\sqrt{n}}$ or SEM $= \sqrt{\dfrac{s^2}{n}}$

Arithmetically, these formulae are the same.

The SEM thus takes into account both the scatter and the sample size, thus allowing for the fact that the mean of a bigger sample will be more representative of the true population mean than will the mean of a smaller sample.

### EXAMPLE 4

▷ Let the mean ($\bar{x}$) booking weight in a sample = 52 kg and the standard deviation ($s$) = 12 kg:

- If $n = 9$, SEM $= 12/\sqrt{9} = 12/3 = 4$ kg.
- If $n = 16$, SEM $= 12/\sqrt{16} = 12/4 = 3$ kg.
- If $n = 100$, SEM $= 12/\sqrt{100} = 12/10 = 1.2$ kg.

## Confidence intervals

For a normally distributed sample with 30 or more observations ($n \geq 30$), the same assumptions about the areas under the normal curve can be used for the sample mean, $\bar{x}$, and standard deviation, $s$, as for the population mean, $\mu$, and standard deviation, $\sigma$. These allow the calculation of confidence intervals describing the distribution of data in the sample.

### EXAMPLE 5

▷ Let the mean booking weight in a sample of $n = 36$ be 52 kg and the SEM be 3 kg:

- 95% CI $= 52 \pm (2 \times 3) = 52 \pm 6 = 46$–58 kg.

The practical interpretation of this is that, in this example, there is a 95% probability that the true population mean lies between 46 and 52 kg (or a 5% probability of the true population mean lying outside this range).

▷ If $n = 100$ and the SEM $= 1.2$ kg:

■ 95% CI $= 52 \pm (2 \times 1.2) = 52 \pm 2.4 = 49.6$–$54.4$ kg.

## SKEWED DATA

The distribution of positively skewed and negatively skewed samples are shown in Figures 33.3 and 33.4. The effect of the skewness is to make the mean less 'typical' than other measures that are less influenced by extreme values, such as the median. However, the SEM can still be used for confidence limits because, even with skewed data, the distribution of sample means approaches a normal distribution.

### EXAMPLE 6

▷ Consider a sample of six women with different parities (number of pregnancies leading to a successful outcome after 20 weeks of gestation): para 4, para 2, para 1, para 3, para 2 and para 3:

■ Mean parity is 2.5.
■ Variance is 1.1.
■ $s$ is 1.05.
■ SEM is 0.43.

▷ If a para 13 is now added to this group:

■ Mean parity becomes 4.0.
■ Variance becomes 16.67.
■ $s$ becomes 4.08.
■ SEM is 1.54.

### EXAMPLE 7

▷ In a larger sample of 53 women (Figure 33.3), 7 were para 0, 23 were para 1, 14 were para 2, 4 were para 3, 2 were para 4, 2 were para 5 and 1 was para 6:

■ Median parity is the $(53 + 1)/2$th value in the ranked set, i.e. the 27th value.
■ Since there are 7 para 0 and 23 para 1, the 27th value must be para 1.

FIGURE 33.3 **Frequency histogram of the data in example 7**

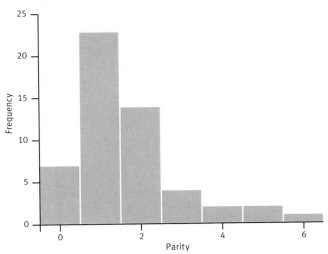

These data have a right-handed tail and are described as positively skewed. The modal group is para 1.

FIGURE 33.4 **Frequency histogram of parity from a sample of women in an area where large family size is the norm**

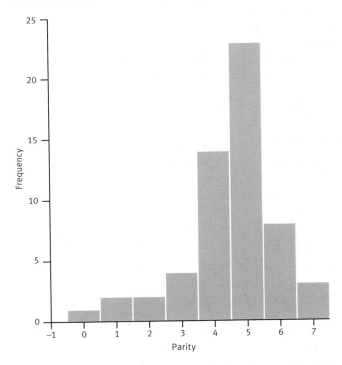

These data have a left-handed tail and are described as negatively skewed. The modal group is para 5.

### Normalising skewed data

When data are not normally distributed, it may be possible to transform them to a normal distribution. This allows the correct use of the mean, standard deviation and standard error of the mean for each sample and thus the calculation of confidence intervals. It also allows the use of more powerful comparative statistics for hypothesis testing.

Endocrine data often follow a positively skewed distribution. This can be normalised by taking the logarithm of the data.

Other commonly used transformations are:

- taking the square root ($\sqrt{x}$)
- squaring ($x^2$)
- taking the reciprocal ($\frac{1}{x}$).

### THE BINOMIAL DISTRIBUTION

The binomial distribution is the simplest form of distribution. It is used for data measured on a discontinuous dichotomous scale (for example, yes/no, alive/dead). With dichotomies, if the proportion ($p$) of subjects falling into one category is known, the proportion in the other, which is ($1-p$) or $q$, is automatically known.

When the number of observations is more than 30 ($n > 30$), the binomial distribution approximates to the normal distribution, which is very useful. Under these circumstances, the standard deviation of $p$ is given by $p \times (1-p)$ and the standard error:

$$\text{SEM} = \sqrt{\frac{p * (1-p)}{n}}$$

This can be used to establish confidence intervals for $p$.

#### EXAMPLE 8

▷ In a sample of 100 pregnant women, 20 admitted smoking; therefore $p = 0.2$ and $(1-p) = 0.8$:

- $\text{SEM} = \sqrt{\dfrac{0.2 * 0.8}{100}} = \sqrt{\dfrac{0.16}{100}} = 0.04$

▷ There is only 1 chance in 20 of the true population proportion of smokers lying outside the range:

- 95% CI $= 0.2 \pm (2 \times 0.04) = 0.12 - 0.28$, or 12–28%.

▷ However, if only 30 women (the lowest acceptable) were sampled and 6 smoked, although the proportion is the same, the SEM is larger and the 95% CI is much wider:

- $\text{SEM} = \sqrt{\dfrac{0.2 * 0.8}{30}} = \sqrt{\dfrac{0.16}{30}} = 0.073$

- 95% CI $= 0.2 \pm (2 \times 0.073) = 0.054 - 0.346$, or 5.4–34.6%.

### THE POISSON DISTRIBUTION

This is another kind of distribution of discrete data, arising when the number of occurrences of an event per unit of time are counted. It therefore relates to integers (whole numbers). This type of distribution was first described by a Prussian army statistician (Figure 33.5). A modern example of the distribution could be the number of admissions to a gynaecological unit from the accident and emergency department each day. Over a period, an average number of admissions can be calculated, but the actual number of admissions each day will be randomly variable. The Poisson distribution allows the calculation of the probability of any specified number of admissions on a single day. Thus this is useful when considering random sums of rare events.

With a Poisson distribution, the distribution is skewed when the mean is close to zero, but the distribution approximates to normal as the mean increases. If the mean number of events is around 9, then the normal approximation is reasonable.

The variance in a Poisson distribution is the same as the mean, so:

- $s = \sqrt{mean}$

FIGURE 33.5 **Frequency histogram of the number of deaths/year in the Prussian Army caused by being kicked by a horse**

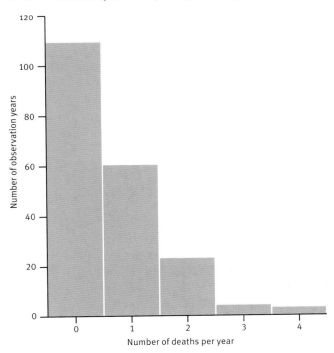

## Probability

The probability of a specific outcome is the proportion of times that the outcome would occur if the observation or experiment was repeated a large number of times.

### THE SHORTHAND OF PROBABILITY

Any probability has to vary between zero and one. A probability of zero means that something cannot happen; a probability of one means that it is certain to happen. For example:

- the proposition that 'all men will die' could be written as $P = 1.0$
- a 50% chance of something happening could be written as $P = 0.5$
- less than one chance in 20 of something happening could be written as $P < 0.05$.

The inequality signs < and > simply mean 'less than' and 'more than'.

## Comparative statistics and hypothesis testing

So far in this chapter, descriptive statistics have been considered. Another important branch of statistics is comparative statistics. These are used when comparing, for example, the effect of a fixed variable, such as gender on a disease or condition, or determining whether some intervention has an effect on a disease or condition. Under both circumstances, hypothesis testing works, by convention, from a null hypothesis (H0), which states that the variable is without effect, and then testing the null hypothesis.

The probability of any observed outcome arising if the null hypothesis is valid is calculated and used to support or reject the hypothesis. This probability is referred to as the $P$ value and the smaller $P$ is, the less can the null hypothesis be supported. The $P$ value can be defined as the probability of having observed any specified outcome (or one more extreme) if the null hypothesis is valid.

By convention (and it is only by convention), H0 is usually rejected if $P < 0.05$. That is, an outcome causing rejection of H0 could occur less than one time in 20 even when the H0 was valid.

The use of $P$ values is open to two main errors:

- alpha (α) or type 1 errors, when H0 is wrongly rejected (on average, once in 20 trials, if $P < 0.05$ is used)
- beta (β) or type 2 errors, when H0 is wrongly not rejected.

Always remember that statistical and biological significance need not be the same. Large studies can make very small differences statistically significant, while even large biological effects can be statistically non-significant in a small study. So do not rely too much on $P$ values. The difference between $P = 0.053$ and $P = 0.047$ may technically be the difference between acceptance and rejection of the null hypothesis but should not constrain thinking about possible implications of erroneously stating that there is no effect.

### SAMPLE SIZE DETERMINATION

When any study is being designed, the size of sample is very important. It must be big enough to give a high chance of any real difference being identified as statistically significant. This should be governed by taking both alpha and beta errors into account.

The power of a study is its ability to detect an effect of a specified size. It is expressed as $(1 - \beta)$ or $100(1 - \beta)\%$.

The sample size ($n$) is usually calculated to give a power of 0.8–0.9 (80–90%). For any hypothesis test, alpha is set in advance (usually 5%) so $P < 0.05$ supports rejection of H0.

## TYPES OF TEST FOR HYPOTHESIS TESTING

The type of data that is collected will determine what forms of analysis it can be subjected to. Are the data nominal (categorical), ordinal, discrete (integers, for example, numbers of children) or continuous? Are they normally distributed? What is the null hypothesis? For example, are two or more groups being compared with each other or with the population? Is the investigation looking for evidence of association between variables? Is the investigation trying to describe or predict the effect of a change in one variable on another? Some of the most commonly used statistical tests are discussed here.

## DISTRIBUTION-FREE (NON-PARAMETRIC) ANALYSES

For non-parametric analysis, minimal assumptions are made about the underlying data distribution. That is, they can be used for data whether or not they are normally distributed.

For comparing groups, the following tests are available:

- sign test
- chi-square ($\chi^2$) test, for $2 \times 2$ and larger contingency tables (be aware of the need for applying Yates' correction factor when the sample size is small)
- McNemar $\chi^2$ test, for 'before' and 'after' categorical data
- Wilcoxon test, for paired data, for the same subject under different conditions
- Mann–Whitney $U$-test, for unpaired data
- Kruskal–Wallis analysis of variance.

The Wilcoxon, Mann–Whitney $U$ and Kruskal–Wallis tests make no assumptions about the underlying data distribution and are the non-parametric equivalent of the Student's paired and unpaired $t$-tests and one-way analysis of variance.

For testing association between groups, the following test is available:

- Spearman's rho ($\rho$).

Again, Spearman's $\rho$ makes no assumption about the underlying data distribution.

### Normally distributed data

Tests for normally distributed data, properly speaking, should only be used when it has been formally confirmed that the data are indeed normally distributed, which may involve normalising skewed data.

For comparing groups, the following tests are available:

- Student's $t$-test, for paired and unpaired data (first check whether the variances differ significantly from each other using the Welch test)
- F test, to determine equality of variances
- analysis of variance (one-way, two or more way, repeated measures).

For testing association between groups, the following tests are available:

- Pearson's $r$
- linear regression analysis
- multiple regression analysis.

For both types of regression analysis, the response variable should be normally distributed; the independent variable need not be and it may have been fixed by the investigator.

## SOME SPECIFIC TESTS

### The chi-square test

In the simplest form of the very useful $\chi^2$ test, the variable under investigation can be only one of two types.

#### EXAMPLE 9

▷ In an investigation concerning the common cold, a GP saw 900 people presenting consecutively at the surgery: 480 were men and 420 were women. Do these data conform to the null hypothesis that the incidence of the common cold is not gender related?

▷ If there were no gender difference, then the expectations (E) would be that 450 of the people are men and 450 are women. Instead the observations (O) are 480 men (an excess of 30) and 420 women (a deficit of 30).

■ Now $\chi^2 = \sum \dfrac{(O-E)^2}{E}$

■ so $\chi^2 = \dfrac{(480-450)^2}{450} + \dfrac{(430-450)^2}{450}$

■ $= \dfrac{+30^2}{450} + \dfrac{-30^2}{450}$

■ $= 4.0$. Consulting a table of $\chi^2$ shows this to be significant ($P < 0.05$).

▷ But if the sample had been only of 90 people, 48 men and 42 women, although the proportions would have been the same, the outcome would be different:

■ $\chi^2 = \dfrac{(48-45)^2}{45} + \dfrac{(43-45)^2}{45}$

■ $= \dfrac{+3^2}{45} + \dfrac{-3^2}{45}$

■ $= 0.4$, which is far from reaching significance.

From example 9, it can be seen that there are instances when $\chi^2$ cannot be used:

■ with proportions
■ when any expected number of observations is less than 5
■ when the total number of observations is less than 20.

The test can be expanded to develop contingency tables, where each cell of the table corresponds to a particular combination of characteristics relating to two or more classifications, which can be categorical.

#### EXAMPLE 10

▷ Table 33.2 is a $2 \times 3$ table. If the null hypothesis is valid and the two variables are unrelated, then the probability of an individual being in a particular row is independent of which column they are in:

■ The proportion of married women is 2787/3438 = 81.1%.
■ The proportion of women who do not drink caffeine is 870/3438 = 25.3%.
■ The expected proportion of married women who don't drink caffeine is 0.811 × 0.253 = 0.205.
■ In terms of the whole sample, the expected number of married women who don't drink caffeine would be 0.205 × 3438 = 705 women.

▷ In fact, the observation was that only 652 married women drank no caffeine. Working through the table, calculating the observed and expected frequencies and then applying the formula for $\chi^2$ will determine whether or not the data fitted the null hypothesis.

TABLE 33.2  **Data relating to daily caffeine consumption and marital status from a sample of 3438 women**

|  |  | Caffeine consumption (mg/day) | | | |
|---|---|---|---|---|---|
|  |  | 0 | 1–150 | 151–300 | Total |
| Marital status | Married | 652 | 1537 | 598 | 2787 |
|  | Single | 218 | 327 | 106 | 651 |
|  | Total | 870 | 1864 | 704 | 3438 |

### t-tests

*t*-tests are very commonly used to compare:

- the mean of a sample with a predicted value, often zero
- the means of two samples.

These can be paired or unpaired samples. Paired samples are those where a measurement(s) is made on the same person under two different conditions, such as the measurement of blood pressure in an antenatal booking clinic and again a month later. It is also sometimes possible to match two groups of subjects very carefully for variables perceived as being important confounders in their own right, such as age or smoking habit, so that each study individual has a matched control. Where observations are made on different groups of subjects without any such careful matching, the data are said to be unpaired. In either case, the underlying population distribution must be normal.

### Different types of t-test

#### EXAMPLE 11

▷ Diastolic blood pressure was measured in 29 women at booking and 3 weeks later and the results ($\bar{x} \pm s$) were as follows:

- booking: $60.5 \pm 7.35$; therefore SEM $= 1.36$ mmHg
- 3/52 later: $57.6 \pm 7.97$; therefore SEM $= 1.48$ mmHg
- change: $-2.9 \pm 6.80$; therefore SEM $= 1.26$ mmHg.

▷ The H0 is that there is no difference (i.e. H0 = 0) between the diastolic blood pressure measured at these two visits. These are properly paired data, which can be compared using the paired *t*-test. This compares the mean difference between blood pressure measured at the first and second visits with (the hypothesised) zero, thus:

- $t$ = (mean change – 0)/SEM of the mean difference
- $t = 2.30$; $P = 0.03$.

### Confidence interval for the difference between two means

The confidence interval specifies a range of values within which the difference between the means of the two populations (or samples) may lie. It contains all the values of $(\mu 1 - \mu 2)$, or (sample mean 1 – sample mean 2), which would not be rejected in a two-tailed hypothesis test. If the confidence interval contains 0, there is no significant difference between the means of the two groups, at the specified level of confidence.

In example 11, the 95% CI of the difference is:

- $-2.9 \pm (1.26 \times 1.96)$
- $= -2.9 \pm 2.47$
- $= -0.43$ to $-5.37$.

This does not include 0 (both values are negative), so the difference is statistically significant at the 5% level.

#### EXAMPLE 12

▷ Suppose now that data on diastolic blood pressure at booking in 30 women from one hospital has been obtained and are to be compared with those from 22 women at booking in another hospital. The results ($\bar{x} \pm s$) were as follows:

- hospital 1: $62.9 \pm 8.44$; therefore SEM $= 1.54$ mmHg
- hospital 2: $67.2 \pm 7.96$; therefore SEM $= 1.70$ mmHg.

▷ An unpaired *t*-test should be used to compare these two samples of booking diastolic blood pressures with respect to place of booking:

- $$t = \frac{\bar{x}_1 - \bar{x}_2}{s\sqrt{\dfrac{1}{n_1} + \dfrac{1}{n_2}}}$$

where *s* is an estimate of the standard deviation for both samples.

- the *t* statistic would be 1.857, which is not statistically significant ($P = 0.069$)
- the 95% CI for the difference would be $-8.94$ to $0.35$, which includes 0.

▷ Therefore, there is no significant difference between the groups at the two hospitals.

## Correlation

Investigators are often interested in whether two variables are associated, such that as one changes, it affects the other. When both variables are measured on a continuous scale and can be assumed to come from a random sample, correlation analysis is used. Pearson's correlation coefficient (r) tests the degree of association between two variables and is a measure of the scatter of the data around an underlying linear trend.

■ $$r = \frac{\Sigma(x-\bar{x})(y-\bar{y})}{\sqrt{\Sigma(x-\bar{x})^2(y-\bar{y})^2}}$$

The data for at least one, and preferably both, of the observations should be normally distributed. If they are not, either try transforming the data or calculate the non-parametric measure of association, Spearman's ρ, which is a ranking test. In either case, tables of r or ρ can be consulted to show whether or not the correlation is statistically significant, although most statistical packages will provide this information automatically.

In Figure 33.6 A, there is a perfect positive correlation between the independent (x) variable and the dependent (y) variable. Pearson's r would therefore be 1.0.

In Figure 33.6 B, there is a perfect negative correlation between the independent and the dependent variables. The correlation coefficient, r, would therefore be –1.0.

A correlation coefficient of about zero means that there is no linear association between the two variables.

### EXAMPLE 13

▷ In this example, a unit change in x is associated with an entirely predictable change in y. Nothing else influences y. To assess the amount of variability of y accounted for by x, simply square the correlation coefficient, r:

■ If r = 0.4, $r^2$ = 0.16, or 16%.

■ In this case, 16% of the variability in y can be accounted for by change in x.

▷ In Figure 33.7, the correlation between the body mass index and booking systolic pressure in 26 women is statistically significant:

■ Pearson's r = 0.504, $r^2$ = 0.254; P = 0.009.

▷ The line of best fit calculated from the regression equation has a slope of 0.254. Of the variation in the booking systolic blood pressure, 25.4% can be accounted for by variation in the body mass index.

Note for example 13 that if Spearman's ρ had been calculated for the same data, it would have been 0.365, which is not statistically significant (P = 0.067). There is considerable scatter around the line and the less sensitive non-parametric test did not therefore identify the association.

FIGURE 33.6 **Scatterplots**

**A** Positive association

**B** Negative association

FIGURE 33.7 **Scatterplot of booking systolic blood pressure in relation to body mass index**

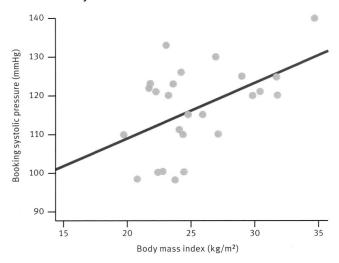

On the other hand, Pearson's correlation is sensitive to outliers, so the rank correlation may have given a truer picture. An awareness of the characteristics of data sets is needed.

It should also never be assumed that, because an association is statistically significant, it is therefore causal. It is always possible that both variables are influenced by something else.

Another technique often used with data on two continuous variables is regression. This allows the value of one variable to be predicted, by knowing the value of the other. It is often possible to describe one as 'independent' and one as 'dependent' by thinking about it. For example, a child's height will be influenced by its age, but its age will not be influenced by its height. Age is therefore the independent variable, plotted, by convention, on the $x$ (horizontal) axis, while height is the dependent variable, plotted on the $y$ (vertical) axis.

Regression calculations allow a 'line of best fit', such as that shown in Figure 33.7, to be calculated, by calculating the slope and the point of intercept on the $y$ axis where $x = 0$. The line of best fit can then be used to predict $y$ for any given $x$.

## Predictive tests

A good predictive test for a disease or condition must be sensitive and specific, with good positive and negative predictive values, which are defined as follows:

- **sensitivity**: the proportion of true positives that are correctly identified by the test
- **specificity**: the proportion of true negatives that are correctly identified by the test
- **positive predictive value**: the proportion of people with positive results who are correctly diagnosed
- **negative predictive value**: the proportion of people with negative results who are correctly diagnosed.

### EXAMPLE 14

▷ Imagine a scenario in which the presence of an abnormal uterine artery resistance index (RI ≥ 0.58) at 24 weeks of gestation is used to predict pre-eclampsia in a group of 144 women:[1]

- 63 women had an RI ≥ 0.58 at 24 weeks; 28 went on to develop pre-eclampsia.
- 81 women had an RI < 0.58 at 24 weeks; 8 went on to develop pre-eclampsia.

▷ This would give the following values:

- true positives (a) = 28
- false positives (b) = 35
- false negatives (c) = 8
- true negatives (d) = 73.

▷ Therefore the sensitivity, specificity and positive and negative predictive values can be calculated:

- sensitivity = a/(a + c) = 28/(28 + 8) = 77.8%
- specificity = d/(b + d) = 73/(35 + 73) = 67.6%
- positive predictive value = a/(a + b) = 28/(28 + 35) = 44.4%
- negative predictive value = d/(c + d) = 73/(8 + 73) = 90.1%.

▷ A caveat is in order here. These formulae for positive and negative predictive values only apply if the proportion of women with pre-eclampsia in the sample accurately reflects the true prevalence of pre-eclampsia in the population. This will not in general be true with case–control type sampling as here.

# Some useful concepts

## INCIDENCE AND PREVALENCE

The incidence ($I$) of a disease is the rate at which new cases of the disease occur in a population previously free of it.

$$I = \frac{r}{N * t}$$

where $r$ = number of new cases, $N$ = population size and $t$ = time interval.

Incidence is often expressed per 1000 or 1 000 000 of the population, to avoid small decimals, and per year, to give the annual incidence rate. The incidence rate is thus the number of new cases per head of the population per unit time.

The prevalence ($P$) of a condition measures the frequency of existing disease at a given time.

$$P = \frac{R}{N}$$

where $R$ = total number of cases at the given time and $N$ = total population at that time.

- In a stable situation, incidence and prevalence are related by:

$$P = I \times D$$

where $D$ is the average duration of the disease.

## CRUDE AND STANDARDISED PROPORTIONS

A crude proportion is one expressed without making any allowance for factors that might influence it. Birth and death rates are crude rates. They are usually expressed per 10 000 or 100 000 of the population, to avoid small decimals.

A standardised proportion is one that has been corrected (standardised) for one or more factors such as smoking, gender, age or race.
When these proportions relate to all events occurring within a specified time, such as a year, they are known as crude and standardised rates.

**TABLE 33.3 Data relating to maternal smoking in pregnancy and outcome (fetal growth restriction) from a sample of 200 pregnancies**

|  |  | Smoker | | |
|---|---|---|---|---|
|  |  | Yes | No | Total |
| Fetal growth restriction | Yes | 11 | 9 | 20 |
|  | No | 59 | 121 | 180 |
|  | Total | 70 | 130 | 200 |

*EXAMPLE 15*

▷ Table 33.3 presents data for a sample of 200 babies, in which 20 had birthweights at or below the 10th centile (fetal growth restriction; FGR):

- The crude proportion of FGR is thus 10%.

▷ Of the mothers, 35% smoked and 11 of these mothers had babies with FGR.

- Proportion of FGR in smokers = 11/70 = 15.7%
- Proportion of FGR in non-smokers = 9/130 = 6.9%
- These are the proportions of FGR standardised for smoking.

## ODDS RATIOS

An odds ratio (OR) gives an estimate, for which a confidence interval can be calculated, for the association between two binary (for example, yes/no) variables and allows testing for the effects of other variables on that association (logistic regression). The odds of an event happening is the ratio of the probability that it does happen to the probability that it does not (for example, if five in 50 people are 'yes', the odds is five in 45 or one in nine).

Table 33.4 shows data from the Genetics of Preeclampsia study.[2] For this retrospective analysis, the outcome of interest was delivery before 34 weeks of gestation, which is displayed in the rows, while the groups were defined on the basis of whether or not the mother had continued to smoke during pregnancy (the columns).

The odds that a woman who delivered before 34 weeks of gestation was also a smoker is calculated as 31/178 (17.42).

TABLE 33.4 **Data relating to maternal smoking in pregnancy and outcome (gestational age at delivery) from a sample of 926 pre-eclamptic pregnancies**

| | | Smoker | | |
|---|---|---|---|---|
| | | Yes | No | Total |
| Delivered before 34 weeks of gestation | Yes | 31 | 178 | 209 |
| | No | 58 | 659 | 717 |
| | Total | 89 | 837 | 926 |

*Source*: Genetics of Preeclampsia Consortium.[2]

The odds that a woman who delivered at or after 34 weeks was also a smoker were 58/659 (8.80). The OR is thus 17.42/8.80, or 1.98. Statistical software will calculate the 95% confidence interval for this ratio, which is 1.24–3.16. The null hypothesis is that there is no difference between the two ORs, that is, that the OR is not significantly different from 1.0. However, in this example, the 95% confidence interval does not cross 1.0, so it can be inferred that continuing to smoke increases the risk of delivery before 34 weeks of gestation.

## RELATIVE RISK

Relative risk (RR) compares the proportions with a particular outcome in two groups selected before the start of a study as differing in one or more features (for example, nulliparous compared with parous, normal build compared with obese). They are thus selected prospectively.

This contrasts with OR, which can be calculated from a prospective or retrospective design.

To illustrate this, imagine that the data in Table 33.4 had come from a study designed to assess whether smoking is associated with very premature delivery. The proportions delivering prematurely are 31/89 (34.83%) in the smoking group and 178/837 (21.27%) in the non-smokers. The relative risk of delivery before 34 weeks of gestation is thus 34.83/21.27, or 1.64. Statistical software will calculate the 95% confidence interval for this ratio, which is 1.20–2.24. The predicted value of the relative risk from H0 is again 1.0. However, in this example, the 95% confidence interval does not cross 1.0, so it can be assumed that smoking is associated with a significantly greater risk of premature delivery.

## QUANTIFICATION OF RISK – THE RISK MATRIX

Clinical risk management is improved when there has been a clear assessment of the likelihood of a risk arising and the consequences if it does. The use of risk matrices such as that shown in Table 33.5 is one way of achieving this. The likelihood of a specified risk arising is shown horizontally and the consequences vertically. The likelihood will be defined from existing data, and there must be agreement as to what each term (Impossible, Unlikely, etc.) means in the context of the risk being assessed. The impact of each is also assigned a score, which should be arrived at as a consensus among experienced staff. Combining these scores, usually by multiplying, allows risks to be described as anything from no risk to high risk and

TABLE 33.5 **Outline example of a risk matrix**

| | | Likelihood | | | | | |
|---|---|---|---|---|---|---|---|
| | | Impossible (0) | Rare (1) | Unlikely (2) | Moderate (3) | Likely (4) | Certain (5) |
| Consequences | Negligible (0) | 0 | 0 | 0 | 0 | 0 | 0 |
| | Minor (1) | 0 | 1 | 2 | 3 | 4 | 5 |
| | Serious (2) | 0 | 2 | 4 | 6 | 8 | 10 |
| | Major (3) | 0 | 3 | 6 | 9 | 12 | 15 |
| | Fatal (4) | 0 | 4 | 8 | 12 | 16 | 20 |

Risk levels: green = minor or negligible | yellow = moderate | orange = major | red = extreme

*Source*: Thompson PJ, Owen JH. (2005).[3]

colour coding is frequently used to alert the users to the overall risk level. An action plan must then be developed for each final risk score category. Another example of an NHS risk score matrix can be found in 'NHS 24 Risk Management Strategy 2009'.[4]

## Levels of evidence

Evidence-based medicine has been described as 'the conscientious, explicit and judicious use of current best evidence in making decisions about the care of individual patients'.[5] To practise evidence-based medicine, the level of evidence needs to be assessed from the type of information that the particular study provides, which may range from a systematic review to the purely anecdotal.

| Level | Evidence |
|---|---|
| 1a | Systematic review and meta-analysis of randomised controlled trials |
| 1b | At least one randomised controlled trial |
| 2a | At least one well-designed controlled study, without randomisation |
| 2b | At least one other type of well-designed, quasi-experimental study |
| 3 | Well-designed descriptive studies |
| 4 | Expert committee reports or opinions and/or clinical experience of respected authorities. |

These levels of evidence have been used by the Clinical Outcomes Group of the National Health Service Executive to develop a slightly simplified grading scheme:

- **Grade A:** requires at least one randomised controlled trial as part of a body of literature of overall good quality and consistency addressing the specific recommendation (evidence levels Ia Ib).
- **Grade B:** requires the availability of well-controlled clinical studies but no randomised clinical trials on the topic of recommendations (evidence levels IIa IIb III).

- **Grade C:** requires evidence obtained from expert committee reports or opinions and/or clinical experiences of respected authorities and indicates an absence of directly applicable clinical studies of good quality (evidence level IV).

## Clinical trials

Clinical trials compare groups of people who differ only with respect to their treatment. In an open trial, both clinician and patient know what treatment the patient is receiving. Allocation to treatment may or may not be random.

It is, however, preferable if allocation to treatment groups is random (to avoid conscious and unconscious bias) and made by those otherwise unconnected with the trial so that neither the patient nor the clinician knows which treatment is being given (a double-blind study). Blinding is less important if the outcome is objective. If only the patient is unaware of the treatment being given, the study is a single-blind study.

However, the Consolidated Standards of Reporting Trials (CONSORT [www.consort-statement.org]) statement suggests that the widely used terms single-blinding and double-blinding should now be avoided as it is clearer to specify who is and who is not blinded.

Outcome measures should be defined before the trial starts. They are usually classified into primary and secondary study outcomes. It is best to concentrate on a single primary outcome, because this is more straightforward to interpret.

### CONTROLS

It is sometimes possible for a person to be their own control. This is optimal, as only one variable differs between 'before' and 'after' treatment or intervention. When this is not possible and allocation to treatment cannot be random and blinded, the control group should be matched for as many variables (for example, age, sex, body mass index, obstetric history) as possible with the treatment group. They should be studied at the same time as the treatment group. If time matching is really impossible, the controls become historical. This is much weaker, because so many underlying variables will have changed.

## Final examples: maternal and neonatal mortality

Around 600 000 women per year die from pregnancy-related causes worldwide, the huge majority in low income countries. Investigators cannot know if mortality rates are falling without baseline data.

### EXAMPLE 16

▷ In Figure 33.8 A and B, note the very different scales on the *y* axes. These scatterplots illustrate the use of simple statistical methods to make numbers more easily assimilable. They show the same worrying trends in both countries. In Jamaica, the rise in indirect deaths is due to HIV/AIDS, cardiac disease and diabetes, while in the UK, the rise in indirect deaths is mainly attributed to cardiac and psychiatric disease.

### EXAMPLE 17

▷ Table 33.6 shows a wide range of neonatal mortality rates across three geographically neighbouring local authorities. The rate in Bromsgrove is statistically significantly different from that in Birmingham because there is no overlap between the lower (5th) percentile for Birmingham and the upper (95th) percentile for Bromsgrove.

Don't forget that there will be many underlying factors affecting the neonatal mortality rates in example 17 and, if interpreted without knowledge of such factors, they could be seriously misinterpreted.

In a placebo-controlled trial of a drug, people are randomly allocated to receive either the active treatment or an apparently identical, but actually inactive, treatment, which may be combined with a standard treatment.

In a crossover trial, the same people are treated in (usually) two different ways (for example, both placebo and active treatment), with a 'washout' period between the two regimes. The order of administration of treatment should be randomised and double-blinded.

FIGURE 33.8 **Scatterplots of maternal mortality rates by triennia with their associated lines of best fit**

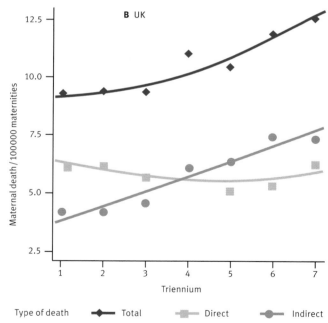

Triennium 1 = 1981–83; 2 = 1993–95; 3 = 1998–2000; 4 = 2001–03;
Triennium 1 = 1985–87; 2 = 1988–90; 3 = 1991–93; 4 = 1994–96;
5 = 1997–99; 6 = 2000–02; 7 = 2003–05.

*Source: Saving Mothers' Lives.*[6]

TABLE 33.6 **Neonatal mortality rates per 1000 live births (2000–02) in the West Midlands**

| Local authority | Rate | 95% confidence interval | |
| --- | --- | --- | --- |
| | | Lower limit | Upper limit |
| Birmingham | 9.19 | 8.31 | 10.13 |
| Lichfield | 6.29 | 3.60 | 10.19 |
| Bromsgrove | 2.45 | 0.90 | 5.32 |

*Source*: University of Birmingham. (2004).[7]

## REFERENCES

1. PARRETTI E, MEALLI F, MAGRINI A, CIONI R, MECACCI F, LA TORRE P, *et al*. Cross-sectional and longitudinal evaluation of uterine artery Doppler velocimetry for the prediction of pre-eclampsia in normotensive women with specific risk factors. *Ultrasound Obstet Gynecol* 2003;22:160–5.

2. BROUGHTON PIPKIN F, The Genetics of Preeclampsia Consortium. Smoking in moderate/severe preeclampsia worsens pregnancy outcome, but smoking cessation limits the damage. *Hypertension* 2008;51:1042–6.

3. THOMPSON PJ, OWEN JH. Risk management in obstetrics; just another inspection or improving patient care? *Fetal Matern Med Rev* 2005;16:195–209.

4. National Health Service. NHS 24 Risk Management Strategy 2009. London: NHS; 2009. [www.nhs24.com/content/mediaassets/board/10.4a%20Risk%20Management%20Strategy.pdf].

5. STRAUSS SE, RICHARDSON WS, GLASZIOU P, HAYNES RB. *Evidence-based Medicine: How to Practice and Teach EBM*. 3rd edition. London: Churchill Livingstone; 2005.

6. LEWIS G, editor. The Confidential Enquiry into Maternal and Child Health. *Saving Mothers' Lives: reviewing maternat deaths to make motherhood safer– 2003–2005*. The Seventh Report on Confidential Enquiries into Maternal Deaths in the United Kingdom. London: CEMACH; 2007.

CHAPTER 34

# Screening and trials statistics

*Andrew H Shennan and Annette Briley*

## Introduction

All clinicians should have a fundamental understanding of statistics as they pertain to screening and clinical trials. Screening is a common phenomenon throughout medicine but particularly in the reproductive sciences.

Research is an organised and systematic process of enquiry. Its aim is to develop concepts and theories and to be able to describe phenomena. It adds to the scientific body of knowledge.[1] Traditionally, knowledge has been gained by experience but by applying research, one can expand and add to the knowledge far more quickly. Research takes the form of many assessments. Each assessment suits a different situation and its quality cannot always be judged by its size or method. For example, a case report may be extremely important in very rare diseases. Clinical trials involving a randomised design are generally viewed as a 'gold standard' for evaluating an intervention. There are a number of types of studies:

- retrospective studies
- systematic research
- qualitative research
- quantitative research
- surveys
- cohort studies
- case–control studies
- randomised control trials.

Statistics are required in clinical investigation to ascertain if events are by chance and to be able to quantify any risk determined.[2] Good clinical practice is now often determined by evidence-based medicine. Although much of knowledge is still based on clinical judgement, increasing amounts of clinical care can be determined by research-acquired evidence. Good clinical care will always be a combination of applying experience with evidence-based knowledge. Whenever possible, clinicians should try to quantify what has previously been qualitative or intuitive decision making. This chapter will outline the principles involved in statistical analysis.

## Determining the size of a study

To answer the research question it addresses, a study must have enough subjects. A study evaluating a single group should have a sample size large enough to give sufficient certainty to influence clinical practice; statistically, this is achieved by a suitably small standard error (SE) for the quantity estimated. When two groups are compared, then a power calculation can be used to give a reasonable certainty (generally 80 or 90%) of detecting a clinically important difference between two groups. It is wise to seek advice from a statistician before commencing any study.

A number of factors must be considered before a sample size can be calculated.

### TYPE OF STUDY

This may range from a single sample study, such as a survey, or be a longitudinal study measuring endpoints at a number of times. When comparing two samples, this could be a case–control or a randomised clinical trial. Once the type of study is known, the sample size will be dependent on a number of other variables.

## PRIMARY OUTCOME MEASURE

This is usually a proportion, that is, a categorical endpoint in a clinical trial (i.e. a yes/no answer). However, it may be the mean of a measurement or a summary score (based on the average of measurements at a number of time points or in different places).

Alternative endpoints may be an ordered scale (for example, worse, no change or better) or a survival time. The choice of endpoint will depend on the clinical situation and the research question. Often, far smaller sample sizes can be obtained from continuous variables (for example, gestational age) rather then categorical variables (for example, proportion of preterm birth). The same question can be answered using different methodology by considering alternative outcome measures, which can influence the feasibility of performing a trial. Equally, with very rare outcomes (for example, perinatal death), clinical trials may simply be impossible because of the inability to recruit sufficient patients; a composite endpoint may therefore be picked. If more then one endpoint is required (for example, if they are equally important or if both maternal and neonatal endpoints are required), then both (or more) can be powered for; $P$-values must take this into account and can be adjusted to account for this 'multiple hypothesis testing'. A secondary endpoint can be powered for, although rarely there is more than one 'primary outcome' – in effect, two or more studies are being performed.

## THE EXPECTED LIKELY VALUES

In new research, pilot data are invaluable in determining likely proportions, or variation in continuous variables (standard deviation). If power is to be calculated from current literature, then, when standard errors are given, standard deviation is calculated as $SE \times \sqrt{n}$ for the standard error of a single mean, or as $SE / (1/\sqrt{n_1} + 1/\sqrt{n_2})$ for the difference between two means. When confidence intervals are given, the SE can be estimated as (upper limit – lower limit)/4 for 30 observations or more.

The difference should be both plausible and clinically important, although economic or scientific importance may be worthwhile, even if not clinically valuable.

When determining the power of a study, one must also determine the size of effect that is clinically important.

Deciding the clinically important size of an effect cannot be done from statistical tables but must be a clinical judgement. The study should be able to determine a difference that is clinically important. There is no point in having a huge study that determines a tiny difference that does not matter. Sometimes it is not possible to carry out a study large enough to determine a clinically important difference and the design accepts that the study is underpowered but may add to new knowledge and possibly to future meta-analyses. It should be called a pilot study.

## Significance level: alpha (*P*-values)

The size and design of a study will determine its ability to get to the truth. The power of the study is the probability that it will detect a difference if there is a real and important effect in reality. The significance level (or alpha) is the probability of falsely detecting a difference when there is in fact no effect. Alpha can be thought of as the target value of the significance test, which is compared with the observed value, also known as the $P$-value, which is found only at the end of the study. Alpha is usually fixed at 0.05 or 5%; so a $P$-value < 0.05 is taken as significant in most studies.

### LIMITATIONS OF *P*-VALUES

The smaller the $P$-value, the stronger the evidence that there is something going on. (The $P$-value actually measures the chance of the observed result if there is in fact nothing going on.) By convention, a value of $P < 0.05$ (one in 20) is generally taken as a significant difference. One in 20 is actually more likely than rolling a double 6 (one in 36); so it can and does happen by chance. So conventional cut-offs (to determine that something is significant), sometimes do get it wrong (that is, a $P$-value < 0.05 when no real difference exists).

$P$-values are not magical or all important. This should not come as a surprise. In all things in medicine, it is not always clear whether something is real or not (for example, a blood pressure of 88 mmHg does not guarantee that a patient does not have hypertension). Equally a $P$-value of 0.051 does not mean that a real difference does not exist. If there are multiple endpoints to a study, then the chance of one of them being significant when there is no real difference is higher than 5%. All these factors must be taken into account when interpreting *P*-values.

When determining the power of a study, a single primary endpoint is generally defined and powered for in the study design. This prevents the problem of multiple hypotheseis testing.

## Power of a study: beta values

At the same time as deciding the alpha value, we need to think about the chance of getting a significant result if there is a real and important effect (also known as the power of the study or beta). The beta value needs to be as high as possible. In an ideal world you would test every patient who had the disease but, in practice, one has to check a sample. The power therefore depends upon how big the sample is. A 90% power would have a 90% chance of finding a clinically important difference between groups. Studies are generally designed with a 90% power where possible, but sometimes 80% or less has to be accepted to make the trial or study feasible.

## Type 1 and type 2 errors

Once results are published, it is clear that they may be misleading (that is, the truth cannot always be determined), depending upon whether a representative sample has been collected or whether you fall on the wrong side of an arbitrary standard by chance. These are known as type 1 or type 2 errors.

A type 1 error occurs when a correct hypothesis is rejected. In practice, a type 1 error means that a difference is found which is not real (for example, a study may be published that shows a drug reduces blood pressure when the truth is that the drug does not but this study showed it by chance). This sometimes occurs because of publication bias (that is, many unpublished studies have been done on the drug but only the one that shows a significant difference is published whereas the others are not). The reason for type 1 errors is that the 5% arbitrary alpha value, determined by the *P*-value, will get it wrong in one in 20 times.

The other type of error, a type 2 error, is more common, which is when an incorrect hypothesis is accepted.

It generally occurs because the sample size is too small (that is, there is a difference but it is not big enough to fall the right side of the *P*-value, for example, a drug affecting blood pressure is not found to do so). The difference in blood pressure may be 10 mmHg, which may be clinically important but, because of the small sample size, it does not have a *P*-value < 0.05 and therefore the study determines that the drug does not make the blood pressure fall.

Using correct power calculations will limit the chance of these errors.

## Generalisability

When planning a study, one must consider if the sample is representative of the whole population. The larger the study, the more likely this will occur; however, in the rarefied environment of research one may select women who are not representative. For example, if you are doing a clinical trial on epidurals, the research team may be more likely to recruit women during the day who have different characteristics to women who present throughout the 24-hour period.

When evaluating the results of studies, one must consider whether those who entered the study were also likely to be from the general population. One way to determine this is to look at the event rates. For example, the normal vaginal delivery rate in women with epidurals may be higher in the general population than in the study. This suggests that women have been recruited who are different and therefore the generalisability, or the ability to apply the findings to all populations, of the results must be questioned.

Statistical packages are readily available to determine power. However, a basic understanding of the determinants of power (that is, the alpha or beta value) is required, together with the clinical factors.

## Analysing the size of an effect: odds ratios and relative risks

A study or clinical trial may show a significant difference. Clinicians must be aware of the importance of this difference and how it applies to their patients or the population they are interested in.

Odds ratios are generally used to determine the difference between groups (for example, exposed to risk factors or not). Odds are calculated by dividing the number of times an event occurs by the number of times it does not. They are calculated by dividing the odds of being exposed to a risk factor with the odds in a controlled group. Therefore an odds ratio of 1 shows no difference between groups. An odds ratio of more or less than 1 demonstrates an increased or reduced effect, respectively. This may not be significant if the confidence limits cross 1.

Relative risk is similar but is calculated by dividing the risk in a treated or exposed group by a risk in a controlled or unexposed group. In a clinical trial, a relative risk reduction is therefore the proportion by which the intervention reduced the event rate. Relative risks are often given in preference to odds ratios when looking at an effect from a clinical trial. A relative risk reduction of 0.5, therefore, means the intervention will reduce the event by a half. The certainty to which this has occurred is determined by 95% confidence intervals. If the confidence intervals cross 1, then there is a higher possibility that the intervention does not work. Equally if the confidence intervals are wide and approach 1, then the effect may not be as certain. Confidence intervals therefore are the percentage of the time that the true value would fall within these limits. 95% is generally accepted as being appropriate and implies that 95% of the time the true effect is within the limits given.

As an example of how to calculate odds ratios and relative risk, imagine a new fertility drug is given to 100 women and in 1 year 12% conceive, whereas 4% conceive in 100 controls. The risk ratio or relative risk (of conceiving) is therefore:

- 12/4 = 3.

Odds ratios can also be used but usually are taken when an accurate denominator is unknown (for example, in a case–control study when the outcome is rare). For the same example as above, it is calculated by:

- 12/88 : 4/96 as a ratio.

In clinical trials, the denominator is known and therefore relative risks are generally used.

## Screening

The National Screening Committee in 2001 described screening as 'a public health service in which members of a defined population, who do not perceive they are at risk of, or already affected by, a disease or its complications, are asked questions or offered a test to identify those individuals who are more likely to be helped than harmed by further tests or treatment to reduce the risks of disease or its complications'.[3]

The aim of all screening programmes is to detect an individual's predisposition for a disease, preferably at an early stage when the person is considered to be disease free and an intervention is possible. The efficacy of a screening test is assessed by the numbers of people screened who go on to develop the disease. It is impossible to determine absolute risk because of the inability to collect sufficient numbers, therefore screening is calculated using a mathematical formula. Because of the distribution of diseases, there is always a false positive rate. Currently, antenatal screening methods for chromosomal abnormalities mean that around 5% of women will be incorrectly identified to achieve approximately an 80% detection rate.[4] Women will also be incorrectly identified at low risk but will have an affected baby. Whether these risks are acceptable depends on the circumstances and higher or lower false detection rates can be accepted depending on the clinical scenario. For example, women will accept an unnecessary amniocentesis but would not want a Down syndrome baby 'missed', whereas a screening test for pre-eclampsia may not detect all cases of pre-eclampsia; this will be identified in most cases through antenatal screening, so it is not as important to detect all cases.

The prerequisites for screening tests are:[5]

- being simple, safe and acceptable
- having a high sensitivity and specificity with good predictor values
- being reproducible
- having limited overlap between affected and non-affected individuals
- having defined cut-off levels
- being cost effective and therefore relatively inexpensive.

In addition, the condition to which the test is applied should have certain characteristics: it should be an important treatable health problem with established diagnostic strategies, which includes an acceptable test. The natural history of the disease should be defined, preferably with a latent stage, and there should be an agreed policy regarding who to treat.

To understand the statistics for screening, one must consider how useful a test is. A test can give a positive or negative result, both of which can be correct or incorrect (that is, there are four possibilities). To calculate the predictive statistics used in screening, one must consider whether the test result is a true or false positive or a true or false negative. The efficiency of a test can be determined by working out sensitivity and specificity or positive and negative predictive values. Other parameters such as relative risk and likelihood ratios can also be determined and will be described. Table 34.1 demonstrates how the clinical efficiency of a test can be calculated.

## SENSITIVITY

Sensitivity is the proportion of all cases that have an abnormal test result. For example, if the detection of umbilical artery notches has a 90% sensitivity to predict pre-eclampsia, it would imply that 90% of women with pre-eclampsia will have an abnormal uterine artery notch.

TABLE 34.1 **Calculating the clinical efficiency of a test**

| Measure | Formula | |
|---|---|---|
| Sensitivity | TP/(TP + FP) | |
| Specificity | TN/(FP + TN) | |
| Predictive values (positive) | TP/(FP + TP) | |
| Predictive values (negative) | TN/(TN + FN) | |
| Relative risk | TP/(TP + FP) | |
| | FN/(FN + TN) | |
| Likelihood ratio | TP/(TP + FN) | Sensitivity |
| | FP/(TN + FP) | or Specificity |
| Odds ratio | Probability/(1 − probability) | |
| Accuracy | (TP + TN)/total | |

T = true | F = false | P = positive | N = negative

## SPECIFICITY

Specificity is the proportion of cases that do not have a clinical abnormality with a normal test result. The equivalent statement would be that 90% of women without pre-eclampsia have a normal uterine artery Doppler result.

## PREDICTIVE VALUES

Although sensitivity and specificity are useful for looking at the entire population, they do not give information about the individual. Predictive values are more applicable for an individual (that is, they give the percentage chance of that individual being affected or unaffected). These are useful to the clinician but are also highly dependent on the prevalence of the disease concerned. If a disease is rare, even a bad test will have a high negative prediction. A positive prediction is a proportion of cases with an abnormal test result that have the clinical abnormality. So, the positive prediction of an abnormal uterine artery Doppler result (where one in five get the disease) for prediction of pre-eclampsia would imply that 20% of women with an abnormal uterine artery Doppler result will get pre-eclampsia. Negative prediction is the proportion of cases with a normal test result that do not have the clinical abnormality. For example, 99% of women with a normal uterine artery Doppler result will not get pre-eclampsia.

## LIKELIHOOD RATIOS

Other tests are sometimes used to look at the efficiency of a test. For example, a likelihood ratio is the effectiveness of a particular diagnostic test to confirm or exclude a particular diagnosis. The likelihood is a ratio of the event rate before and after the test, so therefore a likelihood ratio of 1 means that the patient is no more or less likely to have a condition once she has had the test. A good test will therefore have a high likelihood ratio. The advantage of using the likelihood ratio is that it can be applied to different populations who are at lower and higher risk. Likelihood ratios generally stay the same in high and low risk populations although this cannot be guaranteed. For example, a fetal fibronectin test to predict preterm birth generally has a high likelihood ratio

FIGURE 34.1 **Receiver–operating characteristic curve**

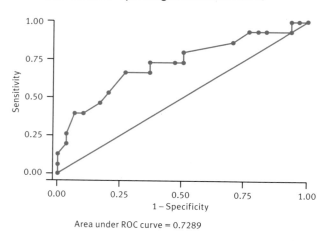

Area under ROC curve = 0.7289

of approximately 10–15. This is similar in a high and low risk population although the absolute risk (that is, the positive prediction) is very different depending on the risk status of the woman.

## Receiver–operating characteristic curves

Figure 34.1 shows a receiver–operating characteristic (ROC) curve. This is a plot of the sensitivity against the false positive rate (also determined as 1 – specificity.) As the sensitivity of a test increases, there will be an inevitable increase in the false positive rate. If there is no discriminatory power, then a ROC curve will effectively be a straight line. This is equivalent to tossing a coin, but a good test will have a high sensitivity with only a small reduction in the false positive rate and therefore the ROC curve will head towards the top left-hand corner of the graph.

ROC curves are useful in determining the best cut-off. For example, a low blood pressure to diagnose pre-eclampsia would have a high sensitivity but clearly there would be a lot of false cases included. Equally, a high blood pressure, say a diastolic over 100 mmHg would ensure that there were very few false determinants of pre-eclampsia but obviously some cases would be missed. A diastolic of 90 mmHg is at the highest point to the top left corner on a graph (that is, the optimal balance between sensitivity and false positive rates) and hence is used as a cut-off for determining risk when diagnosing hypertension in pregnancy. For some tests, sensitivity may be 'sacrificed' at the expense of improving false positive rates depending on the clinical significance. For example, in Down syndrome screening, one accepts very high false positive rates (as the test will be confirmed by amniocentesis) but sensitivity must be as high as possible because 'missed' cases are unacceptable to most women. Down syndrome screening is far from perfect.[6]

## Conclusion

Statistical analysis is just another tool. All clinicians should understand the importance of asking the right question and understand the limitations of statistical analysis. Used correctly, statistics in clinical practice can augment our knowledge and benefit clinical care enormously. Clinicians do not have to be statisticians, but they must engage in the process to understand the best way to inform their practice.

## REFERENCES

1. BOWLING A. *Research Methods in Health*. Buckingham, Philadelphia: Open University Press; 1997.

2. HARRIS M, TAYLOR G. *Medical Statistics Made Easy*. London: Taylor & Francis Group; 2004.

3. National Screening Committee. *Second Report of the UK National Screening Committee*. London: Department of Health; 2001.

4. WALD N J, KENNARD A, HACKSHAW A, MAGUIRE A. Antenatal screening for Down's syndrome. *Health Technol Assess* 1998;2:i–iv,1–112.

5. CUCKLE HS, WALD NJ. Principles of Screening. In: *Antenatal and Neonatal Screening*. Oxford: Oxford University Press; 1984. p.1–22.

6. WHITTLE M. Down's syndrome screening: where to now? *BJOG* 2001;108:559–61.

## USEFUL SOURCES OF INFORMATION

**Centre of Research**: Ethical Campaign [www.corec.org.uk].

**EudraCT**: [https://eudract.emea.europa.eu].

**Institute of Clinical Research**: e-mail: info@ instituteofclinicalresearch.com; Tel: 01628 899755; [www.instituteofclinicalresearch.com].

**Medicines and Healthcare products Regulatory Agency (MHRA)**: e-mail: info@mhra.gsi.gov.uk; Tel: 0207 084 2000; [http://www.mhra.gov.uk/].

**RDDirect**: e-mail: info@rddirect.org.uk; Tel: 0113 295 1122 (Monday to Friday 8.30 a.m. to 5.00 p.m.); [www.rddirect.org.uk].

# CHAPTER 35

# Epidemiology

*Arri Coomarasamy and Khalid S Khan*

## An analytical clinical epidemiologist

Analyses of deaths due to puerperal fever by Ignaz Semmelweiss in Vienna in the early 19th century demonstrated the power of epidemiology. At the age of 28, Semmelweiss deduced that by not washing hands doctors caused or contributed to this deadly disease. In his maternity unit, 20% of the 3000 women who delivered died of puerperal fever. After he commanded that every doctor and nurse on his ward wash their hands with chlorine, the mortality rates from puerperal fever plum-meted down to about 1%! But doctors did not believe Semmelweiss's findings. Rather than being honoured, he was ridiculed and ultimately dismissed from his job.

A dismissed and desperate Semmelweiss stood next to the sink and scolded anyone who forgot to scrub their hands. He wrote to a fellow obstetrician: 'You, Herr Professor, have been a partner in this massacre'. Over time, he began to be considered a lunatic by his own staff. Practice only started to change two decades later when Lister published his seminal work on antisepsis in the medical journal *The Lancet*.

## Introduction

The term 'epidemiology' was conceived to describe the study of epidemics, such as cholera and plague. The term has now acquired a wider meaning to include the study of the distribution of all varieties of diseases in various populations and the factors that influence the occurrence of these diseases. Epidemiology has numerous branches, including those discussed here.

### OBSERVATIONAL EPIDEMIOLOGY

This branch relies on the surveillance of populations and subgroups, using various health statistics and resources. An example would be the study of maternal death rates categorised by age and cause of death. Data are often obtained from national or other registries and other administrative data sources. Analysis for trends, particularly over time, is often an important aspect of observa-tional epidemiology. The Centre for Maternal and Child Enquiries (CMACE) reports represent an exercise in observational epidemiology.

### ANALYTICAL OBSERVATIONAL EPIDEMIOLOGY

Addition of analytical methods to observational epide-miological studies can sometimes allow powerful infer-ences to be drawn about causation and associations. The main analytical methods are the case–control and the cohort study. Influential examples of this branch of epi-demiology are again the CMACE reports, which use quantitative and qualitative methods.

### EXPERIMENTAL EPIDEMIOLOGY

Experimental epidemiology includes studies in which the researcher investigates the effects of intentional inter-vention on the outcome of a disease. A study design that

515

TABLE 35.1 **Definitions of maternal deaths**

| Term | Definition |
| --- | --- |
| Maternal deaths [a] | Deaths of women while pregnant or within 42 days of the end of the pregnancy [b] from any cause related to or aggravated by the pregnancy or its management but not from accidental or incidental causes. |
| Direct [a] | Deaths resulting from obstetric complications of the pregnant state (pregnancy, labour and puerperium), from interventions, omissions, incorrect treatment or from a chain of events resulting from any of the above. |
| Indirect [a] | Deaths resulting from previous existing disease or disease that developed during pregnancy and which was not due to direct obstetric causes but which was aggravated by the physiological effects of pregnancy. |
| Late [c] | Deaths occurring between 42 days and one year after abortion, miscarriage or delivery that are due to *direct* or *indirect* maternal causes. |
| Coincidental (fortuitous) [d] | Deaths from unrelated causes which happen to occur in pregnancy or the puerperium. |
| Pregnancy-related deaths [c] | Deaths occurring in women while pregnant or within 42 days of termination of pregnancy, irrespective of the cause of the death. |

[a] ICD 9  |  [b] This term includes delivery, ectopic pregnancy, miscarriage or termination of pregnancy  |  **c** ICD 10  |
[d] ICD 9/10 classified these deaths as *Fortuitous* but the Enquiry prefers to use the term *Coincidental* as it is a more accurate description  |
The Enquiry also considers deaths from *Late Coincidental* causes

*Reproduced with permission from: Saving Mothers' Lives. London: CEMACH; 2008.* [3]

is often used in this branch of epidemiology is the randomised controlled trial (RCT), which employs random allocation of participants to alternative interventions, with the aim of reducing bias.

## CLINICAL EPIDEMIOLOGY AND EVIDENCE-BASED MEDICINE

More recently, doctors and other healthcare professionals discovered the value of epidemiological methods in enhancing their clinical practice, particularly with regards to their diagnoses and therapies, primarily through meticulous attention to the nature and quality of the evidence on which clinical decisions are based. This discipline has now been given structure and form with the term evidence-based medicine (EBM), which is the conscientious and judicious use of evidence in conjunction with clinical expertise and patients' preferences and values. EBM is now accepted as an essential tool to bring evidence to the bedside and it permeates right through from patient–clinician interaction to healthcare purchasing and policy making. EMB provides hierarchies of evidence to determine what constitutes best available evidence.

## THE ORIGINS OF CLINICAL EPIDEMIOLOGY AND EVIDENCE-BASED MEDICINE

Ancient Greek and Roman philosophers considered health care and medicine to be a stochastic art. This means that it is an art with the peculiar characteristic of unpredictability between means and ends, such that from the outcome of patients it cannot be inferred that the correct principles of management were followed. Because of this unpredictability, healthcare practitioners cannot always infer what will happen to the individual patient before them without reliance on external evidence. The development of numerical methods in conducting patient-centred research (clinical epidemiology) has provided clinicians the tools to deal with unpredictability.

The term EBM was coined in the 1980s to name the clinical strategy of asking questions, finding and appraising relevant data and harnessing this information for everyday clinical practice. Interestingly, it was not until 1992 that this clinical paradigm officially appeared in a peer-reviewed journal, the *Journal of the American Medical Association*.[1] The EBM paradigm asserts that potential advances in health care must be tested and proven to

TABLE 35.2  **Definitions of fetal and neonatal deaths**

| Term | Definition |
|------|------------|
| Late fetal loss | An *in utero* death delivered between $22^{+0}$ and $23^{+6}$ weeks' gestation. |
| Stillbirth | A baby delivered with no signs of life after 24 completed weeks of pregnancy. |
| Early neonatal death | Death of a live born baby occurring less than seven completed days from the time of birth. |
| Late neonatal death | Death of a live born baby occurring after the seventh day and before 28 completed days from the time of birth. |
| Stillbirth rate | Number of stillbirths per 1000 live births and stillbirths. |
| Stillbirth rate (WHO) | Number of late fetal losses and stillbirths per 1000 live births, stillbirths and late fetal losses. |
| Perinatal mortality rate (UK) | Number of stillbirths and early neonatal deaths per 1000 live births and stillbirths. |
| Perinatal mortality rate (WHO) | Number of late fetal losses, stillbirths and early neonatal deaths per 1000 live births and stillbirths. |
| Neonatal mortality rate | Number of neonatal deaths per 1000 live births. |
| Live birth | The complete expulsion or extraction from its mother of a product of conception, irrespective of the duration of pregnancy, which, after such separation, breathes or shows any other evidence of life, such as beating of the heart, pulsation of the umbilical cord or any definite movement of voluntary muscles, whether or not the umbilical cord has been cut or the placenta is attached. |

WHO = World Health Organization

*Reproduced with permission from: Perinatal Mortality 2006. London: CEMACH; 2008.*[6]

do more good than harm before they are incorporated into practice.

## Maternal, neonatal and perinatal mortality

### DEFINITIONS

The International Classification of Diseases (ICD10)[2] defines a maternal death as 'the death of a woman while pregnant or within 42 days of termination of pregnancy, from any cause related to or aggravated by the pregnancy or its management, but not from accidental or incidental causes'. Maternal deaths can be subdivided into various groups, as given in Table 35.1. The definitions relating to fetal and neonatal deaths are summarised in Table 35.2.

### THE CEMACH PROGRAMME

CMACE commenced in April 2003 with a remit to provide reports and analyses on the health of mothers, babies and children carrying out confidential enquiries on a nationwide basis. The Confidential Enquiry into Maternal and Child Health (CEMACH) lies within CMACE and is divided into two sub-programmes: the maternal and perinatal health enquiry (ongoing) and the child health enquiry (scheduled to finish in 2012). Before April 2003, these activities were reported separately by the Confidential Enquiry into Maternal Deaths (CEMD) and the Confidential Enquiry into Stillbirths and Deaths in Infancy (CESDI).

The activities, audits and reports by CMACE are commissioned by the National Patient Safety Agency as part of their responsibility for the national confidential enquiry programme. The Department of Health, Social Services and Public Safety through the Health Promo-

TABLE 35.3 **Trends in maternal deaths in the UK**

| Triennium | Direct deaths known to the Enquiry | | | | Indirect deaths known to the Enquiry | | | | Total direct and indirect deaths known to the Enquiry | | | |
|---|---|---|---|---|---|---|---|---|---|---|---|---|
| | Number | Rate | 95% CI | | Number | Rate | 95% CI | | Number | Rate | 95% CI | |
| 1985–87 | 139 | 6.13 | 5.19 | 7.23 | 84 | 3.70 | 2.99 | 4.58 | 223 | 9.83 | 8.62 | 11.21 |
| 1988–90 | 145 | 6.14 | 5.22 | 7.23 | 93 | 3.94 | 3.22 | 4.83 | 238 | 10.08 | 8.88 | 11.45 |
| 1991–93 | 128 | 5.53 | 4.65 | 6.57 | 100 | 4.32 | 3.55 | 5.25 | 228 | 9.85 | 8.65 | 11.21 |
| 1994–96 | 134 | 6.10 | 5.15 | 7.22 | 134 | 6.10 | 5.15 | 7.22 | 268 | 12.19 | 10.82 | 13.74 |
| 1997–99 | 106 | 4.99 | 4.13 | 6.04 | 136 | 6.40 | 5.41 | 7.57 | 242 | 11.40 | 10.05 | 12.92 |
| 2000–02 | 106 | 5.31 | 4.39 | 6.42 | 155 | 7.76 | 6.63 | 9.08 | 261 | 13.07 | 11.57 | 14.75 |
| 2003–05 | 132 | 6.24 | 5.27 | 7.40 | 163 | 7.71 | 6.61 | 8.99 | 295 | 13.95 | 12.45 | 15.64 |
| Change in rate 2000–02 to 2003–05 | | 0.94 | −0.54 | 2.42 | | 0.05 | −1.66 | 1.77 | | 0.89 | −1.37 | 3.14 |

*Reproduced with permission from: Saving Mothers' Lives. London: CEMACH; 2007.*[3]

tion Agency for Northern Ireland and NHS Quality Improvement Scotland also add to this programme. The various publications by CMACE can be freely accessed at www.cmace.org.uk.

## MATERNAL DEATHS IN THE UK

The CEMD reports are published every 3 years. The seventh report, entitled *Saving Mothers' Lives*,[3] was published in December 2007, covering the triennium 2003–05. During this period, 295 women died from conditions directly or indirectly related to pregnancy out of more than two million births in the UK, giving a maternal mortality rate of 13.95 in 100 000 maternities. This represents a slight but statistically non-significant increase from the previous triennium.[4] Also in common with the previous report, the overall maternal mortality rate from indirect causes is still higher than the deaths from direct causes, although the gap between them has narrowed (Table 35.3).

Despite the multifaceted approaches over the years to reduce maternal mortality in the UK, there is an apparent lack of progress. The reasons for this are thought to be multifactorial, although the following issues have been highlighted to be contributory factors in the CEMD reports:

- **Increasing age of mothers:** The mean age of motherhood is on the increase (although no association between maternal death and age has been shown in the seventh report).[3]
- **Overweight and obesity:** Over 50% of the pregnant women for whom body mass index was known were found to be overweight or obese in the CEMD report. Obesity is associated with a number of complications associated with pregnancy and childbirth, including cardiac disease, pre-eclampsia, gestational diabetes, thromboembolism, post-caesarean wound infection and postpartum haemorrhage.
- **Migrant women:** The number of migrant women in the UK has steadily risen and there are proportionately more deaths among these women. Many migrant women have poor obstetric histories, with complicated pregnancies or serious underlying medical conditions. Black African women, including asylum seekers and newly arrived refugees, have a mortality rate nearly six times higher than white women in the UK. Black Caribbean and Middle Eastern women also have a significantly higher mortality rate, although lower than that of black African women.

TABLE 35.4  **Causes and number and rates of direct deaths in the UK**

| Cause of death | 1985–87 | 1988–90 | 1991–93 | 1994–96 | 1997–99 | 2000–02 | 2003–05 | 1985–87 | 1988–90 | 1991–93 | 1994–96 | 1997–99 | 2000–02 | 2003–05 |
|---|---|---|---|---|---|---|---|---|---|---|---|---|---|---|
| | Deaths | | | | | | | Rates/100 000 maternities | | | | | | |
| Thrombosis and thromboembolism | 32 | 33 | 35 | 48 | 35 | 30 | 41 | 1.41 | 1.40 | 1.51 | 2.18 | 1.65 | 1.50 | 1.94 |
| Pre-eclampsia and eclampsia | 27 | 27 | 20 | 20 | 16 | 14 | 18 | 1.19 | 1.14 | 0.86 | 0.91 | 0.75 | 0.70 | 0.85 |
| Haemorrhage | 10 | 22 | 15 | 12 | 7 | 17 | 14 | 0.44 | 0.93 | 0.65 | 0.55 | 0.33 | 0.85 | 0.66 |
| Amniotic fluid embolism | 9 | 11 | 10 | 17 | 8 | 5 | 17 | 0.40 | 0.47 | 0.43 | 0.77 | 0.38 | 0.25 | 0.80 |
| Early pregnancy deaths | 16 | 24 | 17 | 15 | 17 | 15 | 14 | 0.71 | 1.02 | 0.73 | 0.68 | 0.80 | 0.75 | 0.66 |
| Ectopic | 11 | 15 | 9 | 12 | 13 | 11 | 10 | 0.48 | 0.64 | 0.39 | 0.55 | 0.61 | 0.55 | 0.47 |
| Spontaneous miscarriage | 4 | 6 | 3 | 2 | 2 | 1 | 1 | 0.18 | 0.25 | 0.13 | 0.09 | 0.09 | 0.05 | 0.05 |
| Legal termination | 1 | 3 | 5 | 1 | 2 | 3 | 2 | 0.04 | 0.13 | 0.22 | 0.05 | 0.09 | 0.15 | 0.09 |
| Other | 0 | 0 | 2 | 0 | 0 | 0 | 1 | 0.00 | 0.00 | 0.09 | 0.00 | 0.00 | 0.00 | 0.14 |
| Genital tract sepsis | 9 | 17 | 15 | 16 | 18 | 13 | 18 | 0.40 | 0.72 | 0.65 | 0.73 | 0.85 | 0.65 | 0.85 |
| Other direct | 27 | 17 | 14 | 7 | 7 | 8 | 4 | 1.19 | 0.72 | 0.60 | 0.32 | 0.33 | 0.40 | 0.19 |
| Genital tract trauma | 6 | 3 | 4 | 5 | 2 | 1 | 3 | 0.26 | 0.13 | 0.17 | 0.23 | 0.09 | 0.05 | 0.14 |
| Fatty liver | 6 | 5 | 2 | 2 | 4 | 3 | 1 | 0.26 | 0.21 | 0.09 | 0.09 | 0.19 | 0.15 | 0.05 |
| Other causes | 15 | 9 | 8 | 0 | 1 | 4 | 0 | 0.66 | 0.38 | 0.35 | 0.00 | 0.05 | 0.20 | 0.00 |
| Anaesthetic | 6 | 4 | 8 | 1 | 3 | 6 | 6 | 0.23 | 0.17 | 0.35 | 0.05 | 0.14 | 0.30 | 0.28 |
| All *direct* | 139 | 145 | 128 | 134 | 106 | 106 | 132 | 6.13 | 6.14 | 5.53 | 6.10 | 4.99 | 5.31 | 6.24 |

*Reproduced with permission from: Saving Mothers' Lives. London: CEMACH; 2007.*[3]

## Direct maternal deaths in the UK

Thromboembolism was the most common cause of direct deaths in the seventh CEMD report (Table 35.4).[3] There was a slight rise in deaths from sepsis and pre-eclampsia but reductions in deaths from haemorrhage, anaesthesia and uterine trauma. There was also an unexplained rise in deaths from amniotic fluid embolism.

## Indirect maternal deaths in the UK

Cardiac disease was the most common cause of indirect deaths and maternal deaths overall (Table 35.5). This was primarily due to acquired heart disease in younger women related to obesity, poor diet and smoking.

In the seventh CEMD report for the triennium 2003–05,[3] there was a welcome decrease in the rate of suicide, which was the overall leading cause of death in the previous triennium.[4] If sustained in the next triennium, this decline may indicate that the recommendations made in the last two reports concerning identifying women at potential risk in the antenatal period and developing management plans for them are having a beneficial effect.

TABLE 35.5 **Causes and number and rates of indirect deaths in the UK**

| Cause of death | 1985–87 | 1988–90 | 1991–93 | 1994–96 | 1997–99 | 2000–02 | 2003–05 | 1985–87 | 1988–90 | 1991–93 | 1994–96 | 1997–99 | 2000–02 | 2003–05 |
|---|---|---|---|---|---|---|---|---|---|---|---|---|---|---|
| | Deaths | | | | | | | Rates/100 000 maternities | | | | | | |
| Cardiac | 23 | 18 | 37 | 39 | 35 | 44 | 48 | 1.01 | 0.76 | 1.60 | 1.77 | 1.65 | 2.20 | 2.27 |
| Psychiatric *indirect* | – | – | – | 9 | 15 | 16 | 18 | – | – | – | 0.41 | 0.71 | 0.80 | 0.85 |
| Other *indirect* | 62 | 75 | 63 | 86 | 75 | 90 | 87 | 2.73 | 3.18 | 2.72 | 3.91 | 3.53 | 4.51 | 4.12 |
| *Indirect* malignancies | – | – | – | – | 11 | 5 | 10 | – | – | – | – | 0.52 | 0.25 | 0.47 |
| All *indirect* | 84 | 93 | 100 | 134 | 136 | 155 | 163 | 3.70 | 3.94 | 4.32 | 6.10 | 6.40 | 7.76 | 7.71 |

– = data not previously collected separately

*Reproduced with permission from: Saving Mothers' Lives. London: CEMACH; 2007.*[3]

## Top ten recommendations to reduce maternal mortality in the UK

To ensure that the most crucial messages are not lost, the authors of the seventh CEMD report[3] have compiled a list of top ten recommendations that every commissioner, provider, policy maker and other stakeholder involved in providing maternity services are asked to introduce, implement and audit. This list is reproduced in Box 35.1. The rationale for the recommendations can be found in the full report.[2]

## MATERNAL DEATHS – AN INTERNATIONAL PERSPECTIVE

The maternal deaths in the UK and the rest of the developed world represent less than 1% of the total maternal deaths worldwide. More than 99% of the 500 000 women who die during pregnancy or childbirth do so in the developing world. It is therefore essential to understand the epidemiology of maternal deaths and disability elsewhere in the world, particularly in the developing world. The lifetime risk of death from pregnancy and childbirth may be as high as one in 16 in the developing world, compared with about one in 10 000 in the developed world. The maternal mortality rate is estimated to be about 830 in 100 000 (almost one in 100 mothers) in sub-Saharan Africa, compared with 24 in 100 000 in Europe (Table 35.6). These figures represent the largest public health divergence in the world. However, this is in many ways

only the tip of the iceberg, as it is estimated that: (i) around 20 million women a year are left with serious ill health or disability as a result of pregnancy and childbirth; (ii) millions of children are left motherless; and (iii) an estimated one million young children die as a result of the death of their mother.

## Causes of maternal deaths worldwide

A systematic review consisting of 34 datasets (35 197 maternal deaths) found wide regional variation in the causes of maternal deaths.[5] Some of the main findings are listed below:

- Haemorrhage was the leading cause of death in Africa (point estimate 33.9%, range 13.3–43.6%) and in Asia (30.8%, 5.9–48.5%).
- Hypertensive disorders were responsible for the most deaths in Latin America and the Caribbean (25.7%, 7.9–52.4%).
- Deaths due to abortion were the highest in Latin America and the Caribbean (12%), as high as 30% of all deaths in some countries in this region.
- Deaths due to sepsis were higher in Africa (odds ratio 2.71), Asia (1.91) and Latin America and the Caribbean (2.06) than in developed countries.

It is estimated that approximately 80% of maternal deaths are due to direct obstetric causes and 20% due to indirect causes (Table 35.7). The five leading direct causes are postpartum haemorrhage, sepsis, pre-eclampsia and

BOX 35.1 **The top ten recommendations regarding maternal mortality in the UK**

### PRECONCEPTION CARE

1. Preconception counselling and support, both opportunistic and planned, should be provided for women of childbearing age with pre-existing serious medical or mental health conditions which may be aggravated by pregnancy. This includes obesity. This recommendation especially applies to women prior to having assisted reproduction and other fertility treatments.

### ACCESS TO CARE

2. Maternity service providers should ensure that antenatal services are accessible and welcoming so that all women, including those who currently find it difficult to access maternity care, can reach them easily and earlier in their pregnancy. Women should also have had their first full booking visit and hand-held maternity record completed by 12 completed weeks of pregnancy.

3. Pregnant women who, on referral to maternity services, are already 12 or more weeks pregnant should be seen within 2 weeks of the referral.

### MIGRANT WOMEN

4. All pregnant mothers from countries where women may experience poorer overall general health, and who have not previously had a full medical examination in the United Kingdom, should have a medical history taken and clinical assessment made of their overall health, including a cardiovascular examination at booking, or as soon as possible thereafter. This should be performed by an appropriately trained doctor, who could be their usual GP. Women from countries where genital mutilation, or cutting, is prevalent should be sensitively asked about this during their pregnancy and management plans for delivery agreed during the antenatal period.

### SYSTOLIC HYPERTENSION REQUIRES TREATMENT

5. All pregnant women with a systolic blood pressure of 160 mmHg or more require antihypertensive treatment. Consideration should also be given to initiating treatment at lower pressures if the overall clinical picture suggests rapid deterioration and/or where the development of severe hypertension can be anticipated.

### CAESAREAN SECTION

6.1 While recognising that for some mothers and/or their babies caesarean section may be the safest mode of delivery, mothers must be advised that caesarean section is not a risk-free procedure and can cause problems in current and future pregnancies.

6.2 Women who have had a previous caesarean section must have placental localisation in their current pregnancy to exclude placenta praevia and, if present, to enable further investigation to try to identify praevia accreta and the development of safe management strategies.

### CLINICAL SKILLS

7. Maternity service providers and clinical directors must ensure that all clinical staff caring for pregnant women actually learn from any critical events and serious untoward incidents occurring in their trust or practice. How this is planned to be achieved should be documented at the end of each incident report form.

8. All clinical staff must undertake regular, written, documented and audited training for:

   ■ the identification, initial management and referral for serious medical and mental health conditions which, although unrelated to pregnancy, may affect pregnant women or recently delivered mothers

   ■ the early recognition and management of severely ill pregnant women and impending maternal collapse

   ■ the improvement of basic, immediate and advanced life support skills. A number of courses provide additional training for staff caring for pregnant women and newborn babies.

### EARLY WARNING SCORING SYSTEM

9. There is an urgent need for the routine use of a national obstetric early warning chart, similar to those in use in other areas of clinical practice, which can be used for all obstetric women which will help in the more timely recognition, treatment and referral of women who have, or are developing, a critical illness. It is important these charts are also used for pregnant women being cared for outside the obstetric setting for example in gynaecology, emergency departments and in critical care.

### NATIONAL GUIDELINES

10. Guidelines are urgently required for the management of: the obese pregnant woman; sepsis in pregnancy; pain and bleeding in early pregnancy.

*Reproduced with permission from: Saving Mothers' Lives. London: CEMACH; 2007.[3]*

TABLE 35.6 **Maternal mortality estimates by World Health Organization/United Nations Regions in 2000**

| Region | Maternal mortality ratio (maternal deaths per 100000 live births) | Maternal deaths (n) | Lifetime risk of maternal death |
|---|---|---|---|
| WORLD TOTAL | 400 | 529000 | 74 |
| DEVELOPED REGIONS [a] | 20 | 2500 | 2800 |
| EUROPE | 24 | 1700 | 2400 |
| DEVELOPING REGIONS | 440 | 527000 | 61 |
| AFRICA | 830 | 251000 | 20 |
| Northern Africa | 130 | 4600 | 210 |
| Sub-Saharan Africa | 920 | 247000 | 16 |
| ASIA | 330 | 253000 | 94 |
| Eastern Asia | 55 | 11000 | 840 |
| South-central Asia | 520 | 207000 | 46 |
| South-eastern Asia | 210 | 25000 | 140 |
| Western Asia | 190 | 9800 | 120 |
| LATIN AMERICA AND THE CARIBBEAN | 190 | 22000 | 160 |
| OCEANIA | 240 | 530 | 83 |

[a] Includes UK, Canada, USA, Japan, Australia and New Zealand, which are excluded from the regional totals

*Reproduced with permission from: Why Mothers Die. London: RCOG Press; 2003.* [4]

eclampsia, obstructed labour and abortion. Overall, these comprise around 80% of the deaths. The contribution from HIV and other infections such as malaria is also substantial in the developing world.

Figures 35.1 and 35.2 provide detailed statistics of causes of maternal deaths by regions and countries.

## STILLBIRTHS AND NEONATAL DEATHS

A CEMACH report on stillbirths and neonatal deaths provided information on perinatal deaths at a local, regional and national level. [5]

### Stillbirths

In England, Wales and Northern Ireland, the stillbirth rate was 5.3 (95% CI 5.1–5.5) in 1000 total births in 2006. There was no significant change in the still-

birth rate between 2000 and 2006 (Table 35.8). The la of progress in reducing stillbirth rates is thought to related to demographic factors known to be associat with stillbirths, such as obesity, ethnicity, deprivati and maternal age. One important contributory factor stillbirths is growth restriction: over one-third (40%) unexplained stillbirths had a birthweight below the ten centile for gestation and a quarter (26%) of them we below the third centile.

About 50% of stillbirths were categorised as 'un plained' using the existing Wigglesworth classificati system (Figure 35.3). It is unlikely that this proporti will fall in the future, as autopsy uptake has continu to decline from 48% of all deaths in 2000 to 38% in 20 The most common identifiable causes of stillbirths we congenital malformations and antepartum haemorrha (Figure 35.3).

TABLE 35.7  **Estimated incidence of major global causes of direct maternal deaths in 2000**

| Cause | Incidence of complication (% of live births) | Causes (*n*) | Case fatality rate | Maternal deaths (*n*) | Percentage of all *direct* deaths (%) |
|---|---|---|---|---|---|
| Haemorrhage | 10.5 | 13 795 000 | 1.0 | 132 000 | 28 |
| Sepsis | 4.4 | 576 800 | 1.3 | 79 000 | 16 |
| Pre-eclampsia/eclampsia | 3.2 | 4 152 000 | 1.47 | 63 000 | 13 |
| Obstructed labour | 4.6 | 6 038 000 | 0.7 | 42 000 | 9 |
| Abortion | 14.8 | 19 340 000 | 0.3 | 69 000 | 15 |

These estimates have been developed for the World Health Organization's calculations of the global burden of disease and are based upon both literature review and expert consensus; the full results will be published in future issues of the World Health Report

*Reproduced with permission from: Why Mothers Die. London: RCOG Press; 2003.*[4]

## Neonatal deaths

In England, Wales and Northern Ireland, the neonatal mortality rate was 3.4 in 1000 (95% CI 3.3–3.6) total births in 2006. The most common cause was immaturity (Figure 35.4). Unlike the stillbirth rate, the neonatal mortality rate declined significantly between 2000 and 2006 (Table 35.8, Figure 35.5).

## Perinatal deaths

In England, Wales and Northern Ireland, the perinatal mortality rate was 7.9 in 1000 (95% CI 7.7–8.1) total births in 2006. There was a small reduction in overall perinatal deaths to 2006, although rates actually increased between 2002 and 2004 (Table 35.8).

## Intrapartum-related deaths

The rate of intrapartum-related deaths did not change significantly between 2000 and 2006. In 2006, the proportion of intrapartum-related deaths was 7.6% (269/3531) for stillbirths and 7.7% (165/2154) for neonatal deaths. Half of the intrapartum deaths were classified as 'unexplained' using the Aberdeen obstetric classification. The most common identifiable causes were linked to catastrophic events at delivery, such as placental abruption (20% for stillbirths and 15% for neonatal deaths), cord prolapse and compression (8% for stillbirths and 4% for neonatal deaths) or uterine rupture. Maternal infection and black ethnicity were associated with intrapartum-related stillbirths.

TABLE 35.8  **Stillbirth, perinatal and neonatal death trends in England, Wales and Northern Ireland in 2000–06**

| Measure | Rate (95% CI) | | | | | | |
|---|---|---|---|---|---|---|---|
| | 2000 | 2001 | 2002 | 2003 | 2004 | 2005[A] | 2006 |
| Live births | 625 642 | 616 322 | 617 299 | 642 899 | 662 039 | 668 681 | 693 366 |
| Stillbirths[a] | 5.4 (5.2–5.6) | 5.4 (5.2–5.6) | 5.7 (5.5–5.9) | 5.8 (5.6–6.0) | 5.7 (5.5–5.9) | 5.3 (5.2–5.5) | 5.3 (5.1–5.5) |
| Perinatal deaths (UK)[a] | 8.3 (8.1–8.5) | 8.1 (7.9–8.3) | 8.5 (8.2–8.7) | 8.6 (8.4–8.8) | 8.4 (8.2–8.6) | 8.1 (7.8–8.3) | 7.9 (7.7–8.1) |
| Neonatal deaths[b] | 3.9 (3.7–4.0) | 3.7 (3.6–3.9) | 3.6 (3.5–3.8) | 3.7 (3.6–3.9) | 3.4 (3.3–3.5) | 3.5 (3.4–3.7) | 3.4 (3.3–3.6) |

[a] Rate/1000 total births  |  [b] Rate/1000 live births

*Reproduced with permission from: Perinatal Mortality 2006. London: CEMACH; 2008.*[6]

FIGURE 35.1 **Geographical variation in distribution of causes of maternal deaths**

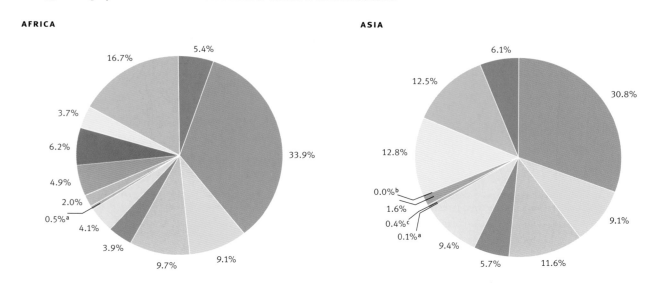

**AFRICA**

5.4%
16.7%
3.7%
6.2%
4.9%
2.0%
0.5%ᵃ
4.1%
3.9%
9.7%
9.1%
33.9%

**ASIA**

6.1%
12.5%
12.8%
0.0%ᵇ
1.6%
0.4%ᶜ
0.1%ᵃ
9.4%
5.7%
11.6%
9.1%
30.8%

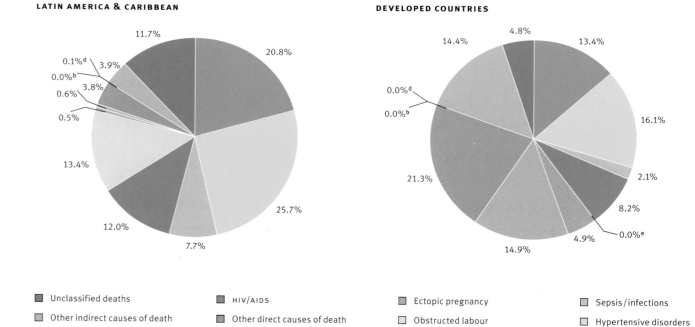

**LATIN AMERICA & CARIBBEAN**

11.7%
0.1%ᵈ
3.9%
0.0%ᵇ
3.8%
0.6%
0.5%
13.4%
12.0%
7.7%
25.7%
20.8%

**DEVELOPED COUNTRIES**

4.8%
14.4%
13.4%
0.0%ᵈ
0.0%ᵇ
16.1%
2.1%
8.2%
0.0%ᵉ
4.9%
14.9%
21.3%

| ■ Unclassified deaths | ■ HIV/AIDS | ■ Ectopic pregnancy | ■ Sepsis/infections |
| ■ Other indirect causes of death | ■ Other direct causes of death | ■ Obstructed labour | ■ Hypertensive disorders |
| ■ Anaemia | ■ Embolism | ■ Abortion | ■ Haemorrhage |

ᵃ Ectopic pregnancy  |  ᵇ HIV/AIDS  |  ᶜ Embolism  |  ᵈ Anaemia  |  ᵉ Obstructed labour

*Reproduced with permission from*: WHO analysis of causes of maternal death: a systematic review. Khan KS, Wojdyla D, Say L, Gülmezoglu AM, Van Look PF. *Lancet* 2006; 367:1066–74.⁵

FIGURE 35.2  **Distribution by country of haemorrhage, hypertensive disorders, sepsis or infection and abortion as causes of maternal deaths**

**A  HAEMORRHAGE**

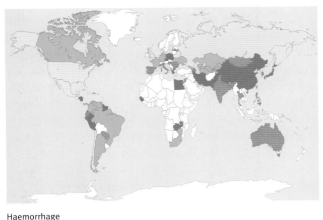

Haemorrhage

- Missing or excluded
- 0.01–10.00%
- 10.01–20.00%
- 20.01–30.00%
- ≥30.01%

**B  HYPERTENSIVE DISORDERS**

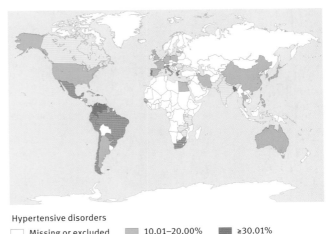

Hypertensive disorders

- Missing or excluded
- 0.01–10.00%
- 10.01–20.00%
- 20.01–30.00%
- ≥30.01%

**C  SEPSIS OR INFECTION**

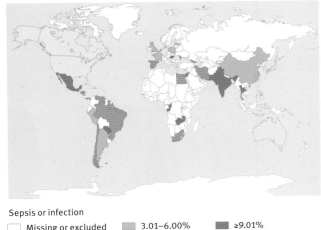

Sepsis or infection

- Missing or excluded
- 0.01–3.00%
- 3.01–6.00%
- 6.01–9.00%
- ≥9.01%

**D  ABORTION**

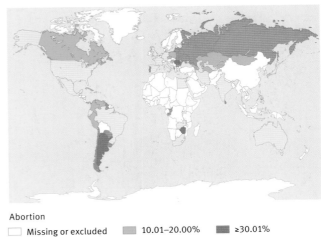

Abortion

- Missing or excluded
- 0.01–10.00%
- 10.01–20.00%
- 20.01–30.00%
- ≥30.01%

*Reproduced with permission from*: WHO analysis of causes of maternal death: a systematic review. Khan KS, Wojdyla D, Say L, Gülmezoglu AM, Van Look PF. *Lancet* 2006; 367:1066–74.[5]

FIGURE 35.3 **Causes of stillbirths in England, Wales and Northern Ireland in 2006**

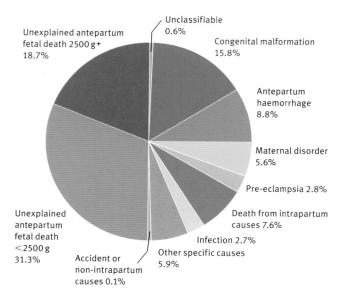

*Reproduced with permission from: Perinatal Mortality 2006. London: CEMACH; 2008.*[6]

FIGURE 35.4 **Causes of neonatal deaths in England, Wales and Northern Ireland in 2006**

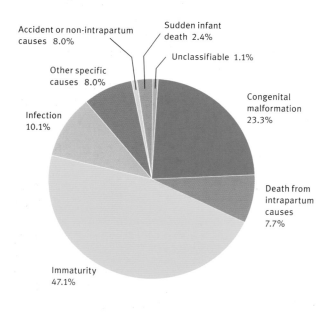

*Reproduced with permission from: Perinatal Mortality 2006. London: CEMACH; 2008.*[6]

### Deaths in twins

In England and Wales, the stillbirth, perinatal and neonatal mortality rates in twin pregnancies decreased significantly between 2000 and 2006. The stillbirth rate in twin pregnancies dropped from 17.7 in 1000 (95% CI 15.8–19.8) total births in 2000 to 12.5 in 1000 (95% CI 11.0–14.1) total births in 2006 ($P < 0.001$). The perinatal death rate in twin pregnancies has dropped from 35.3 in 1000 (95% CI 32.6–38.3) total births in 2000 to 27.2 in 1000 (95% CI 25.0–29.5) total births in 2006. The neonatal death rate in twin pregnancies also dropped from 22.3 in 1000 (95% CI 20.2–24.7) total births in 2000 to 19.3 in 1000 (95% CI 17.5–21.4) total births in 2006.

### Risk factors for stillbirths and neonatal deaths

The main factors associated with stillbirths and neonatal deaths are mother's age, obesity, social deprivation and ethnicity. Mothers aged less than 20 years and over 40 years had the highest rates of stillbirth, neonatal and perinatal deaths. A body mass index over 30 mg / kg$^2$ was associated with stillbirth and neonatal death. In comparison with the expected 20%, over one-third of all stillbirths and neonatal deaths were to mothers in the most deprived quintile. In comparison with women of white ethnicity, women of black and Asian ethnicity had

FIGURE 35.5 **Trend in neonatal deaths, England and Wales in 2000–06**

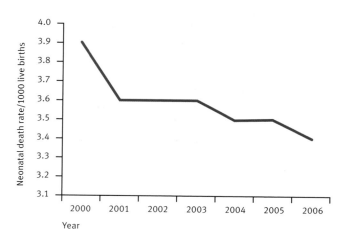

*Reproduced with permission from: Perinatal Mortality 2006. London: CEMACH; 2008.*[6]

approximately twice the rate of stillbirths and neonatal deaths.

## Epidemiology of disorders leading to pregnancy failure

Miscarriages, recurrent miscarriages and ectopic pregnancy are associated with substantial psychological and physical burdens, including death. For instance, the seventh triennial report (2003–05) included six deaths following miscarriage (five from sepsis), ten deaths from ruptured ectopic pregnancies and two deaths after termination of pregnancy. [3]

### MISCARRIAGE

Miscarriage, defined as the spontaneous loss of an intrauterine pregnancy before viability (that is, before 24 completed weeks) is the most common early pregnancy complication and is reported to occur in 15–25% of all pregnancies, accounting for over 50 000 inpatient admissions every year in the UK. This prevalence is likely to be an underestimation, as many miscarriages occur before or with the onset of menstruation and thus are not recognised as 'miscarriages'. The true rate of pregnancy loss after implantation is estimated to be over 50%. The definitions relating to miscarriage are given in Chapter 36, Table 36.6.

### Risk factors and causes

The risk of miscarriage decreases sharply after 10 weeks of gestation, with the risk of miscarriage being less than 2% from 10 weeks to term. The factors associated with miscarriage are described below:

- **Age and chromosomal abnormalities:** Chromosomal abnormalities (such as trisomy, XO and triploidy) are identified in more than 60% of embryos miscarried in the first 13 weeks. Most chromosomal problems are sporadic and are unlikely to recur. However, they are more likely to occur in older women, thus contributing to the increased rates of miscarriages observed in older women (Figure 35.6). Some chromosomal problems, such as balanced translocations in one of the parents, can result in an increased risk of recurrent miscarriages.

- **Thrombophilias:** These include both acquired (antiphospholipid syndrome: lupus anticoagulant and anticardiolipin antibodies) and congenital (such as protein C or S deficiency, activated protein C resistance [factor V Leiden mutation] and antithrombin III deficiency).
- **Anatomic causes:** These include uterine müllerian anomaly, uterine septum (the anomaly most commonly associated with pregnancy loss), unicornuate uterus, diethylstilbestrol-linked condition, acquired defects (for example, Asherman syndrome), cervical weakness, fibroids and uterine polyps.
- **Endocrine factors:** These include polycystic ovary syndrome, diabetes mellitus (particularly if it is poorly controlled), antithyroid antibodies (regardless of thyroid function test abnormalities) and luteal-phase deficiency (although the existence, the definition and diagnosis, and the management of luteal phase deficiency have been and are likely to continue to be a matter of debate).
- **Infectious causes:** These include rubella, cytomegalovirus, malaria, chlamydia, salmonella or any acute pyrexial illness, particularly when the infection involves peritonitis.
- **Smoking:** Maternal and paternal smoking are both associated with miscarriage.
- **Excessive alcohol consumption and drugs:** for example, cocaine and caffeine are associated with risk of miscarriage.
- **Multiple pregnancy:** Higher-order multiples are associated with an increased risk of miscarriages and preterm births.

### RECURRENT MISCARRIAGES

Recurrent miscarriage is defined as the loss of three consecutive pregnancies before viability. It affects approximately 1% of women. If the risk of sporadic miscarriage is about 15%, then the theoretical risk of having three consecutive miscarriages by chance is about 0.34% (15% × 15% × 15%), which is much less than the actual observed rate of 1% and suggests that some women have a predisposition to recurrent miscarriage. This is indeed the case.

FIGURE 35.6  **Risk of miscarriage by maternal age at conception**

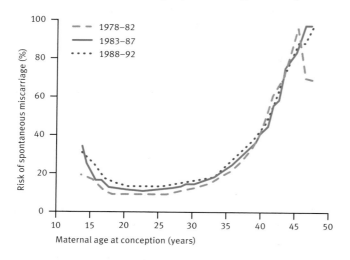

FIGURE 35.7  **Risk of ectopic pregnancy by maternal age at conception**

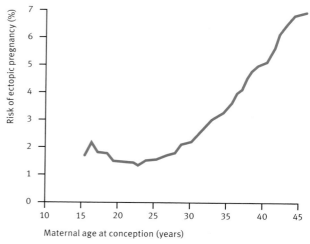

In this large prospective study, a total of 634 272 women and 1 221 546 pregnancy outcomes were studied. Overall, 13.5% of the pregnancies intended to be carried to term ended with fetal loss. At age 42 years, more than 50% of such pregnancies resulted in fetal loss. The risk of a miscarriage was 8.9% in women aged 20–24 years and 74.7% in those aged 45 years or more.

*Reproduced with permission from*: Maternal age and fetal loss: population-based register linkage stude. Nybo Andersen AM, Wohlfahrt J, Christens P, Olsen J, Melbye M. *Br Med J* 2000; 320:1708–12. [7]

*Reproduced with permission from*: Maternal age and fetal loss: population-based register linkage stude. Nybo Andersen AM, Wohlfahrt J, Christens P, Olsen J, Melbye M. *Br Med J* 2000; 320:1708–12. [7]

### Risk factors and causes

- **Chromosomal abnormalities:** 3–5% of screened parents have chromosomal abnormalities, most commonly a balanced reciprocal translocation and less commonly a Robertsonian translocation.
- **Thrombophilias:** In contrast to the 2% prevalence of antiphospholipid antibodies in the low-risk obstetric population, women with a history of recurrent miscarriages have 15% risk of antiphospholipid syndrome (lupus anticoagulant in 9.1% and anticardiolipin antibodies in 5.5%). Women with antiphospholipid syndrome have a 90% risk of miscarriage, which can be reduced with aspirin and heparin therapy. See also section above.
- **Anatomical causes:** See section above.
- **Endocrine causes:** See section above.

The risk of live birth after three consecutive miscarriages is 40–70%. After five consecutive miscarriages, the risk falls to 20–50%.

## ECTOPIC PREGNANCIES

The incidence of ectopic pregnancies (defined as the implantation of pregnancy outside the uterine cavity) can vary with the accuracy of the diagnostic tools, thoroughness of the work-up and the denominators used for the rates. Publications have used number of births, number of pregnancies or number of women of reproductive age as denominators. The number of women aged 15–44 years is commonly used as a denominator and the reported annual incidence rate varies between 100–175 in 100 000 women aged between 15–44 years in the UK (that is, one or two in 1000 women of reproductive age). Taking pregnancies as a denominator, in the 3-year period 2003–05, there were 32 100 ectopic pregnancies in 2 891 892 estimated pregnancies in the UK, giving a rate of 11.1 in 1000 pregnancies or just over 1%. There were 10 ectopic-related deaths in the seventh triennial period, giving a death rate of 0.35 in 100 000 (95% CI 0.19–0.64) ectopic pregnancies. Both the incidence of ectopic pregnancies and the death rate have remained static. Most (98%) ectopic pregnancies occur in the fallopian tubes, with the remainder occuring in the ovary, cervix or abdominal cavity.

**528**

## Risk factors and causes

- Increasing age (see Figure 35.7).
- History of pelvic inflammatory disease.
- Previous ectopic pregnancies.
- History of infertility.
- **Assisted conception (a heterotopic pregnancy):** An intrauterine pregnancy and an extrauterine pregnancy at the same time can be found in up to 2% of *in vitro* fertilisation pregnancies.
- Pelvic surgery.
- Tubal surgery.
- Early age at intercourse.
- **Failure of an intrauterine contraceptive device or progestogen-only oral contraceptive, including emergency contraception:** the risk of a pregnancy being ectopic is greater than with other forms of contraception.

## Epidemiology of infertility

### FERTILITY, INFERTILITY AND CAUSES

The National Institute for Health and Clinical Excellence (NICE) defines infertility as the inability to conceive despite regular unprotected intercourse after 24 months of trying to conceive. About one in seven couples (approximately 3.5 million couples in the UK) is infertile by this definition. It is therefore no surprise that infertility is the second most common reason for women aged 20–45 years to see their general practitioner, the most common reason being pregnancy itself.

The highest conception rate per monthly cycle among couples with proven normal fertility occurs in the first month of trying and is reported to be 33%. The monthly rate (fecundability) then falls quickly over 6 months, to about 5% per month. The cumulative pregnancy rates over various periods of trying to conceive are given in Table 35.9.

The most common single reason for infertility is now recognised to be male factor (32.5%, Table 35.10), which includes men with reduced sperm count (less than 20 million/ml), reduced motility (< 50% motile), poor morphology (less than 15% normal spermatozoa) or azoospermia (absolute lack of spermatozoa in the ejaculate, which is found in 1–2% of infertile couples). The second most

common reason is unexplained, which refers to the situation in which a recognised cause for infertility is not found (in about one in four couples).

### TREATMENT AND SUCCESS

Although various specific therapeutic options may be available for specific causes of infertility, most couples with one or more of the main causes of infertility (male factor, unexplained, tubal factor and ovulatory) would ultimately have *in vitro* fertilisation (IVF) to attempt to achieve a pregnancy. It should therefore come as no surprise that about 1% of all births in the UK are now the result of IVF, although the NHS funds only about 25% of all IVF treatment. In countries where the government provides liberal funding for IVF, as many as 5% of all births may be from IVF. The success rate for IVF depends on various factors, the two most important ones being the woman's age and the choice of clinic. The average live birth rates for IVF treatment (per cycle started) in the UK are:

- 29.6% for women under 35 years
- 23.6% for women aged 35–37 years
- 18.2% for women aged 38–39 years
- 10.0% for women aged 40–42 years
- 3.2% for women aged 43–44 years
- 0.8% for women aged over 44 years.

NICE has recommended that it would be appropriate to fund IVF treatment when the chances of success were more than 10%. Thus, most primary care trusts have an upper age limit of 39 years and offer funding only for one cycle of IVF treatment, even though most couples will need more than one cycle of treatment to achieve a pregnancy.

Currently, over 40 000 IVF cycles are carried out in the UK (Figure 35.8) in 122 clinics licensed by the Human Fertilisation and Embryology Authority. About 50% of IVF is conventional, with the other 50% representing IVF with intracytoplasmic sperm injection (micromanipulation to inject spermatozoa directly into the egg to aid fertilisation).

TABLE 35.9 **Cumulative pregnancy rates over various periods of trying to conceive**

| Time trying to conceive (months) | Cumulative pregnancy rates (%) |
|---|---|
| 1 | 20–33 |
| 3 | 50 |
| 6 | 60–70 |
| 12 | 85 |
| 18 | 90 |
| 24 | 92–95 |

## ASSISTED CONCEPTION AND MATERNAL MORTALITY

In the seventh triennial report CEMD (2003–05),[3] 12 women died from about 120 000 assisted reproduction treatment cycles, thus giving a mortality rate of one in 10 000 treatment cycles. Eight of the deaths were from direct causes, four of which were due to ovarian hyperstimulation syndrome: all four women had substandard care in that they were not treated with thromboprophylaxis. The other four direct deaths were from sepsis, embolism and bleeding and were not directly related to IVF (Table 35.11).

It should be appreciated that, beneath the iceberg of mortality, there is likely to be much greater morbidity. It is now widely accepted that the single most adverse effect from assisted reproduction is multiple pregnancy. Most embryo transfers in the UK are double embryo transfers, resulting in about 25% twin pregnancy rates in those who become pregnant. The seventh triennial report, consistent with other published literature, showed an increase in maternal mortality with multiple pregnancies compared with singleton pregnancies (relative risk 2.5, 95% CI 1.4–4.5). Although these data were not specific to the IVF population, there is no reason to suggest that the increased risk should not apply to the IVF population and thus the current drive to reduce multiple pregnancies in IVF practice with a view to reduce maternal and perinatal risk is likely to continue.

## Epidemiology of cancers affecting women

The majority of cancer registries around the world belong to the International Association of Cancer Registries (IACR) and submit their data routinely to the International Agency for Research on Cancer (www.iarc.fr). Furthermore, as well as belonging to IACR, European cancer registries also belong to the European Network of Cancer Registries (www.encr.com.fr). These organi-

TABLE 35.10 **Reasons for infertility**

| Cause | IVF treatment cycles (%) | | | | | | | |
|---|---|---|---|---|---|---|---|---|
| | 2000 | 2001 | 2002 | 2003 | 2004 | 2005 | 2006 | Change 2000–06 |
| Male factor | 27.6 | 29.7 | 31.5 | 31.8 | 31.9 | 32.6 | 32.5 | +4.9 |
| Tubal disease | 19.1 | 17.6 | 16.7 | 16.1 | 16.2 | 15.7 | 15.3 | −3.8 |
| Multiple male and female factors | 19.1 | 16.1 | 14.6 | 13.4 | 12.2 | 11.5 | 10.8 | −8.3 |
| Unexplained | 17.5 | 19.1 | 19.1 | 19.8 | 21.0 | 21.7 | 23.1 | +5.6 |
| Ovulatory disorder | 7.4 | 7.9 | 8.1 | 8.5 | 8.6 | 8.9 | 8.4 | +1.0 |
| Multiple female factors | 5.7 | 5.6 | 6.0 | 6.5 | 6.2 | 5.9 | 5.5 | −0.2 |
| Endometriosis | 2.5 | 3.0 | 3.0 | 2.8 | 2.8 | 2.9 | 2.9 | +0.4 |
| Other | 0.8 | 0.7 | 0.7 | 0.8 | 0.8 | 0.7 | 1.1 | +0.3 |
| Uterine | 0.2 | 0.3 | 0.3 | 0.3 | 0.3 | 0.3 | 0.4 | +0.2 |

*Source*: Human Fertilisation and Embryology Authority.[8]

FIGURE 35.8 **Numbers of *in vitro* fertilisation and micromanipulation treatments (intracytoplasmic sperm injection and subzonal insemination)**

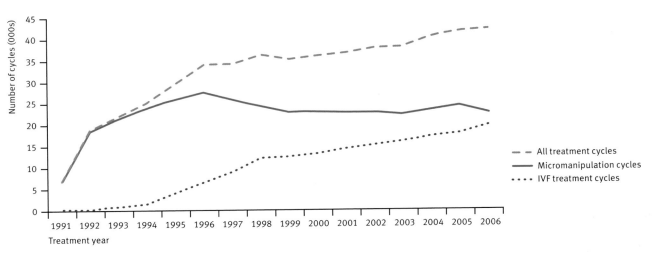

*Source*: Human Fertilisation and Embryology Authority.[9]

sations act as rich resources of epidemiological data on cancers, including the four main cancers in gynaecology: ovarian, cervical, uterine and vulval cancers.

The most common female cancer worldwide is breast cancer. Gynaecological cancers as a group resulted in approximately 6700 deaths in England and Wales in 2005, an overall rate of 24 in 100 000 women, just over half that of breast cancer. The most common gynaecological cancer worldwide is cervical cancer, which is also the second most common female cancer worldwide. The most common gynaecological cancer in the UK is ovarian cancer.

## OVARIAN CANCER

Ovarian cancer is responsible for more deaths per year than all other gynaecological cancers combined, approximately 4500 deaths per year in the UK, ranking fourth after breast, lung and bowel cancer as one of the leading causes of cancer death in women. There are 7000 new cases every year in the UK. The lifetime risk of ovarian cancer is one in 48. The high mortality rate is largely a result of the late presentation of ovarian cancer; over 50% of women will have stage III disease at diagnosis and most will have lymphatic spread. The overall 5-year survival rate is 30%. The majority (85–90%) of malignant ovarian tumours will be epithelial. The peak age for this form of ovarian cancer is 62 years. Up to 5–10% of ovar-

TABLE 35.11 **Maternal deaths and rates per 100 000 assisted reproductive technology procedures, including IVF, UK 1997–2005**

| Years | Deaths | | | | Treatment cycles (*n*) |
| | Number | Rate | 95% CI | | |
| --- | --- | --- | --- | --- | --- |
| 1997–99 | 20 | 19.17 | 12.41 | 29.61 | 104 320 |
| 2000–02 | 8 | 7.32 | 3.71 | 14.44 | 109 308 |
| 2003–05 | 12 | 10.08 | 5.76 | 17.61 | 119 080 |

ian cancer is associated with genetic predisposition from one of three autosomally inherited gene classes: *BRCA1*, *BRCA2* and *HNPCC*.

## UTERINE CANCER

Endometrial cancer is the second most common gynaecological cancer in women in the UK with approximately 6400 cases per year. It is also the second most common gynaecological cancer in Europe after ovarian cancer. In the USA, it has become the most common malignant neoplasm of the female pelvis. The most frequently found histological type of endometrial cancer is adenocarcinoma. The death rate is 2.5 in 100 000, as most cases can be cured. The median age for endometrial cancer is 61 years, with the majority of women presenting in the postmenopausal period. Endometrial cancer commonly presents early in its natural history, 75% of cases having stage I disease at the time of diagnosis. The risk factors include obesity, nulliparity, late menopause, unopposed estrogen therapy, estrogen-secreting tumours, polycystic ovary syndrome and personal or family history of breast or bowel cancer.

## VULVAL CANCER

Vulval cancer is a rare gynaecological malignancy. It accounts for 4% of all female genital tract malignancy, with approximately 1000 new cases per year diagnosed in the UK. Historically, this has been a cancer of the elderly, with approximately one-third of women presenting over the age of 75 years. There is an increasing incidence in younger women, with around 10% of all cases occuring in women under the age of 40 years. Over 90% of vulval cancer is squamous in origin. The risk factors include lichen sclerosus (4–7% risk of developing vulval cancer), vulval intraepithelial neoplasia (5–10% risk of cancer), Paget's disease, melanoma, smoking, immune suppression, advanced age and history of cervical neoplasia.

## CERVICAL CANCER

The incidence of cervical cancer in developed countries has fallen with the advent of the national screening programme and is likely to fall further with human papillomavirus vaccination. The majority of cervical cancer is squamous cell (80–90%) or adenocarcinoma. In the UK, there are approximately 2700 new cases each year and 1300 deaths per year due to cervical cancer. Over 50% of those cases are now diagnosed at an early stage in the disease, with stage I and stage II disease accounting for well over 60% of cases. The mean age of presentation is 52.2 years but the distribution of the disease is bimodal, with peaks at 35–39 years and then again at 60–64 years. The lifetime risk in Europe is 1% and that in Africa, Asia and Latin America is 5%. New cases worldwide are estimated to be around 450 000. Risk factors include early onset of sexual activity, multiple sexual partners, low socioeconomic class, cigarette smoking, use of the oral contraceptive pill, sexually transmitted infections (particularly human papilloma viruses 16 and 18), and immune suppression.

## REFERENCES

1. Evidence-Based Medicine Working Group. Evidence-based medicine: a new approach to teaching the practice of medicine. *JAMA* 1992;268:2420–5.

2. World Health Organization. *International Classification of Diseases, 10th Revision*. Geneva: WHO; 2007 [http://apps.who.int/classification/apps/icd/icd10online/].

3. Lewis G, editor. The Confidential Enquiry into Maternal and Child Health. *Saving Mothers' Lives: reviewing maternal deaths to make motherhood safer – 2003–2005. The Seventh Report on Confidential Enquiries into Maternal Deaths in the United Kingdom*. London: CEMACH; 2007.

4. Lewis G, Drife J, editors. Confidential Enquiry into Maternal and Child Health. *Why Mothers Die: the Sixth Report on Confidential Enquiries into Maternal Deaths in the United Kingdom, 2000–2002*. London: RCOG Press; 2003.

5. Khan K S, Wojdyla D, Say L, Gülmezoglu A M, Van Look P F. WHO analysis of causes of maternal death: a systematic review. *Lancet* 2006;367:1066–74.

6. Confidential Enquiry into Maternal and Child Health. *Perinatal Mortality 2006*. London: CEMACH; 2008.

7. Nybo Andersen A M, Wohlfahrt J, Christens P, Olsen J, Melbye M. Maternal age and fetal loss: population based register linkage study. *Br Med J* 2000;320:1708–12.

8. Human Fertilisation and Embryology Authority. *Facts and Figures 2006: Fertility problems and treatment*. London: HFEA; 2008 [www.hfea.gov.uk/Facts_and_Figures_2006_fertility_probs_and_treatment_2008-10-08.pdf].

9. Human Fertilisation and Embryology Authority. A long term analysis of the HFEA Register data (1991–2006). London: HFEA; 2008 [www.hfea.gov.uk/fertility-treatment-trends.html].

## Sample questions relating to basic statistics and screening and trials statistics

### EXTENDED MATCHING QUESTIONS

#### Questions 1–4

■ *These questions relate to descriptive statistics. For each item below, select the* **single** *best option from the list of options (A–D). Each option may be used once, more than once or not at all.*

OPTIONS

▷ **A**  Mean
▷ **B**  Median
▷ **C**  Mode
▷ **D**  Range

**1** ▶ Represents the spread of data in a sample

**2** ▶ Represents the interval on a frequency histogram within which the greatest number of observations fall

**3** ▶ Represents the average

**4** ▶ Represents the middle value in a ranked data set

#### Questions 5–8

■ *These questions relate to statistical tests. For each item below, select the* **single** *best option from the list above. Each option may be used once, more than once or not at all.*

OPTIONS

▷ **A**  Kruskal–Wallis test
▷ **B**  Mann–Whitney U-test
▷ **C**  McNemar $\chi^2$ test
▷ **D**  Wilcoxon test
▷ **E**  $\chi^2$ test
▷ **F**  Spearman's correlation
▷ **G**  Multiple regression analysis

**5** ▶ A test for unpaired data

**6** ▶ A test for paired data

**7** ▶ An analysis of variance

**8** ▶ A test for before and after categorical data

#### Questions 9–16

■ *These questions relate to a predictive test on the observations given in the table below. For each item below, select the* **single** *best option from the list of options (A–L). Each option may be used once, more than once or not at all.*

|  |  | Disease | | |
|---|---|---|---|---|
|  |  | *Positive* | *Negative* | **Total** |
| **Test result** | *Positive* | 48 | 55 | 103 |
|  | *Negative* | 2 | 45 | 47 |
|  | **Total** | 50 | 100 | 150 |

OPTIONS

▷ **A**   2
▷ **B**   45
▷ **C**   47
▷ **D**   48
▷ **E**   50
▷ **F**   55
▷ **G**   100
▷ **H**   103
▷ **I**   45%
▷ **J**   466%
▷ **K**   957%
▷ **L**   96%

**9** ▶ Number of false negatives

**10** ▶ Number of false positives

**11** ▶ Negative predictive value

**12** ▶ Positive predictive value

**13** ▶ Sensitivity

**14** ▶ Specificity

**15** ▶ True negative

**16** ▶ True positive

## Questions 17 – 20

- *For each description below, select the **single** most appropriate level of evidence fulfilled from the list of options of options (A–F). Each option may be used once, more than once or not at all.*

OPTIONS

▷ **A** Level 1a
▷ **B** Level 1b
▷ **C** Level 2a
▷ **D** Level 2b
▷ **E** Level 3
▷ **F** Level 4

**17** ▶ At least one randomised controlled trial has been carried out

**18** ▶ At least one well-designed controlled study, without randomisation

**19** ▶ At least one other type of well-designed, quasi-experimental study

**20** ▶ Well-designed descriptive study

## MULTIPLE CHOICE QUESTIONS

**21** ▶ When describing a scale of measurement:

**A** ▷ An interval scale is where the interval between any two neighbouring points is the same as that between any other two neighbouring points
**B** ▷ A ratio scale is an interval scale with a fixed zero
**C** ▷ Nominal scales are parametric
**D** ▷ Data from an ordinal scale can be expressed on an interval scale
**E** ▷ Interval scaled data can be added together

**22** ▶ Regarding measurement accuracy and reliability:

**A** ▷ A measurement is accurate if it matches exactly an accepted standard
**B** ▷ Accuracy and precision are the same
**C** ▷ A reliable measurement is one that can be repeated with minimal variation
**D** ▷ A reliable measurement needs to be taken several times
**E** ▷ Valid measurements are always indisputable

**23** ▶ Central tendency can be described by:

**A** ▷ the mean
**B** ▷ the range
**C** ▷ the median
**D** ▷ the mode
**E** ▷ the standard deviation

**24** ▶ A normal distribution:

**A** ▷ is multimodal
**B** ▷ has equal observations either side of the midpoint
**C** ▷ has a mean, median and mode that are all the same
**D** ▷ is characterised by its standard error
**E** ▷ has kurtosis

**25** ▶ Regarding measures of variability:

**A** ▷ Variance is the average amount by which any individual measurement differs from the median
**B** ▷ Standard deviation tells you about the variability in a sample
**C** ▷ 95% of the data are within two standard deviations of the mean
**D** ▷ The coefficient of variation expresses the standard deviation as a percentage of the mean
**E** ▷ The standard error of the mean takes into account the sample size

**26** ▶ In probability and hypothesis testing:

**A** ▷ If $P = 1$, then the chance of something happening is 100%
**B** ▷ If $P < 005$, it is statistically significant
**C** ▷ If $P < 005$, then the outcome has occurred by chance in 19 out of 20 times
**D** ▷ Type 2 errors occur when the null hypothesis is wrongly rejected
**E** ▷ The power of a study is its ability to detect an effect of a specified size

**27** ▶ Chi-squared tests:

**A** ▷ are used to compare distributions
**B** ▷ depend on the observed and expected results only
**C** ▷ are significant if the result is 005 or less
**D** ▷ are used if the expected $n < 5$
**E** ▷ are used with proportions

28 ▶ The *t*-test:

A ▷ is used to compare the difference between two medians

B ▷ is used to compare the mean of a sample with a predicted value

C ▷ can only be used on data that is Normally distributed

D ▷ must have paired samples

E ▷ paired samples are measurements made by the same person under different conditions

29 ▶ When assessing statistical correlations:

A ▷ Pearson's (*r*) correlation tests the association between two variables

B ▷ Pearson's (*r*) correlation relies on all data being Normally distributed

C ▷ If Pearson's $r = 0$, there is a negative correlation

D ▷ A statistically significant association means it is causal

E ▷ Regression allows prediction of a variable

30 ▶ Regarding epidemiology:

A ▷ Specificity is the proportion of true positives that are correctly identified by a test

B ▷ The positive predictive value is the proportion of patients with a positive test result

C ▷ The incidence of a disease is the rate at which new cases of the disease occur in any population

D ▷ The incidence rate is the number of new cases per head of the population per unit time

E ▷ The prevalence of a condition measures the frequency of existing disease at a given time

31 ▶ When evaluating the odds ratio and relative risk:

A ▷ An odds ratio allows a confidence interval to be calculated between two variables

B ▷ An odds ratio allows the effect of other variables on an association to be tested

C ▷ An odds ratio can use groups selected retrospectively

D ▷ If ten in 100 patients have an illness, the odds ratio is 1 : 10

E ▷ Relative risk compares proportions with a particular outcome in two different groups

32 ▶ Regarding the management of clinical trials:

A ▷ A comparison of treatment only is involved

B ▷ Randomisation avoids unconscious bias

C ▷ In a double-blind study, the patient, clinician and assessor are all blinded to the treatment

D ▷ A randomised controlled trial can use historical data for a control group

E ▷ Patients can be their own control

## Sample questions relating to epidemiology

### EXTENDED MATCHING QUESTIONS

### Questions 1–5

■ *These questions relate to maternal mortality. For each item below, select the **single** best option from the list of options (A–K). Each option may be used once, more than once or not at all.*

OPTIONS

▷ **A** Maternal deaths resulting from complications unique to pregnancy

▷ **B** Maternal deaths resulting from previous existing disease or a newly developing medical condition unrelated to pregnancy, aggravated by pregnancy

▷ **C** Maternal deaths from causes unrelated to pregnancy

▷ **D** Direct and indirect deaths occurring between 42 days and 1 year after the end of a pregnancy

▷ **E** Direct deaths per 100 000 maternities

▷ **F** Indirect deaths per 100 000 maternities

▷ **G** Number of maternal deaths in a given time period per 100 000 women of reproductive age

▷ **H** Direct deaths per 100 000 live births

▷ **I** Indirect deaths per 100 000 live births

▷ **J** Direct and indirect deaths per 100 000 live births

▷ **K** The number of mothers delivered of registrable live births at any gestation or stillbirths of 24 weeks of gestation or later

1 ▶ Defines indirect maternal deaths

2 ▶ Defines coincidental maternal deaths

3 ▶ Defines maternal mortality ratio

4 ▶ Defines maternities

5 ▶ Defines maternal mortality rate

## Questions 6−11

- *These questions relate to perinatal mortality. For each item below, select the **single** best option from the list above. Each option may be used once, more than once or not at all.*

OPTIONS

▷ **A** A child delivered between $22^{+0}$ and $23^{+6}$ weeks of gestation that did not show any signs of life

▷ **B** A child delivered between $22^{+0}$ and $23^{+6}$ weeks of gestation that did show signs of life

▷ **C** A child delivered after week 24 of pregnancy that did not show any signs of life

▷ **D** A child delivered after week 24 of pregnancy that did show signs of life

▷ **E** Death of a live born baby occurring less than 7 completed days from the time of birth

▷ **F** Death of a live born baby occurring from day 7 of life and before 28 completed days from the time of birth

▷ **G** Stillbirths per 1000 live births and stillbirths

▷ **H** Stillbirths per 1000 live births

▷ **I** Stillbirths and early neonatal deaths per 1000 live births and stillbirths

▷ **J** Stillbirths, early and late neonatal deaths per 1000 live births and stillbirths

▷ **K** Late fetal losses, stillbirths and early neonatal deaths per 1000 live births and stillbirths

▷ **L** Late fetal losses, stillbirths, early and late neonatal deaths per 1000 live births and stillbirths

▷ **M** Neonatal deaths per 1000 live births

6 ▶ Defines late fetal loss

7 ▶ Defines stillbirth

8 ▶ Defines late neonatal death

9 ▶ Defines stillbirth rate

10 ▶ Defines perinatal mortality rate in the UK

11 ▶ Defines neonatal mortality rate

# Surgery

# CHAPTER 36

# Surgery in obstetrics and gynaecology

*Andrew R Sizer*

## Introduction

A sound knowledge of surgery and its underlying principles remains essential for the aspiring obstetrician and gynaecologist.

## Surgical rates, operative success and complication rates

### SURGICAL RATES

Operative rates in gynaecology have declined in the last 10 years. Some examples of how medical and minimally invasive therapies have impacted on surgical rates are shown in Table 36.1.

TABLE 36.1 **Therapies that have had an impact on surgical rates**

| Surgical procedure affected | Alternative therapy that has reduced surgical rate |
|---|---|
| Hysterectomy | Levonorgestrel-containing intrauterine system |
| | Balloon endometrial ablation |
| | Transcervical resection of endometrium |
| Myomectomy | Fibroid embolisation |
| Colposuspension | Tension-free vaginal tape |
| Tubal surgery for infertility | *In vitro* fertilisation |

There are a number of factors that influence the rate of a particular operation:

- effectiveness of the operation
- availability of non-surgical alternatives
- preference of the surgeon
- cost
- availability of equipment
- length of hospital stay.

In obstetrics, the most important surgical rate that is always under scrutiny is the caesarean section rate. The World Health Organization has suggested that there is no benefit to mother or baby in having a caesarean rate over 15% but some maternity units in the UK have rates that are almost double this.

There are a number of potential factors that may contribute to the high caesarean section rate in the UK. Some of these are outlined in Table 36.2.

### SURGICAL SUCCESS RATES

It is often difficult to define what is meant by a 'successful operation'. To a patient, it could mean several things:

- resolution of symptoms
- a neat cosmetic appearance of the abdominal scar
- a healthy baby following a caesarean section.

To a surgeon, success may be judged by different criteria, but the resolution of a patient's original complaint will obviously be of prime concern. Factors that may influence whether or not an operation has been deemed to be successful are as follows:

TABLE 36.2 **Factors that contribute to high caesarean rates in the UK**

| Factor | Explanation of factor | Contribution to caesarean rate |
|---|---|---|
| Increasing maternal age | The median age at first delivery is slowly rising in the UK | Increased maternal age has been shown to be linked to increased chance of caesarean in a number of studies |
| Previous caesarean | Previous caesarean is the main factor contributing to the rising rate in the UK | Rates of attempting vaginal birth after caesarean are suboptimal in the UK, so repeat caesarean is leading to an exponential rise in caesarean rates |
| Breech | Most breeches at term are now delivered by caesarean | Following publication of the Term Breech Trial,[1] many units have stopped conducting vaginal breech deliveries with a subsequent increase in caesarean rate |
| Obstetric skill of trainees | With decreased hours on the labour ward, there is concern that obstetric skills of trainees are declining | If rotational or instrumental deliveries fail because of lack of skill, then delivery will be by caesarean, increasing the caesarean rate |
| Multiple pregnancy | With the increased use of assisted reproduction, the number of multiple pregnancies has also increased | Multiple pregnancies have always had a high caesarean rate, so their increased numbers will contribute to the overall caesarean rate |

- appropriate choice of surgical procedure for the presenting complaint
- skill of the surgeon
- appropriate preparation, optimising the patient's condition and ensuring that all necessary equipment is available
- good equipment
- good anaesthesia
- good perioperative care.

## SURGICAL COMPLICATIONS

All operations have complications associated with them. Some are minor complications; some are very serious and will include death. Before contemplating any operation, all patients should be informed frankly of the risks and benefits of undergoing the procedure as well as a discussion of all complications with serious sequelae. There is a specific space to record these discussions on the consent form.

In summary, there are many types of complications and they can be classified in different ways. In addition, there are many factors than can influence the rate of complications. However, a good knowledge of the principles of how complications arise and the factors that influence their occurrence should allow one to identify possible complications for any operation.

### Factors affecting complication rates

There are a number of factors that contribute to complication rates and, broadly, these can be divided into patient-related factors and surgery-related factors, as shown in Table 36.3.

### Types of complication

Complications are often described according to the time frame in which they present after a surgical procedure. A common system is to divide complications into immediate, early and late.

Complications can present in varying ways. Post-operative bleeding will present with tachycardia, hypotension and poor urine output. Infection will present with pyrexia, tachycardia and sometimes more vague symptoms like confusion in the elderly. A full description of complications and their management is not within the scope of the Part 1 syllabus, but a general knowledge is essential in clinical practice.

TABLE 36.3  **Patient-related and surgery-related factors affecting complication rates**

| Factor | Example | Complication |
|---|---|---|
| **COMPLICATIONS RELATED TO THE PATIENT** | | |
| Pre-existing medical conditions | Cardiovascular disease | Anaesthesia-related complications |
| Obesity | Body mass index >30 kg/m² | Difficult access leading to suboptimal surgery or unintended damage to other organs |
| | | Poor haemostasis |
| | | Wound breakdown |
| Inadequate starvation prior to surgery | Vomiting during induction of anaesthesia | Aspiration pneumonia |
| **COMPLICATIONS RELATED TO THE SURGEON/PROCEDURE** | | |
| Poor/inadequate surgical technique | Failure to achieve adequate haemostasis | Postoperative bleeding |
| | Inadequate attention to aseptic technique | Postoperative infection |
| | Inadequate training for the procedure that is being undertaken | Failure to resolve symptoms or unintended damage to pelvic/abdominal organs |
| Difficult pathology | Extensive pelvic endometriosis | Unintended damage to ureters |
| Faulty equipment | Failure of insulation on diathermy devices | Damage to surrounding structures and/or burns on patient's skin |

## Common procedures in obstetrics and gynaecology and their complications

Below is a discussion of four common operations in obstetrics and gynaecology, with a brief description of the complications that may be associated with each procedure (see also Table 36.4). Knowledge of these is essential when seeking consent from patients.

### LAPAROSCOPY

Laparoscopy involves the insertion of an endoscope into the peritoneal cavity to inspect the pelvic and abdominal organs. Commonly, a Veress needle is used to inflate the peritoneal cavity with carbon dioxide gas prior to the insertion of operative ports, although other techniques such as open laparoscopy are also used. Laparoscopy is used for both diagnostic and therapeutic purposes. Further ports can be inserted into the peritoneal cavity to introduce additional instruments if required.

Most complications are fortunately rare, with an incidence of less than 1%. As was seen in Table 36.3, the probability of complications depends on many factors. Complications are more likely with operative laparoscopy than a diagnostic procedure.

### HYSTEROSCOPY

Hysteroscopy involves the insertion of an endoscope through the cervical canal into the uterus to view the endometrial cavity. Most commonly the procedure is diagnostic but it is also possible to resect fibroids, polyps and the endometrium with a larger resectoscope. Distension media include fluids and carbon dioxide gas.

### HYSTERECTOMY

Hysterectomy is an operation that involves removal of the uterus. The procedure can be total, where both the uterus and cervix are removed, or subtotal, where only the body of the uterus is removed. The operation can be performed via different routes: abdominal, vaginal or laparoscopic. Different types and different routes all have their own profile and rate of complications.

## CAESAREAN SECTION

Caesarean section is one of the most commonly performed operations. Unfortunately it can be associated with a high incidence of complications. Since caesarean section involves a laparotomy, the complications are similar to those described for hysterectomy (Table 36.4). However, bladder trauma is more common, as are lacerations that extend into the vagina.

There are also obstetric factors that increase the incidence of complications at caesarean section:

- advancing maternal age
- advanced stage of labour
- increased fetal weight
- fetal distress.

## Blood transfusion

In the UK, blood for transfusion is obtained via the National Blood Service. The National Blood Service recruits non-remunerated altruistic adult donors.

TABLE 36.4 **Types of complications after obstetric and gynaecological surgery**

| Immediate | Early | Late |
|---|---|---|
| **LAPAROSCOPY** | | |
| Failed pneumoperitoneum: extraperitoneal emphysema | Pelvic inflammatory disease owing to introduction of organisms by manipulating cannula | Hernia at port sites |
| Bradycardia owing to peritoneal distension | Peritonitis due to unrecognised bowel trauma | Adhesions |
| Bowel injury | Pain | |
| Vessel injury, e.g. iliacs, aorta | | |
| **HYSTEROSCOPY** | | |
| Perforation of the uterus | Bleeding | Intrauterine adhesions following resection |
| Bleeding | Fluid overload | |
| | Hyponatraemia | |
| | Infection due to introduction of organisms into the uterine cavity | |
| | Discharge | |
| **HYSTERECTOMY** | | |
| Bleeding | Pain | Adhesions |
| Damage to adjacent organ, e.g. bladder, bowel, ureter | Chest infection | Fistula |
| | Urinary tract infection | Incisional hernia |
| | Deep-vein thrombosis | |
| | Ileus | |
| | Voiding dysfunction | |

Many donate blood on a regular basis (as often as every 4 months). Some groups are excluded from donating as they are deemed to be high risk for infection. All donated samples are tested for syphilis, HIV-1 and -2 and hepatitis B and C. Obviously there are other viruses (and possibly unknown pathogens) that could be transmitted by blood transfusion.

Blood donations have a shelf life of 42 days, although blood can now be frozen. Blood and blood products are always in short supply and should only be used when essential. Some preparations are very expensive and their use would need to be discussed with a consultant haematologist.

## TYPES OF BLOOD PRODUCTS

### Whole blood

Whole blood is used very rarely, such as in acute haemorrhage. Stored whole blood has some undesirable characteristics, such as the presence of anticoagulant (sodium citrate) and a high level of potassium, because stored cells lyse and release potassium.

In general, whole blood is separated into red cell concentrates and platelet-containing plasma. The plasma is then separated into platelet concentrates and plasma, which is rich in clotting factors. The plasma is then frozen to extend its storage period.

### Packed red cells

Red cells are concentrated so, although they have the same oxygen-carrying capacity as a unit of whole blood, they are in a much smaller volume, reducing the chance of circulatory overload. Packed cells are therefore useful in patients with anaemia who have a normal blood volume. However, other therapies should be tried first before resorting to blood transfusion.

### Frozen red cells

If a cryoprotectant (such as glycerol) is added to blood, it can be frozen successfully. This may be useful when there is blood with unusual antigens. However, frozen blood is very expensive.

### Platelets

Platelets are used in patients with marked thrombocytopenia. One bag of platelets will increase the platelet count by approximately $7 \times 10^9$ per litre. The shelf life of platelets is around 7 days.

### Fresh frozen plasma

Fresh frozen plasma can be stored for up to 1 year. It is rich in clotting factors and may be required in addition to packed cells where there is an acute haemorrhage.

Fresh frozen plasma can be separated into cryoprecipitate and human albumin solution. Cryoprecipitate is particularly rich in factor VIII, von Willebrand factor and fibrinogen and so is useful in the management of clotting disorders. Human albumin solution may be used in situations where there is acute hypoproteinaemia.

## AVOIDANCE OF BLOOD PRODUCTS

Blood and blood products are always in short supply and should only be used when absolutely necessary. In addition, there are situations where blood must not be used, such as the treatment of a Jehovah's Witness.

## ALTERNATIVES TO USING ALLOGENIC BLOOD TRANSFUSION

### Donation of autologous blood preoperatively

Patients can donate blood for their own use preoperatively. This has many advantages, such as the avoidance of alloimmunisation and infection risk. However, the period between the donation and surgery would need to be maximised so that the patient can recover their haemoglobin level before surgery. The procedure is expensive and has not really taken off in the UK.

### Blood salvage

Any blood lost at surgery, or even from surgical drains postoperatively, can be anticoagulated and retrieved. The cells can then be washed, filtered and concentrated and are then available for reinfusion into the patient. This technique is only appropriate when the collection site is free from infection or malignancy.

### Erythropoietin

Recombinant erythropoietin has been developed and, when administered rapidly, increases erythropoiesis, causing a rise in haemoglobin levels. However, this treatment is expensive and should be reserved for exceptional circumstances.

## ADVERSE EFFECTS OF ALLOGENIC BLOOD TRANSFUSION

### Acute reactions

A haemolytic reaction is one caused by incompatibility in antigens (ABO or others) between the transfused blood and the recipient. This is a serious complication and has a high mortality rate. An anaphylactic-type reaction ensues. If there is any reaction at the start of a transfusion, then it must be stopped immediately. Many of these reactions are caused by administrative errors in allocating or transfusing the wrong blood, so it is essential that a robust system of checking is in place. Any such transfused blood will be haemolysed by the recipient's immune system.

A non-haemolytic reaction is a febrile reaction and most commonly occurs because the recipient has antibodies that are directed towards the leucocytes of the transfused blood. It occurs in up to 5% of transfusions. Symptoms are fever and urticarial rash.

### Lung injury

A form of acute respiratory distress syndrome can occur after blood transfusion and cause lung injury. This appears to be a result of antibodies that are directed towards the leucocytes of the transfused blood.

### Circulatory overload

If large volumes are transfused, congestive heart failure can ensue. It is therefore important to transfuse slowly, use diuretics as required and packed cells (with a smaller volume) rather than whole blood.

### Transmission of pathogens

Although blood products are screened, it is still possible to transmit other pathogens with a blood transfusion.

### Immunosuppression

Immunosuppression is a well-recognised feature of blood transfusion. Its cause is a suppression of cell-mediated immunity by allogenic blood.

### Iron overload

Iron overload is a complication of repeated transfusions, such as occurs in thalassaemia. Organs can become damaged by excessive iron stores. Iron chelation therapy with desferrioxamine can reduce this complication.

## Fluid balance in surgery and anaesthesia

Fluid balance has been discussed in some detail in Chapter 7, but the principles will be revisited in this section, in addition to a discussion of the effects of surgery and anaesthesia on fluid and electrolyte balance. Descriptions of the functions, distribution and causes of disturbance for sodium, potassium and the three other most important electrolytes are described in Table 36.5.

### FLUID BALANCE

Fluid balance refers to a state where the required amount of bodily water is present and correctly distributed amongst the body compartments. Fluid balance is directly linked to electrolyte balance.

Total body water constitutes 70% of lean body weight but this varies as a percentage of total body weight according to the amount of adipose tissue. Therefore, an average 70 kg man contains 42 litres of water, whereas a 50 kg woman will contain 27 litres.

Of the total body water, approximately one-third is extracellular, 25% as plasma and 75% as interstitial fluid, in which the most important electrolyte is sodium and approximately two-thirds is intracellular, in which the most important electrolyte is potassium.

TABLE 36.5 **The five most important electrolytes**

| Electrolyte | Function | Distribution | Disturbance and causes |
|---|---|---|---|
| Sodium (Na) | Key role in fluid balance | Predominantly in extracellular fluid | Hyponatraemia: caused by insufficient intake (e.g. inadequate sodium in intravenous fluids), excessive water, diuretic therapy or hypoadrenalism |
| | Contributes half the osmolarity of the extracellular fluid | Regulated by antidiuretic hormone, aldosterone and atrial natriuretic peptide | Hypernatraemia: caused by excessive salt intake, excessive water depletion or hyperaldosteronism |
| Potassium (K) | Maintenance of intracellular fluid volume | Predominantly in intracellular fluid | Hypokalaemia: caused by dietary insufficiency, inadequate intravenous therapy, insulin therapy, beta agonists, vomiting, diarrhoea |
| | Regulation of pH | Serum level regulated by aldosterone | Hyperkalaemia: caused by excessive intravenous administration, blood transfusion, Addison's disease, potassium-sparing diuretics |
| | Establishes resting membrane potential of cells | | |
| Calcium (Ca) | Role in excitable cells, neurotransmitter release and blood clotting | Predominantly in bone | Hypocalcaemia: caused by hypoparathyroidism, inadequate vitamin D intake and renal disease |
| | | Mainly extracellular | Hypercalcaemia: caused by malignancy or hyperparathyroidism |
| | | Regulated by parathyroid hormone | |
| Chloride (Cl) | Balances anions in all fluid compartments | Diffuses easily between extracellular fluid and intracellular fluid | Hypochloraemia: found in pyloric stenosis and respiratory alkalosis |
| | | Levels linked to sodium concentration | Hyperchloraemia: caused by excessive intravenous saline administration or severe dehydration |
| Bicarbonate (HCO$_3$) | Major buffer in plasma | Predominantly in extracellular fluid although small amounts also found in intracellular fluid | Deficit leads to metabolic acidosis; caused by use of carbonic anhydrase inhibitors, diarrhoea, fistulae |
| | Helps maintain balance of anions and cations in all fluid compartments | Serum level controlled by kidneys | Excess leads to metabolic alkalosis; caused by excessive bicarbonate administration, chronic vomiting, diuretic use |

A normal intake of water is 2.5–3.0 litres/day. Most of this is ingested in the form of food and drinks but a small volume is produced as a result of metabolic processes. Fluid loss is in the form of urine (1500 ml), insensible loss (sweat, lungs; 850 ml) and faeces (100 ml).

## MOVEMENT OF FLUID BETWEEN COMPARTMENTS

The movement of fluid between the interstitial fluid and the intracellular fluid is governed by the osmotic forces that the electrolytes sodium and potassium generate. A change in the concentration of either electrolyte will cause water to enter or leave the cell.

The most important factor for the movement of fluid between the capillary and interstitial fluid is bulk flow. The capillary endothelium is freely permeable to water and electrolytes but not to plasma proteins. There are two important pressures to consider:

- hydrostatic forces (blood pressure), which push fluid out of the vessel into the interstitium
- plasma oncotic pressure from plasma proteins, which draws fluid back into the capillary.

At the arteriolar end of the capillary, the hydrostatic force is greater, resulting in net filtration of fluid. At the venous end of the capillary, the plasma oncotic force is greater, resulting in net reabsorption of fluid.

### REGULATION OF FLUID BALANCE

There are three key hormones to consider: antidiuretic hormone (ADH, vasopressin), aldosterone and atrial natriuretic peptide (ANP).

Decreased fluid volume causes the release of renin in the kidney, which has two effects:

- stimulation of the release of ADH from the posterior pituitary
- production of angiotensin I from angiotensinogen: angiotensin I is converted to angiotensin II in the lung and this causes vasoconstriction. Angiotensin II also has the effect of causing aldosterone release from the adrenal cortex, resulting in increased water and sodium absorption in the kidney.

Increased fluid volume inhibits renin and, therefore, ADH release. It also causes the release of ANP from the heart, which increases fluid and sodium loss from the kidney.

### EFFECTS OF ANAESTHESIA AND SURGERY ON FLUID BALANCE

The perioperative period is a slightly unusual situation, where fluid balance can be difficult to maintain or control. Before theatre, patients are often starved for several hours, so there may be up to a litre of fluid deficit before any anaesthesia or surgery commences. Surgery itself is stressful to the body and stress results in steroid release from the adrenal cortex. Steroids such as aldosterone will cause sodium and water retention. There can also be large fluid shifts in the perioperative period (for example, haemorrhage) causing derangement in fluid and electrolyte balance. Intraoperative blood loss is often underestimated, which means that fluid may be under-replaced.

The kidney will be affected by anaesthesia and surgery in several ways:

- Many anaesthetic agents have direct effects on renal blood flow and glomerular filtration rate.
- Hypotension/hypovolaemia will have direct effects on renal function (pre-renal failure).
- Sympathetic tone and circulating catecholamines will cause renal vasoconstriction.

These actions on the kidney will result in increased levels of ADH secretion from the posterior pituitary, and indeed it has been shown that ADH levels may increase by 50–100 times in the immediate perioperative period and may take up to 5 days to return to normal.

The effects on the kidney are all caused by fluid loss and the body responds by effecting sodium and water retention. Therefore oliguria may persist for some days after surgery.

It must also be remembered that tissue injury during surgery results in the release of cytokines and these have the effect of increasing capillary permeability. This can result in the accumulation of fluid in otherwise 'dry' spaces such as the lungs and peritoneal cavity, even though there may be significant hypovolaemia.

## Management of early pregnancy problems

### MISCARRIAGE

Miscarriage is a common event and is estimated to occur in 10–20% of pregnancies, although the incidence may actually be much higher. Miscarriage accounts for approximately 50 000 inpatient admissions a year, predominantly for surgical evacuation, although this number should now fall with the increased availability of expectant and medical management of miscarriage.

Older textbooks will often refer to miscarriage as 'abortion'. This terminology should be avoided owing to its negative connotations. Table 36.6 contains the current definitions of types of miscarriage.

Hospitals should have a dedicated early pregnancy unit for the management of early pregnancy problems. Ideally, this should provide a 7 day service.

## Management of miscarriage

There are three management options for miscarriage, surgical, medical and conservative (also known as expectant management). The complications and advantages of each management option for miscarriages are shown in Table 36.7.

Surgical management of miscarriage involves a procedure known as evacuation of retained products of conception (ERPC). ERPC is one of the most common gynaecological procedures and, in the past, the vast majority of miscarriages were managed this way. Now, there are the medical and conservative alternatives, but ERPC

should be offered to women who prefer to be managed this way and where there is excessive bleeding, infected retained tissue or suspected gestational trophoblastic neoplasia.

ERPC is most commonly carried out under general anaesthesia in the UK, although it is possible to use sedation or local anaesthesia. Vaginal prostaglandins can be administered prior to the procedure to soften the cervix making it easier to dilate. This also reduces trauma. After dilatation of the cervix to an appropriate size, an ERPC is normally performed with a suction catheter that is agitated inside the uterus. Sometimes a sharp metal curette is also used. Intravenous oxytocin can be used to cause the uterus to contract to minimise blood loss. The procedure is complete once the cavity is empty.

Medical management of miscarriage is an effective alternative to surgical evacuation and is increasing in use and popularity. It is predominantly an outpatient procedure. Medical management should be offered to women

TABLE 36.6 **Definitions of types of miscarriage**

| Type | Definition |
|---|---|
| Threatened miscarriage | early pregnancy with bleeding and/or pain but where ultrasound scan subsequently shows the pregnancy to be viable |
| Complete miscarriage | early pregnancy loss where all products of conception have been expelled from the uterus |
| Incomplete miscarriage | early pregnancy loss where a significant amount of products of conception remain within the uterine cavity |
| Inevitable miscarriage | early pregnancy with bleeding and/or pain and where speculum examination shows the cervical os to be open, with or without products of conception passing through: ultrasound may show the fetal heartbeat to be present or absent |
| Missed/silent/delayed miscarriage | either an intrauterine gestational sac with mean diameter 20 mm with no visible fetal pole or a fetal pole with crown–rump length 6 mm or more and no visible fetal heartbeat |
| Miscarriage with infection | early pregnancy loss with retained products of conception within the uterine cavity that have become infected |
| Recurrent miscarriage | three or more consecutive early pregnancy losses |
| Rregnancy of unknown location | a situation where the serum beta human chorionic gonadotrophin (hCG) is above the discriminatory zone for ultrasound detection (usually 1000 or 1500 iu/l), but where no pregnancy, either intrauterine or extrauterine, can be detected |
| Pregnancy of uncertain viability | early intrauterine pregnancy where the mean sac diameter is less then 20 mm or the crown–rump length is less than 6 mm with no visible fetal heartbeat. |
| Retained products of conception | pregnancy tissue remaining in the uterus with an anteroposterior diameter more than 15 mm when measured by ultrasound. |

**TABLE 36.7 Advantages and complications and disadvantages of each management option for miscarriages**

| Advantages over other procedures | Complications or disadvantages |
|---|---|
| **EVACUATION OF RETAINED PRODUCTS OF CONCEPTION** | |
| Quick procedure | Bleeding |
| Minimal follow up | Infection |
| Less pain | Complications of anaesthesia |
| | Perforation of the uterus |
| | Cervical tears |
| | Intra-abdominal trauma |
| | Intrauterine adhesion formation |
| **MEDICAL MANAGEMENT** | |
| Less chance of infection | More painful than ERPC |
| Cheaper than ERPC | Bleeding can last for up to 3 weeks |
| Outpatient-based procedure | ERPC may still be required |
| High patient acceptability | |
| **EXPECTANT MANAGEMENT** | |
| 'Natural' method | May take several weeks to complete |
| Low chance of infection | Medical/surgical management may still be required |
| Cheap | |
| Outpatient-based procedure | |

ERPC = evacuation of retained products of conception

who prefer to be managed this way, who are prepared to accept follow up and who can access hospital easily.

Medical management usually involves the use of the oral antiprogesterone mifepristone, followed 48 hours later by either oral or vaginal misoprostol, a synthetic prostaglandin. After the misoprostol has been given, many women remain in hospital until they have passed tissue vaginally and their bleeding has settled.

Conservative management of miscarriage may be offered to women who do not wish to have any medical or surgical intervention and prefer to wait for any retained products of conception to pass naturally. They should be warned, however, that this may take several weeks if there is an intact pregnancy sac inside the uterus. Expectant management is highly effective in incomplete miscarriage.

### Other points

Where tissue is expelled from the uterus or obtained by ERPC, it is useful to send it for histological examination to confirm intrauterine pregnancy and to exclude gestational trophoblastic neoplasia.

Women who are rhesus negative need to be administered with 250 iu anti-D antibodies when the uterus has been medically or surgically evacuated.

### GESTATIONAL TROPHOBLASTIC NEOPLASIA

Gestational trophoblastic neoplasia includes a group of pathologies – some benign, some malignant – that are abnormalities of trophoblastic tissue. This group includes hydatidiform mole, invasive mole, choriocarcinoma and placental-site trophoblastic tumour. Of these, hydatidiform mole is seen most frequently, and this is subdivided into two main types:

- **Complete hydatidiform mole:** genetically, the tissue is diploid and the genetic material is paternal in origin. A complete mole most commonly occurs after duplication of a haploid sperm that has fertilised a genetically 'empty' ovum but can also occur after dispermic fertilisation of an empty ovum. Histologically, there is no fetal tissue within the mole.
- **Partial hydatidiform mole:** genetically, the tissue is triploid and results from dispermic fertilisation of a normal ovum. Histologically, there is usually a fetus or fetal tissue present.

Although a complete mole has a fairly characteristic appearance on ultrasound, it can be difficult to diagnose a partial mole. Often, all that can be seen are some cystic spaces within the placental tissue.

### Management of hydatidiform mole

The treatment of choice for hydatidiform mole is surgical evacuation of the uterus. Cervical priming with prostaglandins or use of oxytocin should be avoided since these will cause the uterus to contract and may disseminate trophoblastic tissue through the bloodstream.

Histological examination of the tissue is essential to confirm the diagnosis. A partial mole may not be diagnosed until the pregnancy is too advanced for safe surgical evacuation. In this case, medical management may be required.

It is extremely important that any woman who is found to have gestational trophoblastic neoplasia is registered with a trophoblastic tumour and screening centre. There are two in England and one in Scotland. The centre will arrange all relevant follow up after a diagnosis of gestational trophoblastic neoplasia and will arrange any chemotherapy for persistent neoplasia that may be required.

Further pregnancy is not advised until at least 6 months after serum hCG levels have returned to normal. The risk of a future molar pregnancy is one in 80 pregnancies.

## ECTOPIC PREGNANCY

An ectopic pregnancy is a pregnancy that has implanted outside the endometrial cavity. The most common site is the fallopian tube but other sites include the cervix, uterine cornua, ovary and abdominal cavity. The incidence of ectopic pregnancy is just over 1% of all pregnancies and it can present at any gestation. The classic presentation of a ruptured tubal ectopic is severe pain and collapse after approximately 8 weeks of amenorrhoea with a positive pregnancy test.

### Management of ectopic pregnancy

There are three management options for ectopic pregnancy, surgical, medical and conservative, according to the presentation, symptoms and other findings, such as ultrasound scan and serum hCG level. Comparison of the advantages of management options for ectopic pregnancy are shown in Table 36.8.

TABLE 36.8 **Comparisons of the management options for ectopic pregnancy**

| Advantages of laparotomy | Advantages of laparoscopy |
|---|---|
| Quicker entry in acute situation | More appropriate in stable situation |
| More appropriate when large haemoperitoneum | Shorter operating time |
| Less specialised surgical skills | Less blood loss |
| No need for specialised equipment | Shorter stay in hospital |
| | Less need for analgesia |
| **Advantages of salpingectomy** | **Advantages of salpingotomy** |
| Less chance of persistent trophoblast | May preserve tube so that it can continue to function |
| Better haemostasis | |
| Possibly reduced risk of future ectopic | |
| Less/shorter follow up | |
| **Advantages of methotrexate** | **Disadvantages of methotrexate** |
| Avoid risks of surgery | Side effects |
| Cheaper | Need for long-term follow-up |
| Fallopian tubes remain intact | Cannot try for further pregnancy for 3 months |
| | May still need surgical management |

Surgery by laparotomy is required immediately for the acute state, when a woman presents with a ruptured ectopic pregnancy. This is an emergency and immediate laparotomy is required to remove the tube and arrest the bleeding. Every year there are maternal deaths from ruptured ectopic pregnancy.

In the non-acute state, where an ectopic pregnancy has been diagnosed but the woman is stable, the surgical treatment of choice would be laparoscopic salpingectomy or salpingotomy: the decision then being whether to remove the tube containing the ectopic pregnancy (salpingectomy) or to open the tube and remove the pregnancy, leaving the tube in place (salpingotomy). At the moment, common practice would be to perform a salpingectomy if the contralateral tube looks healthy. However, if the contralateral tube looks damaged or diseased, then a salpingotomy could be performed, provided that there is adequate haemostasis. The options would, of course, be discussed with the woman beforehand so that a management plan is in place.

Medical management can be as effective as surgery in women with an ectopic pregnancy who are stable. Treatment is normally via a single intramuscular injection of methotrexate, the dose of which is calculated from the body surface area. Fourteen percent of women will need more than one dose of methotrexate. Less than 10% will ultimately need surgery.

The suitability criteria for medical management of ectopic pregnancy are:

- normal renal and liver function tests
- serum hCG less than 3000 iu/l
- minimal or mild symptoms only
- no evidence of haemoperitoneum on ultrasound
- ectopic mass less than 5 cm diameter
- no evidence of fetal heartbeat.

Conservative management can be appropriate in very small ectopic pregnancies, where the serum hCG levels are falling, and in pregnancies of unknown location. For conservative management to be considered, the initial serum hCG should be less than 1500 iu/l and there should be minimal fluid in the pouch of Douglas on pelvic ultrasound. Serum hCG should be measured twice weekly until levels have fallen by 50%. Once this has been achieved, then weekly checks are appropriate. Follow up should continue until serum hCG levels are lower than 20 iu/l. Should the woman become symptomatic, or the hCG levels plateau or rise, active management would be required.

## REFERENCE

1. HANNAH ME, HANNAH WJ, HEWSON SA, HODNETT ED, SAIGAL S, WILLIAM AR. Planned caesarean section versus planned vaginal birth for breech presentation at term: arandomised multicentre trial. Term Breech Trial Collaborative Group. *Lancet* 2000;356:1375–83.

## FURTHER READING

National Blood Service [www.blood.co.uk].

RASSAM SS, COUNSELL DJ, Perioperative electrolyte and fluid balance. *Continuing Education in Anaesthesia, Critical Care and Pain* 2005;5:157–60.

Royal College of Obstetricians and Gynaecologists. *RCOG Greentop Guideline No. 21. The Management of Tubal Pregnancy.* London: RCOG; 2004.

Royal College of Obstetricians and Gynaecologists. *RCOG Greentop Guideline No. 38. The Management of Gestational Trophoblastic Neoplasia.* London: RCOG; 2010.

Royal College of Obstetricians and Gynaecologists. *RCOG Greentop Guideline No. 25. The Management of Early Pregnancy Loss.* London: RCOG; 2006.

# Sample questions relating to surgery in obstetrics and gynaecology

## EXTENDED MATCHING QUESTIONS

### Questions 1–12

■ *These questions relate to types of blood products. For each item below, select the* **single** *best option from the list of options (A–E). Each option may be used once, more than once or not at all.*

OPTIONS

▷ **A** Whole blood
▷ **B** Packed red cells
▷ **C** Frozen red cells
▷ **D** Platelets
▷ **E** Fresh frozen plasma

1 ▶ Is used in thrombocytopenia

2 ▶ Is used in anaemia

3 ▶ Is used to reduce infused fluid volume

4 ▶ Is used if blood with rare antigens is required

5 ▶ Is rarely used

6 ▶ Is rich in clotting factors

7 ▶ Has a high level of potassium

8 ▶ Contains an anticoagulant

9 ▶ Contains glycerol

10 ▶ Has a 1-year shelf life

11 ▶ Has a 7-day shelf life

12 ▶ Is expensive

### Questions 13–22

■ *These questions relate to key blood electrolytes. For each item below, select the* **single** *best option from the list of options (A–H). Each option may be used once, more than once or not at all.*

OPTIONS

▷ **A** Sodium
▷ **B** Potassium
▷ **C** Calcium
▷ **D** Chloride
▷ **E** Bicarbonate
▷ **F** Urea
▷ **G** Creatinine
▷ **H** Albumin

13 ▶ Balances anions and cations in all compartments

14 ▶ Balances anions in all compartments

15 ▶ Contributes half the osmolarity of the extracellular fluid

16 ▶ Is involved in membrane resting potential

17 ▶ Is involved in blood clotting

18 ▶ Is involved in neurotransmitter release

19 ▶ Maintains intracellular fluid volumes

20 ▶ Moves easily between all compartments

21 ▶ Is regulated by antidiuretic hormone

22 ▶ Regulates pH

**Questions 23–36**

- *These questions relate to electrolyte disturbances. For each item below, select the **single** best option from the list of options (A–H). Each option may be used once, more than once or not at all.*

OPTIONS

▷ **A** Hyponatraemia
▷ **B** Hypernatraemia
▷ **C** Hypokalaemia
▷ **D** Hyperkalaemia
▷ **E** Hypocalcaemia
▷ **F** Hypercalcaemia
▷ **G** Hypochloraemia
▷ **H** Hyperchloraemia

23 ▶ Is caused by water depletion

24 ▶ Is caused by excessive water

25 ▶ Is caused by vomiting

26 ▶ Is caused by diarrhoea

27 ▶ Is caused by hyperparathyroidism

28 ▶ Is caused by Addison disease

29 ▶ Is caused by severe dehydration

30 ▶ Is caused by poor vitamin D intake

31 ▶ Is found in respiratory alkalosis

32 ▶ Is caused by hypoadrenalism

33 ▶ Is caused by insulin therapy

34 ▶ Is caused by diuretic therapy

35 ▶ Is caused by blood transfusion

36 ▶ Is caused by beta agonists

## MULTIPLE CHOICE QUESTIONS

37 ▶ Rates of gynaecological surgery:

   **A** ▷ have decreased over the last 10 years
   **B** ▷ have been affected by medical management of conditions
   **C** ▷ specifically, hysterectomies, have been reduced due to the use of levonorgestrel-containing intrauterine system
   **D** ▷ are influenced by the age of the patient
   **E** ▷ are influenced by the length of hospital stay

38 ▶ Surgical success rates:

   **A** ▷ have the same criteria for surgeons and for patients
   **B** ▷ consider a neat cosmetic appearance of the abdominal scar a success
   **C** ▷ are increased with good anaesthesia
   **D** ▷ are unrelated to the equipment used
   **E** ▷ are increased with optimisation of the patient's condition

39 ▶ Regarding surgical complications:

   **A** ▷ All operations have complications associated with them
   **B** ▷ A body mass index of $> 25\,kg/m^2$ leads to poor haemostasis
   **C** ▷ A faulty diathermy device can cause serious burns to patients
   **D** ▷ Haemorrhage is an immediate complication
   **E** ▷ A deep vein thrombosis is a late complication

40 ▶ Adverse reactions of blood transfusion include:

   **A** ▷ acute haemolytic reactions due to antigen incompatibility
   **B** ▷ acute nonhaemolytic reactions that are usually fatal
   **C** ▷ lung injury due to a clot formation on the lung
   **D** ▷ immunosuppression
   **E** ▷ iron overload

**41** ▶ Regarding body fluid balance:

    **A** ▷ The most important intracellular electrolyte is potassium

    **B** ▷ The body produces water internally as a result of metabolic processes

    **C** ▷ Movement of fluid between the interstitial and intracellular compartments is due to osmotic pressure generated by protein

    **D** ▷ Hydrostatic forces are due to blood pressure

    **E** ▷ At the arteriolar end of a capillary, plasma osmotic forces are greater

**42** ▶ Regarding effects of anaesthesia and surgery on fluid balance:

    **A** ▷ Preoperatively, most patients have fluid excess

    **B** ▷ Steroids released in surgery cause fluid retention

    **C** ▷ Perioperatively, fluid shifts between compartments is minimal

    **D** ▷ Perioperatively, antidiuretic hormone release is decreased

    **E** ▷ Cytokine release perioperatively causes fluid accumulation in the lungs

**43** ▶ Regarding gestational trophoblastic disease:

    **A** ▷ All gestational trophoblastic disease is malignant

    **B** ▷ Hydatiform mole is the most common

    **C** ▷ A complete mole is maternal in origin

    **D** ▷ A complete mole contains no fetal tissue

    **E** ▷ A partial mole is due to dispermic fertilisation

Answers

# CHAPTER 37

# Answers

## Answers for Chapters 2–4

### EXTENDED MATCHING QUESTIONS

1 ▶ **E** = 5
2 ▶ **D** = 4
3 ▶ **E** = 5
4 ▶ **C** = 3
5 ▶ **C** = 3
6 ▶ **H** = 8
7 ▶ **D** = 4
8 ▶ **M** = S2–4
9 ▶ **H** = S1–2
10 ▶ **D** = L4–S3
11 ▶ **M** = S2–4
12 ▶ **F** = Transitional cells
13 ▶ **A** = Stratified squamous epithelium
14 ▶ **C** = Ciliated cells
15 ▶ **B** = Columnar epithelium
16 ▶ **D** = Secretory cells
17 ▶ **E** = Cuboidal epithelium
18 ▶ **D** = Secretory cells
19 ▶ **A** = Stratified squamous epithelium
20 ▶ **A** = Stratified squamous epithelium

### MULTIPLE CHOICE QUESTIONS

21 ▶ Regarding the pelvic nerves:

    **A = True** ▷ They are part of the autonomic nervous system

    **B = True** ▷ The sacral plexus gives off the pudendal nerve

    **C = False** ▷ The sciatic nerve is formed by the L4–S2 roots

    **D = False** ▷ The sciatic nerve passes through the lesser sciatic foramen

    **E = False** ▷ The sciatic nerve supplies the anterior aspect of the knee

22 ▶ The obturator nerve:

    **A = False** ▷ is formed by the L2–5 roots

    **B = False** ▷ lies along the floor of the pelvis

    **C = True** ▷ exits the pelvis through the obturator canal

    **D = False** ▷ splits into anterior, medial and posterior parts on leaving the pelvis

    **E = False** ▷ supplies muscles of the anterior thigh

23 ▶ Regarding the arteries of the pelvis:

    **A = False** ▷ The umbilical artery supplies the posterior portion of the bladder

    **B = True** ▷ The pelvic ureters are supplied by the superior vesical artery

    **C = False** ▷ The inferior vesicle artery originates from the posterior internal iliac artery

    **D = False** ▷ The vaginal artery originates from the anterior part of the internal iliac artery

    **E = False** ▷ The lower rectum is supplied by the inferior rectal artery

24 ▶ Concerning the urinary system:

    **A = True** ▷ The ureters cross the bifurcation of the common iliac arteries on entering the pelvis

    **B = False** ▷ The ureters are retroperitoneal along their whole length

    **C = False** ▷ The renal arteries supply the ureters along their entire length

    **D = False** ▷ The ureters pass above the uterine artery

    **E = True** ▷ The ureters drain lymph to the internal iliac lymph nodes

25 ▶ Concerning the vagina:

A = **False** ▷ The lateral two walls of the vagina are in contact with each other

B = **True** ▷ The bulbospongiosus muscle compresses the vagina

C = **False** ▷ The superior third of the vagina is supplied by the vaginal arteries

D = **False** ▷ The pudendal nerve provides somatic innervation to the whole vagina

E = **True** ▷ Sympathetic innervation is derived from the lumbar splanchnic nerves

26 ▶ Concerning the female reproductive system:

A = **True** ▷ The cervix drains lymph into to the internal iliac lymph nodes

B = **False** ▷ The cervical canal has its widest part at the internal os

C = **False** ▷ The round ligament is posterior to the ovarian ligament

D = **False** ▷ The cervix is more muscular than the uterus

E = **True** ▷ The broad ligament is formed by peritoneum

27 ▶ Concerning the female reproductive system:

A = **False** ▷ The mesometrium suspends the ovary

B = **True** ▷ The cardinal ligaments provide a major support for the uterus

C = **False** ▷ The uterosacral ligaments attach to the lateral part of the sacrum

D = **True** ▷ The rectouterine pouch (pouch of Douglas) is the lowest part of the pelvis

E = **False** ▷ The uterus drains blood into the external iliac vein

## Answers for Chapter 5

### EXTENDED MATCHING QUESTIONS

1 ▶ **D** = Mitosis
2 ▶ **B** = DNA synthesis
3 ▶ **H** = Resting phase
4 ▶ **E** = Preparation for DNA synthesis
5 ▶ **F** = Preparation for mitosis

### MULTIPLE CHOICE QUESTIONS

6 ▶ Regarding eukaryotic cell membranes:

A = **True** ▷ Cholesterol makes the phospholipid bilayer of the plasma membrane become firm

B = **False** ▷ Receptors for circulating molecules are found on the inside of the plasma membrane

C = **True** ▷ Protein receptors are embedded within the plasma membrane

D = **True** ▷ The Golgi complex has a single membrane surrounding it

E = **True** ▷ The nucleus has a double membrane

7 ▶ Regarding the nucleus of the cell:

A = **False** ▷ It is the second largest organelle

B = **False** ▷ The nuclear envelope is a single membrane

C = **True** ▷ Messenger RNA is transported out of the nucleus

D = **True** ▷ Ribosomal RNA is synthesised entirely within the nucleolus

E = **True** ▷ The nucleus membrane is often continuous with the rough endoplasmic reticulum

8 ▶ The following are synthesised inside the smooth endoplasmic reticulum:

A = **False** ▷ Enzymes
B = **True** ▷ Fatty acids
C = **False** ▷ Glucose
D = **True** ▷ Phospholipids
E = **False** ▷ Proteins

9 ▶ The rough endoplasmic reticulum:

A = **True** ▷ has ribosomes attached to its surface
B = **True** ▷ synthesises cell proteins
C = **False** ▷ retains proteins for several days
D = **True** ▷ is abundant in the pancreatic acinar cells
E = **False** ▷ sends proteins to the smooth endoplasmic reticulum

**10 ▶ Human mitochondria characteristically:**

A = **False** ▷ metabolise proteins
B = **False** ▷ have a smooth inner surface
C = **False** ▷ contain cytosol
D = **True** ▷ have reactions that occur in the intermembrane space
E = **True** ▷ have DNA inherited through the mother only

**11 ▶ Regarding the cell's 'disposal system':**

A = **False** ▷ Lysosomes and peroxisomes have double membranes
B = **True** ▷ Lysosomes and peroxisomes contain enzymes
C = **False** ▷ Lysosomes have an internal pH of 3.0
D = **True** ▷ Peroxisomes remove toxic molecules from the blood
E = **True** ▷ Peroxisomes are the main organelle for oxidising fatty acids

**12 ▶ Regarding cell–cell signalling:**

A = **True** ▷ Endocrine signalling always relies on the bloodstream for transport
B = **False** ▷ Neurotransmitters are a form of autocrine transmission
C = **True** ▷ Self-signalling is known as autocrine signalling
D = **True** ▷ Membrane-bound signalling proteins interact with receptors on a neighbouring cell
E = **False** ▷ Gap junctions help retain cell rigidity

**13 ▶ Human eicosanoids**

A = **True** ▷ are cell signalling molecules
B = **False** ▷ are made in the mitochondria
C = **True** ▷ are made by all cells
D = **False** ▷ are all made from arachidonic acid
E = **False** ▷ help myometrial relaxation

**14 ▶ Regarding cyclooxygenase (COX):**

A = **False** ▷ COX-1 is expressed at sites of inflammation
B = **False** ▷ Aspirin temporarily inactivates platelet COX
C = **True** ▷ Aspirin is more active against COX-1 than against COX-2
D = **False** ▷ Aspirin is a COX antagonist
E = **True** ▷ Fetal membranes release COX-2 during labour

**15 ▶ Regarding $Ca^{2+}$ as an intracellular messenger:**

A = **False** ▷ The intracellular concentration of free $Ca^{2+}$ is higher than the $Ca^{2+}$ concentration of the extracellular fluid
B = **True** ▷ The endoplasmic reticulum has high levels of free $Ca^{2+}$
C = **True** ▷ Mitochondria pump $Ca^{2+}$ in from the cytosol
D = **True** ▷ $Ca^{2+}$-ATPases pump $Ca^{2+}$ out of cells
E = **False** ▷ the $Ca^{2+}$–calmodulin complex directly activates smooth muscle contraction

**16 ▶ Regarding the molecular basis of cancer:**

A = **False** ▷ Oncogenes are present in tumour cells only
B = **True** ▷ Proto-oncogenes are required for normal cell growth
E = **False** ▷ Tumour cells have less mitotic activity than normal cells
D = **True** ▷ *p53* mutations are present in half of all cancers
E = **False** ▷ Presence of the protein adenomatous polyposis coli (APC) is a cause of colorectal cancer

**17 ▶ Regarding neoplastic cells:**

A = **False** ▷ They are usually well differentiated
B = **True** ▷ Carcinomas can be derived from endoderm
C = **False** ▷ Sarcomas are derived from ectoderm
D = **True** ▷ Metastatic tumour cells break down the basal lamina
E = **False** ▷ Tumour masses of more than 1 mm need their own blood supply

**18 ▶ Regarding nucleic acids:**

A = **True** ▷ DNA is longer than RNA
B = **True** ▷ RNA is single-stranded
C = **False** ▷ DNA strands are held together by ionic bonds
D = **False** ▷ uracil replaces guanine in RNA
E = **False** ▷ DNA and RNA contain the same pentose sugar

19 ▶ Regarding the synthesis of messenger RNA (mRNA):

A = **False** ▷ The process is called translation
B = **True** ▷ RNA polymerase is the main enzyme of this process
C = **False** ▷ The base sequence of the mRNA transcript matches that of the template strand
D = **False** ▷ Only one mRNA copy is produced from each part of DNA
E = **False** ▷ Exons are removed from the mRNA

20 ▶ Regarding protein synthesis:

A = **False** ▷ The final step of forming proteins from messenger RNA is called transcription
B = **True** ▷ The whole process requires mRNA, ribosomal RNA and transfer RNA
C = **True** ▷ Transer RNA carries three amino acids
D = **False** ▷ Ribosomes have no role in the final part of protein synthesis, where messenger RNA acts as a blueprint for the sequence of amino acids
E = **False** ▷ The tertiary structure of a protein depends on hydrophilic interactions between different parts of the amino acid sequence

## Answers for Chapter 6

### EXTENDED MATCHING QUESTIONS

1 ▶ **C** = Increases the concentration of cyclic adenosine monophosphate (cAMP)
2 ▶ **A** = Several effects
3 ▶ **D** = Increases the concentrations of inositol trisphosphate and $Ca^{2+}$
4 ▶ **C** = Increases the concentration of cAMP

### MULTIPLE CHOICE QUESTIONS

5 ▶ Regarding the synthesis of steroids:

A = **True** ▷ The process involves two classes of enzyme
B = **True** ▷ Cytochrome P450 increases steroid solubility
C = **True** ▷ The pattern of enzyme expression determines the type of steroid produced
D = **False** ▷ The placenta can form the full range of steroids
E = **False** ▷ Estriol is unique to the fetus

6 ▶ Regarding steroid hormone receptors:

A = **False** ▷ Steroids cannot pass through the plasma membrane
B = **False** ▷ The ligand-binding domain has a hydrophilic binding site
C = **False** ▷ The DNA-binding domain contains sulphur bridges
D = **False** ▷ Steroid receptors exist on the plasma membrane and the nucleus membrane
E = **True** ▷ An activated steroid receptor translocates into the nucleus

7 ▶ The following are steroid receptors:

A = **False** ▷ Aldosterone receptor
B = **True** ▷ Androgen receptor
C = **False** ▷ Cortisol receptor
D = **True** ▷ Estrogen receptor
E = **True** ▷ Progesterone receptor

8 ▶ Regarding the synthesis of prostaglandins:

A = **True** ▷ All prostaglandins are synthesised from arachidonic acid
B = **False** ▷ Arachidonic acid is found in the cytosol
C = **False** ▷ Phospholipase $A_1$ releases free arachidonate
D = **True** ▷ Cyclooxygenase enzymes act on the free arachidonate
E = **True** ▷ Prostaglandin $G_2$ is the first prostaglandin formed

**9 ▶ Regarding prostaglandins:**

A = **True** ▷ They act via G proteins
B = **False** ▷ They act by freely transcending the plasma membrane
C = **True** ▷ They have fast response times
D = **False** ▷ Prostaglandin $F_{2\alpha}$ exerts its cellular effects via $Ca^{2+}$ signalling
E = **True** ▷ Prostaglandin $E_2$ transduces its signals via changes in the intracellular concentration of cyclic adenosine monophosphate (cAMP)

**10 ▶ Regarding myometrial contractions:**

A = **True** ▷ They are caused by oxytocin
B = **False** ▷ They are caused by prostaglandin $F_2$
C = **False** ▷ They are caused by hormones that increase the concentration of cyclic adenosine monophosphate (cAMP)
D = **False** ▷ Oxytocin suppresses uterine prostaglandin synthesis
E = **True** ▷ Prostaglandin $F_2$ increases the number of oxytocin receptors on the uterus

**11 ▶ Regarding progesterone:**

A = **True** ▷ It is the most important myometrial relaxant
B = **True** ▷ It increases the intracellular concentration of cyclic adenosine monophosphate (cAMP)
C = **False** ▷ It influences the action of oxytocin only
D = **False** ▷ Placental output is stable throughout pregnancy
E = **False** ▷ Prostacyclin opposes its actions

**12 ▶ Regarding prostaglandins:**

A = **False** ▷ They are a class of leucotrienes
B = **True** ▷ They share the common precursor arachidonic acid
C = **False** ▷ They increase the flux of $Ca^{2+}$ from the extracellular fluid into myometrial muscle to cause myometrial contractility
D = **False** ▷ Only prostaglandin $E_2$ can ripen the cervix
E = **False** ▷ During labour, the cervix is the most important location of prostaglandin release

**Answers for Chapter 7**

**EXTENDED MATCHING QUESTIONS**

1 ▶ A = Acidosis
2 ▶ E = Respiratory alkalosis
3 ▶ B = Alkalosis
4 ▶ E = Respiratory alkalosis
5 ▶ G = Metabolic alkalosis
6 ▶ F = Respiratory acidosis

**MULTIPLE CHOICE QUESTIONS**

**7 ▶ During pregnancy:**

A = **False** ▷ the $Na^+$ plasma concentration decreases
B = **True** ▷ the plasma volume increases from 3 to 4.5 l
C = **False** ▷ the interstitial-fluid volume remains unchanged
D = **False** ▷ the intracellular-fluid volume remains the same
E = **False** ▷ there is no change in the colloid osmotic pressure of plasma

**8 ▶ Regarding the acid–base balance of the extracellular fluid:**

A = **False** ▷ Acidosis occurs when the blood is more acidic than normal
B = **False** ▷ Buffers readjust the pH value of the extracellular fluid over a few hours
C = **False** ▷ Renal mechanisms that adjust $H^+$ excretion begin to work within minutes
D = **False** ▷ The buffer capacity of a buffer is greatest when it is all in either a weak alkaline or a weak acidic form
E = **False** ▷ The bicarbonate system is a strong buffer

**9** ▶ Regarding the acid–base balance:

A = **True** ▷ Haemoglobin has multiple acidic and basic groups

B = **False** ▷ Oxygenated haemoglobin is a better buffer then deoxygenated haemoglobin

C = **False** ▷ $CO_2$ dissolves better in plasma if haemoglobin is oxygenated

D = **True** ▷ $CO_2$ that enters red blood cells can be catalysed by carbonic anhydrase to form carbonic acid

E = **True** ▷ Bicarbonate ions diffuse out of red blood cells in exchange for $Cl^-$ ions

**10** ▶ In labour:

A = **False** ▷ the mother tends to have an uncompensated respiratory acidosis

B = **True** ▷ maternal haemoglobin has an increased affinity for $O_2$

C = **False** ▷ there is a decrease in the concentration of deoxygenated haemoglobin in the fetus

D = **True** ▷ the fetus becomes acidotic because of its metabolism

E = **False** ▷ respiratory acidosis does not occur in the fetus

# Answers for Chapter 8

## MULTIPLE CHOICE QUESTIONS

**1** ▶ The body uses $Ca^{2+}$ for the following processes:

A = **True** ▷ Muscle contraction

B = **True** ▷ Extracellular messenger

C = **True** ▷ Intracellular messenger

D = **True** ▷ Enzyme co-factor

E = **True** ▷ Stabilisation of membrane potentials

**2** ▶ The following play a role in $Ca^{2+}$ homeostasis:

A = **True** ▷ Bone

B = **True** ▷ Kidney

C = **True** ▷ Parathyroid glands

D = **True** ▷ Thyroid gland

E = **True** ▷ Gastrointestinal tract

**3** ▶ Regarding parathyroid hormone (PTH):

A = **False** ▷ Primary hyperparathyroidism is characterised by low serum concentrations of PTH and $Ca^{2+}$

B = **True** ▷ It promotes the renal excretion of phosphate

C = **False** ▷ It decreases the renal synthesis of calcitriol

D = **False** ▷ It is not synthesised by the fetus

E = **True** ▷ Secretion of PTH is increased by a decrease in serum $Ca^{2+}$

**4** ▶ Regarding vitamin D:

A = **False** ▷ It is a polypeptide

B = **False** ▷ Fifty percent is acquired from the diet

C = **False** ▷ It is activated in the liver by $1\alpha$-hydroxylase

D = **False** ▷ It increases serum levels of $Ca^{2+}$ and $PO_4^{3-}$ by decreasing the rate of active secretion

E = **True** ▷ The major circulating form of vitamin D is 25-hydroxvitamin $D_3$ (calcidiol)

**5** ▶ Regarding vitamin D:

A = **False** ▷ It decreases the serum $Ca^{2+}$ concentration

B = **False** ▷ It decreases the serum phosphate concentration

C = **True** ▷ Calcitriol is metabolically active

D = **True** ▷ Calcidiol is metabolically active

E = **True** ▷ It is transported in the blood bound to vitamin-D-binding protein

**6** ▶ Regarding the synthesis of vitamin D:

A = **True** ▷ It requires ultraviolet light

B = **False** ▷ The first precursor to vitamin D is hydrocholesterol

C = **True** ▷ Vitamin $D_2$ and vitamin $D_3$ are hydroxylated to the same product

D = **False** ▷ Active vitamin D is formed in the distal convoluted tubule

E = **True** ▷ It is increased by low serum concentrations of phosphate

7 ▶ Regarding the maternal and fetal Ca²⁺ balance:

**A = False** ▷ In the fetus, 80% of Ca²⁺ accumulation occurs in the first trimester
**B = False** ▷ Maternal bone mineral density decreases continually through pregnancy
**C = True** ▷ Low maternal vitamin D levels mean that the fetus is more likely to develop diabetes
**D = False** ▷ The neonate has low serum calcitonin
**E = False** ▷ The mother has high levels of parathyroid hormone

8 ▶ Regarding the structure of bone:

**A = False** ▷ Seventy-five percent is matrix
**B = True** ▷ Ninety percent of matrix is type 1 collagen
**C = True** ▷ The mineral component contains Ca²⁺
**D = False** ▷ The mineral component provides resilience
**E = False** ▷ Collagen provides rigidity

9 ▶ Trabecular bone:

**A = True** ▷ is strong
**B = False** ▷ is heavy
**C = False** ▷ forms the outer part of bone
**D = True** ▷ is spongy in appearance
**E = True** ▷ has a high surface area

10 ▶ In the metabolism of bone:

**A = True** ▷ osteoblasts produce bone
**B = False** ▷ osteoblasts respond to mechanical strain
**C = False** ▷ each osteoblast is constantly active
**D = True** ▷ osteoclasts reabsorb bone
**E = False** ▷ osteocytes produce matrix

11 ▶ Regarding bone remodelling:

**A = False** ▷ A complete cycle takes 180 days
**B = False** ▷ The process takes place deep in the bone
**C = True** ▷ The process involves both osteoblast and osteoclasts
**D = False** ▷ Hydroxyapatite is not destroyed
**E = False** ▷ Gaps left by osteoclasts are filled with hydroxyapatite

12 ▶ Osteoporosis:

**A = True** ▷ is associated with underactive osteoblasts
**B = False** ▷ is only caused by a loss of estrogen
**C = True** ▷ is diagnosed by a low score following a dual energy X-ray absorptiometry scan
**D = False** ▷ does not occur in women below the age of 65 years
**E = True** ▷ is associated with low body weight, cigarette smoking, alcohol consumption, poor nutrition and physical inactivity

13 ▶ Regarding osteopenia:

**A = False** ▷ It is diagnosed if the bone mineral density is more than 2.5 standard deviations away from the mean value for a young healthy adult
**B = False** ▷ The loss of bone mineral is greater than in osteoporosis
**C = True** ▷ Increasing Ca²⁺ intake is essential to prevent progression
**D = True** ▷ It is more common in women with prolonged secondary amenorrhoea
**E = True** ▷ It is more common in people with long-term steroid use

14 ▶ The following are true regarding osteoporosis:

**A = False** ▷ Maximum bone mass is reached in puberty
**B = True** ▷ Men have a higher maximum bone mass than women
**C = False** ▷ Any decrease in bone mineral density is dangerous
**D = False** ▷ Bone mass remains constant until the age of around 50 years
**E = False** ▷ Excluding the menopause, women still have a faster loss in bone mineral density than men

15 ▶ The following are true regarding osteoporosis:

**A = False** ▷ Hypogonadism is the most common cause of osteoporosis in men
**B = False** ▷ An increase in body weight makes osteoporotic fractures more common
**C = True** ▷ Heparin increases the risk of osteoporotic fractures
**D = True** ▷ It is more common in hyperthyroidism
**E = True** ▷ It is more common in Cushing syndrome

## Answers for Chapter 9

### EXTENDED MATCHING QUESTIONS

1 ▶ **A** = Chylomicron
2 ▶ **D** = High-density lipoprotein
3 ▶ **B** = Very-low-density lipoprotein
4 ▶ **B** = Very-low-density lipoprotein
5 ▶ **C** = Low-density lipoprotein
6 ▶ **E** = Fatty acid–albumin
7 ▶ **D** = High-density lipoprotein
8 ▶ **A** = Chylomicron
9 ▶ **C** = Low-density lipoprotein

### MULTIPLE CHOICE QUESTIONS

10 ▶ Regarding metabolism:

**A** = **False** ▷ All reactions are reversible
**B** = **False** ▷ All pathways run at the same speed
**C** = **True** ▷ Triacylglycerols are broken down to free fatty acids
**D** = **True** ▷ All substances are eventually converted to acetyl coenzyme A
**E** = **False** ▷ Acetyl coenzyme A is hydrolysed

11 ▶ Regarding the metabolism of carbohydrates:

**A** = **True** ▷ They can be ingested as huge polymers
**B** = **True** ▷ Disaccharides are a readily available glucose source
**C** = **False** ▷ Sucrose produces a slow rise in blood sugar
**D** = **True** ▷ Glucose polymers are slow to be digested
**E** = **True** ▷ All dietary carbohydrate can be converted to glucose

12 ▶ Regarding the metabolism of glucose:

**A** = **True** ▷ Aerobic glucose metabolism yields more ATP than anaerobic metabolism
**B** = **False** ▷ Under anaerobical conditions, glucose is converted into pyruvate
**C** = **True** ▷ All tissues can consume glucose
**D** = **True** ▷ Glucose is quickly replenished in the blood after it has been removed
**E** = **True** ▷ Glucose is the only fuel that can be respired anaerobically

13 ▶ Regarding the anaerobic metabolism of glucose:

**A** = **True** ▷ The presence of lactate confirms anaerobic glucose metabolism
**B** = **True** ▷ Lactate is a metabolic dead end
**C** = **False** ▷ Lactate cannot be reduced back to pyruvate
**D** = **False** ▷ The formation of lactate from pyruvate requires oxidised nicotinamide adenine dinucleotide (NAD⁺)
**E** = **True** ▷ Glucose can be formed from lactate

14 ▶ Regarding the homeostasis of blood glucose:

**A** = **False** ▷ In people without diabetes, the fasting blood glucose concentration can be as low as 3 mmol/l
**B** = **True** ▷ In people without diabetes, the postprandial blood glucose concentration can be as high as 8 mmol/l
**C** = **True** ▷ Pregnant women tolerate lower fasting blood glucose concentrations than nonpregnant women
**D** = **False** ▷ Glucose only appears in the urine if the blood glucose concentration rises above 9 mmol/l
**E** = **True** ▷ Hypoglycaemic coma can result from overconsumption of alcohol

15 ▶ The following increase the breakdown of triacylglycerols:

**A** = **True** ▷ Adrenaline
**B** = **True** ▷ Diabetic coma
**C** = **True** ▷ Glucagon
**D** = **False** ▷ Insulin
**E** = **True** ▷ Noradrenaline

16 ▶ Regarding the plasma concentration of triacylglycerols:

**A** = **False** ▷ It is lowered in exercise
**B** = **False** ▷ It is lowered in stress
**C** = **True** ▷ It is raised in people with diabetes
**D** = **True** ▷ If elevated, this increases the risk of coronary heart disease
**E** = **True** ▷ It is at its lowest in the normal fed state

**17** ► Regarding diabetic ketoacidosis:

**A** = **False** ▷ It occurs predominantly in type 2 diabetes
**B** = **True** ▷ It causes a hypoxic coma
**C** = **True** ▷ It occurs in people with diabetes who have a concurrent illness
**D** = **True** ▷ There is a decrease in the affinity of haemoglobin for $O_2$
**E** = **False** ▷ Treatment is by rapid infusion of insulin

**18** ► The following are signs of diabetic ketoacidosis:

**A** = **True** ▷ Hyperglycaemia
**B** = **True** ▷ Glycosuria
**C** = **False** ▷ Hyperkalaemia
**D** = **True** ▷ Low partial pressure of $O_2$
**E** = **False** ▷ High partial pressure of $CO_2$

**19** ► The following are related to the development of diabetic ketoacidosis:

**A** = **True** ▷ Dehydration
**B** = **True** ▷ Hypoxia
**C** = **False** ▷ Low fatty acids
**D** = **False** ▷ Low kidney excretion of $H^+$
**E** = **True** ▷ Osmotic diuresis

**20** ► Regarding gestational diabetes:

**A** = **True** ▷ All women have some insulin resistance in pregnancy
**B** = **True** ▷ Blood levels of insulin are high
**C** = **False** ▷ Blood levels of fatty acids are low
**D** = **False** ▷ It is diagnosed using a random blood sugar test
**E** = **True** ▷ It lasts for the duration of pregnancy only

**21** ► The following elements form parts of proteins:

**A** = **True** ▷ Carbon
**B** = **True** ▷ Hydrogen
**C** = **True** ▷ Nitrogen
**D** = **True** ▷ Oxygen
**E** = **False** ▷ Silicon

**22** ► The following increase protein breakdown:

**A** = **False** ▷ Exercise
**B** = **False** ▷ Growth
**C** = **True** ▷ High-protein diet
**D** = **False** ▷ Pregnancy
**E** = **True** ▷ Starvation

**23** ► Regarding the urea cycle:

**A** = **False** ▷ It incorporates 1 mole of nitrogen into 1 mole of urea
**B** = **True** ▷ Its dysfunction causes brain oedema in newborn babies
**C** = **False** ▷ It produces energy
**D** = **True** ▷ It occurs in the liver
**E** = **False** ▷ Its product (urea) is nonsoluble

**24** ► Regarding amino acids:

**A** = **False** ▷ They all enter the tricarboxylic acid cycle
**B** = **False** ▷ They can all be used to form glucose
**C** = **False** ▷ Some amino acids can produce both glucose and ketones
**D** = **True** ▷ Alanine and glutamine represent 70% of the amino acids released by muscle to produce glucose
**E** = **True** ▷ Tyrosine is ketogenic

**25** ► The following are end products of the metabolism of phenylalanine by phenylalanine hydroxylase:

**A** = **True** ▷ Thyroxine
**B** = **True** ▷ Melanin
**C** = **False** ▷ Oxygen
**D** = **True** ▷ Water
**E** = **False** ▷ Phenylacetate

**26** ► Regarding phenylketonuria:

**A** = **False** ▷ The accumulation of phenylalanine increases the uptake of other amino acids by the brain
**B** = **False** ▷ Affected people have mild mental restriction
**C** = **True** ▷ Screening involves the Guthrie test
**D** = **False** ▷ Screening should take place within 3 days of birth
**E** = **False** ▷ Treatment is with a special diet until the age of 5 years

**27 ▶** Regarding the complex metabolism of the maternal and fetal unit:

**A = False** ▷ There is insulin resistance in maternal tissues throughout pregnancy

**B = True** ▷ Maternal insulin sensitivity is reduced by at least 50% in pregnancy

**C = True** ▷ Maternal anabolic activities are increased in the first trimester

**D = False** ▷ Fetal nutrient uptake is favoured throughout pregnancy

**E = False** ▷ The fetus oxidises ketone bodies and fatty acids

**28 ▶** Regarding metabolism of glucose and fats in the newborn baby:

**A = True** ▷ Gluconeogenesis is inactive in the fetus

**B = True** ▷ The newborn baby activates the ketogenic pathway

**C = True** ▷ There is little lipogenic capacity

**D = False** ▷ Newborns have a low-fat diet

**E = True** ▷ Lipoprotein lipase activity increases in the newborn's heart

## Answers for Chapter 10

### EXTENDED MATCHING QUESTIONS

**1 ▶ D =** Cutting current
**2 ▶ D =** Cutting current
**3 ▶ C =** Coagulation current
**4 ▶ C =** Coagulation current
**5 ▶ B =** Blended waveform
**6 ▶ E =** Desiccation
**7 ▶ F =** Fulguration

### MULTIPLE CHOICE QUESTIONS

**8 ▶** Ultrasound can be used for the following:

**A = False** ▷ Fetal therapy
**B = True** ▷ To determine the nature of a tissue
**C = True** ▷ To assess the movement of tissues
**D = True** ▷ To measure blood flow
**E = True** ▷ To measure structures

**9 ▶** The following are ultrasound interactions with tissues:

**A = True** ▷ Reflection
**B = True** ▷ Scatter
**C = True** ▷ Absorption
**D = False** ▷ Refraction
**E = False** ▷ Radiation

**10 ▶** Regarding the detrimental effects of diagnostic ultrasound:

**A = False** ▷ It has proven harmful adverse effects
**B = True** ▷ The main safety issue concerns the heating of tissues
**C = False** ▷ Soft tissues are at greatest risk of heating
**D = True** ▷ Soft tissues experience secondary heating
**E = False** ▷ The thermal index is the same for all tissues

**11 ▶** X-rays:

**A = True** ▷ are a form of electromagnetic radiation
**B = False** ▷ are shorter than gamma rays
**C = False** ▷ are measured in candela
**D = True** ▷ are very energy-inefficient to produce
**E = True** ▷ are formed by the acceleration of electrons

**12 ▶** Regarding X-rays:

**A = True** ▷ They pass easily through soft tissues
**B = False** ▷ Structures that let most of the X-rays pass through appear white on film
**C = True** ▷ They can be used to produce real-time images
**D = True** ▷ They are used to embolise the uterine artery for the treatment of fibroids
**E = False** ▷ They are useful in imaging the brain

**13 ▶** Hysterosalpingography:

**A = False** ▷ is usually performed in the second half of the menstrual cycle
**B = True** ▷ leaves no radiation after the procedure has ended
**C = False** ▷ involves an effective radiation dose that is equivalent to 1 month's background radiation
**D = True** ▷ can cause a flare-up of untreated sexually transmitted disease
**E = True** ▷ carries a small teratogenic risk owing to ovarian irradiation

14 ▶ Regarding dual energy X-ray absorptiometry:

A = **True** ▷ It allows the calculation of bone mineral density

B = **False** ▷ It involves the firing of three different energy beams at bone

C = **True** ▷ The T score predicts the risk of developing a fracture

D = **True** ▷ A T score of −1 is normal

E = **False** ▷ It underestimates the bone mineral density of tall people

15 ▶ Magnetic resonance imaging

A = **True** ▷ provides high contrast between different soft tissues

B = **False** ▷ produces the same amount of ionising radiation as computed tomography

C = **True** ▷ affects all protons in the body

D = **True** ▷ works by emitting a radiofrequency pulse as protons move between magnetic fields

E = **True** ▷ is used to characterise pathological tissue

16 ▶ Regarding magnetic resonance imaging:

A = **True** ▷ There are no harmful effects on the developing fetus

B = **False** ▷ Contrast agents do not cross the placenta

C = **True** ▷ It is contraindicated in people with metal fragments in the eyes

D = **False** ▷ It is contraindicated in claustrophobic people

E = **True** ▷ It is a very noisy procedure

17 ▶ Regarding electrosurgery:

A = **True** ▷ The electric current during monopolar diathermy runs from the generator to the person being treated and back

B = **False** ▷ The electric current used in monopolar diathermy has a lower frequency than the current of the mains supply

C = **False** ▷ Low-frequency currents have no effect on cells

D = **False** ▷ High-frequency currents directly produce heat

E = **True** ▷ Bipolar diathermy does not allow cutting

18 ▶ Regarding radiotherapy:

A = **False** ▷ The radiation used is measured in sievert

B = **False** ▷ Its use is widespread in malignant and nonmalignant conditions

C = **False** ▷ The process entails damaging malignant cell walls

D = **False** ▷ Tissue hypoxia decreases the resistance to radiation

E = **True** ▷ Using protons rather than X-rays decreases the adverse effects of radiotherapy

19 ▶ Regarding radiotherapy:

A = **True** ▷ It can be used as primary or adjuvant therapy

B = **False** ▷ It is best used prior to surgery if used as an adjuvant

C = **True** ▷ It can be used prior to surgery to reduce the tumour size

D = **False** ▷ A linear accelerator uses only one two-dimensional beam

E = **True** ▷ With internal-beam radiotherapy, the dose of radiation to the tumour is increased while the dose to surrounding tissues is decreased

20 ▶ The following are recognised medium- and long-term adverse effects of radiotherapy:

A = **False** ▷ Oedema

B = **True** ▷ Fatigue

C = **True** ▷ Fibrosis

D = **True** ▷ Hair loss

E = **True** ▷ Dryness due to gland damage

## Answers for Chapter 11

### EXTENDED MATCHING QUESTIONS

1 ▶ **G** = Surface ectoderm
2 ▶ **A** = Endoderm
3 ▶ **B** = Intermediate mesoderm
4 ▶ **A** = Endoderm

### MULTIPLE CHOICE QUESTIONS

5 ▶ Regarding fertilisation and implantation:

**A = False** ▷ Fertilisation occurs in the fimbrial end of the fallopian tube
**B = True** ▷ Capacitation is necessary prior to fertilisation
**C = True** ▷ The acrosome enzymes allow the spermatozoon to penetrate the zona pellucida
**D = False** ▷ Fertilisation begins the resumption of the second mitotic division
**E = False** ▷ The embryo implants during the proliferative phase of the endometrium

6 ▶ Regarding implantation and placentation:

**A = False** ▷ Implantation usually occurs on day 4 after fertilisation
**B = False** ▷ Cells for the syncytiotrophoblast are derived from the inner cell mass
**C = True** ▷ By day 12, the uteroplacental circulation has formed
**D = False** ▷ The decidual reaction occurs only at the site of implantation
**E = False** ▷ Beta human chorionic gonadotrophin is produced by the cytotrophoblast

7 ▶ Regarding the amnion and chorion:

**A = False** ▷ The amniotic cavity begins to develop on day 9
**B = False** ▷ The amniotic cavity is formed between cells of the hypoblast
**C = True** ▷ The trophoblast lines the blastocyst cavity
**D = True** ▷ The chorion begins to form in the extraembryonic mesoderm
**E = True** ▷ By week 2, the embryo is connected to the cytotrophoblast by a connecting stalk of extraembryonic mesoderm

8 ▶ Regarding neural development:

**A = True** ▷ The primitive streak starts to form by the end of the second week
**B = False** ▷ The primitive pit represents the caudal end of the fetus
**C = False** ▷ Cells that displace the hypoblast form the mesoderm
**D = True** ▷ The notochord is the basis of the formation of the skeleton
**E = True** ▷ The neural plate derives from the ectoderm

9 ▶ Regarding fertilisation:

**A = True** ▷ The process usually takes place within 24 hours of ovulation
**B = True** ▷ Capacitation is aided by secretions of the uterine wall
**C = False** ▷ The acrosome reaction occurs when the spermatozoon comes into contact with the zona pellucida
**D = True** ▷ Pronuclei are formed by condensation of the chromosome of the gametes
**E = True** ▷ A zygote is formed when the male and female pronuclei meet

10 ▶ Regarding blastocyst formation:

**A = True** ▷ Cleavage begins after completion of the second meiotic division
**B = True** ▷ Cleavage occurs by mitosis
**C = False** ▷ After 3 days, there are 32 cells
**D = True** ▷ The morula is a solid sphere of cells
**E = False** ▷ A blastomere forms when there is a cavity in the morula

11 ▶ Regarding the first week of development:

**A = True** ▷ The blastocoele is a cavity within the blastocyst
**B = False** ▷ The wall surrounding the blastocoele is two cells thick
**C = True** ▷ The cells surrounding the blastocoele becomes the trophoblast
**D = False** ▷ The blastocyst enters the lumen of the uterus on day 6
**E = False** ▷ The inner cell mass is formed from the cells on the outer surface of the blastocoele

**12 ▶** Regarding week 2 of development:

**A = False** ▷ Fertilisation initiates the decidual reaction

**B = True** ▷ Cells of the decidual reaction form part of the placenta

**C = True** ▷ The syncytiotrophoblast is invasive

**D = True** ▷ The primary yolk sac is the source of nutrition for early embryos

**E = False** ▷ Hypoblast cells adapt to produce amniotic fluid

**13 ▶** Regarding week 2 of development:

**A = False** ▷ Maternal sinusoids are small veins

**B = False** ▷ Maternal sinusoids connect the lacunae in the cytotrophoblast

**C = True** ▷ Primary chorionic villi are formed from the cytotrophoblast

**D = False** ▷ The umbilical cord is a stalk of epiblast

**E = True** ▷ Uterine epithelium eventually reforms to cover the conceptus

**14 ▶** Regarding week 3 of development:

**A = True** ▷ The bilaminar disc is made up of the epiblast and hypoblast

**B = False** ▷ The formation of the early gut is called gastrulation

**C = False** ▷ The hypoblast becomes the ectoderm

**D = False** ▷ The middle layer is formed from the hypoblast

**E = True** ▷ The mesoderm forms muscles

**15 ▶** Regarding week 3 of development:

**A = True** ▷ The cloacal plate is made of two germ cell layers

**B = True** ▷ The gut is continuous with the amniotic cavity from week 4

**C = False** ▷ Cells for neurulation are derived from the endoderm

**D = False** ▷ The neural plate enlarges to fill most of the caudal end of the bilaminar disc

**E = False** ▷ The neural fold forms the spinal cord

**16 ▶** The neural crest cells form:

**A = True** ▷ the dorsal root

**B = False** ▷ sympathetic ganglia

**C = False** ▷ adrenal cortex

**D = True** ▷ glial cells

**E = True** ▷ melanocytes

**17 ▶** Regarding mesoderm segmentation:

**A = True** ▷ Somites are formed from the paraxial mesoderm

**B = False** ▷ Forty pairs of somites are formed in total

**C = True** ▷ Dermomyotomes form connective tissue

**D = False** ▷ Sclerotomes form skeletal muscles

**E = True** ▷ Somites carry with them the innervations from the spinal cord

## Answers for Chapter 12

### EXTENDED MATCHING QUESTIONS

1 ▶ **E** = Paramesonephric ducts
2 ▶ **C** = Mesonephric ducts
3 ▶ **D** = Mesonephric tubules
4 ▶ **D** = Mesonephric tubules
5 ▶ **H** = Urogenital sinus
6 ▶ **F** = Phallus
7 ▶ **F** = True hermaphrodite
8 ▶ **E** = Androgen insensitivity syndrome
9 ▶ **B** = Hypospadias
10 ▶ **A** = Female pseudohermaphrodite
11 ▶ **D** = Pseudohermaphroditism
12 ▶ **E** = Pelvic kidney
13 ▶ **B** = Duplication of the ureters
14 ▶ **F** = Renal agenesis
15 ▶ **A** = Autosomal recessive polycystic kidney disease
16 ▶ **A** = Gonads
17 ▶ **A** = Gonads
18 ▶ **E** = Paramesonephric ducts
19 ▶ **C** = Mesonephric ducts
20 ▶ **G** = Urogenital folds

## MULTIPLE CHOICE QUESTIONS

**21** ▶ During the development of the urinary system from the nephrogenic cord of the urogenital ridge:

- **A = True** ▷ There are three types of kidneys during embryonic life
- **B = True** ▷ The kidneys develop from the intermediate mesoderm
- **C = False** ▷ The mesonephros appears during week 5 of development
- **D = True** ▷ The mesonephric tubules are involved in renal corpuscle formation
- **E = False** ▷ The mesonephros has stopped functioning by week 9

**22** ▶ During the development of the urinary system from the nephrogenic cord of the urogenital ridge:

- **A = True** ▷ The ureteric buds form from intermediate mesoderm
- **B = True** ▷ Expansion of the ureteric bud forms the renal pelvis
- **C = False** ▷ The metanephric blastema forms the collecting ducts
- **D = False** ▷ The proximal and distal convoluted tubules meet at week 10
- **E = True** ▷ Urine production starts during week 12

**23** ▶ During development of the metanephros:

- **A = True** ▷ The metanephros starts off as a pelvic organ
- **B = False** ▷ The metanephric mesoderm forms the minor calyces
- **C = True** ▷ The metanephric vesicles differentiate into the renal tubules
- **D = True** ▷ The metanephric vesicles form glomeruli
- **E = False** ▷ All nephrons are formed by 20 weeks

**24** ▶ During development of the bladder from the urogenital sinus:

- **A = True** ▷ The urogenital septum is derived from mesoderm
- **B = True** ▷ The cranial part of the urogenital septum forms the bladder
- **C = False** ▷ The middle part forms the whole urethra in males
- **D = False** ▷ The caudal part forms the prostate in males
- **E = True** ▷ The mucosa is mesodermal in origin

**25** ▶ During development of the bladder from the urogenital sinus:

- **A = False** ▷ The cloaca is divided by the endodermal urorectal septum
- **B = True** ▷ The allantois persists into adult life as the urachus
- **C = False** ▷ The bladder is lined with mesodermal epithelium
- **D = True** ▷ In females, the urogenital sinus becomes the vaginal vestibule
- **E = True** ▷ Urethral epithelium is endodermal in origin

**26** ▶ During the development of the urethra:

- **A = True** ▷ The epithelium is derived from the endoderm
- **B = True** ▷ The smooth muscle is derived from mesoderm
- **C = False** ▷ In males, the urethral epithelium gives rise to paraurethral glands
- **D = False** ▷ Urachal fistulas drain urine into the vagina
- **E = False** ▷ The base of the bladder is exposed in bladder exstrophy

**27** ▶ Regarding gonadogenesis:

- **A = True** ▷ Gonadal development begins in week 4
- **B = False** ▷ The gonads are undifferentiated until week 8
- **C = False** ▷ The gonadal ridges form laterally to the mesonephros
- **D = False** ▷ The sex-determining region is located on the long arm of chromosome Y
- **E = True** ▷ The gonadal cords divide the gonadal ridges

**28** ▶ Regarding gonadogenesis:

- **A = True** ▷ The seminiferous cords develop in the rete testis
- **B = False** ▷ Sertoli cells are formed from the mesenchyme of the gonadal ridge
- **C = False** ▷ The seminiferous tubules are patent from week 12
- **D = True** ▷ In the ovary, the medullary sex cords degenerate
- **E = False** ▷ The primordial germ cells originate from the intermediate mesoderm

29 ▶ During the process of external genital development:

A = **True** ▷ The genital tubercle forms from the cloacal folds

B = **False** ▷ In males, the external urethral meatus is derived from the same epithelium as the rest of the urethral lining

C = **True** ▷ The corpora cavernosa develops from mesenchyme in the phallus

D = **True** ▷ The vaginal fornices develop from the paramesonephric ducts

E = **False** ▷ The urethral folds meet to form the clitoris

30 ▶ The following pairs of structures are derived from the same embryonic structure:

A = **False** ▷ The epoophoron and the gubernaculum

B = **True** ▷ The efferent ductules and the paraoophoron

C = **True** ▷ The ductus deferens and the duct of Gartner

D = **True** ▷ The appendix of the testis and the uterus

E = **False** ▷ The ventral aspect of the penis and the labia majora

31 ▶ During the development of the male genital tract:

A = **False** ▷ Sertoli cells begin to form in the mesonephric duct

B = **True** ▷ Sertoli cells form testis cords that become the seminiferous tubules

C = **True** ▷ The vas deferens is formed by the mesonephric ducts

D = **True** ▷ Leydig cells produce testosterone

E = **False** ▷ The prostate develops independently from the urethra

32 ▶ In the male embryo, the mesonephric ducts form:

A = **False** ▷ appendix of testes

B = **True** ▷ ductus deferens

C = **False** ▷ efferent ductules

D = **True** ▷ ejaculatory duct

E = **True** ▷ epididymis

33 ▶ The following structures form a layer of the covering of the testis:

A = **False** ▷ Gubernaculum

B = **True** ▷ Processus vaginalis

C = **True** ▷ Transversalis fascia

D = **True** ▷ Internal abdominal oblique muscle

E = **True** ▷ External abdominal oblique muscle

34 ▶ During the development of the female genital tract:

A = **True** ▷ The primitive sex cords form clusters

B = **False** ▷ The oogonia enter and are inhibited at the first mitotic stage

C = **False** ▷ The mesonephric ducts form the fallopian tubes, uterus and upper one-third of the vagina

D = **True** ▷ The lower part of the vagina is formed by the vaginal plate

E = **False** ▷ The epoophoron and paroophoron are remnants of the mesonephric and paramesonephric ducts respectively

35 ▶ In the female embryo, the mesonephric ducts form:

A = **True** ▷ appendix vesiculosa

B = **True** ▷ duct of epoophoron

C = **True** ▷ duct of Gartner

D = **False** ▷ epoophoron

E = **False** ▷ paroophoron

## Answers for Chapters 13 and 14

### EXTENDED MATCHING QUESTIONS

1 ▶ **E** = Sinus venosus atrial septal defect
2 ▶ **C** = Ostium secundum atrial septal defect
3 ▶ **B** = Endocardial cushion defects with foramen primum atrial septal defect
4 ▶ **C** = Ostium secundum atrial septal defect
5 ▶ **A** = Common atrium (cor triloculare biventriculare)
6 ▶ **A** = Common atrium (cor triloculare biventriculare)
7 ▶ **E** = Sinus venosus atrial septal defect
8 ▶ **A** = Common atrium (cor triloculare biventriculare)
9 ▶ **B** = Membranous ventricular septal defect
10 ▶ **D** = Single ventricle (cor triloculare biatriatum)
11 ▶ **A** = Atrioventricular septal defect
12 ▶ **B** = Membranous ventricular septal defect
13 ▶ **A** = Atrioventricular septal defect
14 ▶ **D** = Single ventricle (cor triloculare biatriatum)
15 ▶ **B** = Membranous ventricular septal defect
16 ▶ **D** = Ductus venosus
17 ▶ **L** = Umbilical vein
18 ▶ **K** = Umbilical arteries
19 ▶ **L** = Umbilical vein
20 ▶ **C** = Ductus arteriosus
21 ▶ **I** = Right atrium
22 ▶ **D** = Ductus venosus

## MULTIPLE CHOICE QUESTIONS

23 ▶ Regarding the development of the fetal heart:

**A = True** ▷ The primordial heart and vascular system appears in the middle of week 3

**B = True** ▷ The cardiac jelly separates the myoblasts from the endothelial tube

**C = True** ▷ The endocardium is formed by the endothelial lining in the cardiac loop

**D = False** ▷ The pericardium is formed from the outermost myoblasts

**E = True** ▷ The coronary arteries are formed from the mesothelial cells covering the myocardium

24 ▶ Regarding the process of cardiac looping:

**A = True** ▷ The truncus arteriosus connects to the aortic sac

**B = True** ▷ The sinus venosus receives the umbilical blood supply

**C = True** ▷ The ventricle and bulbus cordis are the fastest growing parts of the fetal heart

**D = False** ▷ Is completed by day 35

**E = False** ▷ The heart is in contact with the pericardium until week 8

25 ▶ Regarding cardiac partitioning:

**A = True** ▷ The atria are separated from the ventricles first

**B = True** ▷ The septum primum separates the atria into two

**C = False** ▷ The foramen primum remains patent

**D = False** ▷ The foramen ovale forms in the septum primum

**E = False** ▷ The foramen secundum forms around the foramen ovale

26 ▶ During partitioning of the sinus venosus:

**A = True** ▷ There are left and right sinus horns

**B = True** ▷ The left sinus horn becomes obliterated

**C = True** ▷ The right sinus horn receives all blood from the entire body

**D = False** ▷ The right sinus horn becomes the right atrium

**E = False** ▷ The sulcus terminalis is the internal wall of the sinus venosus

27 ▶ During partitioning of the heart:

**A = False** ▷ The interventricular septum grows as a continuation of the septum primum

**B = False** ▷ The interventricular septum closes in week 9

**C = True** ▷ Bulbar ridges form during week 5

**D = False** ▷ The bulbus cordis and truncus arteriosus forms the descending aorta

**E = True** ▷ The bulbus cordis and truncus arteriosus forms the pulmonary trunk

28 ▶ Regarding the formation of heart valves:

**A = True** ▷ The atrioventricular valves are formed by hollowing of the ventricle by the bloodstream

**B = False** ▷ The valves are formed from the thick muscular wall

**C = True** ▷ The valves are covered in endocardium

**D = False** ▷ The semilunar valves form from four swellings around the aorta and pulmonary trunk

**E = False** ▷ The semilunar valves form by rotation of the great vessels

29 ▶ Congenital heart defects:

**A = True** ▷ are the most common birth defects

**B = False** ▷ account for 10% of malformations in live births

**C = False** ▷ account for 10% of malformations in still births

**D = False** ▷ are genetic in 20% of cases

**E = True** ▷ affect one-third of children with chromosomal abnormalities

30 ▶ Regarding congenital heart defects:

**A = True** ▷ Almost all children with Edwards syndrome (trisomy 18) have a heart defect

**B = False** ▷ They are not associated with DiGeorge syndrome

**C = False** ▷ 5% are due to environmental factors

**D = False** ▷ Gestational diet-controlled diabetes increases the incidence of congenital heart effects

**E = True** ▷ Isotretinoin (vitamin A) is a known cardiovascular teratogen

**31** ▶ Regarding cardiac anomalies:

**A** = **True** ▷ In dextrocardia, the heart lies on the right side of the thorax

**B** = **True** ▷ Dextrocardia is associated with situs inversus

**C** = **False** ▷ Ectopia cordis is the most frequent cardiac positional anomaly

**D** = **True** ▷ In ectopia cordis, the heart is exposed on the surface of the thorax

**E** = **False** ▷ Ectopia cordis is due to abnormal cardiac development

**32** ▶ Regarding atrial septal defect:

**A** = **True** ▷ Incidence is about six in 10 000

**B** = **False** ▷ Incidence in males is equal to that in females

**C** = **True** ▷ Patent foramen ovale is the most common type

**D** = **False** ▷ Patent foramen ovale occurs in 10% of neonates

**E** = **True** ▷ Foramen secundum atrial septal defect often leads to pulmonary hypertension after the third decade of life

**33** ▶ Tetralogy of Fallot:

**A** = **True** ▷ is the most common abnormality of the conotruncal region

**B** = **False** ▷ is usually fatal

**C** = **True** ▷ causes a ventricular septal defect

**D** = **False** ▷ causes left ventricular hypertrophy

**E** = **True** ▷ causes right ventricular outflow obstruction

**34** ▶ Regarding the conducting system of the heart:

**A** = **True** ▷ The atrium is the initial pacemaker of the heart

**B** = **False** ▷ The sinoatrial node is formed in week 6 of life

**C** = **False** ▷ The bundle of His forms in the ventricle and passes up towards the atrioventricular node

**D** = **False** ▷ Nerve supply to the heart develops before the conducting system

**E** = **True** ▷ 50% of sudden infant deaths are due to abnormalities of the conducting system

**35** ▶ Mixing of oxygenated and deoxygenated fetal blood takes place in:

**A** = **True** ▷ the inferior vena cava

**B** = **True** ▷ the left atrium

**C** = **True** ▷ the liver

**D** = **True** ▷ the right atrium

**E** = **False** ▷ the superior vena cava

**36** ▶ During the formation of the stomach:

**A** = **False** ▷ The stomach rotates 90° anticlockwise around its longitudinal axis

**B** = **True** ▷ The left side rotates to face anteriorly

**C** = **True** ▷ The posterior wall grows faster than the anterior wall

**D** = **True** ▷ The ventral mesogastrium forms the lesser omentum

**E** = **False** ▷ The caudal mesogastrium forms the greater omentum

**37** ▶ During the development of the liver and biliary apparatus:

**A** = **False** ▷ The bile duct arises from the duodenum

**B** = **False** ▷ The bile duct originally enters the duodenum posteriorly

**C** = **True** ▷ The gallbladder and cystic duct develop from the same outgrowth

**D** = **False** ▷ Bile formation begins during week 10

**E** = **True** ▷ Hepatic sinusoids are made up of, amongst others, umbilical veins

**38** ▶ During the development of the liver:

**A** = **False** ▷ The septum transversum provides mesodermal cells for the liver parenchyma

**B** = **True** ▷ The septum transversum provides mesodermal cells for connective tissue

**C** = **False** ▷ The entire surface of the liver differentiates into visceral peritoneum

**D** = **True** ▷ The central tendon of the diaphragm is formed from the embryological liver

**E** = **True** ▷ Haematopoiesis begins during week 6

**39** ▶ During development of the midgut:

A = **True** ▷ The superior mesenteric artery supplies the entire midgut

B = **True** ▷ The vitelline duct is an open connection between the midgut and the yolk sac

C = **False** ▷ The midgut forms the proximal one-third of the transverse colon

D = **True** ▷ The primary loop of bowel rotates around an axis by 270°

E = **False** ▷ The primary intestinal loop rotation occurs during the bowel herniation time only

**40** ▶ During development of the midgut:

A = **False** ▷ The midgut enters the umbilical cord in week 8

B = **False** ▷ Herniated bowel begins to return to the abdomen by week 12

C = **True** ▷ On returning to the abdomen, the caecum lies below the liver

D = **True** ▷ The appendix is relatively large in the neonate

E = **True** ▷ The pancreas becomes retroperitoneal by being pressed by the colon to the posterior abdominal wall

**41** ▶ During development of the hindgut:

A = **False** ▷ The hindgut is supplied by the middle mesenteric artery

B = **False** ▷ The cloaca is lined with mesoderm

C = **True** ▷ The urorectal septum is made of mesoderm

D = **False** ▷ The urorectal septum comes into contact with the cloacal membrane

E = **True** ▷ The tip of the urorectal septum forms the perineal body

**42** ▶ Regarding the development of the anal canal:

A = **True** ▷ The junction between the superior and inferior anal canal is marked by the pectinate line

B = **False** ▷ Above the pectinate line, the epithelium is stratified squamous

C = **False** ▷ Below the pectinate line, the epithelium is keratinised

D = **False** ▷ The lymphatic drainage is the same for the entire anal canal

E = **False** ▷ Carcinomas from the upper two-thirds are painful

**43** ▶ The inferior two-thirds of the anal canal:

A = **False** ▷ are derived from endoderm

B = **True** ▷ are 13 mm long

C = **False** ▷ receive blood from arteries originating from the inferior mesenteric artery

D = **True** ▷ drain to the superficial inguinal nodes

E = **False** ▷ have a nerve supply from the autonomic nervous system

**44** ▶ Regarding omphalocele:

A = **False** ▷ Incidence is one in 10 000 births

B = **True** ▷ Omphalocele is caused by failure of the bowel to return to the abdomen

C = **False** ▷ Diagnosis can be from week 9 onwards

D = **False** ▷ The viscera are uncovered

E = **True** ▷ Mortality rate is 25%

**45** ▶ Gastroschisis:

A = **True** ▷ occurs in one in 10 000 births

B = **False** ▷ occurs in older mothers

C = **False** ▷ is equally spread between male and female fetuses

D = **True** ▷ herniation occurs through a weakness owing to regression of the right umbilical vein

E = **False** ▷ is associated with chromosomal abnormalities

## Answers for Chapter 15

### EXTENDED MATCHING QUESTIONS

1 ▶ **G** = Morula
2 ▶ **B** = Blastocyst
3 ▶ **C** = Blastomere
4 ▶ **L** = Zona pellucida
5 ▶ **I** = Trophoblast
6 ▶ **F** = Decidua

## MULTIPLE CHOICE QUESTIONS

**7** ▶ During early development of an embryo from the fertilisation of the oocyte:

A = **True** ▷ First cleavage division takes place in the ampulla

B = **False** ▷ First cleavage occurs within 12 hours

C = **False** ▷ Cell divisions are regular at every 6 hours

D = **True** ▷ All blastomeres are totipotent

E = **False** ▷ The embryo enters the uterus at the 16-cell stage

**8** ▶ During early development of an embryo from the fertilisation of the oocyte:

A = **True** ▷ The outer cell mass forms the placenta

B = **True** ▷ The inner cell mass develops into the fetus

C = **False** ▷ In the preimplantation phase, new trophoblast develops from the outer cell mass

D = **False** ▷ The inner and outer cell masses are in direct contact

E = **False** ▷ The process is driven by glucose

**9** ▶ Regarding decidualisation:

A = **False** ▷ The process occurs when the embryo enters the uterine cavity

B = **False** ▷ Decidualisation entails local change only

C = **False** ▷ There is suppression of the maternal defence system

D = **True** ▷ Decidualisation regulates trophoblast invasion

E = **False** ▷ The uterine cavity becomes fluid filled

**10** ▶ Regarding the process of attachment of the embryo:

A = **False** ▷ The zona pellucida is retained

B = **True** ▷ The endometrial epithelium is destroyed

C = **True** ▷ Attachment is complete by day 12

D = **False** ▷ Trophoblast cells destroy endometrial cells with which they come into contact

E = **False** ▷ Vascular endothelial growth factor is made by the trophoblast

**11** ▶ Regarding the placenta:

A = **False** ▷ The cytotrophoblast is the outer cell layer

B = **False** ▷ The syncytiotrophoblast has distinct cells

C = **False** ▷ The cytotrophoblast has multinucleated cells

D = **True** ▷ Lacunae form before implantation is complete

E = **True** ▷ The trophoblast penetrates into the myometrium

**12** ▶ The placenta:

A = **True** ▷ has an anchoring role from day 13

B = **True** ▷ reaches its ultimate form by week 12

C = **False** ▷ reaches full thickness by week 10

D = **False** ▷ weighs less than the fetus from week 12 onwards

E = **False** ▷ weighs one-quarter of the fetus at term

**13** ▶ Regarding placental development:

A = **True** ▷ The extraembryonic mesoderm of the primary stem villi vascularises

B = **True** ▷ Villi forming from a primary villous are collectively known as a lobule

C = **False** ▷ There are 100 lobules in a placenta

D = **False** ▷ Twenty-five lobules make up one cotyledon

E = **True** ▷ All lobules are formed by week 10

**14** ▶ Regarding immunotolerance of pregnancy:

A = **True** ▷ Trophoblastic cells are exposed to maternal allogenic immune responses

B = **True** ▷ There is enlargement of the uterine stromal cells

C = **True** ▷ There is a uterine-specific population of natural killer cells

D = **False** ▷ Tubal ectopic pregnancies show poor trophoblast invasion

E = **False** ▷ Deficient decidua produces poor trophoblastic invasion

**15** ▶ Regarding immunotolerance of pregnancy:

A = **False** ▷ Fetal cells that enter the maternal circulation do not provoke a reaction

B = **False** ▷ Trophoblast is always negative for major histocompatibility complex class 1 expression

C = **False** ▷ Syncytiotrophoblast expresses major histocompatibility complex class 2

D = **True** ▷ Human leucocyte antigen G expression is only expressed by trophoblast invading the decidua

E = **False** ▷ CD8+ regulatory T-cells are not present in the pregnant uterus

**16** ▶ Regarding perfusion of the intervillous spaces of the placenta with maternal blood:

A = **False** ▷ Simple diffusion is more efficient in early pregnancy than in late pregnancy

B = **True** ▷ Nonpolar molecules diffuse across the placenta

C = **True** ▷ Urea diffuses across the placenta

D = **False** ▷ Diffusion of oxygen across the placenta is dependent on the thickness of the terminal villi

E = **False** ▷ Only the maternal side changes as pregnancy progresses

**17** ▶ Regarding perfusion of the intervillous spaces of the placenta with maternal blood:

A = **True** ▷ Oxygen transfer is promoted by a rise in fetal pH

B = **True** ▷ Blood flow through the placenta increases transport of oxygen across the placenta

C = **True** ▷ Glucose is transported across the placenta by specific carriers

D = **True** ▷ Some amino acids are synthesised within the trophoblast

E = **False** ▷ All amino acid uptake by the placenta is used for fetal growth

**18** ▶ Regarding perfusion of the intervillous spaces of the placenta with maternal blood:

A = **False** ▷ Water is exchanged at the placenta only

B = **False** ▷ There is a large hydrostatic force pushing water from the mother to the fetus

C = **False** ▷ Iron diffuses down its concentration gradient

D = **False** ▷ Calcium diffuses down its concentration gradient

E = **False** ▷ Sodium diffuses across in a co-transport system only

**19** ▶ Regarding amniotic fluid:

A = **False** ▷ It has a volume of 50 ml at week 8

B = **True** ▷ There is no production after week 34

C = **True** ▷ The creatinine concentration of amniotic fluid increases towards term

D = **False** ▷ The amnion arises between the ectodermal and endodermal layers

E = **False** ▷ The amnion contains lymphatics

**20** ▶ Human chorionic gonadotrophin:

A = **False** ▷ is secreted by the cytotrophoblast

B = **True** ▷ is secreted from day 7 post fertilisation

C = **False** ▷ has three amino acid chains

D = **True** ▷ rises rapidly until week 12

E = **True** ▷ binds to luteinising hormone receptors in the corpus luteum

**21** ▶ Regarding molar pregnancies:

A = **False** ▷ They contain no fetal tissue

B = **True** ▷ A complete mole has 46 chromosomes in each cell

C = **True** ▷ A complete mole contains maternally derived chromosomes

D = **False** ▷ A partial mole has 23 chromosomes in each cell

E = **True** ▷ Moles contain highly invasive placental tissue

# Answers for Chapters 16 and 17

## EXTENDED MATCHING QUESTIONS

1 ▶ **C** = Growth hormone
2 ▶ **F** = Thyroid-stimulating hormone
3 ▶ **C** = Growth hormone
4 ▶ **E** = Prolactin
5 ▶ **E** = Prolactin
6 ▶ **A** = Adrenocorticotrophin
7 ▶ **F** = Thyroid-stimulating hormone
8 ▶ **D** = Luteinising hormone
9 ▶ **B** = Follicle-stimulating hormone

## MULTIPLE CHOICE QUESTIONS

10 ▶ Regarding hypothalamic hormones:

**A** = **True** ▷ They are all peptides
**B** = **True** ▷ Only the release of corticotrophin-releasing hormone follows a circadian rhythm
**C** = **False** ▷ They have a long half-life
**D** = **True** ▷ Thyrotrophin-releasing hormone (TRH) increases prolactin release
**E** = **True** ▷ TRH stimulates the release of thyrotrophin-stimulating hormone

11 ▶ Regarding the adrenal gland:

**A** = **False** ▷ Norepinephrine mainly increases glycogenolysis
**B** = **True** ▷ Cortisol stimulates gluconeogenesis
**C** = **False** ▷ Ninety-five percent of cortisol is bound to albumin
**D** = **True** ▷ The zona reticularis secretes androgenic hormones
**E** = **False** ▷ Epinephrine is released on stimulation by sympathetic postganglionic cholinergic neurons

12 ▶ Regarding aldosterone:

**A** = **True** ▷ Angiotensinogen stimulates aldosterone production
**B** = **False** ▷ Aldosterone decreases the excretion of $K^+$
**C** = **True** ▷ The plasma $K^+$ concentration directly stimulates aldosterone production
**D** = **False** ▷ Aldosterone mainly acts in the proximal convoluted tubule
**E** = **True** ▷ Aldosterone increases the excretion of $H_2O$

# Answers for Chapter 18

## EXTENDED MATCHING QUESTIONS

1 ▶ **B** = Neurofibromatosis type 1
2 ▶ **A** = Marfan syndrome
3 ▶ **E** = Autosomal dominant polycystic kidney disease

## MULTIPLE CHOICE QUESTIONS

4 ▶ Regarding chromosomes:

**A** = **False** ▷ Humans have 23 pairs of autosomal chromosomes
**B** = **False** ▷ The centromere always lies at the centre of each chromosome
**C** = **False** ▷ The p arm is the long arm
**D** = **False** ▷ Submetacentric chromosomes have the centromere at the top of the chromosome
**E** = **True** ▷ The numbering of chromosomes is done according to their length

5 ▶ Nondisjunction:

**A** = **True** ▷ results in aneuploidy
**B** = **False** ▷ occurs because of chromosome nonseparation in meiosis II
**C** = **True** ▷ occurs because sister chromatids fail to separate during mitotic anaphase
**D** = **True** ▷ causes trisomies
**E** = **True** ▷ causes monosomies

6 ▶ The following pregnancy outcomes are possible if a parent has a balanced reciprocal translocation:

**A** = **True** ▷ A normal pregnancy with the child having a normal karyotype
**B** = **True** ▷ A normal pregnancy with the child having a balanced translocation
**C** = **False** ▷ A spontaneous miscarriage because the child has a balanced translocation
**D** = **False** ▷ A term pregnancy with the child having an increased chance of developmental delay because of a balanced translocation
**E** = **True** ▷ A term pregnancy with the child having an increased chance of developmental delay because of an unbalanced translocation

**7** ▶ Regarding common trisomic conditions:

**A** = **True** ▷ Ninety-five percent of Down syndrome occurrences are caused by nondisjunction

**B** = **True** ▷ All individuals with Down syndrome have some learning difficulties

**C** = **True** ▷ Patau syndrome is associated with holoprosencephaly

**D** = **False** ▷ Patau syndrome is associated with diaphragmatic hernias

**E** = **False** ▷ Edwards syndrome is associated with blindness

**8** ▶ Regarding common trisomic conditions:

**A** = **False** ▷ Individuals with Down syndrome have a ten-fold increased risk of atrioventricular septal defect

**B** = **False** ▷ People with Down syndrome are scaphocephalic

**C** = **True** ▷ Patau syndrome is associated with polydactyly

**D** = **False** ▷ Patau syndrome is associated with duodenal atresia

**E** = **False** ▷ Edwards syndrome is associated with acute lymphoblastic anaemia

**9** ▶ Regarding Klinefelter syndrome:

**A** = **False** ▷ It is usually picked up on ultrasound
**B** = **False** ▷ It is associated with short stature
**C** = **True** ▷ Those affected are infertile
**D** = **True** ▷ Those affected develop gynaecomastia
**E** = **False** ▷ Those affected are more likely to be homosexual

**10** ▶ Regarding autosomal recessive diseases:

**A** = **True** ▷ Both inherited genes are affected
**B** = **False** ▷ If both parents are carriers, then 50% of children will have the condition
**C** = **True** ▷ If both parents are carriers, then 75% of children will be normal or carriers
**D** = **True** ▷ There is an increased risk of these diseases in consanguineous marriages
**E** = **True** ▷ They usually skip a generation

**11** ▶ Regarding screening tests for trisomy 21:

**A** = **False** ▷ The triple test has a trisomy 21 detection rate of 60%

**B** = **True** ▷ The combined test includes a nuchal translucency scan and measurement of beta-human chorionic gonadotrophin and pregnancy-associated plasma protein A (PaPP-A)

**C** = **False** ▷ The combined test has a trisomy 21 detection rate of 80%

**D** = **False** ▷ The quadruple test includes a measurement of PaPP-A

**E** = **False** ▷ The quadruple test is carried out in the first trimester

**12** ▶ Regarding diagnostic tests:

**A** = **True** ▷ Cell-free fetal DNA is measured to determine the rhesus status of the fetus

**B** = **False** ▷ Chorionic villus sampling is best carried out after week 13 of gestation

**C** = **False** ▷ Cytotrophoblast cells are more representative of fetal cells than the placental mesechyme

**D** = **False** ▷ Direct cell preparation is used in amniocentesis

**E** = **False** ▷ Cordocentesis is only done after week 22 of gestation

## Answers for Chapter 19

### EXTENDED MATCHING QUESTIONS

1 ▶ **H** = Natural killer cells
2 ▶ **C** = Dendritic cells
3 ▶ **H** = Natural killer cells
4 ▶ **C** = Immunoglobulin A
5 ▶ **G** = Complement protein 3
6 ▶ **D** = Immunoglobulin
7 ▶ **D** = Interleukin-10
8 ▶ **I** = Interferon gamma
9 ▶ **J** = Granulocyte–macrophage colony-stimulating factor
10 ▶ **C** = Eosinophils
11 ▶ **E** = Monocytes
12 ▶ **F** = Neutrophils
13 ▶ **E** = Monocytes
14 ▶ **D** = Mast cells
15 ▶ **G** = Tissue macrophages

16 ▶ **B** = Dendritic cells
17 ▶ **E** = Monocytes
18 ▶ **G** = Tissue macrophages
19 ▶ **D** = Mast cells
20 ▶ **F** = Neutrophils
21 ▶ **D** = Mast cells
22 ▶ **D** = Immunoglobulin G
23 ▶ **C** = Immunoglobulin E
24 ▶ **D** = Immunoglobulin G
25 ▶ **E** = Immunoglobulin M
26 ▶ **D** = Immunoglobulin G
27 ▶ **C** = Immunoglobulin E
28 ▶ **C** = Immunoglobulin E
29 ▶ **D** = Immunoglobulin G
30 ▶ **A** = Immunoglobulin A
31 ▶ **E** = Immunoglobulin M
32 ▶ **E** = Immunoglobulin M
33 ▶ **A** = Immunoglobulin A

## MULTIPLE CHOICE QUESTIONS

34 ▶ When comparing the innate and adaptive immune responses:

    **A** = **False** ▷ The innate response has some memory
    **B** = **False** ▷ Natural killer cells belong to the adaptive immune response
    **C** = **True** ▷ The innate response to repeat infection is identical to the primary innate response
    **D** = **True** ▷ The adaptive response requires several days to become effective
    **E** = **True** ▷ Complement is the humoral component of the innate response

35 ▶ Phagocytes

    **A** = **False** ▷ are derived from the spleen
    **B** = **True** ▷ are divided into two categories
    **C** = **True** ▷ act on endogenous and exogenous particles
    **D** = **True** ▷ are released upon activation by cytokines
    **E** = **False** ▷ work independently of the adaptive immune response

36 ▶ Natural killer cells

    **A** = **False** ▷ are phagocytes of the macrophage lineage
    **B** = **True** ▷ play a role in both the adaptive and the innate immune responses
    **C** = **True** ▷ are cytotoxic against tumour cells and virally infected cells
    **D** = **False** ▷ attack cells that express an excess of major histocompatibility complex class I molecules
    **E** = **True** ▷ are activated by cytokines

37 ▶ The complement system:

    **A** = **True** ▷ is made up of 20 proteins
    **B** = **False** ▷ constitutes 1% of the serum proteins
    **C** = **True** ▷ causes damage to bacterial cell walls
    **D** = **True** ▷ is activated by the adaptive immune response
    **E** = **False** ▷ contains major fragments designated the suffix 'a'

38 ▶ Regarding the complement system:

    **A** = **True** ▷ All pathways require the cleavage of complement protein C3
    **B** = **False** ▷ The classic pathway is activated by antibodies to immunoglobulin G only
    **C** = **False** ▷ In the classic pathway, an antigen–antibody complex causes increased release of complement component C1q
    **D** = **True** ▷ The classic pathway requires previous encounter with the antigen
    **E** = **False** ▷ Deficiencies in the classic pathway result in overwhelming bacterial infections

39 ▶ Regarding the complement system:

    **A** = **True** ▷ The alternative pathway is activated by complement binding to antigens
    **B** = **False** ▷ The alternative pathway requires antibody for activation
    **C** = **False** ▷ The mannose-binding lectin pathway is part of the adaptive immune response
    **D** = **True** ▷ In the final lytic sequence, all three pathways converge
    **E** = **True** ▷ The final lytic sequence creates a channel in the membrane of the target cell through which salts and water can flow

**40** ▶ Antibodies:

A = **True** ▷ are effective against bacteria
B = **False** ▷ are not effective against viruses
C = **False** ▷ are divided into six classes
D = **True** ▷ have two light chains
E = **False** ▷ have one heavy chain

**41** ▶ Regarding antibodies:

A = **True** ▷ The type of heavy chain determines the class of antibody
B = **False** ▷ The carboxy terminus is the antigen-binding site
C = **False** ▷ All immunoglobulins are bifunctional
D = **True** ▷ Immunoglobulin G has four heavy chain subtypes
E = **False** ▷ Immunoglobulin E has two different heavy chain subtypes

**42** ▶ Immunoglobulin M:

A = **False** ▷ comprises 30% of the serum immunoglobulin pool
B = **True** ▷ is the first antibody formed in a primary response
C = **False** ▷ exists in mucosal membranes
D = **False** ▷ activates the alternative complement pathway
E = **False** ▷ crosses the placenta

**43** ▶ Regarding immunoglobulin G (IgG):

A = **True** ▷ It is the most common serum immunoglobulin
B = **False** ▷ It has six subclasses
C = **False** ▷ IgG2 crosses the placenta
D = **True** ▷ IgG4 activates complement via the classic pathway
E = **True** ▷ IgG1 mediates opsonisation

**44** ▶ Immunoglobulin A:

A = **False** ▷ is characteristic of a primary immune response
B = **True** ▷ induces phagocytosis
C = **True** ▷ is secreted into the saliva
D = **False** ▷ crosses the placenta
E = **True** ▷ is secreted into breast milk

**45** ▶ Regarding T cells:

A = **True** ▷ They mediate the adaptive immune response
B = **True** ▷ They mediate antigen recognition
C = **False** ▷ They have three classes of receptors
D = **True** ▷ Ninety-five percent of T cells express the alpha/beta T cell receptor
E = **True** ▷ Beta/gamma T cell receptors are present on the pregnant uterus

**46** ▶ Regarding T cells:

A = **True** ▷ They recognise antigens presented by major histocompatibility complex (MHC) class II molecules
B = **False** ▷ Thymocytes are selected if they recognise nonself-MHC molecules in the thymus
C = **False** ▷ Negative selection is used against all nonselected thymocytes
D = **False** ▷ CD4-positive cells remain in the thymus
E = **False** ▷ Gamma/delta T cells express CD8

**47** ▶ Regarding single-positive (CD4- or CD8-positive) T cells:

A = **True** ▷ CD4 is a transmembrane protein
B = **False** ▷ They recognise major histocompatibility complex class I molecules
C = **False** ▷ CD4 type 2 T helper cells release interferon
D = **True** ▷ CD8 cells kill tumour cells
E = **True** ▷ CD8 cells kill virally infected cells

**48** ▶ Regarding interferons (IFNs):

A = **True** ▷ They are proteins
B = **False** ▷ They inhibit bacteria
C = **True** ▷ They are produced early in infection
D = **False** ▷ IFN-$\alpha$ is produced by fibroblasts
E = **False** ▷ IFN-$\beta$ is produced by natural killer cells

**49** ▶ Regarding interleukins (ILs):

A = **True** ▷ They are secreted by leucocytes
B = **True** ▷ IL-2 stimulates proliferation and differentiation of T cells
C = **False** ▷ IL-4 is produced by type 1 T helper cells
D = **True** ▷ IL-10 is secreted by mast cells
E = **False** ▷ IL-12 enhances the cytolytic activity of CD4-positive T cells

**50** ► Regarding cytokines:

**A = False** ▷ Interleukin-1 activates complement
**B = True** ▷ Activated T cells produce tumour necrosis factor alpha (TNF-α)
**C = True** ▷ TNF-α production is stimulated by endotoxins
**D = False** ▷ CD8-positive cells are categorised into type 1 and type 2 T helper cells
**E = True** ▷ Type 2 T helper cells promote the antibody response to bacterial infection

**51** ► Regarding cytokines:

**A = True** ▷ Granulocyte–macrophage colony-stimulating factor induces the development of nonlymphoid cells
**B = False** ▷ Transforming growth factor beta activates the proliferation of T cells
**C = True** ▷ Chemokines are involved in cell migration
**D = False** ▷ Chemokines attract complement
**E = False** ▷ Chemokines are equally distributed in a given tissue

**52** ► Class II major histocompatibility complex molecules:

**A = False** ▷ have limited polymorphism
**B = True** ▷ present longer peptides than class I molecules do
**C = True** ▷ are expressed on B cells
**D = False** ▷ present antigen to CD8-positive cells
**E = True** ▷ present peptides that are mostly exogenous antigens

**53** ► Regarding maternal and fetal immune interactions:

**A = True** ▷ There is an interface between the extravillous cytotrophoblast and the myometrium
**B = True** ▷ There are specialised natural killer cells in the maternal decidua
**C = False** ▷ Decidual natural killer cells are cytotoxic
**D = False** ▷ T cells make up the majority of decidual cells
**E = False** ▷ Passive maternal immunity is important to the fetus in the third trimester

**54** ► Regarding the interface between chorionic villi and maternal blood:

**A = True** ▷ It is important in the third trimester
**B = False** ▷ It allows passage of nonblood fetal cells into the maternal system
**C = True** ▷ It is the site of maternal–fetal haemorrhage
**D = False** ▷ Fetal leucocytes are found in the maternal system from the second trimester on
**E = True** ▷ It leaves the placenta in contact with all maternal blood cells

**55** ► Regarding the expression of major histocompatibility complex (MHC) antigens by trophoblasts:

**A = False** ▷ Class I MHC expression is found on the syncytiotrophoblast
**B = True** ▷ Class I MHC expression is found on the invasive extravillous cytotrophoblast
**C = False** ▷ Class II MHC expression is found on the syncytiotrophoblast
**D = False** ▷ Class II MHC expression is found on the invasive extravillous cytotrophoblast
**E = True** ▷ Extravillous cytotrophoblasts are unique in not expressing class I human leucocyte antigen A

**56** ► Regarding trophoblast human leucocyte antigen G (HLA-G):

**A = False** ▷ It has a similar structure to other major histocompatibility complex class II molecules
**B = False** ▷ There are four types
**C = False** ▷ It displays extensive polymorphism
**D = True** ▷ Paternal and maternal HLA-G molecules are very similar
**E = False** ▷ It induces the proliferation of CD4-positive T cells

**57** ► Regarding trophoblast human leucocyte antigens (HLAs):

**A = False** ▷ HLA-G molecules present peptides in a similar way to classic major histocompatibility complex class II molecules
**B = False** ▷ HLA-G induces CD8-positive T cells
**C = True** ▷ HLA-E is expressed on the invasive extravillous cytotrophoblast
**D = True** ▷ HLA-C is polymorphic
**E = True** ▷ HLA-C is expressed on the extravillous trophoblast

**58** ▶ Regarding abnormal maternal immune responses to a pregnancy:

A = **True** ▷ Human leucocyte antigen G is poorly expressed on the invasive extravillous cytotrophoblast in women with recurrent miscarriages

B = **False** ▷ In pre-eclampsia, there is a greater shift to the production of CD4-positive type 2 T helper cells than normal

C = **False** ▷ The maternal systemic inflammatory processes are decreased in pre-eclamptic pregnancies

D = **True** ▷ The presence of maternal lupus anticoagulant antibodies is associated with an 85–95% risk of fetal mortality

E = **True** ▷ Maternal anticardiolipin antibodies cause poor placentation

## Answers for Chapter 20

### MULTIPLE CHOICE QUESTIONS

**1** ▶ Streptococcaceae:

A = **True** ▷ are Gram-positive
B = **False** ▷ are obligate anaerobes
C = **False** ▷ grow individually
D = **False** ▷ are positive for the catalase test
E = **True** ▷ fall into two main groups

**2** ▶ Necrotising fasciitis:

A = **True** ▷ is caused by streptococcal infection
B = **True** ▷ involves the fat and fascia
C = **True** ▷ can rapidly lead to death
D = **False** ▷ is not associated with pain
E = **True** ▷ requires immediate surgical debridement

**3** ▶ Regarding *Streptococcus agalactiae* (group B streptococcus or GBS):

A = **False** ▷ It is not normally found in the female genital tract
B = **False** ▷ Ninety percent of babies born to GBS-positive mothers are infected
C = **True** ▷ Premature delivery increases the risk of GBS infection
D = **True** ▷ Prolonged rupture of membranes increases the risk of GBS infection
E = **False** ▷ Intrapartum maternal fever does not alter the risk of GBS infection

**4** ▶ *Streptococcus agalactiae* (group B streptococcus):

A = **False** ▷ should be screened for in all pregnant women
B = **True** ▷ can cause miscarriage in pregnancy
C = **True** ▷ can cause postpartum sepsis
D = **False** ▷ causes infection in otherwise healthy men
E = **False** ▷ is more common in the young than the old

**5** ▶ Staphylococci:

A = **False** ▷ are Gram-negative
B = **False** ▷ are facultative aerobes
C = **True** ▷ form clusters
D = **False** ▷ are commensals of the gastrointestinal tract
E = **True** ▷ are treated with flucloxacillin

**6** ▶ Regarding meticillin-resistant *Staphylococcus aureus*:

A = **True** ▷ It is resistant to all beta-lactam antibiotics only
B = **True** ▷ It is spread by direct contact
C = **True** ▷ Infected people are usually asymptomatic
D = **True** ▷ The infection is cleared by nasal mupirocin
E = **False** ▷ It is more common in the community than in hospitals

**7** ▶ Meticillin-resistant *Staphylococcus aureus* responds to the following antibiotics:

A = **False** ▷ Cephalosporins
B = **False** ▷ Flucloxacillin
C = **True** ▷ Rifampicin
D = **True** ▷ Tetracyclines
E = **True** ▷ Vancomycin

**8** ▶ *Listeria monocytogenes*:

A = **False** ▷ is Gram-negative
B = **False** ▷ is spore-forming
C = **False** ▷ is a coccus
D = **False** ▷ is an aerobe organism
E = **False** ▷ is alpha-haemolytic

9 ▶ *Listeria monocytogenes*:

    **A** = **True** ▷ is found in soil

    **B** = **True** ▷ can tolerate a wide range of temperatures

    **C** = **False** ▷ is an extracellular pathogen

    **D** = **False** ▷ causes encephalitis

    **E** = **False** ▷ is best treated with oral amoxicillin

10 ▶ Regarding the consequences of *Listeria monocytogenes* infection during pregnancy:

    **A** = **False** ▷ Ninety-five percent of maternal infection results in fetal infection

    **B** = **True** ▷ Infected pregnant women usually remain asymptomatic

    **C** = **True** ▷ The infection is known to cause preterm labour

    **D** = **True** ▷ The mortality rate of early neonatal listeriosis is higher than 50%

    **E** = **False** ▷ Late neonatal listeriosis often presents with septicaemia

11 ▶ Enterobacteriaceae:

    **A** = **False** ▷ are Gram-positive

    **B** = **True** ▷ are bacilli

    **C** = **True** ▷ ferment glucose

    **D** = **False** ▷ are aerobe organisms

    **E** = **False** ▷ are all overt pathogens

12 ▶ Regarding urinary tract infections (UTIs) caused by Enterobacteriaceae:

    **A** = **True** ▷ *Escherichia coli* is the most common cause of community-acquired UTI

    **B** = **False** ▷ A dipstick positive for leucocytes and nitrite is diagnostic of a UTI

    **C** = **False** ▷ Cefalexin is the treatment of choice for community-acquired UTI

    **D** = **True** ▷ Pregnancy increases the risk of asymptomatic UTI

    **E** = **True** ▷ A UTI increases the risk of preterm labour

13 ▶ Regarding enterobacterial infections:

    **A** = **False** ▷ Enterobacteriaceae only cause cholecystitis if biliary calculi are present

    **B** = **False** ▷ Enterobacteriaceae are common causes of wound infection in thoracic surgery

    **C** = **True** ▷ *Escherichia coli* is the most common cause of bacteraemia

    **D** = **True** ▷ Treatment of bacteraemia should include a cephalosporin

    **E** = **True** ▷ *E. coli* is the most common cause of neonatal sepsis

14 ▶ Regarding Gram-negative glucose-nonfermenting bacilli:

    **A** = **False** ▷ They are rare in the hospital environment

    **B** = **False** ▷ They are highly pathogenic

    **C** = **True** ▷ *Pseudomonas aeruginosa* causes ventilator-associated pneumonia

    **D** = **False** ▷ *P. aeruginosa* causes wound infections in people with impaired immunity

    **E** = **True** ▷ *Burkholderia cepacia* causes lower respiratory tract infection in people with cystic fibrosis

15 ▶ The neisseriae:

    **A** = **True** ▷ are Gram-negative

    **B** = **False** ▷ are bacilli

    **C** = **False** ▷ form clusters

    **D** = **True** ▷ are obligate aerobes

    **E** = **False** ▷ are negative for the catalase test

16 ▶ Regarding *Neisseria meningitidis* (meningococcus):

    **A** = **False** ▷ It is not part of the normal flora in humans

    **B** = **False** ▷ Infected people develop a slow-spreading petechial rash

    **C** = **False** ▷ People with meningitis typically have co-existing septicaemia

    **D** = **False** ▷ The cerebrospinal fluid glucose concentration of infected persons is increased

    **E** = **True** ▷ Treatment is with penicillin

**17** ▶ *Neisseria gonorrhoeae* (gonococcus):

    **A = False** ▷ is the most common cause of sexually transmitted bacterial infection in the UK

    **B = True** ▷ is not part of the normal human flora

    **C = True** ▷ does not always cause symptoms in men

    **D = False** ▷ causes nondischarging urethritis in men

    **E = True** ▷ causes proctitis after receptive anal intercourse

**18** ▶ Regarding the Spirochaetaceae:

    **A = False** ▷ They are visible on Gram staining

    **B = True** ▷ They have axial filaments that allow them to rotate lengthwise

    **C = True** ▷ They are notoriously difficult to culture

    **D = True** ▷ *Leptospira interrogans* is found in animal urine

    **E = False** ▷ *Borrelia burgdorferi* causes Weil disease

**19** ▶ *Mycobacteria*:

    **A = True** ▷ are obligate aerobes

    **B = False** ▷ are motile

    **C = True** ▷ are nonsporing organisms

    **D = True** ▷ are rod-shaped

    **E = False** ▷ have cell walls that have a lipid content of 90%

**20** ▶ Regarding tuberculosis:

    **A = True** ▷ The incidence is rising in the UK

    **B = False** ▷ It is ten times more likely to occur in people born outside the UK

    **C = False** ▷ It is pulmonary in 90% of cases

    **D = True** ▷ The diagnosis requires a Ziehl–Neelsen stain

    **E = True** ▷ Histologically, it is characterised by caseating granulomas

**21** ▶ Regarding the treatment of tuberculosis:

    **A = True** ▷ Four drugs are now the standard treatment

    **B = False** ▷ It continues unaltered for 6 months

    **C = False** ▷ Rifampicin can cause peripheral neuropathy

    **D = True** ▷ Ethambutol can cause optic neuritis

    **E = True** ▷ People with open pulmonary tuberculosis should be admitted as inpatients

**22** ▶ Regarding actinomycosis:

    **A = True** ▷ It is caused by Gram-positive organisms

    **B = False** ▷ It is most commonly caused by the genus *Actinobaculum*

    **C = False** ▷ It is more common in women than in men

    **D = False** ▷ Pelvic infection is almost always associated with an intrauterine contraceptive device (IUCD)

    **E = False** ▷ First-line treatment is with long-term cephalosporins

**23** ▶ Regarding the genus *Candida*:

    **A = True** ▷ It includes more than 100 species

    **B = True** ▷ It can infect all mucous membranes

    **C = False** ▷ Infections are less likely to occur in people using inhaled steroids

    **D = True** ▷ Infections rarely involve an internal organ

    **E = False** ▷ All infections respond to azole therapy

**24** ▶ Regarding malaria:

    **A = True** ▷ Plasmodium falciparum causes the majority of malaria deaths

    **B = True** ▷ The disease is carried by Anopheles mosquitoes only

    **C = False** ▷ The sporozoite multiplies in the bloodstream

    **D = False** ▷ The life cycle is completed in hepatocytes

    **E = True** ▷ One million people a year die from the disease

**25** ▶ The following reduce the risk of contracting malaria:

    **A = True** ▷ Absence of Duffy factor

    **B = True** ▷ Alpha thalassaemia

    **C = True** ▷ Beta thalassaemia

    **D = False** ▷ HIV

    **E = True** ▷ Sickle-cell trait

**26** ▶ Regarding malaria and pregnancy:

**A = True** ▷ Pregnant women are more likely than nonpregnant women to contract malaria

**B = False** ▷ Malaria is less likely to recur in pregnant women than in nonpregnant women

**C = True** ▷ The disease causes a low birth weight

**D = True** ▷ The disease causes severe maternal anaemia

**E = True** ▷ The disease causes preterm labour

**27** ▶ Regarding infection control:

**A = True** ▷ If a microorganism is transmitted by droplets, then a negative-pressure room is required

**B = False** ▷ If a microorganism is transmitted by droplets, aprons and gloves should be worn when seeing the infected person

**C = True** ▷ Alcohol gel should be used after every contact with an infected person

**D = False** ▷ The 'bare below the elbows' policy has not been proven to prevent cross-infection

**E = False** ▷ Stethoscopes need not be cleaned between use

## Answers for Chapter 21

### EXTENDED MATCHING QUESTIONS

1 ▶ **E** = Rubella virus
2 ▶ **E** = Rubella virus
3 ▶ **C** = Parvovirus B19
4 ▶ **B** = Cytomegalovirus
5 ▶ **B** = Cytomegalovirus
6 ▶ **A** = Varicella zoster virus
7 ▶ **A** = Varicella zoster virus
8 ▶ **B** = Cytomegalovirus
9 ▶ **C** = Parvovirus B19
10 ▶ **D** = Herpes simplex virus

### MULTIPLE CHOICE QUESTIONS

**11** ▶ Regarding varicella zoster virus:

**A = True** ▷ The primary infection is also known as chickenpox

**B = False** ▷ It presents with a rash covering the entire body

**C = False** ▷ Lifelong immunity occurs after a second infection

**D = False** ▷ Re-infection is common

**E = True** ▷ Virus reactivation is known as shingles

**12** ▶ Regarding varicella zoster virus:

**A = True** ▷ It is a single-strain herpes virus

**B = False** ▷ It contains single-stranded DNA

**C = True** ▷ It is spread by person-to-person contact

**D = False** ▷ The incubation period lasts 1 week

**E = False** ▷ Infections are preventable by a killed vaccine

**13** ▶ Regarding varicella zoster and pregnancy:

**A = False** ▷ Infection of the fetus is most likely in the first trimester

**B = True** ▷ Infection of the fetus is most likely in the second trimester

**C = False** ▷ Detection of the virus in maternal blood confirms the diagnosis

**D = True** ▷ If a child presents before the age of 1 year with clinical zoster reactivation, then in utero infection must have occurred

**E = True** ▷ Varicella zoster immunoglobulin can be given during pregnancy

**14** ▶ The following are features of fetal varicella infection:

**A = True** ▷ Skin scarring
**B = False** ▷ Limb hyperplasia
**C = True** ▷ Chorioretinitis
**D = True** ▷ Cortical atrophy
**E = False** ▷ Liver fibrosis

**15** ▶ Regarding cytomegalovirus:

**A** = **False** ▷ It is the second most common congenital infection
**B** = **False** ▷ Only recurrent infection causes congenital abnormalities
**C** = **False** ▷ First-time mothers are at the highest risk
**D** = **True** ▷ Breastfeeding is the most effective mode of transmission
**E** = **False** ▷ Re-infection is most common in Caucasian women

**16** ▶ Cytomegalovirus:

**A** = **True** ▷ is a herpes virus
**B** = **True** ▷ contains double-stranded DNA
**C** = **False** ▷ has an incubation period of 14 days
**D** = **False** ▷ has a live attenuated vaccine
**E** = **True** ▷ is treatable with antivirals

**17** ▶ Regarding cytomegalovirus:

**A** = **False** ▷ Previous infection affords complete immunity against a different strain
**B** = **True** ▷ There is an increased risk of placental transmission if conception occurs within 6 months of a primary infection
**C** = **True** ▷ It is usually asymptomatic
**D** = **True** ▷ Fever can last for 3 weeks
**E** = **False** ▷ The monospot test is positive

**18** ▶ Regarding fetal cytomegalovirus infection:

**A** = **False** ▷ The infection is usually symptomatic at birth
**B** = **True** ▷ Microcephaly is a common finding
**C** = **True** ▷ Sixty percent of those presenting at birth have hearing loss
**D** = **False** ▷ Cerebral palsy is rare in symptomatic babies
**E** = **True** ▷ Up to 10% of asymptomatic babies are restricted in their mental development

**19** ▶ Regarding parvovirus B19:

**A** = **False** ▷ It occurs in summer epidemics
**B** = **True** ▷ Infected individuals who have developed the typical parvovirus rash are not infectious
**C** = **True** ▷ It deposits antigen–antibody complexes into the synovial joints
**D** = **True** ▷ It causes a slapped-cheek-like rash
**E** = **False** ▷ It causes arthralgia, usually of the neck

**20** ▶ Parvovirus B19:

**A** = **False** ▷ contains double-stranded DNA
**B** = **True** ▷ is spread by droplets
**C** = **False** ▷ has an incubation period of 21 days
**D** = **True** ▷ has no vaccine
**E** = **True** ▷ is treated *in utero* by a fetal blood transfusion

**21** ▶ Parvovirus B19 infection in pregnancy:

**A** = **True** ▷ causes fetal anaemia
**B** = **True** ▷ causes fetal hydrops
**C** = **False** ▷ causes fetal immune suppression
**D** = **True** ▷ causes fetal loss
**E** = **False** ▷ causes mental restriction in the newborn baby

**22** ▶ Herpes simplex virus:

**A** = **True** ▷ contains double-stranded DNA
**B** = **True** ▷ is spread via infected body fluids only
**C** = **True** ▷ has an incubation period of up to 2 weeks
**D** = **True** ▷ does not have a vaccine
**E** = **True** ▷ is treatable with antivirals

**23** ▶ The rubella virus:

**A** = **False** ▷ contains double-stranded DNA
**B** = **True** ▷ is spread by person-to-person contact
**C** = **True** ▷ has an incubation period of 13–20 days
**D** = **False** ▷ has a killed vaccine
**E** = **False** ▷ is treated with antivirals

**24** ▶ Regarding rubella and pregnancy:

**A** = **True** ▷ Infection should be considered in all women with a viral-type exanthema
**B** = **True** ▷ All women with symptoms should have an immunoglobulin G (IgG) test even if they have previously had a positive IgG test
**C** = **False** ▷ The first symptom is a maculopapular rash
**D** = **True** ▷ Maternal lymphadenopathy is usually present
**E** = **False** ▷ On presentation, most infected women have a positive IgG result

**25** ▶ Regarding first-trimester rubella infections:

- **A = True** ▷ Fetal hearing loss is common
- **B = True** ▷ Sixty percent of infected fetuses develop a heart defect
- **C = False** ▷ Half of infected fetuses develop cataracts
- **D = False** ▷ Fetal neurological defects are rare
- **E = False** ▷ Prenatal diagnosis is most important during this trimester

## Answers for Chapter 22

### EXTENDED MATCHING QUESTIONS

1 ▶ **O** = Syphilis
2 ▶ **A** = Actinomycosis
3 ▶ **D** = Chancroid
4 ▶ **E** = *Chlamydia trachomatis*
5 ▶ **L** = Human papillomavirus
6 ▶ **F** = *Escherichia coli*
7 ▶ **B** = Bacterial vaginosis
8 ▶ **Q** = Tuberculosis
9 ▶ **C** = *Candida albicans*
10 ▶ **P** = Trichomoniasis
11 ▶ **J** = Herpes simplex virus

### MULTIPLE CHOICE QUESTIONS

**12** ▶ Physiological vaginal discharge:

- **A = True** ▷ becomes yellow on contact with air
- **B = False** ▷ contains 99% lactobacilli
- **C = True** ▷ contains epithelial cells from the vaginal walls
- **D = True** ▷ always has an acidic pH
- **E = False** ▷ decreases in amount midcycle

**13** ▶ Vaginal candidiasis:

- **A = False** ▷ is caused by *Candida albicans* in 95% of presenting women
- **B = True** ▷ is estrogen-dependent
- **C = False** ▷ is common in prepubertal girls
- **D = True** ▷ is more common in women who wear tights
- **E = True** ▷ is common in patients who use steroids

**14** ▶ Regarding vaginal candidiasis:

- **A = True** ▷ The vulva is red
- **B = False** ▷ Discharge is usually offensive
- **C = False** ▷ Recurrent infections not responding to treatment are common
- **D = True** ▷ In pregnancy, topical treatment for 7 days is best used
- **E = False** ▷ If untreated in pregnancy, it is proven to cause preterm delivery

**15** ▶ Regarding bacterial vaginosis:

- **A = False** ▷ It is caused by aerobic organisms
- **B = True** ▷ *Gardnerella vaginalis* is a common cause
- **C = True** ▷ The discharge is offensive
- **D = True** ▷ Clue cells are seen on microscopy
- **E = True** ▷ There is an increased risk of second-trimester miscarriage in pregnant women

**16** ▶ Trichomoniasis:

- **A = True** ▷ causes a green/yellow discharge
- **B = False** ▷ does not affect the cervix
- **C = True** ▷ co-exists with bacterial vaginosis
- **D = False** ▷ is diagnosed microscopically
- **E = False** ▷ is treated with topical clindamycin

**17** ▶ Regarding infections of the cervix:

- **A = True** ▷ Human papillomavirus is a sexually transmitted infection
- **B = False** ▷ Herpes simplex virus 2 leads to wart formation on the cervix
- **C = False** ▷ *Neisseria gonorrhoeae* affects the squamous epithelium of the cervix
- **D = True** ▷ *Chlamydia trachomatis* causes follicular cervicitis
- **E = True** ▷ *Trichomonas vaginalis* causes a strawberry cervix

**18** ▶ Regarding infection of the fallopian tubes:

**A** = **False** ▷ The most common route of infection is via the local lymphatics

**B** = **True** ▷ Tuberculosis invades by the blood-borne route

**C** = **True** ▷ During acute salpingitis, pus forms within the lumen

**D** = **True** ▷ Hydrosalpinx is a long-term consequence of infection

**E** = **False** ▷ Mild inflammation tends to lead to a tubo-ovarian abscess

**19** ▶ *Chlamydia trachomatis*:

**A** = **True** ▷ is the most common cause of sexually transmitted bacterial infection in the UK

**B** = **False** ▷ is more likely to be asymptomatic in men than in women

**C** = **False** ▷ is restricted to the genital tract

**D** = **True** ▷ is the most important cause of nongonococcal urethritis in men

**E** = **True** ▷ causes cervicitis in women

**20** ▶ Regarding *Chlamydia trachomatis*:

**A** = **True** ▷ It is an obligate intracellular pathogen

**B** = **False** ▷ It directly damages epithelial cells by releasing toxic particles

**C** = **True** ▷ Self-collected swabs are as sensitive for the diagnosis as endocervical swabs

**D** = **False** ▷ The infection is treated with metronidazole

**E** = **False** ▷ It is a known cause of preterm labour in pregnant women

**21** ▶ Regarding gonorrhoea:

**A** = **False** ▷ The incidence is increasing in the developed world

**B** = **True** ▷ It is symptomatic in 90% of men

**C** = **False** ▷ It is not known to cause chronic infection in women

**D** = **False** ▷ It causes a yellow urethral discharge in men

**E** = **True** ▷ It is a known cause of proctitis

**22** ▶ Regarding *Neisseria gonorrhoeae*:

**A** = **False** ▷ It is a Gram-positive diplococcus

**B** = **False** ▷ It is diagnosed microscopically

**C** = **False** ▷ Treatment is standardised to a single dose of cefixime

**D** = **True** ▷ Fifty percent of women with *Neisseria gonorrhoeae* also have a *Chlamydia* infection

**E** = **True** ▷ Post-treatment swabs should be carried out

**23** ▶ Cervicitis:

**A** = **True** ▷ is a clinical diagnosis

**B** = **True** ▷ causes purulent discharge seen at the cervical os

**C** = **False** ▷ only bleeds if swabbed vigorously

**D** = **False** ▷ is rarely caused by a sexually transmitted infection

**E** = **True** ▷ causes nabothian follicles if it becomes chronic

**24** ▶ Regarding pelvic inflammatory disease:

**A** = **True** ▷ Plasma cells are seen on endometrial biopsy

**B** = **True** ▷ It is associated with intermenstrual bleeding

**C** = **False** ▷ In salpingitis, plasma cells are the first leucocytes to enter

**D** = **True** ▷ Pus leaking from the tubes causes them to adhere to the ovaries

**E** = **False** ▷ The omentum is usually unable to confine the infection to the pelvis

**25** ▶ Regarding pelvic inflammatory disease in pregnancy:

**A** = **False** ▷ *Chlamydia* infection increases the risk of preterm birth five-fold

**B** = **True** ▷ Gonorrhoea can cause chorioamnionitis

**C** = **True** ▷ *Chlamydia trachomatis* causes ophthalmia neonatorum

**D** = **False** ▷ *Neisseria gonorrhoeae* causes pneumonitis in the first few months of life

**E** = **False** ▷ Azithromycin is used to treat gonorrhoea in pregnancy

ANSWERS

15 | EMQs and MCQs

**26** ▶ Regarding nonherpes genital ulcers:

**A = True** ▷ Lymphogranuloma venereum is caused by specific serovars of *Chlamydia trachomatis*

**B = True** ▷ Lymphogranuloma venereum causes severe proctocolitis

**C = False** ▷ Chancroid is an infection caused by *Klebsiella granulomatis*

**D = True** ▷ Chancroid causes inflamed lymph nodes to weep through the skin

**E = True** ▷ Granuloma inguinale causes elephantiasis

**27** ▶ Regarding syphilis:

**A = False** ▷ The incidence is decreasing in the UK
**B = False** ▷ It is most common in women with multiple partners
**C = True** ▷ It is caused by *Treponema pallidum*
**D = True** ▷ It produces chancres
**E = True** ▷ In women it most often causes lesions of the cervix

**28** ▶ Regarding syphilis:

**A = False** ▷ Chancres require treatment to resolve
**B = False** ▷ Condylomata lata are perianal lesions of primary syphilis
**C = True** ▷ Secondary syphilis presents with a systemic rash
**D = True** ▷ It causes alopecia
**E = True** ▷ It causes sensorineural deafness

**29** ▶ Syphilis:

**A = True** ▷ affects the central nervous system (neurosyphilis) twice as often in men as in women
**B = True** ▷ causes strokes
**C = False** ▷ causes myocardial infarction
**D = True** ▷ causes miscarriage in pregnant women
**E = True** ▷ causes fetal deafness if transmitted during pregnancy

**30** ▶ Regarding syphilis:

**A = True** ▷ It is caused by *Treponema pallidum* subspecies *pallidum*
**B = True** ▷ It is usually contracted through sexual contact
**C = False** ▷ The first-line antibiotic is doxycycline
**D = True** ▷ It produces a chancre
**E = True** ▷ Lesions only arise at the site of entry of *Treponema pallidum*

**31** ▶ Regarding syphilis:

**A = False** ▷ Primary syphilis has an incubation period of 28 days
**B = False** ▷ Primary syphilis produces a painful ulcer
**C = True** ▷ Secondary syphilis presents as a systemic disease
**D = False** ▷ People with secondary syphilis have a localised rash on their genitals
**E = True** ▷ The latent phase can last years

**32** ▶ Regarding syphilis:

**A = False** ▷ Secondary syphilis presents up to 6 months after healing of the primary chancre
**B = True** ▷ The infected person is asymptomatic during the latent phase
**C = False** ▷ Latent syphilis eventually progresses to tertiary syphilis
**D = False** ▷ Tertiary syphilis is associated with a dissecting aorta
**E = True** ▷ Tertiary syphilis is associated with tabes dorsalis

**33** ▶ Regarding the human papillomavirus:

**A = True** ▷ There are more than 100 types
**B = False** ▷ Penetrative intercourse is required for infection
**C = True** ▷ In developed countries the lifetime risk of infection is 70–80%
**D = False** ▷ Infected women usually have genital warts
**E = False** ▷ The immune system is inefficient at clearing the virus completely

**34** ▶ The following types of human papillomavirus (HPV) have a low oncogenic potential:

**A = True** ▷ HPV-6
**B = True** ▷ HPV-11
**C = False** ▷ HPV-16
**D = False** ▷ HPV-18
**E = False** ▷ HPV-31

**35** ▶ Regarding human papillomavirus (HPV) and cervical cancer:

**A = True** ▷ The majority (99.7%) of squamous cell carcinomas of the cervix contain HPV DNA

**B = False** ▷ In unscreened populations, 25% of women with HPV of high oncogenic potential develop cervical cancer

**C = True** ▷ In screened populations, 1% of women with HPV of high oncogenic potential develop cervical cancer

**D = False** ▷ Smoking is a greater risk factor for cervical cancer than HPV

**E = True** ▷ All women with cervical warts should be sent for colposcopy

**36** ▶ Molluscum contagiosum:

**A = True** ▷ is a poxvirus
**B = False** ▷ causes red lesions
**C = False** ▷ does not occur in children
**D = True** ▷ requires cryotherapy for treatment
**E = False** ▷ is no longer infectious once the lesions have burst

**37** ▶ Regarding HIV infection:

**A = True** ▷ HIV is a retrovirus

**B = False** ▷ Acute seroconversion in the first few weeks of HIV infection is rare

**C = True** ▷ There are often several opportunistic infections as the immune system weakens

**D = True** ▷ AIDS is defined by the onset of life-threatening opportunistic infections or of malignancies associated with immunodeficiency

**E = False** ▷ Without antiretroviral treatment the median time to the development of AIDS is 5 years

**38** ▶ The following are common AIDS-presenting illnesses:

**A = True** ▷ *Pneumocystis* pneumonia
**B = True** ▷ Cerebral toxoplasmosis
**C = True** ▷ Cytomegalovirus retinitis
**D = True** ▷ Kaposi sarcoma
**E = True** ▷ *Mycobacterium avium* complex infection

**39** ▶ Regarding the treatment of HIV infection:

**A = False** ▷ First-line drug treatment involves the use of a nucleoside or nucleotide reverse transcriptase inhibitor and a nonnucleoside reverse transcriptase inhibitor (NNRTI)

**B = True** ▷ Protease inhibitors are used if there is resistance to NNRTIs

**C = False** ▷ A rise in the CD8 count is a sign that treatment is successful

**D = False** ▷ Clotrimazole is used to prevent *Pneumocystis* pneumonia

**E = False** ▷ Antifungals are of limited use in people with severe immunodeficiency

**40** ▶ Regarding HIV:

**A = False** ▷ The diagnosis is based on finding HIV RNA in the plasma

**B = True** ▷ Homosexual intercourse is the most common form of transmission in developed countries

**C = False** ▷ In developing countries more men are infected than women

**D = True** ▷ Genital infections are more common in HIV-positive people

**E = True** ▷ Bacterial vaginosis is a risk factor for transmission

**41** ▶ Regarding vertical HIV transmission:

**A = False** ▷ Without intervention this occurs in 50% of pregnancies

**B = False** ▷ Infection *in utero* is impossible

**C = True** ▷ Babies can present with AIDS in the neonatal period

**D = False** ▷ All mothers with HIV or AIDS should have a caesarean section

**E = False** ▷ Breastfeeding is permissible in mothers with HIV or AIDS

**42** ▶ Regarding urinary tract infection (UTI):

**A = True** ▷ In young girls UTIs need investigation to exclude congenital abnormalities

**B = True** ▷ *Escherichia coli* is the most common pathogen in UTIs

**C = False** ▷ Sexual intercourse does not increase the risk of a UTI

**D = False** ▷ Antibiotics for UTIs stop periurethral infection

**E = False** ▷ Amoxicillin has no affect on the lactobacilli in the vagina

43 ▶ Regarding urinary tract infection:

A = **False** ▷ External dysuria is a symptom
B = **True** ▷ Haematuria is a sign of severe disease
C = **False** ▷ Symptomatic women should be treated without delay
D = **False** ▷ Treatment should be commenced based on a dipstick test that is positive for nitrites only
E = **True** ▷ A pure growth of at least $10^8$ organisms/l is interpreted as confirming an infection

## Answers for chapters 23–25

### EXTENDED MATCHING QUESTIONS

1 ▶ **D** = Cytokines
2 ▶ **A** = Histamine
3 ▶ **E** = Kinins
4 ▶ **B** = Partial hydatidiform mole
5 ▶ **D** = Choriocarcinoma
6 ▶ **C** = Invasive hydatidiform mole
7 ▶ **A** = Complete hydatidiform mole
8 ▶ **A** = Human chorionic gonadotrophin
9 ▶ **H** = CA19-9
10 ▶ **G** = CA125
11 ▶ **F** = Prostate-specific antigen
12 ▶ **G** = CA125
13 ▶ **D** = Alphafetoprotein

### MULTIPLE CHOICE QUESTIONS

14 ▶ Regarding wound healing:

A = **True** ▷ Granulation tissue is a mixture of myofibroblasts and capillaries only
B = **True** ▷ Healing by first intention occurs only if there is close approximation of the tissue edges
C = **False** ▷ A keloid scar is caused by excessive epithelial regeneration
D = **False** ▷ Granulation is the main process of organisation in the healing of bone
E = **False** ▷ The hepatic architecture is easily rebuilt after being damaged

15 ▶ Regarding inflammation:

A = **True** ▷ The aim of it is to repair tissues
B = **False** ▷ Vascular dilatation is the first response
C = **False** ▷ White blood cells diffuse through the cell walls
D = **False** ▷ Neutrophils cannot cross the vessel walls
E = **False** ▷ Mononuclear cells are the first cells to cross the vessel walls

16 ▶ Regarding inflammation:

A = **True** ▷ Acute inflammation may result in the formation of an abscess
B = **False** ▷ Acute inflammation becomes chronic inflammation after 1 week
C = **True** ▷ Chronic inflammation can occur as a result of acute inflammation
D = **False** ▷ Chronic inflammation involves mast cell infiltration
E = **True** ▷ Granulomas are collections of epithelioid cells

17 ▶ Regarding malignant spread:

A = **True** ▷ Carcinomas spread to lymph nodes
B = **True** ▷ Osteosarcomas spread through the blood
C = **False** ▷ Renal cancer spreads through lymph nodes
D = **True** ▷ Lobular breast cancer spreads to serous cavities
E = **False** ▷ Basal cell carcinomas spread through the blood

18 ▶ Regarding gynaecological neoplasias:

A = **False** ▷ Malignant tumours of the vulva are associated with herpes simplex virus
B = **False** ▷ Lymph node spread is not a prognostic factor in malignant tumours of the vulva
C = **False** ▷ The number of partners a woman has had does not alter her risk of cervical intraepithelial neoplasia
D = **False** ▷ Krukenberg tumours arise from the breast
E = **True** ▷ Choricarcinomas are trophoblastic

**19** ▶ Regarding gynaecological neoplasias:

    **A = False** ▷ The most important human papillomavirus types in the aetiology of cervical intraepithelial neoplasia (CIN) are types 14 and 16

    **B = False** ▷ Smoking is not an independent risk factor for CIN

    **C = False** ▷ Leiomyosarcomas arise from the stromal cells of the uterus

    **D = True** ▷ Metastatic ovarian cancer is histologically similar to primary tissue

    **E = False** ▷ Krukenberg tumours are cystic

## Answers for Chapter 26

### EXTENDED MATCHING QUESTIONS

1 ▶ **K** = Ranitidine
2 ▶ **L** = Cyproterone acetate
3 ▶ **F** = Cabergoline
4 ▶ **M** = Metoclopramide
5 ▶ **D** = Pilocarpine
6 ▶ **J** = Tolterodine
7 ▶ **G** = Atenolol
8 ▶ **A** = Salbutamol
9 ▶ **B** = Methyldopa
10 ▶ **C** = Chloramphenicol
11 ▶ **E** = Nitrofurantoin
12 ▶ **D** = Macrolides
13 ▶ **F** = Penicillins
14 ▶ **I** = Tetracyclines
15 ▶ **I** = Tetracyclines
16 ▶ **A** = Aminoglycosides
17 ▶ **H** = Sulphonamides
18 ▶ **H** = Sulphonamides
19 ▶ **A** = Aminoglycosides
20 ▶ **G** = Tetracyclines
21 ▶ **J** = Aspirin
22 ▶ **A** = Angiotensin-converting enzyme inhibitors
23 ▶ **E** = Carbamazepine
24 ▶ **O** = Warfarin
25 ▶ **D** = Nitrofurantoin
26 ▶ **O** = Warfarin
27 ▶ **C** = Beta blockers

### MULTIPLE CHOICE QUESTIONS

**28** ▶ A drug's absorption rate is increased by:

    **A = True** ▷ lipid solubility
    **B = False** ▷ high polarity
    **C = True** ▷ attaching to a specific carrier
    **D = True** ▷ accelerating gastric emptying
    **E = False** ▷ rectal rather than oral administration

**29** ▶ Regarding renal clearance:

    **A = True** ▷ Large drugs are not renally excreted
    **B = True** ▷ Protein-bound drugs are poorly excreted
    **C = False** ▷ Excretion is passive in the proximal convoluted tubule
    **D = False** ▷ Excretion is active in the descending loops of Henle
    **E = False** ▷ Acidic drugs use cation transporters

**30** ▶ Regarding kidney excretion:

    **A = False** ▷ Polar drugs are distributed over a large volume
    **B = True** ▷ Polar drugs are easily cleared by the kidney
    **C = False** ▷ Albumin-bound drugs are easily cleared
    **D = False** ▷ Acidic drugs are not secreted into the proximal tubule
    **E = False** ▷ Tubular reabsorption rates are the same for all drugs

**31** ▶ Regarding drug pharmacokinetics:

    **A = True** ▷ There is an increase in volume of the third space
    **B = False** ▷ There is an increase in serum concentration of drugs
    **C = True** ▷ There is an increase in clearance of drugs
    **D = True** ▷ Liver metabolism is increased
    **E = False** ▷ Fat-soluble drugs are more affected by pregnancy changes

**32** ▶ Regarding drug interactions:

    **A = False** ▷ Enzyme inducers cause an increase in serum concentration of other drugs
    **B = True** ▷ Enzyme inhibitors increase the risk of drug toxicity
    **C = True** ▷ Phenytoin is an enzyme inducer
    **D = False** ▷ Sulphonamides are an enzyme inducer
    **E = False** ▷ Ampicillin increases the effects of oral estrogens

**33** ▶ Regarding the effects of drugs on enzyme expression:

A = False ▷ Smoking decreases enzyme induction
B = False ▷ Alcohol decreases enzyme induction
C = False ▷ Enzyme induction is usually due to a decrease in enzyme breakdown
D = True ▷ Enzyme inhibition can increase the action of other drugs
E = True ▷ Phenytoin leads to reduced efficiency of warfarin

**34** ▶ Regarding drug prescription in relation to pregnancy and lactation:

A = True ▷ All women of reproductive age might be pregnant
B = True ▷ Drugs should be avoided in the first trimester if possible
C = False ▷ Known teratogenic anticonvulsant drugs should be stopped in pregnancy
D = True ▷ Most drugs cross the placenta
E = False ▷ Large doses should be used for the shortest possible time

**35** ▶ Regarding prenatal exposure to a teratogen:

A = True ▷ Up to day 17, any teratogenic effect results in miscarriage
B = True ▷ The earlier the exposure, the more marked the effect
C = False ▷ All organs are sensitive for the same period of time
D = False ▷ There is no risk of teratogenicity after week 8
E = True ▷ Anencephaly is most likely to occur with exposure to tetratogens around day 24

**36** ▶ Miscarriage can be caused by:

A = True ▷ ergotamine
B = False ▷ gabapentin
C = True ▷ mifepristone
D = True ▷ thrombolytics
E = False ▷ carbamazepine

**37** ▶ Regarding the use of anticonvulsants:

A = False ▷ Risks of teratogenicity decrease if folic acid is given at the start of pregnancy
B = False ▷ Women who have not had a fit for more than a year should stop taking them
C = True ▷ Polypharmacy increases the risks of teratogenicity
D = True ▷ Sodium valproate is the most teratogenic anticonvulsant
E = False ▷ Phenytoin has dose-related effect on verbal IQ

**38** ▶ Phenytoin is associated with:

A = True ▷ cleft lip/palate
B = True ▷ microcephaly
C = True ▷ cardiac abnormalities
D = True ▷ mental retardation
E = False ▷ neural tube defects

**39** ▶ Antibiotics contraindicated in pregnancy are:

A = False ▷ macrolides
B = False ▷ penicillins
C = False ▷ quinolones
D = True ▷ sulphonamides
E = True ▷ tetracyclines

**40** ▶ Antibiotics used with caution in pregnancy are:

A = False ▷ macrolides
B = False ▷ cephalosporins
C = True ▷ quinolones
D = True ▷ nitrofurantoin
E = True ▷ aminoglycosides

**41** ▶ Regarding the use of anticonvulsants in pregnancy:

A = True ▷ Of the anticonvulsants sodium valproate has the highest risk of teratogenesis
B = True ▷ Carbamazepine causes neural tube defects
C = True ▷ Folic acid should always be given as well
D = True ▷ There is a five-fold increase in fetal malformations
E = False ▷ Teratogenicity is a more important consideration than good seizure control

42 ▶ Regarding the use of anticoagulants in pregnancy:

    **A** = **False** ▷ Warfarin causes nasal hypoplasia in the second trimester

    **B** = **False** ▷ Heparin use in the first trimester causes chondroplasia

    **C** = **True** ▷ Warfarin may cause major haemorrhage towards the end of pregnancy

    **D** = **True** ▷ There are no common fetal abnormalities with the use of heparin in pregnancy

    **E** = **False** ▷ Warfarin must be exchanged for heparin by week 8

## Answers for Chapter 27

### EXTENDED MATCHING QUESTIONS

  1 ▶ **A** = Angiotensin-converting enzyme inhibitors
  2 ▶ **G** = Thiazides
  3 ▶ **E** = Methyldopa
  4 ▶ **E** = Methyldopa
  5 ▶ **E** = Methyldopa
  6 ▶ **B** = Beta blockers
  7 ▶ **B** = Beta blockers
  8 ▶ **F** = Nifedipine
  9 ▶ **C** = Hydralazine
10 ▶ **D** = Magnesium sulphate
11 ▶ **B** = Beta mimetics
12 ▶ **A** = Atosiban
13 ▶ **D** = Magnesium sulphate
14 ▶ **A** = Atosiban
15 ▶ **B** = Beta mimetics
16 ▶ **C** = Misoprostol
17 ▶ **A** = Carboprost
18 ▶ **B** = Ergometrine
19 ▶ **D** = Syntocinon
20 ▶ **C** = Misoprostol
21 ▶ **A** = Carboprost
22 ▶ **B** = Ergometrine
23 ▶ **C** = Cyclophosphamide
24 ▶ **A** = Fluorouracil
25 ▶ **F** = Paclitaxel
26 ▶ **E** = Methotrexate
27 ▶ **B** = Cisplatin
28 ▶ **C** = Cyclophosphamide
29 ▶ **D** = Doxorubicin
30 ▶ **B** = Cisplatin

### MULTIPLE CHOICE QUESTIONS

31 ▷ Methyldopa:

    **A** = **True** ▷ is safe in pregnancy
    **B** = **True** ▷ acts centrally
    **C** = **False** ▷ has no effect on sympathetic outflow
    **D** = **True** ▷ causes depression
    **E** = **False** ▷ causes a drop in baseline on cardiotocograph

32 ▷ Nifedipine:

    **A** = **True** ▷ is a calcium channel blocker
    **B** = **False** ▷ is licensed in pregnancy
    **C** = **True** ▷ is a tocolytic
    **D** = **True** ▷ causes peripheral oedema
    **E** = **False** ▷ causes arrhythmia

33 ▷ Regarding intravenous antihypertensives:

    **A** = **False** ▷ Hydralazine acts centrally
    **B** = **True** ▷ Hydralazine is known to cause lupus-like events
    **C** = **True** ▷ Magnesium sulphate is a membrane stabiliser
    **D** = **True** ▷ Magnesium sulphate is the best antihypertensive at reducing eclamptic fits
    **E** = **True** ▷ Magnesium sulphate causes cardiorespiratory arrest

34 ▷ Drugs to treat detrusor overactivity:

    **A** = **True** ▷ include antimuscarinics
    **B** = **True** ▷ include desmopressin
    **C** = **False** ▷ include duloxetine
    **D** = **True** ▷ cause a dry mouth
    **E** = **False** ▷ cause diarrhoea

35 ▷ Regarding chemotheraputic drugs used in gynaecological oncology:

    **A** = **True** ▷ Platinum agents are used in ovarian cancer
    **B** = **True** ▷ Cisplatin is used in cervical cancer
    **C** = **True** ▷ Methotrexate has a use in metastatic cervical cancer
    **D** = **False** ▷ Folate antagonists are used in vulval cancer
    **E** = **False** ▷ Methotrexate alone is used in high-risk trophoblastic disease

# Answers for Chapter 28

## MULTIPLE CHOICE QUESTIONS

### 1 ▶ Regarding estrogens:

**A = True** ▷ During the childbearing years, estradiol is the most potent estrogen
**B = False** ▷ After the menopause, estriol is the most abundant estrogen
**C = True** ▷ After the menopause, the ovaries stop producing estrogens completely
**D = True** ▷ Estrogens terminate the pubertal growth spurt in women
**E = False** ▷ The hypothalamus and the heart contain the same type of estrogen receptor

### 2 ▶ Regarding pharmacological estrogens:

**A = False** ▷ Pharmacological estrogens contain an ethinyl group to prevent first-pass metabolism
**B = True** ▷ Pharmacological estrogens are usually estradiols
**C = False** ▷ Plant estrogens are used in the combined oral contraceptive
**D = False** ▷ Clomiphene citrate acts by replicating the actions of estrogen
**E = True** ▷ Tamoxifen is an estrogen antagonist in the breast but an agonist in the skeleton

### 3 ▶ Regarding endogenous progesterone:

**A = False** ▷ Outside of pregnancy, progesterone is mainly produced by the adrenal cortex
**B = True** ▷ Progesterone production is at its peak during the luteal phase
**C = True** ▷ Progesterone causes an increase in body temperature
**D = True** ▷ Progesterone is responsible for decidual development
**E = False** ▷ Progesterone is an antagonistic estrogen on the uterus

### 4 ▶ Regarding pharmacological progestogens:

**A = True** ▷ Large doses need to be given orally
**B = False** ▷ Medroxyprogesterone acetate is a 19-carbon steroid
**C = True** ▷ Medroxyprogesterone acetate is used for the treatment of endometriosis
**D = True** ▷ Norethisterone has androgenic properties
**E = False** ▷ In hormone replacement therapy, progesterone is given at constant doses

### 5 ▶ Adverse effects of progesterone treatment are:

**A = False** ▷ loss of libido
**B = True** ▷ acne
**C = True** ▷ mood swings
**D = False** ▷ insomnia
**E = True** ▷ hirsutism

### 6 ▶ Gonadotrophin-releasing hormone analogues:

**A = True** ▷ are used for oestrogen suppression
**B = True** ▷ when used, may cause a worsening of symptoms before improvement
**C = True** ▷ are well known to cause insomnia
**D = False** ▷ produce long-lasting adverse effects
**E = False** ▷ have no effect on bone density

### 7 ▶ Regarding hormone replacement therapy:

**A = True** ▷ Progesterone produces a dose-dependent histological change
**B = False** ▷ Progesterone must be used for at least 7 days a month to reduce the risk of endometrial cancer
**C = True** ▷ Transdermal patches use estradiol
**D = True** ▷ Estrogen levels should be checked prior to each subcutaneous insertion of an implant, regardless of the patient's symptoms
**E = False** ▷ Tibolone should not be given unopposed

### 8 ▶ Regarding hormone replacement therapy:

**A = True** ▷ The risk of deep vein thrombosis is increased
**B = True** ▷ The therapy is a well-known treatment for osteoporosis
**C = True** ▷ If unopposed estrogen is used, there is a relative risk of endometrial cancer of 95
**D = False** ▷ Tibolone is an estrogen and progesterone preparation
**E = False** ▷ Tibolone produces a withdrawal bleed

## Answers for Chapters 29 and 30

### MULTIPLE CHOICE QUESTIONS

**1** ▶ During female fetal reproductive development:

**A** = **True** ▷ Oogonia develop from germ cells

**B** = **False** ▷ The number of oogonia entering the fetal gonad is the number of oocytes that a female will have

**C** = **False** ▷ The oocyte completes the first meiotic division

**D** = **False** ▷ The oocytes are stored in the medulla of the ovary

**E** = **False** ▷ Oocytes are lost from the first trimester onwards

**2** ▶ During the process of follicle growth:

**A** = **False** ▷ Follicle-stimulating hormone is required to begin growth

**B** = **False** ▷ Follicles grow by increasing fluid in the oocyte

**C** = **False** ▷ Capillaries for follicular growth form in the granulosa layer

**D** = **False** ▷ The follicle grows for 45 days from initiation to selection

**E** = **False** ▷ An antral follicle contains a fluid-filled cavity within the oocyte

**3** ▶ Regarding follicular selection:

**A** = **True** ▷ Follicle-stimulating hormone is required for follicular growth from the antral stage onwards only

**B** = **False** ▷ Estrogen is formed in the thecal cells

**C** = **False** ▷ As the corpus luteum of the previous cycle fails, there is a fall in follicle-stimulating hormone

**D** = **True** ▷ As the follicle's granulosa cells increase, serum inhibin increases

**E** = **True** ▷ Follicle-stimulating hormone causes the granulosa cells to develop luteinising hormone receptors

**4** ▶ During ovulation:

**A** = **True** ▷ The antral pressure rises prior to ovulation

**B** = **False** ▷ There is a rise in steroid production directly after ovulation

**C** = **True** ▷ Luteinising hormone causes the first meiotic division to be completed

**D** = **False** ▷ After moving into the fallopian tube, the oocyte completes the second meiotic division

**E** = **True** ▷ Estradiol causes the cilia in the fallopian tube to be produced

**5** ▶ Regarding the uterus:

**A** = **True** ▷ During the follicular phase, the endometrial cells divide

**B** = **False** ▷ The glands multiply in number in the proliferative phase

**C** = **False** ▷ After ovulation, the endometrial layer thickens by further hyperplasia

**D** = **True** ▷ Prostaglandins cause constriction of the spiral arterioles

**E** = **True** ▷ Necrosis of the endometrial layer is initially due to hypoxia

**6** ▶ Regarding the development of the vagina and cervix:

**A** = **False** ▷ The vagina is lined with keratinised squamous epithelium

**B** = **True** ▷ Cell shedding from the vagina helps to inhibit infection

**C** = **True** ▷ The vagina is always acidic

**D** = **True** ▷ The cervix becomes more oedematous during the follicular phase

**E** = **True** ▷ Glycoproteins form channels in the cervical mucus to assist fertilisation

**7** ▶ Regarding the testes:

**A** = **False** ▷ The normal volume of each testis is 30–40 ml

**B** = **False** ▷ The seminiferous tubules are the sites of sperm storage

**C** = **False** ▷ Spermatogenesis takes place in Sertoli cells

**D** = **True** ▷ Spermatogonia are only laid down in fetal life

**E** = **False** ▷ There is good blood flow through the basal lamina to the Sertoli cells

**8 ▶** Regarding spermatogenesis:

**A = False** ▷ There is a wave of mitotic division of spermatogonia every 28 days

**B = False** ▷ Daughter spermatogonia are to become spermatozoa

**C = False** ▷ Primary spermatocytes have 23 chromosomes

**D = True** ▷ Each spermatocyte gives four spermatids

**E = True** ▷ Normal spermatogenesis requires the presence of testosterone and follicle-stimulating hormone

**9 ▶** Regarding spermatogenesis:

**A = True** ▷ Each meiotic division moves the spermatids towards the lumen of the seminiferous tubule

**B = False** ▷ The process of spermatogenesis takes 80 days

**C = True** ▷ The tubules all open in the rete

**D = True** ▷ The epididymis is 5 m long

**E = False** ▷ Spermatozoa for intracytoplasmic sperm injection are removed from the rete

**10 ▶** Regarding androgen synthesis in males:

**A = True** ▷ The process occurs mainly in the Leydig cells

**B = False** ▷ The process is under the control of follicle-stimulating hormone

**C = True** ▷ Testosterone is converted to estradiol in the Sertoli cells

**D = True** ▷ In the male fetus, testosterone production is under the control of human chorionic gonadotrophin

**E = True** ▷ The level of testosterone falls in the male from fetal life until adrenarche

**11 ▶** Regarding the deposition of sperm in the female genital tract:

**A = False** ▷ Only the parasympathetic pelvic nerves influence erection

**B = False** ▷ Blood flow mainly into the corpus spongiosum causes an erection

**C = True** ▷ The vas deferens contracts

**D = True** ▷ About 120 million spermatozoa are normally deposited

**E = True** ▷ The ejaculate coagulates within 1 minute of entry into the vagina

**12 ▶** The following statements regarding fertilisation and the oocyte are correct:

**A = True** ▷ The oocyte completes the second meiotic division

**B = False** ▷ The first polar body is formed

**C = True** ▷ The cortical granules release their contents to prevent polyspermy

**D = False** ▷ There is a further meiotic cell division

**E = True** ▷ Blastocyst cells begin to produce human chorionic gonadotrophin

## Answers for Chapter 31

### MULTIPLE CHOICE QUESTIONS

**1 ▶** Regarding maternal cardiac output in pregnancy:

**A = False** ▷ Cardiac output increases by 25%

**B = False** ▷ Cardiac output continues to rise until term

**C = False** ▷ Increase occurs by increasing the heart rate only

**D = True** ▷ The breasts receive much of the early extra cardiac output

**E = True** ▷ At term, the skin receives 500 ml per minute (18% of cardiac output)

**2 ▶** Regarding maternal cardiovascular physiology in pregnancy:

**A = True** ▷ Peripheral vascular resistance is reduced in pregnancy

**B = False** ▷ Blood pressure falls to its lowest at week 20

**C = True** ▷ The diastolic blood pressure falls by 10 mmHg

**D = True** ▷ Maternal electrocardiogram shows left axis deviation

**E = False** ▷ Maternal electrocardiogram shows Q waves in lead II

**3 ▶** Regarding maternal cardiovascular physiology in pregnancy:

**A = True** ▷ Blood volume increases by 30%

**B = False** ▷ Plasma volume increase by 30%

**C = False** ▷ Stroke volume increases by 25%

**D = False** ▷ The heart rate increases by 20%

**E = True** ▷ There is left ventricular hypertrophy

**4** ▶ Regarding the maternal respiratory system in pregnancy:

**A** = **True** ▷ Progesterone increases ventilation
**B** = **False** ▷ Ventilation increases by 25%
**C** = **True** ▷ $PCO_2$ falls during pregnancy
**D** = **False** ▷ There is a decrease in the calibre of the tracheobronchial tree
**E** = **False** ▷ Respiratory rate increases

**5** ▶ Regarding the maternal respiratory system in pregnancy:

**A** = **False** ▷ Breathing becomes increasingly thoracic
**B** = **False** ▷ Tidal volume doubles
**C** = **False** ▷ Forced expiratory volume increases
**D** = **True** ▷ Dyspnoea is experienced in 70% of cases
**E** = **True** ▷ 40% of increased oxygen consumption is for the fetus

**6** ▶ During pregnancy:

**A** = **True** ▷ The kidneys increase in size
**B** = **False** ▷ The ureters dilate owing to the size of the uterus only
**C** = **False** ▷ Renal blood flow doubles
**D** = **True** ▷ The glomerular filtration rate increases by 50%
**E** = **True** ▷ There is increased excretion of bicarbonate

**7** ▶ Regarding the maternal gastrointestinal tract and nutrition in pregnancy:

**A** = **False** ▷ Progesterone increases gastric emptying
**B** = **True** ▷ 80% of women suffer from acid reflux
**C** = **True** ▷ Gastric contents are more acidic
**D** = **False** ▷ Gallbladder emptying is increased
**E** = **True** ▷ Women with obstetric cholestasis are more likely to have fetal distress in labour

**8** ▶ Lactating women require higher amounts than pregnant women of:

**A** = **True** ▷ vitamin A
**B** = **True** ▷ vitamin $B_2$
**C** = **True** ▷ vitamin C
**D** = **True** ▷ vitamin E
**E** = **False** ▷ vitamin K

**9** ▶ Regarding haematological system changes in concert with cardiovascular adaptations:

**A** = **False** ▷ The plasma volume expands by 30%
**B** = **False** ▷ Red cell mass increases until week 32
**C** = **False** ▷ Physiological anaemia is at its worst at week 28
**D** = **False** ▷ Platelets decrease in size in pregnancy
**E** = **True** ▷ White cell count increases predominantly due to neutrophils

**10** ▶ Regarding changes in the haematological system in pregnancy:

**A** = **False** ▷ The pregnant woman requires an extra 600 mg of iron per day
**B** = **False** ▷ Iron absorption is increased due to decreased gastric motility
**C** = **False** ▷ Fibrinolytic activity increases during pregnancy
**D** = **False** ▷ Concentrations of factor XI increase in pregnancy
**E** = **False** ▷ The activity of the fibrinolytic system returns to normal 6 weeks post delivery

**11** ▶ Regarding lactation:

**A** = **False** ▷ The alveolar cells undergo hyperplasia in the third trimester
**B** = **True** ▷ Human placental lactogen causes lactiferous duct hyperplasia
**C** = **True** ▷ High pregnancy levels of progesterone prevent milk production
**D** = **False** ▷ The combined oral contraceptive taken during breastfeeding has no effect on milk production
**E** = **False** ▷ Colostrum has high concentrations of lactose

**12** ▶ Regarding lactation:

**A** = **False** ▷ The amount of protein in milk decreases with time
**B** = **True** ▷ Suckling produces oxytocin
**C** = **True** ▷ Milk production doubles in twin-feeding mothers
**D** = **False** ▷ Extra energy for breast milk production is achieved from greater consumption of food
**E** = **False** ▷ Breast milk is the same in all women

13 ▶ Regarding lactation:

A = **True** ▷ Prolactin is released from the hypothalamus

B = **False** ▷ Prolactin surges immediately after suckling begins

C = **True** ▷ Dopamine suppresses milk production

D = **False** ▷ Metoclopramide suppresses milk production

E = **False** ▷ Prolactin levels naturally decrease 28 days after delivery

14 ▶ Oxytocin:

A = **True** ▷ release is stimulated by suckling

B = **False** ▷ is released by the anterior pituitary

C = **True** ▷ is released if the mother hears the baby crying

D = **True** ▷ acts on myoepithelial cells

E = **False** ▷ is central to milk production

15 ▶ Breast milk:

A = **False** ▷ has galactose as its main carbohydrate

B = **False** ▷ contains more casein than cow's milk

C = **True** ▷ carries vitamin E

D = **True** ▷ contains high amounts of IgA

E = **False** ▷ contains high prolactin levels to suppress ovulation

16 ▶ Regarding the third stage of labour and uterine involution:

A = **False** ▷ There are multiple uterine contractions after delivery of the baby

B = **False** ▷ Oxytocin levels increase dramatically during the third stage of labour

C = **True** ▷ The uterus halves its weight in the first 7 days post delivery

D = **False** ▷ The decidua is shed over the first 6 weeks post delivery

E = **True** ▷ Lochia alba is yellow

17 ▶ During human parturition:

A = **True** ▷ Progesterone suppresses the formation of myometrial gap junctions

B = **True** ▷ Estradiol increases the oxytocin receptors in the myometrium

C = **False** ▷ Oxytocin release is increased prior to labour

D = **True** ▷ The fetus releases oxytocin

E = **False** ▷ The decidua releases prostaglandin 2

18 ▶ During human parturition:

A = **True** ▷ Neutrophils destroy collagen fibres in the cervix

B = **False** ▷ Increasing numbers of myometrial gap junctions increases contraction strength

C = **True** ▷ Magnesium sulphate causes uterine relaxation

D = **False** ▷ Salbutamol causes uterine relaxation by inhibiting calcium influx into myometrial cells

E = **True** ▷ Commencement of labour increases prostaglandin release

## Answers for Chapter 32

### MULTIPLE CHOICE QUESTIONS

1 ▶ In fetal cardiovascular physiology:

A = **False** ▷ Blood circulation is established in week 5

B = **True** ▷ In the fetus, it is the total ventricular output that is important

C = **True** ▷ The heart grows by hyperplasia during fetal life

D = **False** ▷ The fetus has a large stroke volume reserve

E = **False** ▷ Fatty acids are the main cardiac fuel

2 ▶ In the normal regulation of the fetal heart rate:

A = **True** ▷ Sympathetic influence is via the sinoatrial node

B = **False** ▷ The adrenal medulla plays no role in fetal heart rate

C = **True** ▷ Baroreceptors act through the autonomic nervous system in response to blood pressure

D = **False** ▷ The fetal heart rate increases with gestation

E = **True** ▷ The variability of the fetal heart is a direct indication of the status of the fetal brain stem's medulla oblongata

**3 ▶ Regarding abnormal fetal heart rates:**

**A** = **True** ▷ Tachycardia can be caused by the use of beta-sympathomimetic tocolytics

**B** = **True** ▷ Tachycardia can be caused by fetal hypoxia

**C** = **True** ▷ Bradycardia can be caused by fetal hypoxia

**D** = **True** ▷ A baseline rate of less than 110 beats per minute can be normal

**E** = **False** ▷ Fetal heart block is a common cause of bradycardia

**4 ▶ Regarding fetal heart rate variability:**

**A** = **True** ▷ It is defined as fluctuation in the fetal heart rate of at least two cycles per minute

**B** = **False** ▷ It remains stable regardless of gestation

**C** = **False** ▷ Short-term variation measures the time between two T waves on the fetal electrocardiogram

**D** = **True** ▷ The autonomic not the sympathetic nervous system is the cause for variability

**E** = **True** ▷ Magnesium sulphate may cause a decrease in the fetal heart variability

**5 ▶ Regarding the fetal heart:**

**A** = **True** ▷ Accelerations are rare in fetal hypoxia

**B** = **False** ▷ The loss of accelerations for more than 1 hour correlates with increase neonatal morbidity

**C** = **True** ▷ Early decelerations are due to baroreceptor activation

**D** = **True** ▷ Late decelerations begin before the peak of the contractions

**E** = **False** ▷ Late decelerations are due to chemoreceptor stimulation and inhibition of the sympathetic nervous system

**6 ▶ Regarding variable fetal heart decelerations:**

**A** = **True** ▷ Decelerations are variable in terms of relation with uterine contractions, duration and depth

**B** = **True** ▷ Decelerations are due to gradual cord compression

**C** = **False** ▷ Umbilical vein compression causes fetal bradycardia

**D** = **False** ▷ Umbilical artery compression causes a drop in fetal blood pressure

**E** = **False** ▷ The depth of the deceleration is an indication of hypoxaemia

**7 ▶ With reference to the fetal circulation:**

**A** = **False** ▷ The ductus venosus directs blood to the superior vena cava

**B** = **True** ▷ The ductus arteriosus connects the pulmonary artery to the aorta

**C** = **True** ▷ Little blood passes to the lungs

**D** = **False** ▷ Mixing of oxygenated and deoxygenated blood causes mixed blood to flow around the fetus

**E** = **False** ▷ Deoxygenated blood enters the ascending aorta

**8 ▶ Regarding changes to the fetal circulation at birth:**

**A** = **True** ▷ The fetal systemic resistance doubles

**B** = **True** ▷ The pulmonary vascular resistance falls with the first breath

**C** = **True** ▷ The ductus arteriosus closes and seals within 2 days of delivery

**D** = **False** ▷ The ductus venosus closes chemically with prostaglandin

**E** = **False** ▷ The foramen ovale seals closed immediately

**9 ▶ During development of the fetal respiratory system:**

**A** = **True** ▷ The main bronchi develop by week 7

**B** = **True** ▷ Airway branching is complete by week 17

**C** = **False** ▷ The acini develop by week 24

**D** = **True** ▷ Formation of terminal sacs is complete by week 36

**E** = **False** ▷ Alveolar development is complete by term

**10** ▶ Fetal breathing movements:

- **A = True** ▷ begin in the first trimester
- **B = False** ▷ increase in fetal hypoxia
- **C = True** ▷ increase after maternal eating
- **D = False** ▷ do not play a role in lung growth
- **E = False** ▷ cause lung hyperplasia when excessive

**11** ▶ In fetal and neonatal respiratory physiology:

- **A = False** ▷ Fetal lung fluid is mainly swallowed amniotic fluid
- **B = True** ▷ Steroids increase surfactant synthesis
- **C = False** ▷ Maternal diabetes increases lung maturation
- **D = False** ▷ Androgens increase fetal lung maturation
- **E = False** ▷ Labour commences fetal lung fluid reabsorption

**12** ▶ In fetal haematopoiesis:

- **A = False** ▷ The liver is the main source of fetal blood cells until week 24
- **B = True** ▷ Fetal white cells are formed in the liver
- **C = True** ▷ Mature T cells appear in the fetus from week 14
- **D = False** ▷ IgM is of maternal origin
- **E = False** ▷ The immune system is fully functioning by week 24

**13** ▶ Regarding the physiology of the fetal kidneys and skin:

- **A = False** ▷ Fetal urine production begins at week 12
- **B = False** ▷ Fetal urine is isotonic
- **C = False** ▷ The kidneys receive 20% of cardiac output
- **D = False** ▷ Fetal skin is permeable to water
- **E = True** ▷ Fetal skin contributes to amniotic fluid production

**14** ▶ In fetal brain development:

- **A = True** ▷ Neurons proliferate until week 20
- **B = False** ▷ Neurons have completely migrated to the cerebellum by term
- **C = True** ▷ The peripheral nervous system ganglia are derived from cells of the neural crest
- **D = True** ▷ Fetal movements begin at week 7
- **E = False** ▷ Fetuses do not feel pain until week 24

**15** ▶ The fetal baseline heart rate:

- **A = True** ▷ is determined by the sinoatrial node
- **B = True** ▷ is strongly influenced by the sympathetic tone
- **C = True** ▷ decreases with advancing gestation
- **D = False** ▷ is unaffected by catecholamine release
- **E = True** ▷ variability is reduced by alcohol

**16** ▶ In the fetal circulation:

- **A = False** ▷ Homogenously semioxygenated blood circulates through the fetal arteries
- **B = False** ▷ The ductus arteriosus connects the umbilical vein to the inferior vena cava
- **C = True** ▷ Blood flow across the foramen ovale is from right to left
- **D = True** ▷ The patency of the ductus arteriosus is maintained by the vasodilator effects of prostaglandins
- **E = True** ▷ There is a rise in pulmonary pressure at birth

**17** ▶ During development of the fetal lungs:

- **A = False** ▷ Fetal breathing movements begin at about week 32
- **B = True** ▷ Surfactant is produced by type II pneumocytes
- **C = True** ▷ Surfactant is a lipoprotein of which 90% is made of protein
- **D = False** ▷ The saccular phase continues well into the postnatal period
- **E = False** ▷ Initial inflation breaths at birth generate lower pressures than those needed for subsequent breathing

**18** ▶ Fetal haemoglobin:

- **A = True** ▷ consists of two alpha and two delta chains
- **B = True** ▷ is the predominant haemoglobin during fetal life
- **C = False** ▷ is replaced by adult haemoglobin as the predominant haemoglobin during the last trimester
- **D = False** ▷ binds oxygen with lower affinity than adult haemoglobin
- **E = True** ▷ can persist in the adult in haemoglobinopathies

19 ▶ Amniotic fluid volume:

　　A = **False** ▷ measures about 200 ml at week 12
　　B = **False** ▷ is mainly produced by fetal urine at week 10
　　C = **False** ▷ osmolarity increases with advancing gestation as the fetal kidneys mature
　　D = **True** ▷ is meconium stained in about 30% of post-term pregnancies
　　E = **False** ▷ is essential for pulmonary development

## Answers for Chapters 33 and 34

### EXTENDED MATCHING QUESTIONS

1 ▶ **D** = Range
2 ▶ **C** = Mode
3 ▶ **A** = Mean
4 ▶ **B** = Median
5 ▶ **B** = Mann–Whitney U-test
6 ▶ **D** = Wilcoxon test
7 ▶ **A** = Kruskal–Wallis test
8 ▶ **C** = McNemar $x^2$ test
9 ▶ **A** = $x^2$
10 ▶ **F** = 55
11 ▶ **K** = 957%
12 ▶ **J** = 466%
13 ▶ **L** = 96%
14 ▶ **I** = 45%
15 ▶ **B** = 45
16 ▶ **D** = 47
17 ▶ **B** = Level 1b
18 ▶ **C** = Level 2a
19 ▶ **D** = Level 2b
20 ▶ **E** = Level 3

### MULTIPLE CHOICE QUESTIONS

21 ▶ When describing a scale of measurement:

　　A = **True** ▷ An interval scale is where the interval between any two neighbouring points is the same as that between any other two neighbouring points
　　B = **True** ▷ A ratio scale is an interval scale with a fixed zero
　　C = **False** ▷ Nominal scales are parametric
　　D = **False** ▷ Data from an ordinal scale can be expressed on an interval scale
　　E = **True** ▷ Interval scaled data can be added together

22 ▶ Regarding measurement accuracy and reliability:

　　A = **True** ▷ A measurement is accurate if it matches exactly an accepted standard
　　B = **False** ▷ Accuracy and precision are the same
　　C = **True** ▷ A reliable measurement is one that can be repeated with minimal variation
　　D = **False** ▷ A reliable measurement needs to be taken several times
　　E = **True** ▷ Valid measurements are always indisputable

23 ▶ Central tendency can be described by:

　　A = **True** ▷ the mean
　　B = **False** ▷ the range
　　C = **True** ▷ the median
　　D = **True** ▷ the mode
　　E = **False** ▷ the standard deviation

24 ▶ A Normal distribution:

　　A = **False** ▷ is multimodal
　　B = **True** ▷ has equal observations either side of the midpoint
　　C = **True** ▷ has a mean, median and mode that are all the same
　　D = **False** ▷ is characterised by its standard error
　　E = **True** ▷ has kurtosis

**25** ▶ Regarding measures of variability:

**A = False** ▷ Variance is the average amount by which any individual measurement differs from the median

**B = True** ▷ Standard deviation tells you about the variability in a sample

**C = True** ▷ 95% of the data are within two standard deviations of the mean

**D = True** ▷ The coefficient of variation expresses the standard deviation as a percentage of the mean

**E = True** ▷ The standard error of the mean takes into account the sample size

**26** ▶ In probability and hypothesis testing:

**A = True** ▷ If $P = 1$, then the chance of something happening is 100%

**B = True** ▷ If $P < 0.05$, it is statistically significant

**C = False** ▷ If $P < 0.05$, then the outcome has occurred by chance in 19 out of 20 times

**D = False** ▷ Type 2 errors occur when the null hypothesis is wrongly rejected

**E = True** ▷ The power of a study is its ability to detect an effect of a specified size

**27** ▶ Chi-squared tests

**A = True** ▷ are used to compare distributions

**B = True** ▷ depend on the observed and expected results only

**C = True** ▷ are significant if the result is 0.05 or less

**D = False** ▷ are used if the expected $n < 5$

**E = False** ▷ are used with proportions

**28** ▶ The $t$-test

**A = False** ▷ is used to compare the difference between two medians

**B = True** ▷ is used to compare the mean of a sample with a predicted value

**C = True** ▷ can only be used on data that is Normally distributed

**D = False** ▷ must have paired samples

**E = True** ▷ paired samples are measurements made by the same person under different conditions

**29** ▶ When assessing statistical correlations:

**A = True** ▷ Pearson's ($r$) correlation tests the association between two variables

**B = False** ▷ Pearson's ($r$) correlation relies on all data being Normally distributed

**C = False** ▷ If Pearson's $r = 0$, there is a negative correlation

**D = False** ▷ A statistically significant association means it is causal

**E = True** ▷ Regression allows prediction of a variable

**30** ▶ Regarding epidemiology:

**A = False** ▷ Specificity is the proportion of true positives that are correctly identified by a test

**B = False** ▷ The positive predictive value is the proportion of patients with a positive test result

**C = False** ▷ The incidence of a disease is the rate at which new cases of the disease occur in any population

**D = True** ▷ The incidence rate is the number of new cases per head of the population per unit time

**E = True** ▷ The prevalence of a condition measures the frequency of existing disease at a given time

**31** ▶ When evaluating the odds ratio and relative risk:

**A = True** ▷ An odds ratio allows a confidence interval to be calculated between two variables

**B = True** ▷ An odds ratio allows the effect of other variables on an association to be tested

**C = True** ▷ An odds ratio can use groups selected retrospectively

**D = False** ▷ If ten in 100 patients have an illness, the odds ratio is 1:10

**E = True** ▷ Relative risk compares proportions with a particular outcome in two different groups

32 ▶ Regarding the management of clinical trials:

A = **True** ▷ A comparison of treatment only is involved

B = **True** ▷ Randomisation avoids unconscious bias

C = **False** ▷ In a double-blind study, the patient, clinician and assessor are all blinded to the treatment

D = **True** ▷ A randomised controlled trial can use historical data for a control group

E = **True** ▷ Patients can be their own control

## Answers for Chapter 35

### EXTENDED MATCHING QUESTIONS

1 ▶ **B** = Maternal deaths resulting from previous existing disease or a newly developing medical condition unrelated to pregnancy, aggravated by pregnancy

2 ▶ **C** = Maternal deaths from causes unrelated to pregnancy

3 ▶ **J** = Direct and indirect deaths per 100 000 live births

4 ▶ **K** = The number of mothers delivered of registrable live births at any gestation or stillbirths of 24 weeks of gestation or later

5 ▶ **G** = Number of maternal deaths in a given time period per 100 000 women of reproductive age

6 ▶ **A** = A child delivered between $22^{+0}$ and $23^{+6}$ weeks of gestation that did not show any signs of life

7 ▶ **C** = A child delivered after week 24 of pregnancy that did not show any signs of life

8 ▶ **F** = Death of a live born baby occurring from day 7 of life and before 28 completed days from the time of birth

9 ▶ **G** = Stillbirths per 1000 live births and stillbirths

10 ▶ **I** = Stillbirths and early neonatal deaths per 1000 live births and stillbirths

11 ▶ **M** = Neonatal deaths per 1000 live births

## Answers for Chapter 36

### EXTENDED MATCHING QUESTIONS

1 ▶ **D** = Platelets
2 ▶ **B** = Packed red cells
3 ▶ **B** = Packed red cells
4 ▶ **C** = Frozen red cells
5 ▶ **A** = Whole blood
6 ▶ **E** = Fresh frozen plasma
7 ▶ **A** = Whole blood
8 ▶ **A** = Whole blood
9 ▶ **C** = Frozen red cells
10 ▶ **E** = Fresh frozen plasma
11 ▶ **D** = Platelets
12 ▶ **C** = Frozen red cells
13 ▶ **E** = Bicarbonate
14 ▶ **D** = Chloride
15 ▶ **A** = Sodium
16 ▶ **B** = Potassium
17 ▶ **C** = Calcium
18 ▶ **C** = Calcium
19 ▶ **B** = Potassium
20 ▶ **D** = Chloride
21 ▶ **A** = Sodium
22 ▶ **B** = Potassium
23 ▶ **B** = Hypernatraemia
24 ▶ **A** = Hyponatraemia
25 ▶ **C** = Hypokalaemia
26 ▶ **C** = Hypokalaemia
27 ▶ **F** = Hypercalcaemia
28 ▶ **D** = Hyperkalaemia
29 ▶ **H** = Hyperchloraemia
30 ▶ **E** = Hypocalcaemia
31 ▶ **G** = Hypochloraemia
32 ▶ **A** = Hyponatraemia
33 ▶ **C** = Hypokalaemia
34 ▶ **A** = Hyponatraemia
35 ▶ **D** = Hyperkalaemia
36 ▶ **C** = Hypokalaemia

**MULTIPLE CHOICE QUESTIONS**

**37** ▶ Rates of gynaecological surgery:

**A** = **True** ▷ have decreased over the last 10 years

**B** = **True** ▷ have been affected by medical management of conditions

**C** = **True** ▷ specifically hysterectomies, have been reduced due to the use of levonorgestrel-containing intrauterine system

**D** = **False** ▷ are influenced by the age of the patient

**E** = **True** ▷ are influenced by the length of hospital stay

**38** ▶ Surgical success rates:

**A** = **False** ▷ have the same criteria for surgeons and for patients

**B** = **True** ▷ consider a neat cosmetic appearance of the abdominal scar a success

**C** = **True** ▷ are increased with good anaesthesia

**D** = **False** ▷ are unrelated to the equipment used

**E** = **True** ▷ are increased with optimisation of the patient's condition

**39** ▶ Regarding surgical complications:

**A** = **True** ▷ All operations have complications associated with them

**B** = **False** ▷ A body mass index of > 25 kg/m² leads to poor haemostasis

**C** = **True** ▷ A faulty diathermy device can cause serious burns to patients

**D** = **True** ▷ Haemorrhage is an immediate complication

**E** = **False** ▷ A deep vein thrombosis is a late complication

**40** ▶ Adverse reactions of blood transfusion include:

**A** = **True** ▷ acute haemolytic reactions due to antigen incompatibility

**B** = **False** ▷ acute nonhaemolytic reactions that are usually fatal

**C** = **False** ▷ lung injury due to a clot formation on the lung

**D** = **True** ▷ immunosuppression

**E** = **True** ▷ iron overload

**41** ▶ Regarding body fluid balance:

**A** = **True** ▷ The most important intracellular electrolyte is potassium

**B** = **True** ▷ The body produces water internally as a result of metabolic processes

**C** = **False** ▷ Movement of fluid between the interstitial and intracellular compartments is due to osmotic pressure generated by protein

**D** = **True** ▷ Hydrostatic forces are due to blood pressure

**E** = **False** ▷ At the arteriolar end of a capillary, plasma osmotic forces are greater

**42** ▶ Regarding effects of anaesthesia and surgery on fluid balance:

**A** = **False** ▷ Preoperatively, most patients have fluid excess

**B** = **True** ▷ Steroids released in surgery cause fluid retention

**C** = **False** ▷ Perioperatively, fluid shifts between compartments is minimal

**D** = **False** ▷ Perioperatively, antidiuretic hormone release is decreased

**E** = **True** ▷ Cytokine release perioperatively causes fluid accumulation in the lungs

**43** ▶ Regarding gestational trophoblastic disease:

**A** = **False** ▷ All gestational trophoblastic disease is malignant

**B** = **True** ▷ Hydatiform mole is the most common

**C** = **False** ▷ A complete mole is maternal in origin

**D** = **True** ▷ A complete mole contains no fetal tissue

**E** = **True** ▷ A partial mole is due to dispermic fertilisation

# Index